NURSE'S POCKET DRUG GUIDE 2015

EDITORS

Judith A. Barberio, PhD, APN, C, ANP, FNP, GNP
Leonard G. Gomella, MD, FACS
Susan Underwood, RN, MSN, RD, MS
Claudia A. Beck, PhD, ANP-BC

Mc
Graw
Hill
Education

New York Chicago San Francisco Athens
London Madrid Mexico City Milan New Delhi
Singapore Sydney Toronto

Nurse's Pocket Drug Guide 2015

Copyright © 2015 by McGraw-Hill Education. Based on *Clinician's Pocket Drug Reference 2015* Copyright © 2015 by Leonard G. Gomella. Published by the McGraw-Hill Companies, Inc. All rights reserved. Printed in United States. Except as permitted under the United States Copyright Act of 1976, no part of this publication may be reproduced or distributed in any form or by any means, or stored in a data base or retrieval system, without the prior written permission of the publisher.

1 2 3 4 5 6 7 8 9 0   QLM/QLM   19 18 17 16 15 14

ISBN 978-0-07-183518-3
MHID 0-07-183518-0
ISSN 1550-2554

Notice

Medicine is an ever-changing science. As new research and clinical experience broaden our knowledge, changes in treatment and drug therapy are required. The authors and the publisher of this work have checked with sources believed to be reliable in their efforts to provide information that is complete and generally in accord with the standards accepted at the time of publication. However, in view of the possibility of human error or changes in medical sciences, neither the authors nor the publisher nor any other party who has been involved in the preparation or publication of this work warrants that the information contained herein is in every respect accurate or complete, and they disclaim all responsibility for any errors or omissions or for the results obtained from use of the information contained in this work. Readers are encouraged to confirm the information contained herein with other sources. For example and in particular, readers are advised to check the product information sheet included in the package of each drug they plan to administer to be certain that the information contained in this work is accurate and that changes have not been made in the recommended dose or in the contraindications for administration. This recommendation is of particular importance in connection with new or infrequently used drugs.

The book was set in Times by Cenveo® Publisher Services.
The editors were Catherine A. Johnson and Christie Naglieri.
The production supervisor was Richard Ruzycka.
Project management was provided by Kritika Kaushik, Cenveo Publisher Services.
The indexer was Cenveo Publisher Services.
Quad/Graphics Leomminster was printer and binder.
This book is printed on acid-free paper.

McGraw-Hill books are available at special quantity discounts to use as premiums and sales promotions, or for use in corporate training programs. To contact a representative please e-mail us at bulksales@mcgraw-hill.com.

CONTENTS

GENERIC AND SELECTED BRAND DRUG DATA   **37**
COMMONLY USED NATURAL AND HERBAL AGENTS   **417**
TABLES   **433**

INDEX   **463**

EDITORS

Judith A. Barberio, PhD, APN, C, ANP, FNP, GNP
Assistant Clinical Professor
Speciality Director: Adult/Geriatric Nurse Practitioner Track
Rutgers, The State University of New Jersey
College of Nursing
Newark, New Jersey

Leonard G. Gomella, MD, FACS
The Bernard W. Godwin, Jr., Professor
Chairman, Department of Urology
Jefferson Medical College
Associate Director of Clinical Affairs
Kimmel Cancer Center
Thomas Jefferson University
Philadelphia, Pennsylvania

Susan Underwood, RN, MSN, RD, MS
Adjunct, Department of Nutrition, Food Studies and Public Health
New York University
New York, New York

Claudia A. Beck, PhD, ANP-BC

PREFACE

We are pleased to present the ninth 2015 edition of the *Nurse's Pocket Drug Guide*. The goal is to identify the most frequently used and clinically important medications, including branded, generic, and OTC products. The book includes over 1200 generic medications and is designed to represent a cross-section of commonly used products in healthcare practices across the country.

The style of drug presentation includes key "must know" facts of commonly used medications and herbs, essential information for the student, practicing nurse, and healthcare provider. The inclusion of common uses of medications rather than just the official FDA-labeled indications is based on the uses of the medication and herbs supported by publications and community standards of care. All uses have been reviewed by our editorial board.

It is essential that students, registered nurses, and advanced-practice nurses learn more than the name and dose of the medications they administer and prescribe. Certain common side effects and significant warnings and contraindications are associated with prescription medications and herbs. Although nurses and other healthcare providers should ideally be completely familiar with the entire package insert of any medication prescribed, such a requirement is unreasonable. References such as the *Physicians' Desk Reference* and the drug manufacturers' Web sites make package inserts readily available for many medications, but may not highlight clinically significant facts or key data for generic drugs and those available over the counter.

The limitations of difficult-to-read package inserts were acknowledged by the Food and Drug Administration in early 2001, when it noted that healthcare providers do not have time to read the many pages of small print in the typical package insert. Newer drugs are producing more user-friendly package insert summaries that highlight important drug information for easier nursing reference. Although useful, these summaries do not commingle with similarly approved generic or "competing" similar products.

The editorial board has analyzed the information on both brand and generic medications and has made this key prescribing information available in this pocket-sized book. Information in this book is meant for use by healthcare professionals who are familiar with these commonly prescribed medications and herbs.

This 2015 edition has been completely reviewed and updated by our editorial board. Over 110 new drugs and herbs have been added, and dozens of changes in other medications based on FDA actions have been incorporated, including deletions of discontinued brand names and compounds.

Where appropriate, emergency cardiac care (ECC) guidelines are provided based on the latest recommendations for the American Heart Association (*Circulation*, Volume 112, Issue 24 Supplement; December 13, 2005 and Volume 122, Issue 25; December 2010), with the ECC emergency medication summary at the back of the book for rapid reference. Editions of this book are also available in a variety of electronic or eBook formats. Visit www.eDrugbook.com for a link to the electronic versions currently available. Additionally, this Web site has enhanced content features such as a comprehensive listing of "look alike–sound alike" medications that can contribute to prescribing errors.

MEDICATION KEY

Medications are listed by prescribing class, and the individual medications are then listed in alphabetical order by generic name. Some of the more commonly recognized trade names are listed for each medication (in parentheses after the generic name) or if available without prescription, noted as OTC (over the counter).

Generic Drug Name (Selected Common Brand Names [Controlled Substance]) WARNING: Summarized versions of the "Black Box" precautions deemed necessary by the FDA. These are significant precautions and contraindications concerning the individual medication. **Therapeutic and/or Pharmacologic Class:** Class is presented in brackets immediately following the brand name drug. The therapeutic drug class appears first and describes the disease state that the drug treats. The pharmacologic drug class follows and is based on the drug's mechanism of action. **Uses:** This includes both FDA-labeled indications bracketed by * and other "off-label" uses of the medication. Because many medications are used to treat various conditions based on the medical literature and not listed in their package insert, we list common uses of the medication in addition to the official "labeled indications" (FDA approved) based on input from our editorial board. **Action:** How the drug works. This information is helpful in comparing classes of drugs and understanding side effects and contraindications. *Spectrum:* Specifies activity against selected microbes for antimicrobials. **Dose:** *Adults.* Where no specific pediatric dose is given, the implication is that this drug is not commonly used or indicated in that age group. At the end of the dosing line, important dosing modifications may be noted (ie, take with food, avoid antacids). *Peds.* If appropriate dosing for children and infants is included with age ranges as needed. **Caution:** [Pregnancy/fetal risk categories, breast-feeding (as noted above)] cautions concerning the use of the drug in specific settings. **CI:** Contraindications. **Disp:** Common dosing forms. **SE:** Common or significant side effects. **Notes:** Other key information about the drug. **Interactions:** Common drug–drug, drug–herb, and drug–food interactions that may change the drug response. **Labs:** Common laboratory test results that are changed by the drug or significant laboratory monitoring requirements. **NIPE:** (Nursing Indications and/or Patient Education) Significant information that the nurse must be aware of with administration of the drug or information that should be given to any patient taking the drug.

CONTROLLED SUBSTANCE CLASSIFICATION

Medications under the control of the US Drug Enforcement Agency (DEA) (Schedule I–V controlled substances) are indicated by the symbol [C]. Most medications are "uncontrolled" and do not require a DEA prescriber number on the prescription. The following is a general description for the schedules of DEA-controlled substances:

Schedule (C–I) I: All nonresearch use forbidden (eg, heroin, LSD, mescaline).

Schedule (C–II) II: High addictive potential; medical use accepted. No telephone call-in prescriptions; no refills. Some states require special prescription form (eg, cocaine, morphine, methadone).

Schedule (C–III) III: Low to moderate risk of physical dependence, high risk of psychologic dependence; prescription must be rewritten after 6 months or five refills (eg, acetaminophen plus codeine).

Schedule (C–IV) IV: Limited potential for dependence; prescription rules same as for schedule III (eg, benzodiazepines).

Schedule (C–V) V: Very limited abuse potential; prescribing regulations often same as for uncontrolled medications; some states have additional restrictions.

FDA FETAL RISK CATEGORIES

Category A: Adequate studies in pregnant women have not demonstrated a risk to the fetus in the first trimester of pregnancy; there is no evidence of risk in the last two trimesters.

Category B: Animal studies have not demonstrated a risk to the fetus, but no adequate studies have been done in pregnant women.

or

Animal studies have shown an adverse effect, but adequate studies in pregnant women have not demonstrated a risk to the fetus during the first trimester of pregnancy and there is no evidence of risk in the last two trimesters.

Category C: Animal studies have shown an adverse effect on the fetus, but no adequate studies have been done in humans. The benefits from the use of the drug in pregnant women may be acceptable despite its potential risks.

or

No animal reproduction studies and no adequate studies in humans have been done.

Category D: There is evidence of human fetal risk, but the potential benefits from the use of the drug in pregnant women may be acceptable despite its potential risks.

Category X: Studies in animals or humans or adverse reaction reports, or both, have demonstrated fetal abnormalities. The risk of use in pregnant women clearly outweighs any possible benefit.

Category ?: No data available (not a formal FDA classification; included to provide complete data set).

BREAST-FEEDING

No formally recognized classification exists for drugs and breast-feeding. This shorthand was developed for the *Nurse's Pocket Drug Guide*.

+   Compatible with breast-feeding
M   Monitor patient or use with caution
±   Excreted, or likely excreted, with unknown effects or at unknown concentrations
?/–   Unknown excretion, but effects likely to be of concern
–   Contraindicated in breast-feeding
?   No data available

ABBREVIATIONS

▲: change
✓: check, follow, or monitor
↓: decrease/decreased
↑: increase/increased
>: greater than; older than
<: less than; younger than
⊘: not recommended; do not take; avoid
÷/%: divided dose
≠: not equal to; not equivalent to
AA: African American
Ab: antibody
Abd: abdominal
ABGs: arterial blood gases
ABMT: autologous bone marrow
   transplantation
ac: before meals (*ante cibum*)
ACE: angiotensin-converting enzyme
ACEI: angiotensin-converting enzyme
   inhibitor
ACH: acetylcholine
ACLS: advanced cardiac life support
ACS: acute coronary syndrome;
   American Cancer Society;
   American College of Surgeons
ACT: activated coagulation time
ADH: antidiuretic hormone
ADHD: attention-deficit hyperactivity
   disorder
ADR: adverse drug reaction
AF: atrial fibrillation
AF/A flutter: atrial fibrillation/atrial
   flutter
AHA: American Heart Association
Al: aluminum
alk phos: alkaline phosphate

ALL: acute lymphocytic leukemia
ALT: alanine aminotransferase
AMI: acute myocardial infarction
AML: acute myelogenous leukemia
amp: ampule
ANA: antinuclear antibody
ANC: absolute neutrophil count
antiplt: antiplatelet
antiSz: antiseizure
APACHE: acute physiology and
   chronic health evaluation
APAP: acetaminophen (*N*-acetyl-*p*-
   aminophenol)
APN: Advanced Practice Nurse
aPTT: activated partial thromboplastin
   time
ARB: angiotensin II receptor blocker
ARDS: adult respiratory distress
   syndrome
ARF: acute renal failure
AS: aortic stenosis
ASA: aspirin (acetylsalicylic acid)
ASAP: as soon as possible
AST: aspartate aminotransferase
ATP: adenosine triphosphate
AUB: abnormal uterine/vaginal
   bleeding
AUC: area under the curve
AV: atrioventricular
AVM: arteriovenous malformation
BBB: bundle branch block
BBs: beta blockers
BCL: B-cell lymphoma
bid: twice daily
BM: bone marrow; bowel movement

↓ BM: bone marrow suppression, myelosuppression
BMD: bone mineral density
BMI: body mass index
BMT: bone marrow transplantation
BOO: bladder outlet obstruction
BP: blood pressure
↓ BP: hypotension
BPH: benign prostatic hyperplasia
BPM: beats per minute
BS: blood sugar
BSA: body surface area
BUN: blood urea nitrogen
Ca: calcium
CA: cancer
CABG: coronary artery bypass graft
CaCl: calcium chloride
CAD: coronary artery disease
CAP: community-acquired pneumonia
caps: capsule(s)
cardiotox: cardiotoxicity
CBC: complete blood count
CCB: calcium channel blocker
CDC: Centers for Disease Control and Prevention
CF: cystic fibrosis
CHD: coronary heart disease
CHF: congestive heart failure
CI: contraindicated
CIDP: chronic inflammatory demyelinating polyneuropathy
CK: creatine kinase
CLA: *Cis*-linoleic acid
CLL: chronic lymphocytic leukemia
CML: chronic myelogenous leukemia
CMV: cytomegalovirus
CNS: central nervous system
c/o: complains of
combo: combination
comp: complicated

COMT: catechol-*O*-methyltransferase
conc: concentration(s)
cont: continuous
Contra: contraindicated
COPD: chronic obstructive pulmonary disease
COX: cyclooxygenase
CP: chest pain
CPK: creatine phosphokinase
CPP: central precocious puberty
CPR: cardiopulmonary resuscitation
CR: controlled release
CrCl: creatinine clearance
CRF: chronic renal failure
CSF: cerebrospinal fluid
CV: cardiovascular
CVA: cerebrovascular accident; costovertebral angle
CVD: cardiovascular disease
CVH: common variable hypergammaglobulinemia
CYP: cytochrome P-450 enzyme(s)
cytotox: cytotoxicity
CXR: chest X-ray
D: diarrhea
d: day
/d: per day
DA: dopamine
D_5LR: 5% dextrose in lactated Ringer's solution
D_5NS: 5% dextrose in normal saline
D_5W: 5% dextrose in water
DBP: diastolic blood pressure
D/C: discontinue; stop
derm: dermatologic
DI: diabetes insipidus
Disp: dispensed as; how the drug is supplied
DKA: diabetic ketoacidosis
dL: deciliter
DM: diabetes mellitus

DMARD: disease-modifying antirheumatic drug; drugs defined in randomized trials to decrease erosions and joint space narrowing in rheumatoid arthritis (eg, D-penicillamine, methotrexate, azathioprine)
DN: diabetic nephropathy
DOC: drug of choice
DOT: directly observed therapy
dppr: dropper
DR: delayed release
d/t: due to
DVT: deep venous thrombosis
dx: diagnosis
Dz: disease
EC: enteric coated
ECC: emergency cardiac care
ECG: electrocardiogram
ED: erectile dysfunction
EGFR: epidermal growth factor receptor
EIB: exercise-induced bronchoconstriction
ELISA: enzyme-linked immunosorbent assay
EMG: electromyogram
EMIT: enzyme-multiplied immunoassay test
epi: epinephrine
EPS: extrapyramidal symptoms (tardive dyskinesia, tremors and rigidity, restlessness [akathisia], muscle contractions [dystonia], changes in breathing and heart rate)
ER: extended release
ESA: erythropoiesis-stimulating agents
esp: especially
ESR: erythrocyte sedimentation rate
ESRD: end-stage renal disease
ET: endotracheal
EtOH: ethanol

eval: evaluation
exam (s):examination/s
externa: external
extrav: extravasation
FAP: familial adenomatous polyposis
FBS: fasting blood sugar
Fe: iron
fib: fibrillation
FIO_2: fraction of inspired oxygen
FSH: follicle-stimulating hormone
5-FU: fluorouracil
FVC: forced vital capacity
fx: fracture(s)
Fxn: function
g: gram
GABA: gamma-aminobutyric acid
GAD: generalized anxiety disorder
GBM: glioblastoma multiforme
GC: gonorrhea
G-CSF: granulocyte colony-stimulating factor
gen: generation
GERD: gastroesophageal reflux disease
GF: growth factor
GFR: glomerular filtration rate
GGT: gamma-glutamyl transferase
GH: growth hormone
GI: gastrointestinal
GIST: gastrointestinal stromal tumor
GLA: gamma-linoleic acid
GM-CSF: granulocyte-macrophage colony-stimulating factor
GnRH: gonadotropin-releasing hormone
G6PD: glucose-6-phosphate dehydrogenase
gt, gtt: drop, drops (*gutta*)
GTT: glucose tolerance test
GU: genitourinary
GVHD: graft-versus-host disease
h: hour(s)
HA: headache
HBsAg: hepatitis B surface antigen

HBV: hepatitis B virus
HCG: human chorionic gonadotropin
HCL: hairy cell leukemia
Hct: hematocrit
HCTZ: hydrochlorothiazide
HD: hemodialysis
HDAC: histone deacetylase
HDL-C: high-density lipoprotein
　cholesterol
hematotox: hematotoxicity
heme: hemoglobin
hep: hepatitis
hepatotox: hepatotoxicity
HF: heart failure
Hgb: hemoglobin
5-HIAA: 5-hydroxyindoleacetic acid
HIT: heparin-induced
　thrombocytopenia
HITTS: heparin-induced thrombosis-
　thrombocytopenia syndrome
HIV: human immunodeficiency virus
HMG-CoA: hydroxymethylglutaryl
　coenzyme A
H1N1: swine flu strain
h/o: history of
H_2O: water
HPV: human papillomavirus
HR: heart rate
↑ HR: increased heart rate (tachycardia)
hs: at bedtime (*hora somni*)
HSV: herpes simplex virus
5-HT: 5-hydroxytryptamine
HTN: hypertension
Hx: history
IBD: irritable bowel disease
IBS: irritable bowel syndrome
IBW: ideal body weight
ICP: intracranial pressure
I&D: incision & drainage
IFIS: intraoperative floppy iris syndrome
Ig: immunoglobulin

IGF: insulin-like growth factor
IGIV: Immune Globulin, IV
IHSS: idiopathic hypertrophic
　subaortic stenosis
IL: interleukin
IM: intramuscular
impair: impairment
Inf: infusion
info: information
Infxn/Infxns: infection/infections
Inh: inhalation
INH: isoniazid
Inhib/Inhibs: inhibitor(s)
Inj: injection
INR: international normalized ratio
Insuff: insufficiency
intra-Abd: intra-abdominal
intravag: intravaginal
IO: intraosseous
I&O: intake & output
IOP: intraocular pressure
IR: immediate release
ISA: intrinsic sympathomimetic activity
IT: intrathecal
ITP: idiopathic/immune
　thrombocytopenic purpura
IU: international units
IUD: intrauterine device
IV: intravenous
JIA: juvenile idiopathic arthritis
JME: juvenile myoclonic epilepsy
JRA: juvenile rheumatoid arthritis
Jt: joint
K: Klebsiella
K^+: potassium
KCl: potassium chloride
KI: potassium iodide
KOH: potassium hydroxide
L&D: labor and delivery
LA: long acting
L/d: liters per day

LDL: low-density lipoprotein

LDL-C: low-density lipoprotein cholesterol

LFT: liver function test

LH: luteinizing hormone

LHRH: luteinizing hormone–releasing hormone

Li: lithium

Liq: liquid

LMW: low molecular weight

LP: lumbar puncture

LUQ: left upper quadrant

LVD: left ventricular dysfunction

LVEF: left ventricular ejection fraction

LVSD: left ventricular systolic dysfunction

lyte(s): electrolyte(s)

MAC: *Mycobacterium avium* complex

maint: maintenance dose/drug

MAO/MAOI: monoamine oxidase/ inhibitor

max: maximum

mcg: micrograms

mcL: microliter

mcm: micrometer

mcmol: micromole

MDD: major depressive disorder

MDI: multidose inhaler

MDS: myelodysplastic syndrome

meds: medicines

mEq: milliequivalent

met: metastatic

mg: milligram(s)

Mg^{2+}: magnesium

$MgOH_2$: magnesium hydroxide

MI: myocardial infarction; mitral insufficiency

mill: million

min: minute(s)

mL: milliliter

mo: month(s)

MoAb: monoclonal antibody(s)

mod: moderate

MRSA: methicillin-resistant *Staphylococcus aureus*

MS: multiple sclerosis; musculoskeletal

ms: millisecond(s)

MSSA: methicillin-sensitive *Staphylococcus aureus*

MTT: monotetrazolium

MTX: methotrexate

MU: million units

MyG: myasthenia gravis

N: nausea

N/A: not applicable

N/D: nausea/diarrhea

Na: sodium

NA: narrow angle

NAG: narrow angle glaucoma

$NaHCO_3$: sodium bicabonate

NaI: sodium iodide

NEC: necrotizing enterocolitis

nephrotox: nephrotoxicity

neurotox: neurotoxicity

ng: nanogram

NG: nasogastric

NHL: non–Hodgkin lymphoma

NIAON: nonischemic arterial optic neuritis

NIDDM: non–insulin-dependent diabetes mellitus

nl: normal

NMDA: *N*-methyl-D-aspartate

NNRTI: nonnucleoside reverse transcriptase inhibitor

NO: nitric oxide

NPO: nothing by mouth (*nil per os*)

NRTI: nucleoside reverse transcriptase inhibitor

NS: normal saline

NSAID: nonsteroidal anti-inflammatory drug

NSCLC: non–small-cell lung cancer

NSTEMI: Non–ST elevation myocardial infarction

N/V: nausea and vomiting

N/V/D: nausea, vomiting, diarrhea

NYHA: New York Heart Association

OA: osteoarthritis

OAB: overactive bladder

obst: obstruction

OCD: obsessive compulsive disorder

OCP: oral contraceptive pill

OD: overdose

ODT: orally disintegrating tablets

Oint: ointment

OJ: orange juice

OK: recommended

once/wk

ophthal: ophthalmic

OSAHS: obstructive sleep apnea/ hypopnea syndrome

OTC: over the counter

ototox: ototoxicity

oz: ounces

P: phosphorus

PABA: para-amino benzoic acid

PAH: pulmonary arterial hypertension

PAT: paroxysmal atrial tachycardia

pc: after eating (*post cibum*)

PCa: cancer of the prostate

PCI: percutaneous coronary intervention

PCN: penicillin

PCP: *Pneumocystis jiroveci* (formerly *carinii*) pneumonia

PCWP: pulmonary capillary wedge pressure

PDE5: phosphodiesterase type 5

PDGF: platelet-derived growth factor

PE: pulmonary embolus; physical examination; pleural effusion

PEA: pulseless electrical activity

Ped: pediatrics

PFT: pulmonary function test

pg: picogram(s)

Ph: Philadelphia chromosome

Pheo: pheochromocytoma

PHN: post-herpetic neuralgia

photosens: photosensitivity

phototox: phototoxicity

PID: pelvic inflammatory disease

PKU: phenylketonuria

plt(s): platelet(s)

↓ plt: decreased platelets (thrombocytopenia)

PMDD: premenstrual dysphoric disorder

PML: progressive multifocal leukoencephalopathy

PMS: premenstrual syndrome

PNA: penicillin

PO: by mouth (*per os*)

PPD: purified protein derivative

PPI: proton pump inhibitor(s)

PR: by rectum

Prep: preparation(s)

PRG: pregnancy

PRN: as often as needed (*pro re nata*)

PSA: prostate-specific antigen

PSVT: paroxysmal supraventricular tachycardia

pt(s): patient(s)

PT: prothrombin time

PTCA: percutaneous transluminal coronary angioplasty

PTH: parathyroid hormone

PTT: partial thromboplastin time

PUD: peptic ulcer disease

pulm: pulmonary

PVC: premature ventricular contraction

PVD: peripheral vascular disease

PWP: pulmonary wedge pressure

Px: prophylaxis

pyelo: pyelonephritis

q: every (*quaque*)

qd: every day

qh: every hour

q_h: every_hours
qhs: every hour of sleep (before bedtime)
qid: four times a day (*quater in die*)
qmo: every month
q_mo: every_month
qod: every other day
qowk: every other week
qwk: every week
RA: rheumatoid arthritis
RAS: renin–angiotensin system
RBC: red blood cell(s) (count)
RCC: renal cell carcinoma
RDA: recommended dietary allowance
RDS: respiratory distress syndrome
rec: recommends
recons: reconstitution
reeval: reevaluation
REMS: Risk Evaluation and Mitigation Strategy
resp: respiratory
RHuAb: recombinant human antibody
RIA: radioimmune assay
RLS: restless leg syndrome
RR: respiratory rate
RSI: rapid-sequence intubation
RSV: respiratory syncytial virus
RT: reverse transcriptase
RTA: renal tubular acidosis
Rx: prescription
Rxn(s): reaction(s)
s: second(s)
s/p: status/post
SAD: social anxiety disorder or seasonal affective disorder
SAE: serious adverse event
SBE: subacute bacterial endocarditis
SBP: systolic blood pressure
SCLC: small-cell lung cancer
SCr: serum creatinine
SD: single dose
SDV: single-dose vial

SE: side effect(s)
see package insert: see the manufacturer's insert
SIADH: syndrome of inappropriate antidiuretic hormone
sig: significant
SJIA: systemic juvenile idiopathic arthritis
SJS: Stevens–Johnson syndrome
SL: sublingual
SLE: systemic lupus erythematosus
SNRIs: serotonin–norepinephrine reuptake inhibitors
SOB: shortness of breath
Sol/soln: solution
sp: species
SPAG: small particle aerosol generator
SQ: subcutaneous
SR: sustained release
SSRI: selective serotonin reuptake inhibitor
SSS: sick sinus syndrome
S/Sxs: signs & symptoms
stat: immediately (*statim*)
STD: sexually transmitted disease
STEMI: ST elevation myocardial infarction
subsp: subspecies
supl(s): supplement(s)
supp: suppository
susp: suspension
SVR: systemic vascular resistance
SVT: supraventricular tachycardia
SWFI: sterile water for injection
SWSD: shift work sleep disorder
synd: syndrome
synth: synthesis
Sx: symptom(s)
Sz: seizure
tab/tabs: tablet/tablets
TB: tuberculosis
tbsp: tablespoon

TCA: tricyclic antidepressant
TFT: thyroid function test
TIA: transient ischemic attack
tid: three times a day (*ter in die*)
tinc: tincture
TKI: tyrosine kinase inhibitors
TMP: trimethoprim
TMP–SMX: trimethoprim–
   sulfamethoxazole
TNF: tumor necrosis factor
TOUCH: Tysabri Outreach Unified
   Commitment to Health
tox: toxicity
TPA: tissue plasminogen activator
tri: trimester
TSH: thyroid-stimulating hormone
tsp: teaspoon
TRALI: transfusion-related acute
   lung injury
TTP: thrombotic thrombocytopenic
   purpura
TTS: transdermal therapeutic system
Tx: treatment
UC: ulcerative colitis
UGT: uridine 5'
   diphosphoglucuronosyl transferase
ULN: upper limits of normal
uncomp: uncomplicated
UPA: pyrrolizidine alkaloids
URI: upper respiratory infection
UTI: urinary tract infection
UV: ultraviolet

V: vomiting
VAERS: Vaccine Adverse Events
   Reporting System
Vag: vaginal
VEGF: vascular endothelial growth factor
VF: ventricular fibrillation
vit: vitamin
VLDL: very low-density lipoprotein
vol: volume
VPA: valproic acid
VRE: vancomycin-resistant
   Enterococcus
VT: ventricular tachycardia
VTE: venous thromboembolism
w/: with
W/: with
w/hold: withhold
W/P: Warnings and Precautions
WBC: white blood cell(s) (count)
wgt: weight
WHI: Women's Health Initiative
w/in: within
wk: week
/wk: per week
WNL: within normal limits
w/o: without
WPW: Wolff–Parkinson–White
   syndrome
XL: extended release
XR: extended release
ZE: Zollinger–Ellison (syndrome)
Zn^{2+}: zinc

CLASSIFICATION (Generic and common brand names)

ALLERGY

Antihistamines

Azelastine (Astelin, Optivar)
Cetirizine (Zyrtec, Zyrtec D)
Chlorpheniramine (Chlor-Trimeton)

Clemastine Fumarate (Tavist)
Cyproheptadine (Periactin)
Desloratadine (Clarinex)
Diphenhydramine (Benadryl)

Fexofenadine (Allegra, Allegra-D, Generic)
Hydroxyzine (Atarax, Vistaril)
Levocetirizine (Xyzal)
Loratadine (Alavert, Claritin)

Miscellaneous Antiallergy Agents

Budesonide (Rhinocort, Pulmicort)
Cromolyn Sodium (Intal, NasalCrom, Opticrom)
Montelukast (Singulair)
Phenylephrine, Oral (Sudafed, Others [OTC])

Short Ragweed Pollen Allergen Extract (Ragwitek)
Timothy Grass Pollen Allergen Extract (Grastek)
Vernal, Orchard, Perennial Rye, Timothy & Kentucky

Blue Grass Mixed Pollens Allergenic Extract (Oralair)

ANTIDOTES

Acetylcysteine (Acetadote, Mucomyst)
Amifostine (Ethyol)
Atropine/Pralidoxime (DuoDote)
Atropine, Systemic (AtroPen) Auto-Injector
Atropine/Pralidoxime (DuoDote Auto-Injector)

Centruroides (Scorpion) Immune F(ab')2 (Anascorp)
Charcoal (Actidose-Aqua, CharcoCaps, EZ Char, Kerr Insta-Char, Requa Activated Charcoal)
Deferasirox (Exjade)
Dexrazoxane (Totect, Zinecard)

Digoxin Immune Fab (Digibind, DigiFab)
Flumazenil (Romazicon, Generic)
Glucarpidase (Voraxaze)
Hydroxocobalamin (Cyanokit)
Iodine (Potassium Iodide) (Lugol Soln SSKI, Thyro-Block, ThyroSafe, ThyroShield) [OTC]

Ipecac Syrup
(OTC Syrup)
Mesna (Mesnex) [Oral],
Generic [Inf]

Methylene Blue
(Urolene Blue,
Various)

Naloxone (Generic,
Evzio)
Physostigmine (Generic)
Succimer (Chemet)

ANTIMICROBIAL AGENTS

Antibiotics

AMINOGLYCOSIDES

Amikacin (Amikin)
Gentamicin, Injectable
(Generic)

Neomycin Sulfate
(NeoFradin, Generic)
Streptomycin (Generic)
Tobramycin (Nebcin)

Tombramycin, Inhalation
(TOBI, TOBI
Podhaler)

CARBAPENEMS

Doripenem (Doribax)
Ertapenem (Invanz)

Imipenem-Cilastatin
(Primaxin, Generic)

Meropenem (Merrem,
Generic)

CEPHALOSPORINS, FIRST GENERATION

Cefadroxil
(Duricef,
Ultracef)

Cefazolin (Ancef,
Kefzol)

Cephalexin (Keflex,
Generic)
Cephradine (Velosef)

CEPHALOSPORINS, SECOND GENERATION

Cefaclor (Ceclor,
Raniclor)
Cefotetan

Cefoxitin (Mefoxin)
Cefprozil (Cefzil)

Cefuroxime (Ceftin
[Oral], Zinacef
[Parenteral])

CEPHALOSPORINS, THIRD GENERATION

Cefdinir (Omnicef)
Cefditoren (Spectracef)
Cefixime (Suprax)
Cefoperazone (Cefobid)
Cefotaxime (Claforan)

Cefpodoxime (Vantin)
Ceftazidime (Fortaz,
Ceptaz, Tazidime,
Tazicef)
Ceftibuten (Cedax)

Ceftizoxime (Cefizox)
Ceftriaxone (Rocephin)

CEPHALOSPORINS, FOURTH GENERATION

Cefepime (Maxipime)

CEPHALOSPORINS, UNCLASSIFIED ("FIFTH GENERATION")

Ceftaroline (Teflaro)

FLUOROQUINOLONES

Ciprofloxacin
(Cipro, Cipro XR)

Gemifloxacin (Factive)

Levofloxacin (Levaquin,
Generic)

Moxifloxacin (Avelox) Norfloxacin (Noroxin, Chibroxin Ophthalmic) Ofloxacin (Generic)

KETOLIDE

Telithromycin (Ketek)

MACROLIDES

Azithromycin (Zithromax) Erythromycin (E-Mycin, E.E.S., Ery-Tab, EryPed, Ilotycin) Erythromycin & Sulfisoxazole (E.S.P.)

Clarithromycin (Biaxin, Biaxin XL)

PENICILLINS

Amoxicillin (Amoxil, Moxatag) Dicloxacillin (Dynapen, Dycill) Penicillin G Procaine (Wycillin, Others)

Amoxicillin & Clavulanate Potassium (Augmentin, Augmentin ES-600, Augmentin XR) Nafcillin (Nallpen, Generic) Penicillin V (Pen-Vee K Veetids, Others)

Oxacillin (Generic) Piperacillin (Pipracil)

Penicillin G, Aqueous (Potassium or Sodium) (Pfizerpen, Pentids) Piperacillin-Tazobactam (Zosyn, Generic)

Ampicillin Ticarcillin/Potassium Clavulanate (Timentin)

Ampicillin-Sulbactam (Unasyn) Penicillin G Benzathine (Bicillin)

TETRACYCLINES

Doxycycline (Adoxa, Periostat, Oracea, Vibramycin, Vibra-Tabs) Minocycline (Dynacin, Minocin, Solodyn) Tigecycline (Tygacil)

Tetracycline (Generic)

Miscellaneous Antibiotic Agents

Aztreonam (Azactam) [Neosporin Ointment]; Bacitracin/Neomycin/ Polymyxin B/ Hydrocortisone, Topical [Cortisporin]) Telavancin (Vibativ)

Clindamycin (Cleocin, Cleocin-T, Others) Trimethoprim (Primsol, Generic)

Fosfomycin (Monurol) Trimethoprim (TMP)/ Sulfamethoxazole (SMX) [Co-Trimoxazole, TMP-SMX] (Bactrim, Bactrim DS, Septra DS, Generic)

Linezolid (Zyvox) Nitrofurantoin (Furadantin, Macrobid, Macrodantin, Generic)

Metronidazole (Flagyl, MetroGel)

Mupirocin (Bactroban, Bactroban Nasal) Quinupristin/Dalfopristin (Synercid)

Neomycin Topical (see Bacitracin, Neomycin/ Polymyxin B, Topical Retapamulin (Altabax) Vancomycin (Vancocin, Generic)

Rifaximin (Xifaxan)

ANTIFUNGALS

Amphotericin B
(Fungizone)
Amphotericin B
Cholesteryl
(Amphotec)
Amphotericin B Lipid
Complex (Abelcet)
Amphotericin B
Liposomal
(AmBisome)
Anidulafungin (Eraxis)
Caspofungin (Cancidas)
Clotrimazole (Lotrimin,
Mycelex, Others)
[OTC]

Clotrimazole/
Betamethasone
(Lotrisone)
Econazole (Spectazole)
Fluconazole (Diflucan,
Generic)
Itraconazole
(Onmel, Sporanox,
Generic Caps)
Ketoconazole, Oral
(Nizoral)
Ketoconazole, Topical
(Extina, Kuric, Xolegel,
Nizoral A-D Shampoo)
[Shampoo OTC]
Micafungin (Mycamine)

Miconazole (Monistat 1
Combination Pack,
Monistat 3, Monistat 7)
[OTC] (Monistat-Derm)
Miconazole, Buccal
(Oravig)
Nystatin (Mycostatin)
Oxiconazole (Oxistat)
Posaconazole (Noxafil)
Sertaconazole (Ertaczo)
Terbinafine (Lamisil,
Lamisil AT, Generic)
[OTC]
Triamcinolone/Nystatin
(Mycolog-II)
Voriconazole (VFEND,
Generic)

Antimycobacterials

Bedaquiline Fumarate
(Sirturo)
Dapsone, Oral
Ethambutol (Myambutol,
Generic)

Isoniazid (INH)
Pyrazinamide (Generic)
Rifabutin (Mycobutin)
Rifampin (Rifadin,
Rimactane, Generic)

Rifapentine (Priftin)
Streptomycin

Antiparasitics

Benzyl Alcohol (Ulesfia)
Ivermectin, Oral
(Stromectol)

Ivermectin, Topical
(Sklice)
Lindane (Kwell, Others)

Spinosad (Natroba)

Antiprotozoals

Artemether/
Lumefantrine
(Coartem)
Atovaquone (Mepron)

Atovaquone/Proguanil
(Malarone)
Hydroxychloroquine
(Plaquenil, Generic)

Nitazoxanide (Alinia)
Tinidazole (Tindamax,
Generic)

ANTIRETROVIRALS

Abacavir (Ziagen)
Daptomycin (Cubicin)
Darunavir (Prezista)
Delavirdine (Rescriptor)

Didanosine [ddI] (Videx)
Dolutegravir (Tivicay)
Efavirenz (Sustiva)

Efavirenz/Emtricitabine/
Tenofovir (Atripla)
Etravirine (Intelence)
Fosamprenavir (Lexiva)

Indinavir (Crixivan)
Lamivudine (Epivir,
Epivir-HBV, 3TC
[Many Combo
Regimens])
Lopinavir/Ritonavir
(Kaletra)
Maraviroc (Selzentry)
Nelfinavir (Viracept)

Nevirapine (Viramune,
Viramune XR,
Generic)
Raltegravir (Isentress)
Rilpivirine (Edurant)
Ritonavir (Norvir)
Saquinavir (Invirase)
Stavudine (Zerit,
Generic)

Tenofovir (Viread)
Tenofovir/Emtricitabine
(Truvada)
Zidovudine (Retrovir,
Generic)
Zidovudine Lamivudine
(Combivir, Generic)

Antivirals

Acyclovir (Zovirax)
Adefovir (Hepsera)
Amantadine (Symmetrel)
Atazanavir (Reyataz)
Boceprevir (Victrelis)
Cidofovir (Vistide)
Emtricitabine (Emtriva)
Enfuvirtide (Fuzeon)
Famciclovir (Famvir,
Generic)
Foscarnet (Foscavir,
Generic)

Ganciclovir (Cytovene,
Vitrasert)
Interferon Alfa-2b &
Ribavirin Combo
(Rebetron)
Oseltamivir (Tamiflu)
Palivizumab (Synagis)
Peginterferon Alfa-2b
(Peg Intron)
Penciclovir (Denavir)
Ribavirin (Copegus,
Rebetol, Virazole,
Generic)

Rimantadine
(Flumadine, Generic)
Simeprevir (Olysio)
Sofosbuvir (Sovaldi)
Telaprevir (Incivek)
Telbivudine (Tyzeka)
Valacyclovir (Valtrex,
Generic)
Valganciclovir (Valcyte)
Zanamivir (Relenza)

Miscellaneous Antiviral Agents

Daptomycin (Cubicin)
Pentamidine (Pentam
300, NebuPent)

Trimetrexate
(NeuTrexin)

ANTINEOPLASTIC AGENTS

Alkylating Agents

Altretamine (Hexalen)
Bendamustine (Treanda)
Busulfan (Myleran,
Busulfex)
Carboplatin (Paraplatin)
Cisplatin (Platinol,
Platinol AQ)

Oxaliplatin (Eloxatin,
Generic)
Procarbazine (Matulane)
Streptozocin (Zanosar)
Tapentadol (Nucynta)
Temozolomide
(Temodar, Generic)

Triethylene
Thiophosphoramide
(Thiotepa, Thioplex,
Tespa, TSPA)

NITROGEN MUSTARDS

Chlorambucil (Leukeran)
Cyclophosphamide
  (Cytoxan, Neosar)
Ifosfamide (Ifex, Generic)

Mechlorethamine
  (Mustargen); Gel
  Form (Valchlor)

Melphalan [L-PAM]
  (Alkeran, Generic)

NITROSOUREAS

Carmustine [BCNU]
  (BiCNU, Gliadel)

Streptozocin (Zanosar)

Antibiotics

Bleomycin Sulfate
  (Generic)
Dactinomycin
  (Cosmegen)

Daunorubicin
  (Cerubidine)
Doxorubicin
  (Adriamycin, Rubex)
Epirubicin (Ellence)

Idarubicin (Idamycin,
  Generic)
Mitomycin (Mitosol
  [Topical], Generic)

Antimetabolites

Clofarabine (Clolar)
Cytarabine [Ara-C]
  (Cytosar-U)
Cytarabine Liposome
  (DepoCyt)
Floxuridine (Generic)
Fludarabine
  Phosphate (Fludara)

Fluorouracil [5-FU]
  (Generic)
Fluorouracil, Topical [5-
  FU] (Carac, Efudex,
  Fluoroplex, Generic)
Gemcitabine
  (Gemzar, Generic)
Mercaptopurine [6-MP]
  (Purinethol, Generic)

Methotrexate
  (Rheumatrex Dose
  Pack, Trexall)
Nelarabine (Arranon)
Omacetaxine (Synribo)
Pemetrexed (Alimta)
Pralatrexate (Folotyn)
Romidepsin (Istodax)
Thioguanine (Tabloid)

Hedgehog Pathway Inhibitor

Vismodegib (Erivedge)

Hormones

Abiraterone (Zytiga)
Anastrozole (Arimidex)
Bicalutamide (Casodex)
Degarelix (Firmagon)
Enzalutamide (Xtandi)
Estramustine Phosphate
  (Emcyt)
Exemestane (Aromasin,
  Generic)

Flutamide (Generic)
Fulvestrant (Faslodex)
Goserelin (Zoladex)
Histrelin Acetate
  (Supprelin LA, Vantus)
Leuprolide (Eligard,
  Lupron, Lupron
  DEPOT, Lupron
  DEPOT-Ped, Generic)

Levamisole (Ergamisol)
Megestrol Acetate
  (Megace, Megace ES)
Nilutamide (Nilandron)
Tamoxifen
Triptorelin (Trelstar 3.75,
  Trelstar 11.25, Trelstar
  22.5)

Immunotherapy

BCG [Bacillus Calmette-Guérin] (TheraCys, Tice BCG)

Interferon Alfa (Roferon-A, Intron A)

Sipuleucel-T (Provenge)

Mitotic Inhibitors (Vinca Alkaloids)

Etoposide [VP-16] (Etopophos, Toposar, Vepesid, Generic)

Vinblastine (Generic)
Vincristine (Marqibo, Vincasar, Generic)

Vinorelbine (Navelbine, Generic)

Monoclonal Antibodies

Ado-trastuzumab Emtansine (Kadcyla)
Alemtuzumab (Campath relaunch as Lemtrada)
Belimumab (Benlysta)
Bevacizumab (Avastin)

Brentuximab Vedotin (Adcetris)
Cetuximab (Erbitux)
Erlotinib (Tarceva)
Gemtuzumab Ozogamicin (Mylotarg)

Ipilimumab (Yervoy)
Obinutuzumab (Gazyva)
Ofatumumab (Arzerra)
Panitumumab (Vectibix)
Pertuzumab (Perjeta)
Trastuzumab (Herceptin)

Proteasome Inhibitor

Bortezomib (Velcade)

Taxanes

Cabazitaxel (Jevtana)
Docetaxel (Taxotere)

Paclitaxel (Taxol, Abraxane)

Tyrosine Kinase Inhibitors (TKIs)

Afatinib (Gilotrif)
Axitinib (Inlyta)
Baosutinib Monohydrate (Bosulif)
Cabozantinib (Cometriq)
Crizotinib (Xalkori)
Dasatinib (Sprycel)
Erlotinib (Tarceva)

Everolimus (Afinitor)
Gefitinib (Iressa)
Ibrutinib (Imbruvica)
Imatinib (Gleevec)
Lapatinib (Tykerb)
Nilotinib (Tasigna)
Pazopanib (Votrient)
Ponatinib (Clusig)

Regorafenib (Stivarga)
Sorafenib (Nexavar)
Sunitinib (Sutent)
Temsirolimus (Torisel)
Trametinib (Mekinist)
Vandetanib (Caprelsa)

Miscellaneous Antineoplastic Agents

Abiraterone (Zytiga)
Aldesleukin [Interleukin-2, IL-2] (Proleukin)

Aminoglutethimide (Cytadren)
L-Asparaginase (Elspar)

BCG [Bacillus Calmette-Guérin] (TheraCys, Tice BCG)
Carfilzomib (Kyprolis)

Cladribine (Leustatin)
Dacarbazine (DTIC)
Dabrafenib (Tafinlar)
Eribulin (Halaven)
Hydroxyurea (Droxia
  Hydrea, Generic)
Irinotecan (Camptosar,
  Generic)
Ixabepilone (Ixempra
  Kit)
Letrozole (Femara)

Leucovorin (Generic)
Mitoxantrone (Generic)
Panitumumab (Vectibix)
Pemetrexed (Alimta)
Pertuzumab (Perjeta)
Pomalidomide
  (Pomalyst)
Radium-223 Dichloride
  (Xofigo)
Rasburicase (Elitek)
Sipuleucel-T (Provenge)

Thalidomide (Thalomid)
Topotecan (Hycamtin,
  Generic)
Tretinoin, Topical
  [Retinoic Acid]
  (Retin-A, Avita,
  Renova, Retin-A
  Micro)
Ziv-Aflibercept (Zaltrap)

CARDIOVASCULAR (CV) AGENTS

Aldosterone Antagonist

Eplerenone (Inspra)

Spironolactone
  (Aldactone)

Alpha-1-Adrenergic Blockers

Doxazosin (Cardura,
  Cardura XL)

Prazosin (Minipress,
  Generic)

Terazosin (Hytrin,
  Generic)

Angiotensin-Converting Enzyme (ACE) Inhibitors

Benazepril (Lotensin)
Captopril (Capoten,
  Others)
Enalapril (Vasotec)
Fosinopril (Monopril,
  Generic)

Lisinopril (Prinivil,
  Zestril)
Moexipril (Univasc,
  Generic)
Perindopril Erbumine
  (Aceon, Generic)

Quinapril (Accupril,
  Generic)
Ramipril (Altace,
  Generic)
Trandolapril (Mavik,
  Generic)

Angiotensin II Receptor Antagonists/Blockers

Amlodipine/Olmesartan
  (Azor)
Amlodipine/Valsartan
  (Exforge)

Azilsartan (Edarbi)
Candesartan (Atacand)
Eprosartan (Teveten)
Irbesartan (Avapro)

Losartan (Cozaar)
Telmisartan (Micardis)
Valsartan (Diovan)

Antiarrhythmic Agents

Adenosine (Adenocard,
  Adenoscan)
Amiodarone (Cordarone,
  Nexterone, Pacerone)

Atropine, Systemic
  (AtroPen Auto-
  Injector)

Digoxin (Digitek,
  Lanoxin, Lanoxicaps)
Disopyramide (Norpace,
  Norpace CR)

Dofetilide (Tikosyn)
Dronedarone (Multaq)
Esmolol (Brevibloc, Generic)
Flecainide (Tambocor, Generic)

Ibutilide (Corvert, Generic)
Lidocaine, Systemic (Xylocaine, Others)
Mexiletine (Generic)
Procainamide (Generic)

Propafenone (Rythmol, Rhythmol SR, Generic)
Quinidine (Generic)
Sotalol (Betapace, Sorine, Generic)

Beta-Adrenergic Blockers

Acebutolol (Sectral)
Atenolol (Tenormin)
Atenolol/Chlorthalidone (Tenoretic)
Betaxolol (Kerlone)
Bisoprolol (Zebeta)
Carvedilol (Coreg, Coreg CR)

Labetalol (Trandate, Normodyne)
Metoprolol Succinate (Toprol XL, Generic)
Metoprolol Tartrate (Lopressor, Generic)
Nadolol (Corgard)
Nebivolol (Bystolic)

Penbutolol (Levatol)
Pindolol (Generic)
Propranolol (Inderal LA, Innopran XL, Generic)
Timolol (Generic)

Calcium Channel Antagonists/Blockers (CCBs)

Amlodipine (Norvasc)
Amlodipine/Olmesartan (Azor)
Amlodipine/Valsartan (Exforge)
Clevidipine (Cleviprex)
Diltiazem (Cardizem, Cardizem CD, Cardizem LA, Cardizem SR, Cartia XT, Dilacor XR, Diltia

XT, Taztia XT, Tiamate, Tiazac)
Felodipine (Plendil, Generic)
Isradipine (DynaCirc, Generic)
Nicardipine (Cardene, Cardene SR, Generic)
Nifedipine (Adalat CC, Afeditab CR,

Procardia, Procardia XL, Generic)
Nimodipine (Generic)
Nisoldipine (Sular, Generic)
Verapamil (Calan, Caover HS, Isoptin, Verelan, Generic)

Centrally Acting Antihypertensive Agents

Clonidine, Oral (Catapres)

Clonidine, Oral, Extended Release (Kapvay)
Clonidine, Transdermal (Catapres TTS)

Guanfacine (Tenex)
Methyldopa (Generic)

Combination Antihypertensive Agents

Aliskiren/Amlodipine (Tekamlo)

Aliskiren/Amlodipine/ Hydrochlorothiazide (Amturnide)

Aliskirin & Valsartan (Valturna)

Amlodipine/Valsartan/
Hydrochlorothiazide
(Exforge HCT)
Isosorbide Dinitrate
Hydralazine HCl
(BiDil)

Lisinopril/
Hydrochlorothiazide
(Prinzide, Zestoretic,
Generic)
Olmesartan, Amlodipine,
Hydrochlorothiazide
(Tribenzor)

Olmesartan, Olmesartan/
Hydrochlorothiazide
(Benicar, Benicar
HCT)
Telmisartan/Amlodipine
(Twynsta)

Diuretics

Acetazolamide (Diamox)
Amiloride (Midamor)
Bumetanide (Bumex)
Chlorothiazide (Diuril)
Chlorthalidone
Furosemide (Lasix,
Generic)
Hydrochlorothiazide
(HydroDIURIL,
Esidrix, Others)

Hydrochlorothiazide/
Amiloride (Moduretic)
Hydrochlorothiazide/
Spironolactone
(Aldactazide)
Hydrochlorothiazide/
Triamterene (Dyazide,
Maxide)
Indapamide (Lozol)

Mannitol, Intravenous
(Generic)
Metolazone (Zaroxolyn)
Spironolactone
(Aldactone, Generic)
Torsemide (Demadex,
Generic)
Triamterene (Dyrenium)

Inotropic/Pressor Agents

Digoxin (Digitek,
Lanoxin, Lanoxicaps)
Dobutamine (Dobutrex)
Dopamine (Intropin)
Epinephrine (Adrenalin,
EpiPen, EpiPen Jr,
Others)

Inamrinone [Amrinone]
(Inocor)
Isoproterenol (Isuprel)
Milrinone (Primacor,
Generic)
Nesiritide (Natrecor)

Norepinephrine
(Levophed)
Phenylephrine, Systemic
(Generic)

Lipid-Lowering Agents

Cholestyramine
(Questran, Questran
Light, Prevalite)
Colesevelam (WelChol)
Colestipol (Colestid)
Ezetimibe (Zetia)
Ezetimibe/Atorvastatin
(Liptruzet)
Fenofibrate (Antara,
Lipofen, Lofibra,

TriCor, Triglide,
Generic)
Fenofibric Acid
(Fibricor, Trilipix,
Generic)
Gemfibrozil (Lopid,
Generic)
Icosapent Ethyl
(Vascepa)
Mipomersen (Kynamro)

Niacin (Nicotinic Acid)
(Niaspan, Slo-Niacin,
Niacor, Nicolar) [OTC
Forms]
Niacin/Lovastatin
(Advicor)
Niacin/Simvastatin
(Simcor)
Omega-3 Fatty Acid
[Fish Oil] (Lovaza)

Statin/Antihypertensive Combinations

Amlodipine/Atorvastatin
(Caduet)

Statins

Atorvastatin
(Lipitor)
Fluvastatin (Lescol,
Generic)

Lovastatin (Mevacor,
Altoprev)
Pitavastatin (Livalo)

Pravastatin (Pravachol,
Generic)
Rosuvastatin (Crestor)
Simvastatin (Zocor)

Vasodilators

Alprostadil [Prostaglandin
E₁] (Prostin VR)
Epoprostenol (Veletri,
Flolan)
Fenoldopam (Corlopam)
Hydralazine (Apresoline,
Others)
Iloprost (Ventavis)
Isosorbide Dinitrate
(Dilatrate-SR, Isordil,
Sorbitrate, Generic)

Isosorbide Mononitrate
(Ismo, Imdur,
Monoket, Generic)
Macitentan (Opsumit)
Minoxidil, Oral
(Generic)
Nitroglycerin (Nitrostat,
Nitrolingual, Nitro-
Bid Ointment, Nitro-
Bid IV, Nitrodisc,

Transderm-Nitro,
NitroMist, Others)
Nitroprusside
(Nitropress)
Tolazoline (Priscoline)
Treprostinil Sodium
(Remodulin, Tyvaso)
Treprostinil, Extended
Release (Orenitram)

Miscellaneous Cardiovascular Agents

Aliskiren (Tekturna)
Aliskiren/
Hydrochlorothiazide
(Tekturna HCT)
Ambrisentan (Letairis)

Conivaptan (Vaprisol)
Dabigatran (Pradaxa)
Droxidopa (Northera)
Prasugrel (Effient)

Ranolazine (Ranexa)
Sildenafil (Viagra,
Revatio)

CENTRAL NERVOUS SYSTEM AGENTS

Alzheimer Agents

Donepezil (Aricept)
Galantamine
(Razadyne,
RazadyneER)
Memantine (Namenda)

Rivastigmine
(Exelon, Generic)
Rivastigmine
Transdermal
(Exelon Patch,
Generic)

Tacrine (Cognex)

Antianxiety Agents

Alprazolam (Xanax, Niravam)
Buspirone (Generic)
Chlordiazepoxide (Librium) [C-IV]
Clorazepate (Tranxene)

Diazepam (Diastat, Valium)
Doxepin (Sinequan, Adapin)
Hydroxyzine (Atarax, Vistaril, Generic)

Lorazepam (Ativan, Others)
Meprobamate (Generic) [C-IV]
Oxazepam (Generic) [C-IV]

Anticonvulsants

Carbamazepine (Tegretol XR, Carbatrol, Epitol, Equetro)
Clonazepam (Klonopin)
Clobazam (Onfi)
Diazepam (Diastat, Valium)
Ethosuximide (Zarontin)
Eslicarbazepine (Aptiom)
Ezogabine (Potiga)
Fosphenytoin (Cerebyx, Generic)
Gabapentin (Neurontin, Generic)
Lacosamide (Vimpat)

Lamotrigine (Lamictal)
Lamotrigine Extended-Release (Lamictal XR)
Levetiracetam (Keppra, Keppra XR)
Lorazepam (Ativan, Others)
Magnesium Sulfate (Various)
Oxcarbazepine (Oxtellar XR, Trileptal, Generic)
Pentobarbital (Nembutal) [C-II]
Perampanel (Fycompa)

Phenobarbital (Generic) [C-IV]
Phenytoin (Dilantin, Generic)
Rufinamide (Banzel)
Tiagabine (Gabitril, Generic)
Topiramate (Topamax, Generic)
Valproic Acid (Depakene, Depakote, Stavzor, Generic)
Vigabatrin (Sabril)
Zonisamide (Zonegran, Generic)

Antidepressants

Amitriptyline (Elavil)
Bupropion Hydrobromide (Aplenzin)
Bupropion Hydrochloride (Wellbutrin, Wellbutrin SR, Wellbutrin XL, Zyban)
Citalopram (Celexa)
Desipramine (Norpramin)

Desvenlafaxine (Pristiq)
Doxepin (Adapin)
Duloxetine (Cymbalta)
Escitalopram (Lexapro, Generic)
Fluoxetine (Gaboxetine, Prozac, Prozac Weekly, Sarafem, Generic)
Fluvoxamine (Luvox CR, Generic)
Imipramine (Tofranil, Generic)

Levomilnacipran (Fetzima)
Milnacipran (Savella)
Mirtazapine (Remeron, Remeron SolTab, Generic)
Nefazodone (Generic)
Nortriptyline (Aventyl, Pamelor)
Paroxetine (Paxil, Paxis CR, Pexeva, Generic)
Phenelzine (Nardil, Generic)

Selegiline, Oral
(Eldepryl, Zelapar,
Generic)
Selegiline, Transdermal
(Emsam)
Sertraline (Zoloft)

Tranylcypromine
(Parnate)
Trazodone (Desyrel,
Oleptro)
Viibryd (Vilazodone)
Vorapaxar (Zontivity)

Vortioxetine (Brintellix)
Venlafaxine (Effexor,
Effexor XR, Generic)

Antiparkinson Agents

Amantadine (Symmetrel)
Apomorphine (Apokyn)
Benztropine (Cogentin)
Bromocriptine (Parlodel)
Carbidopa/Levodopa
(Parcopa, Sinemet)
Entacapone (Comtan)

Pramipexole (Mirapex,
Mirapex ER, Generic)
Rasagiline (Azilect)
Rivastigmine,
Transdermal
(Exelon Patch)

Ropinirole (Requip,
Requip XL, Generic)
Selegiline (Eldepryl,
Zelapar)
Tolcapone (Tasmar)
Trihexyphenidyl
(Generic)

Antipsychotics

Aripiprazole (Abilify,
Abilify Discmelt)
Asenapine (Saphris)
Chlorpromazine
(Thorazine)
Clozapine (Clozaril,
FazaClo, Versacloz)
Fluphenazine (Prolixin,
Permitil)
Haloperidol (Haldol,
Generic)
Iloperidone (Fanapt)
Lithium Carbonate
Citrate (Generic)

Lurasidone (Latuda)
Molindone (Moban)
Olanzapine (Zyprexa,
Zyprexa Zydis,
Generic)
Olanzapine, LA
Parenteral (Zyprexa
Relprevv)
Paliperidone (Invega,
Invega Sustenna)
Perphenazine (Generic)
Pimozide (Orap)

Prochlorperazine
(Compro, Procomp,
Generic)
Quetiapine (Seroquel,
Seroquel XR, Generic)
Risperidone, Oral
(Risperdal, Risperdal
M-Tab, Generic)
Risperidone, Parenteral
(Risperdal Consta)
Thioridazine (Generic)
Thiothixene (Generic)
Trifluoperazine (Generic)
Ziprasidone (Geodon)

Sedative Hypnotics

Chloral Hydrate
(Aquachloral,
Supprettes)
Dexmedetomidine
(Precedex)
Diphenhydramine
(Benadryl OTC)

Doxepin (Silenor)
Estazolam (ProSom,
Generic) [C-IV]
Eszopiclone (Lunesta)
Etomidate (Amidate)
Flurazepam (Dalmane)
[C-IV]

Hydroxyzine (Atarax,
Vistaril)
Midazolam (Generic)
[C-IV]
Pentobarbital (Nembutal,
Others)
Phenobarbital

Propofol (Diprivan, Generic)
Ramelteon (Rozerem)
Secobarbital (Seconal)
Temazepam (Restoril, Generic) [C-IV]

Thiopental Sodium (Pentothal)
Triazolam (Halcion, Generic)
Zaleplon (Sonata)

Zolpidem (Ambien IR, Ambien CR, Edluar, ZolpiMist, Generic) [C-IV]

Stimulants

Armodafinil (Nuvigil)
Atomoxetine (Strattera)
Dexmethylphenidate (Focalin, Focalin XR)
Dextroamphetamine (Dexedrine, Procentra) [C-II]
Guanfacine (Intuniv)

Lisdexamfetamine (Vyvanse)
Methylphenidate, Oral (Concerta, Metadate CD, Metadate SR, Methylin, Ritalin, Ritalin LA, Ritalin SR, Quillivant XR) [C-II]

Methylphenidate, Transdermal (Daytrana)
Modafinil (Provigil, Generic) [C-IV]
Rivastigmine (Exelon)
Sibutramine (Meridia)

Miscellaneous CNS Agents

Clomipramine (Anafranil)
Clonidine, Oral, Extended-Release (Kapvay)
Dalfampridine (Ampyra)
Fingolimod (Gilenya)
Gabapentin Enacarbil (Horizant)

Interferon Beta-1a (Avonex, Rebif)
Meclizine (Antivert) (Dramamine [OTC])
Natalizumab (Tysabri)
Nimodipine (Nimotop)
Rizatriptan (Maxalt, Maxalt-MLT, Generic)

Sodium Oxybate (Xyrem)
Tasimelteon (Hetlioz)
Teriflunomide (Aubagio)
Tetrabenazine (Xenazine)

DERMATOLOGIC AGENTS

Acitretin (Soriatane)
Acyclovir (Zovirax)
Adapalene (Differin)
Adapalene/Benzoyl Peroxide (Epiduo Gel)
Alefacept (Amevive)
Amphotericin B (Amphocin, Fungizone)

Anthralin (Dritho, Zithranol, Zithranol-RR)
Bacitracin, Topical (Baciguent)
Bacitracin/Polymyxin B, Topical (Polysporin)
Bacitracin/Neomycin/ Polymyxin B, Topical (Neosporin Ointment)

Bacitracin/Neomycin/ Polymyxin B/ Hydrocortisone, Topical (Cortisporin)
Bacitracin, Neomycin, Polymyxin B, & Lidocaine, Topical (Clomycin)

Botulinum Toxin Type A
[Abobotulinumtoxin A]
(Dysport)

Botulinum Toxin Type A
[Incobotulinumtoxin A]
(Xeomin)

Botulinum Toxin Type A
[Onabotulinumtoxin A]
(Botox, Botox
Cosmetic)

Botulinum Toxin Type B
[Rimabotulinumtoxin
B] (Myobloc)

Brimonidine (Mirvaso)

Calcipotriene (Dovonex)

Calcitriol Ointment
(Vectical)

Capsaicin (Capsin,
Zostrix, Others)

Ciclopirox (Ciclodan,
CNL8, Loprox,
Pedipirox-4 Nail Kit,
Penlac)

Ciprofloxacin
(Cipro, Cipro XR,
Proquin XR)

Clindamycin (Cleocin,
Cleocin T, Others)

Clindamycin/Benzoyl
Peroxide (Benzaclin)

Clindamycin/Tretinoin
(Veltin Gel)

Clotrimazole/
Betamethasone
(Lotrisone)

Dapsone Topical
(Aczone)

Dibucaine (Nupercainal)

Diclofenac, Topical
(Solaraze)

Doxepin, Topical
(Zonalon, Prudoxin)

Econazole (Spectazole)

Erythromycin, Topical
(Akne-Mycin, Ery,
Erythra-Derm,
Generic)

Erythromycin/Benzoyl
Peroxide
(Benzamycin)

Finasteride (Propecia)

Fluorouracil, Topical
[5-FU] (Efudex)

Gentamicin, Topical
(Generic)

Imiquimod Cream
(Aldara, Zyclara)

Ingenol Mebutate
(Picato)

Isotretinoin
(Amnesteem, Claravis,
Myorisan, Sotret,
Zentane, Generic)

Ketoconazole (Nizoral,
Generic)

Ketoconazole, Topical
(Extina, Nizoral A-D
Shampoo, Xolegel)
[Shampoo OTC]

Kunecatechins
[Sinecatechins]
(Veregen)

Lactic Acid/Ammonium
Hydroxide
[Ammonium Lactate]
(Lac-Hydrin)

Lindane (Generic)

Lisdexamfetamine
(Vyvanse)

Metronidazole (Flagyl,
Glagyl ER,
Luliconazole [Luzu]
MetroCream,

MetroGel,
MetroLotion)

Miconazole (Monistat 1
Combination Pack,
Monistat 3, Monistat
7) [OTC] (Monistat-
Derm)

Miconazole/Zinc Oxide/
Petrolatum (Vusion)

Minocycline (Arestin,
Dynacin, Minocin,
Solodyn, Generic)

Minoxidil, Topical
(Theroxidil, Rogaine)
[OTC]

Mupirocin (Bactroban,
Bactroban Nasal)

Naftifine (Naftin)

Nystatin (Mycostatin)

Oxiconazole (Oxistat)

Penciclovir (Denavir)

Permethrin (Elimite,
Nix, [OTC])

Pimecrolimus (Elidel)

Podophyllin (Condylox,
Condylox Gel 0.5%,
Podocon-25)

Pramoxine (Anusol
Ointment,
ProctoFoam NS)

Pramoxine &
Hydrocortisone
(Proctofoam-HC)

Selenium Sulfide (Exsel
Shampoo, Selsun Blue
Shampoo, Selsun
Shampoo)

Silver Sulfadiazine
(Silvadene,
Thermazene, Generic)

Steroids, Topical
(see Table 3)

Tacrolimus, Ointment (Protopic)
Tazarotene (Tazorac, Avage)
Terbinafine (Lamisil, Lamisil AT [OTC])

Tolnaftate (Tinactin, Generic [OTC])
Tretinoin, Topical [Retinoic Acid] (Avita, Retin-A, Retin-A Micro, Renova)

Ustekinumab (Stelara)
Vorinostat (Zolinza)

DIETARY SUPPLEMENTS

Calcium Acetate (Calphron, Phos-Ex, PhosLo)
Calcium Glubionate (Calcionate)
Calcium Salts (Chloride, Gluconate, Gluceptate)
Cholecalciferol [Vitamin D_3] (Delta-D)
Cyanocobalamin [Vitamin B_{12}] (Nascobal)
Ferric Carboxymaltose (Injectafer)
Ferric Gluconate Complex (Ferrlecit)

Ferrous Gluconate (Fergon [OTC], Others)
Ferrous Sulfate
Ferumoxytol (Feraheme)
Fish Oil (Lovaza, Others [OTC])
Folic Acid, Injectable, Oral (Generic)
Iron Dextran (Dexferrum, INFeD)
Iron Sucrose (Venofer)
Magnesium Oxide (Mag-Ox 400, Others [OTC])
Magnesium Sulfate (Various)

Multivitamins, Oral [OTC] (see Table 12)
Phytonadione [Vitamin K] (Mephyton, Generic)
Potassium Supplements (see Table 6)
Pyridoxine [Vitamin B_6] (Generic)
Sodium Bicarbonate [NaHCO$_3$] (Generic)
Thiamine [Vitamin B_1] (Generic)

EAR (OTIC) AGENTS

Acetic Acid/Aluminum Acetate, Otic (Domeboro Otic)
Benzocaine/Antipyrine (Auralgan)
Ciprofloxacin, Otic (Cetraxal)
Ciprofloxacin/ Dexamethasone, Otic (Ciprodex)
Ciprofloxacin/ Hydrocortisone, Otic (Cipro HC Otic)

Neomycin/Colistin/ Hydrocortisone (Cortisporin-TC Otic Drops)
Neomycin/Colistin, Hydrocortisone/ Thonzonium (Cortisporin-TC Otic Suspension)
Ofloxacin Otic (Floxin Otic, Floxin Otic Singles)

Polymyxin B & Hydrocortisone (Otobiotic Otic)
Sulfacetamide (Bleph-10, Cetamide, Klaron, Generic)
Sulfacetamide/ Prednisolone (Blephamide)
Triethanolamine (Cerumenex [OTC])

ENDOCRINE SYSTEM AGENTS

Antidiabetic Agents

Acarbose (Precose)
Bromocriptine
  Mesylate
  (Cycloset)
Chlorpropamide
  (Diabinese)
Dapagliflozin (Farxiga)
Exenatide (Byetta)
Glimepiride (Amaryl,
  Generic)
Glimepiride/Pioglitazone
  (Duetact)
Glipizide (Glucotrol,
  Glucotrol XL,
  Generic)
Glyburide (DiaBeta,
  Glynase, Generic)

Glyburide/Metformin
  (Glucovance, Generic)
Insulins, Injectable (see
  Table 4)
Linagliptin/Metformin
  (Jentadueto)
Liraglutide Recombinant
  (Victoza)
Metformin
  (Fortmet, Glucophage,
  Glucophage XR,
  Glumetza, Riomet,
  Generic)
Miglitol (Glyset)
Nateglinide (Starlix,
  Generic)

Pioglitazone (Actos,
  Generic)
Pioglitazone/Metformin
  (ACTOplus Met,
  ACTOplus MET XR,
  Generic)
Repaglinide (Prandin)
Repaglinide/Metformin
  (PrandiMet)
Rosiglitazone (Avandia)
Rosiglitazone/Metformin
  (Avandamet)
Sitagliptin (Januvia)
Sitagliptin & Metformin
  (Janumet)
Tolazamide (Generic)
Tolbutamide (Generic)

Dipepidyl Peptidase-4 (DPP-4) Inhibitors

Alogliptin (Nesina)
Alogliptin/Metformin
  (Kazano)
Alogliptin/Pioglitazone
  (Oseni)

Linagliptin
  (Tradjenta)
Saxagliptin (Onglyza)
Saxagliptin/Metformin
  (Kombiglyze XR)
Sitagliptin (Januvia)

Sitagliptin/Metformin
  (Janumet)
Sitagliptin/Simvastatin
  (Juvisync)

Glucagon-Like Peptide-1 (GLP-1) Receptor Agonists

Exenatide (Byetta)
Exenatide ER
  (Bydureon)

Liraglutide Recombinant
  (Victoza)

Sodium-Glucose Co-Transporter 2 (SGLT2) Inhibitors

Canagliflozin (Invokana)

Hormone & Synthetic Substitutes

Calcitonin (Fortical, Miacalcin)

Calcitriol (Rocaltrol, Calcijex)

Cortisone Systemic & Topical (see Table 2 & Table 3)

Desmopressin (DDAVP, Stimate)

Dexamethasone, Systemic & Topical (Decadron)

Fludrocortisone (Florinef, Generic)

Fluoxymesterone (Androxy) [C-III]

Glucagon, Recombinant (GlucaGen)

Hydrocortisone, Topical/ Systemic (Cortef, Solu-Cortef, Generic)

Methylprednisolone (A-Methapred, Depo-Medrol, Medrol, Medrol Dosepak, Solu-Medrol, Generic) (see Steroids & Table 2)

Prednisolone (Flo-Pred, Omnipred, Orapred, Pediapred, Generic) (see Steroids & Table 2)

Prednisone (Generic) (see Steroids & Table 2)

Testosterone (AndroGel 1%, AndroGel 1.62%, Androderm, Axiron, Fortesta, Striant, Testim, Testopel)

Testosterone, Nasal Gel (Natesto)

Testosterone Undecanoate, Injectable (Aveed)

Vasopressin

Vasopressin [Antidiuretic Hormone. ADH] (Pitressin)

Hypercalcemia/Osteoporosis Agents

Alendronate (Fosamax, Fosamax Plus D)

Denosumab (Prolia, Xgeva)

Etidronate (Didronel)

Gallium Nitrate (Ganite)

Ibandronate (Boniva, Generic)

Pamidronate (Generic)

Raloxifene (Evista)

Risedronate (Actonel, Actonel w/ Calcium, Generic)

Risedronate, Delayed-Release (Atelvia)

Teriparatide (Forteo)

Zoledronic Acid (Zometa, Generic)

Obesity

Lorcaserin (Belviq)

Orlistat (Xenical, Alli [OTC])

Phentermine (Adipex-P, Surenza, Generic)

Phentermine/Topiramate (Qsymia) [C-IV]

Thyroid/Antithyroid

Levothyroxine (Synthroid, Levoxyl, Others)

Liothyronine [T_3] (Cytomel, Triostat)

Methimazole (Tapazole, Generic)

Potassium Iodide (Lugol Soln, Iosat, SSKI, ThyroBlock,

ThyroSafe, ThyroShield) [OTC]

Propylthiouracil (Generic)

Miscellaneous Endocrine Agents

Cinacalcet (Sensipar)
Demeclocycline
 (Declomycin)
Diazoxide (Proglycem)

Mifepristone (Korlym)
Pasireotide (Signifor)
Somatropin (Genotropin,
 Nutropin AQ,

Omnitrope, Saizen,
 Serostim, Zorbtive)
Tesamorelin (Egrifta)

EYE (OPHTHALMIC) AGENTS

Glaucoma Agents

Acetazolamide
 (Diamox)
Apraclonidine (Iopidine)
Betaxolol, Ophthalmic
 (Betoptic)
Brimonidine
 (Alphagan P)
Brimonidine/Timolol
 (Combigan)
Brinzolamide (Azopt)

Brinzolamide/
 Brimonidine
 (Simbrinza)
Bromfenac (Prolensa)
Carteolol, Ophthalmic
Dipivefrin (Propine)
Dorzolamide (Trusopt)
Dorzolamide/Timolol
 (Cosopt)
Echothiophate Iodine,
 Ophthalmic
 (Phospholine Iodide)

Latanoprost (Xalatan)
Levobunolol (AK-Beta,
 Betagan)
Lodoxamide (Alomide)
Rimexolone (Vexol
 Ophthalmic)
Tafluprost (Zioptan)
Timolol, Ophthalmic
 (Betimol, Timoptic,
 Timoptic XE, Generic)
Trifluridine, Ophthalmic
 (Viroptic)

Ophthalmic Antibiotics

Azithromycin,
 Ophthalmic 1%
 (AzaSite)
Bacitracin, Ophthalmic
 (AK-Tracin
 Ophthalmic)
Bacitracin/Neomycin/
 Polymyxin B (Neo-
 polycin, Neosporin
 Ophthalmic)
Bacitracin/Neomycin/
 Polymyxin B/
 Hydrocortisone
 (Neo-polycin HC
 Cortisporin
 Ophthalmic)

Bacitracin/Polymyxin B,
 Ophthalmic (AK-
 Poly-Bac Ophthalmic,
 Polysporin
 Ophthalmic)
Besifloxacin (Besivance)
Ciprofloxacin,
 Ophthalmic (Ciloxan)
Erythromycin,
 Ophthalmic (Ilotycin)
Gentamicin, Ophthalmic
 (Garamycin, Genoptic,
 Gentak, Generic)
Gentamicin/
 Prednisolone,
 Ophthalmic (Pred-G
 Ophthalmic)

Levofloxacin
 Ophthalmic (Quixin,
 Iquix)
Moxifloxacin Ophthalmic
 (Vigamox)
Neomycin/Polymyxin B/
 Hydrocortisone
 (Cortisporin
 Ophthalmic,
 Cortisporin Otic)
Neomycin/
 Dexamethasone (AK-
 Neo-Dex Ophthalmic,
 NeoDecadron
 Ophthalmic)

Neomycin/Polymyxin B/
Dexamethasone,
Ophthalmic (Maxitrol)
Neomycin/Polymyxin B/
Prednisolone (Poly-
Pred Ophthalmic)
Norfloxacin, Ophthalmic
(Chibroxin)
Ofloxacin, Ophthalmic
(Ocuflox)

Silver Nitrate (Generic)
Sulfacetamide,
Ophthalmic (Bleph-
10, Cetamide, Sodium
Sulamyd)
Sulfacetamide/
Prednisolone,
Ophthalmic
(Blephamide, Others)

Tobramycin, Ophthalmic
(AKTob, Tobrex,
Generic)
Tobramycin/
Dexamethasone,
Ophthalmic
(TobraDex)
Trifluridine, Ophthalmic
(Viroptic)

Miscellaneous Ophthalmic Agents

Aflibercept (Eylea)
Alcaftadine, Ophthalmic
(Lastacaft)
Artificial Tears (Tears
Naturale [OTC])
Atropine (Isopto
Atropine, Generic)
Bepotastine Besilate
(Bepreve)
Cidofovir (Vistide)
Cromolyn Sodium
(Opticrom)
Cyclopentolate
(Cyclogyl, Cyclate)
Cyclopentolate/
Phenylephrine
(Cyclomydril)
Cyclosporine (Restasis)

Dexamethasone,
Ophthalmic (AK-Dex
Ophthalmic, Decadron
Ophthalmic, Maxidex)
Diclofenac (Voltaren)
Emedastine (Emadine)
Epinastine (Elestat)
Ganciclovir, Ophthalmic
Gel (Zirgan)
Ketotifen, Ophthalmic
(Alaway, Claritin Eye,
Zaditor, Zyrtec Itchy
Eye) [OTC]
Ketorolac (Acular,
Acular LS, Acular PF)
Levocabastine (Livostin)
Lodoxamide (Alomide)
Loteprednol (Alrex,
Lotemax)

Naphazoline (Albalon,
Naphcon, Generic)
Naphazoline/
Pheniramine
(Naphcon A, Visine A,
Generic)
Nepafenac (Nevanac)
Olopatadine (Patanol,
Pataday)
Pemirolast (Alamast)
Phenylephrine
(Neo-Synephrine
Ophthalmic,
AK-Dilate, Zincfrin
[OTC])
Ranibizumab (Lucentis)
Rimexolone (Vexol)
Scopolamine,
Ophthalmic

GASTROINTESTINAL (GI) AGENTS

Antacids

Alginic Acid/Aluminum
Hydroxide/
Magnesium Trisilicate
(Gaviscon) [OTC]

Aluminum Hydroxide
(Amphojel,
AlternaGEL,
Dermagran) [OTC]

Aluminum Hydroxide/
Magnesium Carbonate
(Gaviscon Extra
Strength, Liquid)
[OTC]

Aluminum Hydroxide/
  Magnesium
  Hydroxide (Maalox)
Aluminum Hydroxide/
  Magnesium
  Hydroxide/
  Simethicone (Mylanta,

Mylanta II, Maalox
  Plus) [OTC]
Aluminum Hydroxide/
  Magnesium Trisilicate
  (Gaviscon, Regular
  Strength) [OTC]

Calcium Carbonate
  (Tums, Alka-Mints)
  [OTC]
Magaldrate (Riopan
  Plus) [OTC]
Simethicone (Generic)
  [OTC]

Antidiarrheals

Bismuth Subsalicylate
  (Pepto-Bismol)
Diphenoxylate/Atropine
  (Lomotil, Lonox)
Kaolin-Pectin (Kaodene,
  Kao-Spen,
  Kapectolin)

Lactobacillus (Lactinex
  Granules) [OTC]
Loperamide (Diamode,
  Imodium) [OTC]
Octreotide (Sandostatin,
  Sandostatin LAR,
  Generic)

Paregoric (Camphorated
  Tincture of Opium)
Rifaximin (Xifaxan,
  Xifaxan550)

Antiemetics

Aprepitant (Emend)
Chlorpromazine
  (Thorazine)
Dimenhydrinate
  (Dramamine, Others)
  [OTC]
Dolasetron (Anzemet)
Dronabinol (Marinol)
  [C-III]
Droperidol (Inapsine)
Fosaprepitant (Emend,
  Injection)

Granisetron (Generic)
Meclizine (Antivert,
  Bonine, Dramamine
  [OTC])
Metoclopramide
  (Reglan, Clopra,
  Octamide)
Nabilone (Cesamet)
Ondansetron (Zofran,
  Zofran ODT)
Ondansetron, Oral
  Soluble Film (Zuplenz)

Palonosetron (Aloxi)
Prochlorperazine
  (Compazine)
Promethazine
  (Promethegan,
  Generic)
Scopolamine (Transderm
  Scop)
Thiethylperazine
  (Torecan)
Trimethobenzamide
  (Tigan, Generic)

Antiulcer Agents

Bismuth Subcitrate/
  Metronidazole/
  Tetracycline (Pylera)
Cimetidine (Tagamet,
  Tagamet HB 200,
  [OTC])

Dexlansoprazole
  (Dexilant, Kapidex)
Esomeprazole (Nexium)
Famotidine (Fluxid,
  Pepcid, Pepcid AC,
  Generic, [OTC])

Lansoprazole (Prevacid,
  Prevacid 24HR
  [OTC])
Nizatidine (Axid, Axid
  AR [OTC], Generic)

Omeprazole (Prilosec, Prilosec [OTC], Generic)
Omeprazole/Sodium Bicarbonate (Zegerid, Zegerid [OTC])
Omeprazole, Sodium Bicarbonate,

Magnesium Hydroxide (Zegerid w/ Magnesium Hydroxide)
Pantoprazole (Protonix, Generic)
Rabeprazole (AcipHex)

Ranitidine (Zantac, Zantac EFFERDose [OTC], Generic)
Sucralfate (Carafate, Generic)

Cathartics/Laxatives

Bisacodyl (Dulcolax [OTC])
Citric Acid/Magnesium Oxide/Sodium Picosulfate (Prepopik)
Docusate Calcium (Surfak)
Docusate Potassium (Dialose)
Docusate Sodium (DOSS, Colace)
Glycerin Suppository
Lactulose (Constulose, Generlac, Chronulac,

Cephulac, Enulose, Others)
Magnesium Citrate (Citroma, Others) [OTC]
Magnesium Hydroxide (Milk of Magnesia) [OTC]
Mineral Oil [OTC]
Mineral Oil Enema (Fleet Mineral Oil) [OTC]
Mineral Oil-Pramoxine HCl-Zinc Oxide [OTC]

Polyethylene Glycol Electrolyte Solution [PEG-ES] (GoLYTELY, CoLyte)
Polyethylene Glycol (PEG) 3350 (MiraLAX) [OTC]
Psyllium (Konsyl, Metamucil, Generic)
Sodium Phosphate (OsmoPrep, Visicol)
Sorbitol (Generic)

Enzymes

Pancrelipase (Creon, Pancreaze, Panakare Plus, Pertzye, Ultresa,

Voikace, Zenpep, Generic)

Miscellaneous GI Agents

Alosetron (Lotronex)
Alvimopan (Entereg)
Apriso (Salix)
Balsalazide (Colazal)
Budesonide (Entocort EC)
Certolizumab Pegol (Cimzia)
Crofelemer (Fulyzaq)

Dexpanthenol (Ilopan-Choline Oral, Ilopan)
Dibucaine (Nupercainal)
Dicyclomine (Bentyl)
Fidaxomicin (Dificid)
Hydrocortisone, Rectal (Anusol-HC Suppository, Cortifoam Rectal,

Proctocort, Others, Generic)
Hyoscyamine (Anaspaz, Cystospaz, Levsin, Others, Generic)
Hyoscyamine/Atropine/ Scopolamine Phenobarbital (Donnatal, Others)
Infliximab (Remicade)

Linaclotide (Linzess)
Lubiprostone (Amitiza)
Mesalamine (Apriso,
    Asacol, Asacol HD,
    Canasa, Lialda,
    Pentasa, Rowasa,
    Generic)
Methylnaltrexone
    Bromide (Relistor)
Metoclopramide
    (Reglan, Clopra,
    Octamide)
Mineral Oil/Pramoxine
    HCl/Zinc Oxide
    (Tucks Ointment)
    [OTC]

Misoprostol (Cytotec)
Neomycin (Neo-Fradin,
    Generic)
Olsalazine (Dipentum)
Oxandrolone (Oxandrin,
    Generic) [C-III]
Pramoxine (Anusol
    Ointment, ProctoFoam
    NS, Others)
Pramoxine/
    Hydrocortisone
    (Enzone,
    ProctoFoam-HC)
Propantheline (Pro-
    Banthine, Generic)

Starch, Topical, Rectal
    (Tucks Suppositories)
    [OTC]
Sulfasalazine
    (Azulfidine,
    Azulfidine EN,
    Generic)
Teduglutide [rDNA
    Origin] (Gattex)
Vasopressin [Antidiuretic
    Hormone (ADH)]
    (Pitressin)
Witch Hazel (Tucks
    Pads, Others [OTC])

HEMATOLOGIC AGENTS

Anticoagulants

Antithrombin,
    Recombinant (ATryn)
Argatroban (Generic)
Bivalirudin (Angiomax)
Dabigatran (Pradaxa)
Dalteparin (Fragmin)

Desirudin (Iprivask)
Enoxaparin (Lovenox)
Fondaparinux (Arixtra,
    Generic)
Heparin (Generic)
Lepirudin (Refludan)

Protamine (Generic)
Tinzaparin (Innohep)
Warfarin (Coumadin,
    Jantoven, Generic)

Antiplatelet Agents

Abciximab (ReoPro)
Aspirin (Bayer, Ecotrin,
    St. Joseph's [OTC])
Cilostazol (Pletal)
Clopidogrel (Plavix)

Dipyridamole
    (Persantine)
Dipyridamole/Aspirin
    (Aggrenox)
Eptifibatide (Integrilin)
Prasugrel (Effient)

Rivaroxaban (Xarelto)
Ticagrelor (Brilinta)
Ticlopidine (Ticlid)
Tirofiban (Aggrastat)

Antithrombotic Agents

Alteplase, Recombinant
    [tPA] (Activase)
Aminocaproic Acid
    (Amicar)

Anistreplase (Eminase)
Apixaban (Eliquis)
Dextran 40 (Gentran 40,
    Rheomacrodex)

Reteplase (Retavase)
Streptokinase (Generic)
Tenecteplase (TNKase)
Urokinase (Abbokinase)

Hematinic Stimulants

Darbepoetin Alfa
(Aranesp)
Eltrombopag (Promacta)
Epoetin Alfa
[Erythropoietin, EPO]
(Epogen, Procrit)

Filgrastim [G-CSF]
(Neupogen)
Iron Dextran
(Dexferrum, INFeD)
Iron Sucrose (Venofer)
Oprelvekin (Neumega)

Pegfilgrastim (Neulasta)
Plerixafor (Mozobil)
Romiplostim (Nplate)
Sargramostim [GM-
CSF] (Leukine)

Volume Expanders

Albumin (Albuked,
Albuminar 20, AlbuRx
25, Albutein,

Buminate, Kedbumin,
Plabumin)
Dextran 40 (Gentran 40,
Rheomacrodex)

Hetastarch (Hespan)
Plasma Protein Fraction
(Plasmanate, Others)

Miscellaneous Hematologic Agents

Antihemophilic
Factor VIII
(Monoclate-P)
Antihemophilic Factor
[Recombinant]
(Advate, Hexilate FS,
Kogenate FS,
Recombinate, Xyntha)
Decitabine (Dacogen)

Deferiprone (Ferriprox)
Desmopressin (DDAVP,
Stimate)
Fibrinogen Concentrate,
Human (Riastap)
Lenalidomide (Revlimid)
Pentoxifylline (Trental,
Generic)

Prothrombin Complex
Concentrate (Human)
(Keentra)
Ruxolitinib (Jakafi)

IMMUNE SYSTEM AGENTS

Immunomodulators

Dimethyl Fumarate
(Tecfidera)
Icatibant (Firazyr)
Interferon Alfa
(Roferon-A, Intron A)
Interferon Alfacon-1
(Infergen)

Interferon Beta-1a
(Rebif)
Interferon Beta-1b
(Betaseron, Extavia)
Interferon Gamma-1b
(Actimmune)
Natalizumab
(Tysabri)

Peginterferon Alfa-2a
[Pegylated Interferon]
(Pegasys)
Peginterferon Alfa-2b
[Pegylated Interferon]
(PegIntron)

Immunomodulators: Disease-Modifying Antirheumatic Drugs (DMARDs)

Abatacept (Orencia)
Adalimumab (Humira)
Anakinra (Kineret)

Certolizumab Pegol (Cimzia)
Etanercept (Enbrel)
Golimumab (Simponi)

Infliximab (Remicade)
Tocilizumab (Actemra)
Tofacitinib (Xeljanz)

Immunosuppressive Agents

Azathioprine (Imuran)
Basiliximab (Simulect)
Belatacept (Nulojix)
Cyclosporine (Gengraf, Neoral, Sandimmune)
Daclizumab (Zenapax)
Everolimus (Zortress)
Lymphocyte Immune Globulin

[Antithymocyte Globulin (ATG)] (Atgam)
Muromonab-CD3 (Orthoclone OKT3)
Mycophenolate Mofetil (CellCept, Generic)
Mycophenolic Acid (Myfortic, Generic)

Sirolimus [Rapamycin] (Rapamune)
Steroids, Systemic (see Table 2)
Tacrolimus (Prograf, Generic)

Vaccines/Serums/Toxoids

Cytomegalovirus Immune Globulin [CMV-IG IV] (CytoGam)
Diphtheria & Tetanus Toxoids (Td) (Decavac for > 7 y)
Diphtheria & Tetanus Toxoids (DT) (Generic Only for < 7 y)
Diphtheria, Tetanus Toxoids, & Acellular Pertussis Adsorbed (DTaP) (Ages < 7 y) (Daptacel, Infanrix, Tripedia)
Diphtheria, Tetanus Toxoids, & Acellular Pertussis Adsorbed

(Tdap) (Ages > 10–11 y) (Boosters: Adacel, Boostrix)
Diphtheria, Tetanus Toxoids, Acellular Pertussis Adsorbed, Hep B (Recombinant), & Inactivated Poliovirus Vaccine (IPV) Combined (Pediarix)
Haemophilus B Conjugate Vaccine (ActHIB, HibTITER, PedvaxHIB, Prohibit, TriHIBit, Others)
Hepatitis A (Inactivated) & Hepatitis B Recombinant Vaccine (Twinrix)

Hepatitis A Vaccine (Havrix, Vaqta)
Hepatitis B Immune Globulin (HyperHep, HepaGam B, Nabi-HB, H-BIG)
Hepatitis B Vaccine (Engerix-B, Recombivax HB)
Human Papillomavirus (Types 6, 11, 16, 18) Recombinant Vaccine (Gardasil)
Immune Globulin, IV (Gamimune N, Sandoglobulin, Gammar IV)
Immune Globulin, Subcutaneous (Vivaglobin)

Influenza Monovalent Vaccine (H1N1), Inactivated (CSL, Novartis, Sanofi, Pasteur)

Influenza Vaccine, Inactivated (Afluria, Fluarix, FluLaval, Fluvirin, Fluzone)

Influenza Virus Vaccine Live, Intranasal (FluMist)

Measles, Mumps, & Rubella Vaccine Live [MMR] (M-M-R II)

Measles, Mumps, Rubella, & Varicella

Virus Vaccine Live [MMRV] (ProQuad)

Meningococcal Conjugate Vaccine [Quadrivalent, MCV4] (Menactra)

Meningococcal Polysaccharide Vaccine [MPSV4] (Menomune A/C/Y/W-135)

Pneumococcal 7-Valent Conjugate Vaccine (Prevnar)

Pneumococcal Vaccine, Polyvalent (Pneumovax-23)

Rotavirus Vaccine, Live, Oral, Monovalent (Rotarix)

Rotavirus Vaccine, Live, Oral, Pentavalent (RotaTeq)

Smallpox Vaccine (Dryvax)

Tetanus Immune Globulin

Tetanus Toxoid (TT)

Varicella Immune Globulin (VarZIG)

Varicella Virus Vaccine (Varivax)

Zoster Vaccine, Live (Zostavax)

MUSCULOSKELETAL AGENTS

Antigout Agents

Allopurinol (Zyloprim, Lopurin, Aloprim)

Colchicine

Febuxostat (Uloric)

Pegloticase (Krystexxa)

Probenecid (Probalan, Generic)

Sulfinpyrazone

Muscle Relaxants

Baclofen (Lioresal Intrathecal, Gablofen)

Carisoprodol (Soma)

Chlorzoxazone (Parafon Forte DSC, Others)

Cyclobenzaprine (Flexeril)

Cyclobenzaprine, Extended-Release (Amrix)

Dantrolene (Dantrium, Revonto)

Diazepam (Diastat, Valium)

Metaxalone (Skelaxin)

Methocarbamol (Robaxin, Generic)

Orphenadrine (Norflex, Generic)

Tizanidine Hydrochloride (Zanaflex)

Neuromuscular Blockers

Atracurium (Tracrium)

Botulinum Toxin Type A [Incobotulinumtoxin A] (Xeomin)

Botulinum Toxin Type A [Onabotulinumtoxin A] (Botox, Botox Cosmetic)

Botulinum Toxin Type B [Rimabotulinumtoxin B] (Myobloc)

Pancuronium (Generic)

| Rocuronium (Zemuron, Generic) | Succinylcholine (Anectine, Quelicin, Generic) | Vecuronium (Generic) |

Miscellaneous Musculoskeletal Agents

Edrophonium (Enlon)
Leflunomide (Arava)
Methotrexate (Rheumatrex Dose Pack, Trexall, Generic)

Sulfasalazine (Azulfidine, Azulfidine EN)
Tizanidine (Zanaflex, Generic)

OB/GYN AGENTS

Contraceptives

Copper Intrauterine Device (IUD) (ParaGard T380A)
Estradiol Cypionate & Medroxyprogesterone Acetate (Lunelle)
Ethinyl Estradiol/ Norelgestromin (Ortho Evra)
Etonogestrel, Implant (Implanon)

Etonogestrel/Ethinyl Estradiol Vaginal Insert (NuvaRing)
Levonorgestrel Intrauterine Device (IUD) (Mirena)
Medroxyprogesterone (Provera, Depo Provera, Depo-Sub Q Provera, Generic)

Oral Contraceptives (see Table 5)
Extended Cycle Combination (Table 5)
Oral Contraceptives, Monophasic (Table 5)
Oral Contraceptives, Multiphasic (Table 5)
Oral Contraceptives, Progestin-Only (Table 5)

Emergency Contraceptives

Levonorgestrel (Next Choice, Plan B, One Step, Generic [OTC])

Ulipristal Acetate (Ella)

Estrogen Supplementation

ESTROGEN ONLY

Estradiol, Oral (Delestrogen, Estrace, Femtrace, Others)
Estradiol (Estrace, Femtrace, Delestrogen)

Estradiol, Metered Gel (Elestrin, Estrogel)
Estradiol Gel (Divigel)
Estradiol, Spray (Evamist)
Estradiol, Transdermal (Alora, Climara,

Estraderm, Vivelle Dot)
Estradiol, Vaginal (Estring, Femring, Vagifem)
Estrogen, Conjugated (Premarin)

Estrogen, Conjugated-
    Synthetic (Cenestin,
    Enjuvia)

Esterified Estrogens
    (Estratab)

Ethinyl Estradiol
    (Estinyl, Feminone)

COMBINATION ESTROGEN/PROGESTIN

Ethinyl Estradiol &
    Drospirenone (YAZ)
Ethinyl Estradiol/
    Levonorgestrel
    (Seasonale)
Ethinyl Estradiol &
    Norelgestromin
    (Ortho Evra)
Esterified Estrogens w/
    Methyltestosterone
    (Estratest, Estratest
    HS, Syntest DS, HS)

Estrogen, Conjugated w/
    Methylprogesterone
    (Premarin w/ Methyl
    Progesterone)
Estrogen, Conjugated w/
    Methyltestosterone
    (Premarin w/
    Methyltestosterone)
Estradiol/Levonorgestrel,
    Transdermal
    (Climara Pro)

Estradiol/
    Medroxyprogesterone
    (Lunelle)
Estradiol/Norethindrone
    (Activella, Generic)
Estrogen, Conjugated/
    Medroxyprogesterone
    (Prempro, Premphase)
Norethindrone Acetate/
    Ethinyl Estradiol
    (Femhrt, Activella)

Vaginal Preparations

Amino-Cerv pH 5.5
    Cream
Miconazole (Monistat 1
    Combination Pack,
    Monistat 3, Monistat

7) [OTC] (Monistat-
    Derm)
Nystatin (Mycostatin)

Terconazole (Terazol 3,
    Terazol 7, Generic)
Tioconazole (Generic
    [OTC])

Miscellaneous OB/GYN Agents

Clomiphene (Clomid)
Conjugated Estrogens/
    Bazedoxifene
    (Duavee)
Dinoprostone (Cervidil
    Vaginal Insert, Prepidil
    Gel, Prostin E2)
Doxylamine/Pyridoxine
    (Diclegis)
Gonadorelin (Factrel)
Leuprolide (Lupron)

Leuprolide Acetate/
    Norethindrone Acetate
    Kit (Lupaneta Pack)
Lutropin Alfa (Luveris)
Lysteda (Tranexamic
    Acid)
Magnesium Sulfate
    (Various)
Medroxyprogesterone
    (Provera, Depo
    Provera, Depo-Sub Q
    Provera)

Methylergonovine
    (Methergine)
Mifepristone [RU 486]
    (Mifeprex)
Nafarelin, Metered
    Spray (SYNAREL)
Ospemifene (Osphena)
Oxytocin (Pitocin,
    Generic)
Paroxetine (Brisdelle)
Terbutaline (Generic)
Tranexamic Acid
    (Lysteda, Generic)

PAIN MEDICATIONS

Local Anesthetics (see also Local Anesthetics Table 1)

Benzocaine (Americaine, Lanacaine, Hurricane, Various [OTC])
Benzocaine/Antipyrine (Auralgan)
Bupivacaine (Marcaine)
Capsaicin (Capsin, Zostrix, Others [OTC])
Cocaine
Dibucaine (Nupercainal)

Lidocaine; Lidocaine/ Epinephrine (Anestacon Topical, Xylocaine, Xylocaine Viscous, Xylocaine MPF, Others)
Lidocaine, Powder Intradermal Injection System (Zingo)
Lidocaine/Prilocaine (EMLA, LMX)

Lidocaine/Tetracaine, Transdermal (Synera); Cream (Pliaglis)
Mepivacaine (Carbocaine)
Pramoxine (Anusol Ointment, ProctoFoam NS, Others)
Procaine (Novocaine)

Migraine Headache

Acetaminophen/Butalbital w/ & w/o Caffeine (Fioricet, Medigesic, Esgic, Dologic Plus, Bupap, Sedapap, Phrenilin)
Almotriptan (Axert)
Aspirin/Butalbital/ Caffeine Compound (Fiorinal)

Aspirin/Butalbital/ Caffeine/Codeine (Fiorinal w/ Codeine)
Eletriptan (Relpax)
Frovatriptan (Frova)
Naratriptan (Amerge, Generic)
Sumatriptan (Alsuma, Imitrex, Imitrex

Statdose, Imitrex Nasal Spray, Generic)
Sumatriptan/Naproxen Sodium (Treximet)
Sumatriptan Needleless System (Sumavel DosePro)
Zolmitriptan (Zomig, Zomig ZMT, Zomig Nasal)

Narcotic Analgesics

Acetaminophen/Codeine (Tylenol 2, 3, 4)
Alfentanil (Alfenta)
Aspirin w/ Codeine (Empirin No. 2, 3, 4)
Buprenorphine (Buprenex)
Buprenorphine/Naloxone (Suboxone)
Buprenorphine, Transdermal (Butrans)
Butorphanol (Stadol)
Codeine

Fentanyl (Sublimaze)
Fentanyl Iontophoretic Transdermal System (Ionsys)
Fentanyl, Transdermal (Duragesic, Generic) [C-II]
Fentanyl, Transmucosal (Abstral, Actiq, Fentora, Lazanda, Onsolis, Generic) [C-II]
Hydrocodone (Zohydro)

Hydrocodone/ Acetaminophen (Lorcet, Vicodin, Hycet, Others)
Hydrocodone & Aspirin (Lortab ASA, Others)
Hydrocodone/Ibuprofen (Vicoprofen, Generic)
Hydromorphone (Dilaudid, Dilaudid HP, Generic) [C-II]

Hydromorphone, Extended-Release (Exalgo)

Levorphanol (Levo-Dromoran)

Meperidine (Demerol, Meperitab, Generic) [C–II]

Methadone (Dolophine, Methadose, Generic) [C-II]

Morphine (Avinza XR, Astramorph/PF, Duramorph, Infumorph, MS Contin, Kadian SR,

Oramorph SR, Roxanol) [C-II]

Morphine, Liposomal (DepoDur)

Morphine/Naltrexone (Embeda)

Nalbuphine (Generic)

Oxycodone (OxyContin, Roxicodone, Generic) [C-II]

Oxycodone/ Acetaminophen (Percocet, Tylox)

Oxycodone/ Acetaminophen ER (Xartemis XR)

Oxycodone/Aspirin (Percodan)

Oxycodone/Ibuprofen (Combunox)

Oxymorphone (Opana, Opana ER)

Pentazocine (Talwin, Talwin Compound, Talwin NX) [C-IV]

Propoxyphene (Darvon-N), Propoxyphene/ Acetaminophen (Generic), Propoxyphene/Aspirin (Generic) [C-IV]

Nonnarcotic Analgesics

Acetaminophen, Injection (Ofirmev)

Acetaminophen, Oral [*N*-Acetyl-*p*-aminophenol (APAP)] (Acephen, Tylenol, Other Generic)

Acetaminophen/ Butalbital/±Caffeine (Fioricet, Medigesic, Repan, Sedapap-10, Two-Dyne, Triapin, Axocet, Phrenilin Forte)

Aspirin (Bayer, Ecotrin, St. Joseph's) [OTC]

Tramadol (Rybix ODT, Ryzolt ER, Ultram, Ultram ER, Generic)

Tramadol/ Acetaminophen (Ultracet)

Nonsteroidal Anti-Inflammatory Agents (NSAIDs)

Celecoxib (Celebrex)

Diclofenac, Oral (Cataflam, Voltaren, Voltaren XR)

Diclofenac, Topical (Flector Patch, Pennsaid, Voltaren Gel)

Diclofenac/Misoprostol (Arthrotec)

Diflunisal (Dolobid)

Etodolac

Fenoprofen (Nalfon, Generic)

Flurbiprofen (Ansaid, Ocufen, Generic)

Ibuprofen, Oral (Advil, Motrin, Motin IB, Rufen, Others, Generic) [OTC]

Ibuprofen, Parenteral (Caldolor)

Indomethacin (Indocin, Generic)

Ketoprofen (Orudis, Oruvail)

Ketorolac (Toradol)

Ketorolac, Nasal (Sprix)

Meloxicam (Mobic, Generic)

Nabumetone (Relafen, Generic)

Naproxen (Aleve [OTC], Anaprox, Anaprox DS, EC-Naprosyn

Naprelan, Naprosyn, Generic)
Naproxen/Esomeprazole (Vimovo)

Oxaprozin (Daypro, Daypro ALTA)
Piroxicam (Feldene, Generic)

Sulindac (Clinoril, Generic)
Tolmetin (Generic)

Miscellaneous Pain Medications

Amitriptyline (Elavil)
Clonidine, Epidural (Duraclon)
Imipramine (Tofranil)

Pregabalin (Lyrica, Generic)
Tapentadol (Nucynta)

Tramadol (Ultram, Ultram ER)
Ziconotide (Prialt)

RESPIRATORY AGENTS

Antitussives, Decongestants, & Expectorants

Acetylcysteine (Acetadote, Mucomyst)
Benzonatate (Tessalon, Zonatuss)
Codeine
Dextromethorphan (Benylin DM, Delsym, Mediquell, PediaCare 1, Others) [OTC]
Guaifenesin (Robitussin, Others, Generic)

Guaifenesin/Codeine (Robafen AC, Others, Generic)
Guaifenesin/ Dextromethorphan (Many OTC Brands)
Hydrocodone/ Guaifenesin (Hycotuss Expectorant)
Hydrocodone/ Homatropine (Hycodan, Hydromet, Others, Generic)
Hydrocodone/ Pseudoephedrine

(Detussin, Histussin-D, Others, Generic) [C-III]
Hydrocodone, Chlorpheniramine, Phenylephrine, Acetaminophen, & Caffeine (Hycomine Compound)
Potassium Iodide (Lugol Soln SSKI)
Pseudoephedrine (Many Mono & Combination Brands [OTC])

Bronchodilators

Albuterol (Proventil, Ventolin, Proair)
Albuterol/Ipratropium (Combivent, DuoNeb)
Aminophylline (Generic)
Arformoterol (Brovana)
Ephedrine (Generic)

Epinephrine (Adrenalin, Sus-Phrine, EpiPen, EpiPen Jr, Others)
Formoterol Fumarate (Foradil, Performist)
Indacaterol (Arcapta Neohaler)

Isoproterenol (Isuprel)
Levalbuterol (Xopenex, Xopenex HFA)
Metaproterenol (Alupent, Metaprel)
Pirbuterol (Maxair, Generic)

Salmeterol (Serevent, Serevent Diskus)

Terbutaline (Brethine, Bricanyl)

Theophylline (Theo24, Theochron, Theolair, Generic)

Respiratory Inhalants

Acetylcysteine (Acetadote, Mucomyst)
Beclomethasone (QVAR)
Beclomethasone, Nasal (Beconase AQ)
Beractant (Survanta)
Budesonide (Rhinocort Aqua, Pulmicort)
Budesonide/Formoterol (Symbicort)
Calfactant (Infasurf)
Ciclesonide, Inhaled (Alvesco)
Ciclesonide, Nasal (Omnaris, Zettona)
Cromolyn Sodium (Intal, NasalCrom, Opticrom, Others)
Dexamethasone, Nasal (Dexacort Phosphate Turbinaire)

Fluticasone Furoate, Nasal (Veramyst)
Fluticasone Propionate, Nasal (Flonase, Generic)
Fluticasone Propionate, Inhaled (Flovent HFA, Flovent Diskus)
Fluticasone & Vilanterol (Breo Ellipta)
Flunisolide (AeroBid, Aerospan, Nasarel)
Fluticasone Furoate
Fluticasone Propionate/Salmeterol Xinafoate (Advair Diskus, Advair HFA)
Formoterol Fumarate (Foradil Aerolizer, Perforomist)
Ipratropium (Atrovent HFA, Atrovent Nasal, Generic)

Mometasone/Formoterol (Dulera)
Mometasone, Inhaled (Asmanex Twisthaler)
Mometasone, Nasal (Nasonex)
Olopatadine, Nasal (Patanase)
Phenylepherine, Nasal (Neo-Synephrine Nasal [OTC])
Tiotropium (Spiriva)
Tobramycin, Inhalation (TOBI, TOBI Podhaler)
Triamcinolone (Azmacort)
Umeclidinium/Vilanterol (Anoro Ellipta)

Surfactants

Beractant (Survanta)

Calfactant (Infasurf)

Lucinactant (Surfaxin)

Miscellaneous Respiratory Agents

Alpha-1-Protease Inhibitor (Glassia, Prolastin C)
Aztreonam, Inhaled
Dornase Alfa (Pulmozyme, DNase)

Mannitol, Inhalation (Aridol)
Montelukast (Singulair)
Omalizumab (Xolair)
Tadalafil (Adcirca)

Zafirlukast (Accolate, Generic)
Zileuton (Zyflo, Zyflo CR)

URINARY/GENITOURINARY AGENTS

Benign Prostatic Hyperplasia

Alfuzosin (Uroxatral)
Doxazosin (Cardura, Cardura XL)
Dutasteride (Avodart)

Dutasteride & Tamsulosin (Jalyn)
Finasteride (Proscar, Generic)
Silodosin (Rapaflo)

Tamsulosin (Flomax, Generic)
Terazosin (Hytrin, Generic)

Bladder Agents

Belladonna/Opium Suppositories (B&O) (Generic)
Bethanechol (Urecholine)
Butabarbital/ Hyoscyamine Phenazopyridine (Pyridium Plus)
Darifenacin (Enablex)
Fesoterodine (Toviaz)
Flavoxate (Generic)
Hyoscyamine (Anaspaz, Cystospaz, Levsin)

Hyoscyamine, Atropine, Scopolamine/ Phenobarbital (Donnatal, Others, Generic)
Methenamine Hippurate (Hiprex), Methenamin Mandelate (Urex, Uroquid-Acid No. 2)
Mirabegron (Myrbetriq)
Oxybutynin (Ditropan, Ditropan XL, Generic)
Oxybutynin Transdermal System (Oxytrol)

Oxybutynin, Topical (Gelnique)
Phenazopyridine (Pyridium, Azo-Standard, Urogesic, Many Others [OTC])
Solifenacin (VESIcare)
Tolterodine (Detrol, Detrol LA, Generic)
Trospium (Sanctura, Sanctura XR, Generic)

Erectile Dysfunction

Alprostadil, Intracavernosal (Caverject, Edex)
Alprostadil, Urethral Suppository (Muse)

Avandafil (Stendra)
Sildenafil (Viagra, Revatio)
Tadalafil (Cialis)

Vardenafil (Levitra, Stayxn)
Yohimbine (Yocon, Yohimex)

Urolithiasis

Potassium Citrate (Urocit-K, Generic)
Potassium Citrate & Citric Acid (Polycitra-K, Generic)

Sodium Citrate/Citric Acid (Bicitra, Oracit)

Trimethoprim (Trimpex, Proloprim)

Miscellaneous Urology Agents

Ammonium Aluminum Sulfate [Alum] [OTC]
BCG [Bacillus Calmette-Guérin] (TheraCys, Tice BCG)
Dimethyl Sulfoxide [DMSO] (Rimso-50)
Methenamine, Phenyl Salicylate, Methylene Blue, Benzoic Acid, Hyoscyamine (Prosed)
Atropine, Sulfate (Urised)
Neomycin/Polymyxin Bladder Irrigant (Neosporin GU Irrigant)
Nitrofurantoin (Furadantin, Macrobid, Macrodantin, Generic)
Pentosan Polysulfate Sodium (Elmiron)
Trimethoprim (Trimpex, Proloprim)

VACCINES/SERUMS/TOXOIDS

Cytomegalovirus Immune Globulin [CMV-IG IV] (CytoGam)
Diphtheria & Tetanus Toxoids (Td) (Decavac, Tenivac for > 7 y)
Diphtheria/Tetanus Toxoids [DT] (Generic Only, for < 7 y)
Diphtheria/Tetanus Toxoids/Acellular Pertussis, Adsorbed [DTaP; for < 7 y] (Daptacel, Infanrix, Tripedia)
Diphtheria/Tetanus Toxoids/Acellular Pertussis, Adsorbed [Tdap; for > 10–11 y] (Boosters: Adacel, Boostrix)
Diphtheria/Tetanus Toxoids/Acellular Pertussis, Adsorbed/
Inactivated Poliovirus Vaccine [IPV]/ Haemophilus b Conjugate Vaccine Combined (Pentacel)
Diphtheria/Tetanus Toxoids/Acellular Pertussis, Adsorbed, Hepatitis B [Recombinant], & Inactivated Poliovirus Vaccine [IPV] Combined (Pediarix)
Haemophilus b Conjugate Vaccine (ActHIB, HibTITER, PedvaxHIB, others)
Hepatitis A [Inactivated] & Hepatitis B [Recombinant] Vaccine (Twinrix)
Hepatitis A Vaccine (Havrix, Vaqta)
Hepatitis B Immune Globulin (HyperHep B, HepaGam B, Nabi-HB, H-BIG)
Hepatitis B Vaccine (Engerix-B, Recombivax HB)
Human Papillomavirus Recombinant Vaccine (Cervarix [Types 16, 18], Gardasil [Types 6, 11, 16, 18])
Immune Globulin, IV (Gamimune N, Gammaplex, Gammar IV, Sandoglobulin, Others)
Immune Globulin, Subcutaneous (Vivaglobin)
Influenza Vaccine, Inactivated, Trivalent (IIV3) (Afluria, Fluarix, Flucelvax, FluLaval, Fluvirin, Fluzone, Fluzone High Dose, Fluzone Intradermal)
Influenza Vaccine, Inactivated, Quadrivalent (IIV4)

(Fluarix Quadrivalent,
Fluzone Quadrivalent)
Influenza Vaccine, Live-
Attenuated,
Quadrivalent (LAIV4)
(FluMist)
Influenza Vaccine,
Recombinant,
Trivalent (RIV3)
(FluBlok)
Measles/Mumps/Rubella
Vaccine, Live [MMR]
(M-M-R II)
Measles/Mumps/
Rubella/Varicella
Virus Vaccine, Live
[MMRV] (ProQuad)

Meningococcal
Conjugate Vaccine
[Quadrivalent, MCV4]
(Menactra, Menveo)
Meningococcal Groups
C & Y & Haemophilus
b Tetanus Toxoid
Conjugate Vaccine
(Menhibrix)
Meningococcal
Polysaccharide
Vaccine [MPSV4]
(Menomune A/C/
Y/W-135)
Pneumococcal 13-Valent
Conjugate Vaccine
(Prevnar 13)

Pneumococcal Vaccine,
Polyvalent
(Pneumovax-23)
Rotavirus Vaccine, Live,
Oral, Pentavalent
(RotaTeq)
Smallpox Vaccine
(ACAM2000)
Tetanus Immune
Globulin (Generic)
Tetanus Toxoid (TT)
(Generic)
Varicella Immune
Globulin (VarZIG)
Varicella Virus Vaccine
(Varivax)
Zoster Vaccine, Live
(Zostavax)

WOUND CARE

Becaplermin
(Regranex Gel)

Silver Nitrate
(Dey-Drop, Others)

MISCELLANEOUS THERAPEUTIC AGENTS

Acamprosate (Campral)
Alglucosidase Alfa
(Lumizyme,
Myozyme)
Apremilast (Otezla)
C1 Esterase Inhibitor
[Human] (Berinert,
Cinryze)
Cilostazol (Pletal)
Dextrose 50%/25%
Drotrecogin Alfa
(Xigris)
Ecallantide
(Kalbitor)
Eculizumab (Soliris)
Ivacaftor (Kalydeco)

Lanthanum Carbonate
(Fosrenol)
Mecasermin (Increlex)
Megestrol Acetate
(Megace, Megace-ES,
Generic)
Methylene Blue (Urolene
Blue, Various)
Naltrexone (ReVia,
Vivitrol, Generic)
Nicotine, Gum
(Nicorette, Others)
Nicotine, Nasal Spray
(Nicotrol NS)
Nicotine, Transdermal
(Habitrol, NicoDerm
CQ [OTC], Others)

Palifermin (Kepivance)
Potassium iodide (Lugol
Soln, SSKI, Thyro-
Block, ThyroSafe,
ThyroShield) [OTC]
Sevelamer Carbonate
(Renvela)
Sevelamer
Hydrochloride
(Renagel)
Sodium Polystyrene
Sulfonate (Kayexalate,
Kionex, Generic)
Sucroferric
Oxyhydroxide
(Velphoro)

Talc (Sterile Talc Powder)

Taliglucerase Alfa (Elelyso)

Varenicline (Chantix)

NATURAL & HERBAL AGENTS

Aloe Vera (*Aloe barbadensis*)
Arnica (*Arnica montana*)
Bilberry (*Vaccinium myrtillus*)
Black Cohosh
Bogbean (*Menyanthes trifoliate*)
Borage (*Borago officinalis*)
Bugleweed (*Lycopus virginicus*)
Butcher's Broom (*Ruscus aculeatus*)
Capsicum (*Capsicum frutescens*)
Cascara Sagrada (*Rhamnus purshiana*)
Chamomile
Chondroitin Sulfate
Comfrey (*Symphytum officinale*)
Coriander (*Coriandrum sativum*)
Cranberry (*Vaccinium macrocarpon*)

Dong Quai (*Angelica polymorpha, sinensis*)
Echinacea (*Echinacea purpurea*)
Ephedra/Ma Huang
Evening Primrose Oil
Feverfew (*Tanacetum parthenium*)
Fish Oil Supplements (Omega-3 Polyunsaturated Fatty Acid)
Garlic (*Allium sativum*)
Gentian (*Gentiana lutea*)
Ginger (*Zingiber officinale*)
Ginkgo Biloba
Ginseng
Glucosamine Sulfate (Chitosamine) & Chondroitin Sulfate
Green Tea (*Camellia sinensis*)
Guarana (*Paullinia cupana*)
Hawthorn (*Crataegus laevigata*)
Horsetail (*Equisetum arvense*)

Kava Kava (Kava Kava Root Extract, *Piper methysticum*)
Licorice (*Glycyrrhiza glabra*)
Melatonin
Milk Thistle (*Silybum marianum*)
Nettle (*Urtica dioica*)
Red Yeast Rice
Resveratrol
Rue (*Ruta graveolens*)
Saw Palmetto (*Serenoa repens*)
Spirulina (*Spirulina* spp)
Stevia (*Stevia rebaudiana*)
St. John's Wort (*Hypericum perforatum*)
Tea Tree (*Melaleuca alternifolia*)
Valerian (*Valeriana officinalis*)
Yohimbine (*Pausinystalia yohimbe*) (Yocon, Yohimex)

GENERIC AND SELECTED BRAND DRUG DATA

Abacavir (Ziagen) [Antiretroviral/NRTI] **WARNING:** Allergy (fever, rash, fatigue, GI, resp) reported; D/C drug stat & do not rechallenge; lactic acidosis & hepatomegaly/steatosis reported **Uses:** *HIV Infxn* **Action:** NRTI **Dose:** *Adults.* 300 mg PO bid or 600 mg PO daily *Peds.* 8 mg/kg bid, 16–20 mg/kg (stable CD4, undetectable VRL) 300 mg bid max **Caution:** [C, –] CDC rec: HIV-infected mothers not breast-feed (transmission risk) **Disp:** Tabs 300 mg; soln 20 mg/mL **CI:** Mod-severe hepatic impair, hypersens **SE:** See Warning **Interactions:** EtOH ↓ drug elimination & ↑ drug exposure; many drug interactions; ↓ methadone levels **Labs:** ↑ LFTs, fat redistribution, N, V, HA, chills; monitor; ↑ GGT, glucose, triglycerides **NIPE:** ⊘ EtOH; monitor & teach pt about hypersensitivity Rxns; HLA-B*5701 at ↑ risk for fatal hypersensitivity Rxn, genetic screen before use; allergic Rxn usually appears w/in first 6 wk of Tx if pt is allergic; D/C drug stat if hypersensitivity Rxn occurs and ⊘ rechallenge; take w/ or w/o food

Abatacept (Orencia) [Immunomodulator] **Uses:** *Mod/severe RA, JIA* **Action:** Selective costimulation modulator, ↓ T-cell activation **Dose:** *Adults.* Initial 500 mg (< 60 kg), 750 mg (60–100 kg); 1 g (> 100 kg) IV over 30 min; repeat at 2 & 4 wk, then q4wk; SQ regimen: after IV dose, 125 mg SQ within 24 h of Inf, then 125 SQ weekly *Peds. 6–17 y.* 10 mg/kg (< 75 kg), 750 mg (75–100 kg), IV over 30 min; repeat at 2 and 4 wks then q4wk (> 100 kg, adult dose) **Caution:** [C,?/–] w/ TNF blockers; anakinra; COPD; h/o predisposition to Infxn; w/ immunosuppressants **CI:** w/Live vaccines w/in 3 mo of D/C abatacept **Disp:** IV soln 125 mg/ml **SE:** HA, URI, N, nasopharyngitis, Infxn, malignancy, Inf Rxns /hypersens (dizziness, HA, HTN), COPD exacerbations, cough, dyspnea **Interactions:** ↑ risk of infection W/ anakinra & TNF antagonists; ↓ effectiveness of vaccines **Labs:** Falsely ↑ blood glucose **NIPE:** Screen for TB prior to use; D/C if serious Infxn occurs; may worsen COPD Sxs

Abciximab (ReoPro) [Platelet-Aggregation Inhibitor/Antiplatelet] **Uses:** *Prevent acute ischemic comps in PCP*, MI Infxn* **Action:** ↓ plt aggregation (glycoprotein IIb/IIIa inhib) **Dose:** *ECC 2010:* ACS w/ immediate PCI: 0.25 mg/kg IV bolus 10–60 min before PCI, then 0.125 mcg/kg/min max 10 mcg/min IV for 12 h; w/ heparin ACS w/ planned PCI w/in 24 h: 0.25 mg/kg IV bolus, then 10 mcg/min IV over 18–24 h concluding 1 h post PCI; *PCI:* 0.25 mg/kg bolus 10–60 min pre-PTCA, then 0.125 mcg/kg/min (max 10 mcg/min) cont Inf for 12 h **Caution:** [C, ?/–] **CI:** Active/ recent (w/in 6 wk) internal hemorrhage, CVA

38 Abiraterone

w/in 2 y or CVA w/ sig neuro deficit, bleeding diathesis or PO anticoagulants w/in 7 d (unless PT < 1.2 × control), ↓ plt (< 100,000 cells/mcL), recent trauma or major surgery (w/in 6 wk), CNS tumor, AVM, aneurysm, severe uncontrolled HTN, vasculitis, dextran use w/ PTCA, murine protein allergy, w/ other glycoprotein IIb/IIIa inhib **Disp:** Inj 2 mg/mL **SE:** Back pain, ↓ BP, CP, allergic Rxns, bleeding **Interactions:** May ↑ risk of bleeding **W/** anticoagulants, antiplts, NSAIDs, thrombolytics **Labs:** ↓ hgb, plt; monitor CBC, PT, PTT, INR, guaiac stools, urine for blood; ↑ WBC **NIPE:** Monitor for ↑ bleeding & bruising; ⊘ shake vial or mix w/ another drug, ⊘ contact sports. Use w/ heparin/ASA

Abiraterone (Zytiga) [CYP17 Inhibitor] **Uses:** *Castrate-resistant metastatic PCa* **Action:** CYP17 inhibitor; ↓ testosterone precursors **Dose:** 1000 mg PO qd w/ 5 mg prednisone bid; w/o food 2 h ac and 1 h pc; ↓ w/ hepatic impair **Caution:** [X, N/A] w/ Severe CHF, monitor for adrenocortical Insuff/ excess, w/ CYP2D6 substrate /CYP3A4 inhib or inducers **CI:** PRG **Disp:** Tabs 250 mg **SE:** Jt swell, edema, muscle pain, hot flush, D, UTI, cough, ↑ BP, ↑ URI, urinary frequency, dyspepsia **Interactions:** ↓ metabolism of CYP2D6 drugs (Table 10) **W/** abiraterone; caution **W/** strong CYP3A4 inducers & inhibitors (Table 10) **Labs:** ↑ LFTs – ↑ LFTs, ↑ TG; ↓ K+, ↓ PO₄⁻³ **NIPE:** CYP17 inhib may ↑ mineralocorticoid SEs; prednisone; ↓ ACTH-limiting SEs

Acamprosate (Campral) [Hypoglycemic/Alpha-Glucosidase Inhibitor] **Uses:** *Maintain abstinence from EtOH* **Action:** ↓ Glutamatergic transmission; ↓ NMDA receptors; related to GABA **Dose:** 666 mg PO tid; CrCl 30–50 mL/min: 333 mg PO tid **Caution:** [C, ?/–] **CI:** CrCl < 30 mL/min **Disp:** Tabs 333 mg EC **SE:** N/D, depression, anxiety, insomnia **Interactions:** None **Labs:** ↑ BS, LFTs, uricacid; ↑ Hgb, Hct; ↓ plts **NIPE:** Does not eliminate EtOH withdrawal Sx; continue even if relapse occurs; caution w/ elderly & pts w/ h/o suicide ideations or depression; take w/o regard to food & swallow whole; ⊘ make up missed dose or take > 3 doses in 24 h

Acarbose (Precose) [Hypoglycemic/Alpha-Glucosidase Inhibitor] **Uses:** *Type 2 DM* **Action:** α-Glucosidase inhib; delays carbohydrate digestion to ↓ glucose **Dose:** 25–100 mg PO tid w/1st bite each meal; 50 mg tid (< 60kg); 100 mg tid (> 60 kg); usual maint 50–100 mg PO tid **Caution:** [B, ?] w/ SCr > 2 mg/dL **CI:** IBD, colonic ulceration, partial intestinal obst; cirrhosis **Disp:** Tabs 25, 50, 100 mg **SE:** Abd pain, D, flatulence, hypersens Rxns **Interactions:** OK **W/** sulfonylureas; ↑ hypoglycemic effect **W/** juniper berries, ginseng, garlic, coriander, celery; ↓ effects **W/** intestinal absorbents, digestive enzyme preps, diuretics, corticosteroids, phenothiazines, estrogens, phenytoin, INH, sympathomimetics, CCBs, thyroid hormones; ↓ conc **OF** digoxin levels **Labs:** ↑ LFTs, ✓ LFTs q3mo for 1st y, ↑ FBS, HbA1c; ↓ Ca, Hgb & Hct, vit B₆; monitor digoxin levels **NIPE:** Take drug tid w/ 1st bite of food, ↓ GISE by ↓ dietary starch, treat hypoglycemia w/ dextrose instead of sucrose, continue diet & exercise program

Acebutolol (Sectral) [Antihypertensive, Antiarrhythmic/Beta-Blocker] Uses: *HTN, arrhythmias* chronic stable angina **Action:** Blocks β-adrenergic receptors, β₁, & ISA **Dose:** *HTN:* 400–800 mg/d 2 ÷ doses *Arrhythmia:* 400–1200 mg/d 2 ÷ doses; ↓ 50% w/ CrCl < 50 mL/min or elderly; max 800 mg/d ↓ 75% w/CrCl < 25 mL/min; max 400 mg/d **Caution:** [B, + M] Can exacerbate ischemic heart Dz **CI:** 2nd-, 3rd-degree heart block, cardiac failure, cardiogenic shock **Disp:** Caps 200, 400 mg **SE:** Fatigue, HA, dizziness, ↓ HR **Interactions:** ↓ antihypertensive effect *W/* NSAIDs, salicylates, thyroid preps, anesthetics, antacids, α-adrenergic stimulants, ma huang, ephedra, licorice; ↓ hypoglycemic effect *OF* glyburide; ↑ hypotensive response *W/* other antihypertensives, nitrates, EtOH, diuretics, black cohosh, hawthorn, goldenseal, parsley; ↑ bradycardia *W/* digoxin, amiodarone; ↓ hypoglycemic effect *OF* insulin **Labs:** ↑ ANA titers; monitor ECG **NIPE:** Teach pt to monitor BP, pulse, S/Sxs CHF; ⊘ D/C abruptly—can ↑ angina or cause MI

Acetaminophen [APAP, N-Acetyl-p-Aminophenol] (Acephen, Ofirmev, IV [Rx], Tylenol, Other Generic) [OTC] WARNING: May cause acute liver failure; associated w/ doses > 4000 mg/d & taking APAP in > 1 product **Uses:** *Mild–mod pain, HA, fever* **Acts:** Nonnarcotic analgesic; ↓ CNS synth of prostaglandins & hypothalamic heat-regulating center **Dose:** *Adults.* 325–650 mg PO or PR q4–6h or 1000 mg PO 3–4 ×/d; max 4 g/d *IV:* < 50 kg: 15 mg/kg IV q6h or 12.5 mg/kg IV q4h; max 75 mg/kg/d. ≥ 50 kg: 650 mg IV q4h or 1000 mg IV q6h; max 4 g/d *Peds < 12 y.* 10–15 mg/kg/dose PO or PR q4–6h; max 5 doses/24 h. Administer q6h if CrCl 10–50 mL/min & q8h if CrCl < 10 mL/min. *IV:* 15 mg/kg IV q6h or 12.5 mg/kg IV q4h; max 75 mg/kg/d **W/P:** [C, +] w/ Hepatic/renal impair in elderly & w/ EtOH use (> 3 drinks/d); w/ > 4 g/d; EtOH liver Dz, G6PD deficiency; w/ warfarin; serious skin rxns (SJS, TEN, AGEP) **CI:** Hypersens **Disp:** Tabs meltaway/dissolving 80, 160 mg; tabs: 325, 500, 650 mg; chew tabs 80, 160 mg; gel caps 500 mg; liq 160 mg/5 mL, 500 mg/15 mL; drops 80 mg/0.8 mL; *Acephen* supp 80, 120, 325, 650 mL; Inj 10 mg/mL **SE:** hepatotoxic; OD hepatotoxic at 10 g; 15 g can be lethal; Rx w/ N-acetylcysteine **Notes:** No anti-inflammatory or plt-inhibiting action; 2014 MedWatch Safety Alert: FDA recommends providers stop using combo products w/> 325 mg APAP/dosage unit. No data that taking > 325 mg APAP/dose is beneficial and this ↑ liver injury risk. ↓ Dose also ↓ risk of inadvertent APAP overdose. Most manufacturers have complied with the 2011 FDA request to limit APAP to 325 mg/dosage unit; however, some Rx combo products w/ > 325 mg of APAP/ dosage unit remain available. An FDA advisory group has recommended a ↓ in max dose to 3000 mg/d **NIPE:** ⊘ETOH; teach S/Sxs hepatotox; ↑ risk if exceed max dose of 3 g/24 h; consult healthcare provider if temp ↑ 103°F/> 3 d; delayed absorption if given w/ food.

Acetaminophen, Injection (Ofirmev) [Analgesic/Antipyretic] Uses: *Mild–mod pain, fever* **Acts:** Nonnarcotic analgesic; CNS synth of prostaglandins & hypothalamic heat-regulating center **Dose:** *Adults & peds > 50 kg.* 1000 mg q6h or 650 mg q4h IV; 4000 mg max/day. < 50 kg: 15 mg/kg q6h or 12.5 mg/kg q4h, 75 mg/kg/day max. **Peds ≥ 2–12 y**: 15 mg/kg q6h or 12.5 mg/kg q4h IV, 75 mg/kg/day max. Min. interval of 4 h **Caution**: [C, +] Excess dose can cause hepatic injury; caution w/ liver Dz, alcoholism, malnutrition, hypovolemia, CrCl < 30 g/min **CI**: Hypersens to components, severe/active liver Dz **Disp**: IV 1000 mg (10 mg/mL) **SE**: N/V, HA, insomnia (adults); N/V, constipation, pruritus, agitation, atelectasis (peds) **Interactions**: Caution W/ CYP2E1 inhibitors & inducers (Table 10); dose ↑ 4000 mg/d may ↑ INR **Labs**: Monitor warfarin **NIPE**: Min dosing interval 4 h; infuse over 15 min. No anti-inflammatory or plt-inhibiting action

Acetaminophen + Butalbital ± Caffeine (Fioricet, Margesic, Esgic, Repan, Sedapap, Dolgic Plus, Bupap, Phrenilin Forte) [C-III] [Analgesic, Antipyretic/Barbiturate] **Uses**: *Tension HA*, mild pain **Action**: Nonnarcotic analgesic w/ barbiturate **Dose**: 1–2 tabs or caps PO q4–6h PRN; ↓ in renal/ hepatic impair; 3 g/24 h APAP max **Caution**: [C, ?/–] Alcoholic liver Dz, G6PD deficiency **CI**: Hypersens **Disp**: Caps: *DolgicPlus:* ↑ butalbital 50 mg, caffeine 40 mg, APAP 750 mg Caps: *Margesic, Esgic:* butalbital 50 mg, caffeine 40 mg, APAP 325 mg Caps: *Phrenilin Forte:* butalbital 50 mg + APAP 650 mg Caps: *Esgic-Plus, Zebutal:* butalbital 50 mg, caffeine 40 mg, APAP 500 mg Liq: *Dolgic LQ:* butalbital 50 mg, caffeine 40 mg, APAP 325 mg/15 mL Tabs: *Medigesic, Fioricet, Repan:* butalbital 50 mg, caffeine 40 mg, APAP 325 mg; *Phrenilin:* butalbital 50 mg + APAP 325 mg; *Sedapap:* butalbital 50 mg + APAP 650 mg **SE**: Drowsiness, dizziness, "hangover" effect, N/V **Interactions**: ↑ Effects *OF* benzodiazepines, opiate analgesics, sedatives/ hypnotics, EtOH, methylphenidate hydrochloride; ↓ effects *OF* MAOIs, TCAs, corticosteroids, theophylline, OCPs, BBs, doxycycline **NIPE**: ⊘ EtOH & CNS depressants, may impair coordination, monitor for depression, use barrier protection contraception; butalbital is habit forming

Acetaminophen + Codeine (Tylenol No. 2, 3, No. 4) [C-III, C-V] [Analgesic, Antipyretic/Opiate] **Uses**: *Mild–mod pain (No. 2–3); mod–severe pain (No. 4)* **Action**: Combined APAP & narcotic analgesic **Dose**: *Adults*. 1–2 tabs q4–6h PRN or 30–60 mg/codeine q4–6h based on codeine content (max dose APAP = 4 g/d) *Peds*. APAP 10–15 mg/kg/dose; codeine 0.5–1 mg/kg dose q4–6h (*guide*: 3–6 y, 5 mL/dose; 7–12 y, 10 mL/dose) max 2.6 g/d if < 12 y; ↓ in renal/ hepatic impair **Caution**: [C, ?] Alcoholic liver Dz; G6PD deficiency **CI**: Hypersens **Disp**: Tabs 300 mg APAP + codeine (No. 2 = 15 mg, No. 3 = 30 mg, No. 4 = 60 mg); susp (C-V) APAP 120 mg + codeine 12 mg/5 mL **SE**: Drowsiness, dizziness, N/V **Interactions**: ↑ Effects *OF* benzodiazepines, opiate analgesics, sedatives/hypnotics, EtOH, methylphenidate hydrochloride; ↓ effects *OF* MAOIs, TCAs, corticosteroids, theophylline, OCPs, BBs, doxycycline **NIPE**: ⊘ EtOH & CNS depressants, may impair coordination, monitor for depression, use barrier protection contraception; codeine may be habit forming

Acetazolamide (Diamox) [Anticonvulsant, Diuretic/Carbonic Anhydrase Inhibitor] Uses: *Diuresis, drug and CHF edema, glaucoma, prevent high-altitude sickness, refractory epilepsy* metabolic alkalosis, resp stimulant in COPD **Action:** Carbonican hydrase inhib; ↓ renal excretion of hydrogen & ↑ renal excretion of Na^+, K^+, HCO_3^-, & H_2O **Dose:** *Adults. Diuretic:* 250–375 mg IV or PO q24h *Glaucoma:* 250–1000 mg PO q24h in ÷ doses *Epilepsy:* 8–30 mg/kg/d PO in ÷ doses *Altitude sickness:* 500–1000 mg/d ÷ dose q8–12 h or SR q12–24 h start 24 h before & 48–72 h after highest ascent *Metabolic alkalosis:* 500 mg IV × 1 *Peds. Epilepsy:* 8–30 mg/kg/24 h PO in ÷ doses; max 1 g/d *Diuretic:* 5 mg/kg/ 24h PO or IV *Alkalinization of urine:* 5 mg/kg/dose PO bid–tid *Glaucoma:* 8–30 mg/kg/24 h PO in 3 ÷ doses; max 1 g/d; ↓ dose w/ CrCl 10–50 mL/min; avoid if CrCl < 10 mL/min **Caution:** [C, +/–] **CI:** Renal/ hepatic/ adrenal failure, sulfa allergy, hyperchloremic acidosis **Disp:** Tabs 125, 250 mg; ER caps 500 mg; Inj 00 mg/vial, powder for recons **SE:** Malaise, metallic taste, drowsiness, photosens, hyperglycemia **Interactions:** Causes ↑ effects *OF* amphetamines, quinidine, procainamide, TCAs, ephedrine; ↓ effects *OF* Li, phenobarbital, salicylates, barbiturates; ↑ K^+ loss *W/* corticosteroids and amphotericin B **Labs:** ↑ uric acid; ↓ K^+, Hgb, Hct, WBC, plt; Monitor serum lytes esp Na^+ & K^+, ✓ CBC, plt, false(+) for urinary protein, urinary urobilinogen; ↓ I uptake **NIPE:** ↓ GI distress w/ food, monitor for S/Sxs metabolic acidosis, ↑ fluid to ↓ risk of kidney stones; SR forms not for epilepsy

Acetic Acid & Aluminum Acetate (Otic Domeboro) [Astringent/ Anti-Infective] Uses: *Otitis externa* **Action:** Anti-infective **Dose:** 4–6 gtt in ear(s) q2–3h **Caution:** [C, ?] **CI:** Perforated tympanic membranes **Disp:** 2% otic soln **SE:** Local irritation **NIPE:** Burning w/ instillation or irrigation

Acetylcysteine (Acetadote, Mucomyst) [Mucolytic/Amino Acid Derivative] Uses: *Mucolytic, antidote to APAP hepatotox/OD* adjuvant Rx chronic bronchopulmonary Dzs & CF* prevent contrast-induced renal dysfunction **Action:** Splits mucoprotein disulfide linkages; restores glutathione in APAP OD to protect liver **Dose:** *Adults & Peds. Nebulizer:* 3–5 mL of 20% soln diluted w/ equal vol of H_2O or NS tid–qid *Antidote:* PO or NG: 140 mg/kg load, then 70 mg/kg q4h × 17 doses (dilute 1:3 in carbonated beverage or OJ), repeat if emesis w/in 1 h of dosing *Acetadote:* 150 mg/kg IV over 60 min, then 50 mg/kg over 4 h, then 100 mg/kg over 16 h; prevent renal dysfunction: 600–1200 mg PO bid × 2 d **Caution:** [B, ?] **Disp:** Soln, inhaled and oral 10%, 20%; Acetadote IV soln 20% **SE:** Bronchospasm (inhaled), N/V, drowsiness, anaphylactoid Rxns w/IV **Interactions:** Discolors rubber, Fe, Cu, Ag; ↓ effect *W/* activated charcoal **Labs:** Monitor ABGs & pulse oximetry w/ bronchospasm **NIPE:** Inform pt of ↑ productive cough; clear airway before aerosol administration; ↑ fluids to liquefy secretions; unpleasant odor will disappear & may cause N/V; activated charcoal absorbs PO acetylcysteine for APAP ingestion; start Rx for APAP OD w/in 6–8 h

Acitretin (Soriatane) [Retinoid] **WARNING:** Not to be used by women who are PRG or who intend to become PRG during/for 3 y following drug D/C; no EtOH during/2 mo following D/C; no blood donation for 3 y following D/C; hepatotoxic **Uses:** *Severe psoriasis*; other keratinization Dz (lichen planus, etc.) **Action:** Retinoid-like activity **Dose:** 25–50 mg/d PO, w/main meal **Caution:** [X, ?/–] Renal/ hepatic impair; in women of reproductive potential **CI:** See Warning; ↑ serum lipids; w/ MTX or tetracyclines **Disp:** Caps 10, 17.5, 25 mg **SE:** Hyperesthesia, cheilitis, skin peeling, alopecia, pruritus, rash, arthralgia, GI upset, photosens, thrombocytosis **Interactions:** ↑ risk of hep W/ methotrexate; ↑ risk of ICP W/ tetracycline; EtOH prolongs teratogenic potential for 2 mo > therapy; ↑ effects OF phenytoin, sulfonylureas; ↓ effects OF progestin OC and possibly all OC **Labs:** ↑ triglycerides, ↑ Na, K, PO_4; ✓ LFTs/lytes/lipids **NIPE:** Response takes up to 2–3 mo; informed consent & FDA guide w/ each Rx required

Aclidinium Bromide (Tudorza Pressair) [Anticholinergic] **Uses:** *Bronchospasm w/ COPD* **Acts:** LA anticholinergic, blocks ACH receptors **Dose:** 400 mcg/inhal, 1 inhal bid; **Caution:** [C, ?] w/ Atropine hypersens, NAG, BPH, or MG; avoid w/ milk allergy **CI:** None **Disp:** Inhal powder, 30/60 doses **SE:** HA, D, nasopharyngitis, cough **Interactions:** ⊘ Concomitant anticholinergic drugs **NIPE:** Not for acute exacerbation; lactose in powder, avoid w/ milk allergy; OK w/ renal impair

Acyclovir (Zovirax) [Antiviral/Synthetic Purine Nucleoside] **Uses:** *Herpes simplex (HSV) (genital/ mucocutaneous, encephalitis, keratitis), Varicella zoster, Herpes zoster (shingles) Infxns* **Action:** Interferes w/ viral DNA synth **Dose: Adults.** *Dose on IBW if obese (> 125% IBW) PO: Initial genital HSV:* 200 mg PO q4h while awake (5 caps/d) × 10 d or 400 mg PO tid × 7–10 d *Chronic HSV suppression:* 400 mg PO bid *Intermittent HSV Rx:* As initial, except Rx for 5 d, or 800 mg PO bid, at prodrome *Topical: Initial herpes genitalis:* Apply q3h (6×/d) for 7 d *HSV encephalitis:* 10 mg/kg IV q8h × 10 d *Herpes zoster:* 800 mg PO 5×/d for 7–10 d *IV:* 10 mg/kg/dose IV q8h × 7 d **Peds.** *Genital HSV:* **3 mo–12 y:** 40–80 mg/kg/d ÷ 3–4 doses (max 1 g); ≥ 12 y: 200 mg 5×/d or 400 mg 3×/d × 5–10 d; *IV:* 5 mg/kg/dose q8h × 5–7 d *HSV encephalitis:* **3 mo–12y:** 60 mg/kg/d IV ÷ q8h ×14–21 d > **12 y:** 30 mg/kg/d IV ÷ q8h × 14–21 d *Chickenpox:* **≥ 2 y:** 20 mg/kg/ dose PO qid × 5 d *Shingles:* **< 12 y:** 30 mg/kg/d PO or 1500 mg/m²/d IV ÷ q8h × 7–10 d; ↓ w/ CrCl < 50 mL/min **Caution:** [B, +] **CI:** Component hypersens **Disp:** Caps 200 mg; tabs 400, 800 mg; susp 200 mg/5 mL; Inj 500 & 1000 mg/vial; Inj soln 50 mg/mL oint 5%, and cream 5% **SE:** Dizziness, lethargy, malaise, confusion, rash, IV site inflammation **Interactions:** ↑ CNS SE W/ MTX & zidovudine, ↑ blood levels W/ probenecid **Labs:** Monitor BUN, SCr, LFTs, CBC; transient ↑ Cr/BUN **NIPE:** Start stat w/Sxs; ↑ hydration w/IV dose; ↑ risk cervical CA w/ genital herpes; ↑ length of Rx in immunocompromised pts; PO better than topical for herpes genitalis

Adalimumab (Humira) [Antirheumatic/TNF Alpha-Blocker] **WARNING:** Cases of TB have been observed; ✓ TB skin test prior to use; hep B reactivation possible, invasive fungal and other opportunistic Infxns reported; lymphoma/other CAs possible in children and adolescents **Uses:** *Mod–severe RA w/ an inadequate response to one or more DMARDs, psoriatic arthritis (PA), juvenile idiopathic arthritis (JIA), plaque psoriasis, ankylosing spondylitis (AS), Crohn Dz, ulcerative colitis* **Action:** TNF-α inhib **Dose:** *RA, PA, AS:* 40 mg SQ qowk; may ↑ 40 mg qwk if not on MTX *JIA:* 15–30 kg 20 mg qowk *Crohn Dz/ ulcerative colitis:* 160 mg d 1, 80 mg 2 wk later, then 2 wk later start maint 40 mg qowk **Caution:** [B, ?/–] See Warning, do not use w/live vaccines **CI:** None **Disp:** Prefilled 0.4 mL (20 mg) & 0.8 mL (40 mg) syringe **SE:** Inj site Rxns, HA, rash, ↑ CHF, anaphylaxis, pancytopenia (aplastic anemia), demyelinating Dz, new -onset psoriasis **Interactions:** ↑ Effects *W/* MTX; ↑ risk of inf/neutropenia *W/* anakinra, TNF blocking agents **Labs:** May ↑ lipids, alk phos **NIPE:** ⊘ Exposure to Infxn; ⊘ admin live virus vaccines; refrigerate prefilled syringe, rotate Inj sites, OK w/ other DMARDs

Adapalene (Differin) [Retinoid]
Uses: *Acne vulgaris* **Action:** Retinoid-like, modulates cell differentiation/keratinization/inflammation **Dose:** *Adults & Peds > 12 y.* Apply 1 × daily to clean/dry skin QHS **Caution:** [C, ?/–] Products w/ sulfur/resorcinol/salicylic acid ↑ irritation **CI:** Component hypersens **Disp:** Top lotion, gel, cream 0.1%; gel 0.3% **SE:** Skin redness, dryness, burning, stinging, scaling, itching, sunburn **NIPE:** Avoid exposure to sunlight/ sunlamps; wear sunscreen; avoid waxing treated areas

Adapalene & Benzoyl Peroxide (Epiduo) [Retinoid + Antibacterial/Keratolytic]
Uses: *Acne vulgaris* **Action:** Retinoid-like, modulates cell differentiation, keratinization, and inflammation w/ antibacterial. **Dose:** *Adults & Peds >12 y.* Apply 1 × daily to clean/dry skin **Caution:** [C, ?/–] Bleaching effects, photosensitivity **CI:** Component hypersens **Disp:** Topical gel adapalene 0.1% and benzoyl peroxide 2.5% (45 g) **SE:** Local irritation, dryness **Interactions:** ⊘ Concomitantly *W/* topical irritants and waxed areas; ↑ risk of irritation w/ sulfur, resorcinol, salicylic acid, and other topical acne meds **NIPE:** Vit A may ↑ SE; ⊘ use on open skin/ wounds or sunburned areas. Avoid eyes, lips, mucous membranes

Adefovir (Hepsera) [Antiviral/Acyclic Nucleotide Analogue]
WARNING: Acute exacerbations of hep B seen after D/C therapy (monitor LFTs); nephrotoxic w/ underlying renal impair w/ chronic use (monitor renal Fxn); HIV resistance/ untreated may emerge; lactic acidosis & severe hepatomegaly w/ steatosis reported **Uses:** *Chronic active hep B* **Action:** Nucleotide analog **Dose:** *CrCl > 50 mL/min:* 10 mg PO daily *CrCl 20–49 mL/min:* 10 mg PO q48h; *CrCl 10–19 mL/min:* 10 mg PO q72h; *HD:* 10 mg PO q7d post dialysis **Caution:** [C, ?/–] **Disp:** Tabs 10 mg **SE:** Asthenia, HA, D, hematuria, Abd pain; see Warning **Interactions:** ↑ Risk of nephrotoxicity *W/* aminoglycosides, cyclosporine, NSAIDs, tacrolimus, vancomycin **Labs:** ↑ LFTs, Cr, CK, amylase, lactate levels **NIPE:** Effects on fetus & baby not known; ⊘ breast-feed; use barrier contraception; ✓ HIV status before using; may take without regard to food

Adenosine (Adenocard, Adenoscan) [Antiarrhythmic/Nucleoside] Uses: *Adenocard* *PSVT*; including w/ WPW; *Adenoscan* pharmacologic stress testing **Action:** Class IV antiarrhythmic; slows AV node conduction **Dose: Stress test:** 140 mcg/kg/min × 6 min cont Inf *Adults.* ECC 2010: 6-mg rapid IV push, then 20-mL NS bolus. Elevate extremity; repeat 12 mg in 1–2 min PRN. *Peds.* ECC 2010: **Symptomatic SVT:** 0.1 mg/kg rapid IV/ IO push (max dose 6 mg); can follow w/0.2 mg/kg rapid IV/ IO push (max dose 12 mg); follow each dose w/ ≥ 5 mL NS flush **Caution:** [C, ?] Hx bronchospasm **CI:** 2nd-/3rd-degree AV block or SSS (w/o pacemaker); Afib/flutter, AF w/ WPW, V, tachycardia, recent MI or CNS bleed **Disp:** Inj 3 mg/mL **SE:** Facial flushing, HA, dyspnea, chest pressure, ↓ BP, proarrhythmic **Interactions:** ↓ Effects *W/* guarana; ↑ effects *W/* dipyridamole, theophylline, caffeine; ↑ risk of hypotension & CP *W/* nicotine; ↑ risk of bradycardia *W/* BBs; ↑ risk of heart block *W/* carbamazepine; ↑ risk of VF *W/* digitalis glycosides **Labs:** Monitor ECG during administration **NIPE:** Monitor BP & pulse during therapy; monitor resp status ↑ risk of bronchospasm in asthmatics; discard unused or unclear soln; doses > 12 mg not OK; can cause momentary asystole when administered; caffeine, theophylline antagonize effects

Ado-trastuzumab Emtansine (Kadcyla) **WARNING:** Do not substitute for trastuzumab; hepatotox (liver failure & death) reported (monitor LFTs/bili prior to initiation & each dose); cardiac tox: may ↓ LVEF (assess LVEF prior to/during tx); embryo-fetal tox **Uses:** *Tx of HER2-positive, metastatic breast CA in pts previously treated w/ trastuzumab and/or taxane* **Acts:** HER2-targeted Ab and microtubule inhibitor conjugate **Dose:** 3.6 mg/kg IV inf q 3 wk until progression or toxicity; do not use dextrose 5% soln; see label for tox dosage mods **NIPE:** [D, –] Interruption of Tx, ↓ dose, or D/C may be necessary due to ADRs (see SE); avoid w/ strong CYP3A4 inhib **CI:** None **Disp:** Lyo ph powder 100, 160 mg/vial **SE:** See Warning; fatigue, N/V/D, constipation, HA, ↑ LFTs, ↓ plts, ↓ WBC, musculoskeletal pain, Inf-related Rxns, hypersens Rxns, neurotox, pulmonary tox, pyrexia **Notes:** Monitor for tox; counsel on PRG prevention/planning (MotHER Pregnancy Registry) **NIPE:** ⊘ PRG; ✓ hepatic function; ✓ K$^+$ prior to and during Tx; use contraception during Tx and 6 mo after D/C; ✓ neurotoxicity (peripheral neuropathy)

Afatinib (Gilotrif) Uses: *Tx NSCLC w/ EGFR exon 19 del or exon 21 (L858R) subs* **Acts:** TKI **Dose:** 40 mg PO 1 × day; 1 h ac or 2 h pc; see label for tox dosage modifications for **W/P:** [D, –] Embryo-fetal tox; severe D, interstitial lung Dz, hepatotox, keratitis, bullous & exfoliative skin disorders; interruption of Tx, ↓ dose, or Tx D/C may be necessary due to ADRs; w/ P-gp inhibitors/inducers (adjust dose) **CI:** None **Disp:** Tabs 20, 30, 40 mg **SE:** V/D, rash/dermatitis acneiform, pruritus, stomatitis, paronychia, dry skin, ↓ appetite, ↓ wgt, conjunctivitis, epistaxis, rhinorrhea, dyspnea, fatigue, ↓ LVEF, pyrexia, cystitis **NIPE:** ✓ Renal/hepatic function; ⊘ food 1 h before or 2 h after taking; ⊘ PRG; use contraception during and up to 2 wk after Tx; ensure adeq hydration; report eye problems immediately (pain, swelling, vision chgs); ⊘ contact lenses

Aflibercept (Eylea) [Recombinant Fusion Protein] Uses: *Neovascular age-related macular degeneration* Acts: Binds VEGF-A & placental growth factor; ↓ neovascularization & vascular permeability Dose: *Adults.* 2 mg (0.05 mL) intravitreal Inj q4 wk × 3 mo, then q8 wk Caution: [C, ?] May cause endophthalmitis or retinal detachment CI: Ocular or periocular Infxn, active intraocular inflammation, hypersens Disp: Inj 40 mg/mL/vial SE: Blurred vision, eye pain, conjunctival hemorrhage, cataract, ↑ IOP, vitreous detachment, floaters, arterial thrombosis NIPE: For ophthalmic intravitreal inj only; may cause inj site pain

Albumin (Albuked, Albuminar 20, AlbuRx 25, Albutein, Buminate, Kedbumin, Plasbumin) [Plasma Volume Expander] Uses: *Plasma vol expansion for shock (eg, burns, hemorrhage),* others based on specific product label: ovarian hyperstimulation synd, CABG support, hypoalbuminemia Action: ↑ intravascular oncotic pressure Dose: *Adults.* Initial 25 g IV; then based on response; 250 g/48 h max Peds. 0.5–1 g/kg/dose; max 6 g/kg/d Caution: [C, ?] Severe anemia; cardiac, renal, or hepatic Insuff d/t protein load & hypervolemia, avoid 25% albumin in preterm infants CI: CHF, severe anemia Disp: Soln 5%, 20%, 25% SE: Chills, fever, CHF, tachycardia, ↑↓ BP, hypervolemia Interactions: Atypical Rxns W/ ACEI withhold 24 h prior to plasma administration Labs: ↑ albumin level NIPE: Monitor BP & D/C if hypotensive; monitor I&O; admin to all blood types; contains 130–160 mEq Na⁺/L; may cause pulm edema; monitor resp status & lung sounds; max Inf rates: 25% vial: 2–3 mL/min; 5% soln: 5–10 mL/min

Albuterol (Proventil, Ventolin, Proair) [Bronchodilator/ Adrenergic] Uses: *Asthma, COPD, prevent exercise-induced bronchospasm* Action: β-Adrenergic sympathomimetic bronchodilator; relaxes bronchial smooth muscle Dose: *Adults. Inhaler:* 2 Inh q4–6h PRN; q4–6h *PO:* 2–4 mg PO tid–qid *Nebulizer:* 1.25–5 mg (0.25–1 mL of 0.5% soln in 2–3 mL of NS) q4–8h PRN *Prevent exercise-induced asthma:* 2 puffs 5–30 min prior to activity Peds. *Inhaler:* 2 Inh q4–6h. *PO:* 0.1–0.2 mg/kg/dose PO; max 2–4 mg PO tid *Nebulizer:* 0.63–5 mg in 2–3 mL of NS q4–8h PRN Caution: [C, ?] Disp: Tabs: 2, 4 mg; XR tabs: 4, 8 mg; syrup: 2 mg/5 mL; 90 mcg/dose metered-dose inhaler; soln for nebulizer 0.083, 0.5% SE: Palpitations, tachycardia, nervousness, GI upset Interactions: ↑ Effects W/ other sympathomimetics; ↑ CV effects W/ MAOI, TCA, inhaled anesthetics; ↑ stimulant effect with caffeine products (cola, tea, coffee, guarana) ↓ effects W/ BBs; ↓ effectiveness OF insulin, oral hypoglycemics, digoxin Labs: Transient ↑ in serum glucose after Inh; transient ↓ K⁺ after Inh NIPE: Monitor HR, BP, ABGs, S/Sxs bronchospasm & CNS stimulation; instruct on use of inhaler; must use as 1st inhaled & rinse mouth after use

Albuterol & Ipratropium (Combivent, DuoNeb) [Bronchodilator/ Adrenergic, Anticholinergic] Uses: *COPD* Action: Combo of β-adrenergic bronchodilator & quaternary anticholinergic Dose: 2 Inh qid; nebulizer 3 mL q6h; max 3 mL q4h Caution: [C, ?] CI: Peanut/soybean allergy Disp:

Metered-dose inhaler, 18 mcg ipratropium & 90 mcg albuterol/puff (contains ozone-depleting CFCs; will be gradually removed from US market); nebulization soln (DuoNeb) ipratropium 0.5 mg & albuterol 2.5 mg/3 mL **SE:** Palpitations, tachycardia, nervousness, GI upset, dizziness, blurred vision **Interactions:** ↑ Effects **W/** anticholinergics, including ophthal meds; ↓ effects **W/** herb jaborandi tree, pill-bearing spurge **NIPE:** See Albuterol; may cause transient blurred vision/irritation or urinary changes

Alcaftadine (Lastacaft) [Antihistamine/Mast Cell Stabilizer]
Uses: *Allergic conjunctivitis* **Action:** Histamine H_1-receptor antag **Dose:** 1 gtt in eye(s) daily **Caution:** [B, ?] **Disp:** Ophth soln 0.25% **SE:** Eye irritation **NIPE:** Remove contacts before use

Aldesleukin [IL-2] (Proleukin) [Immunomodulator/Antineoplastic]
WARNING: Restrict to pts w/ nl cardiac/pulmonary Fxns as defined by formal testing. Caution w/ Hx of cardiac/pulmonary Dz. Administer in hospital setting w/ provider experienced w/ anticancer agents. Assoc w/ capillary leak syndrome (CLS) characterized by ↓ BP and organ perfusion with potential for cardiac/ respiratory tox, GI bleed/infarction, renal insufficiency, edema, and mental status changes. Increased risk of sepsis and bacterial endocarditis. Treat bacterial Infxn before use. Pts w/ central lines are at risk for Infxn. Prophylaxis w/ oxacillin, nafcillin, ciprofloxacin, or vancomycin may reduce staphylococcal Infxn. Hold w/ mod-severe lethargy or somnolence; continued use may result in coma. **Uses:** *Met RCC & melanoma* **Action:** Acts via IL-2 receptor; many immunomodulatory effects **Dose:** 600,000 IU/kg q8h × max 14 doses d 1–5 & d 15–19 of 28-d cycle (FDA-approved dose/schedule for RCC); other schedules (eg, "high dose" 720,000 IU/kg IV q8h up to 12 doses, repeat 10–15 d later) **Caution:** [C, ?/–] **CI:** Organ allografts; abnormal thallium stress test or PFT **Disp:** Powder for recons 22×10^6 IU, when reconstituted 18 mIU IU/mL = 1.1 mg/mL **SE:** Flu-like synd (malaise, fever, chills), N/V/D, ↑ bilirubin; capillary leak synd; ↓ BP, tachycardia, pulm & peripheral edema, fluid retention, & wgt gain; renal & mild hematologic tox, eosinophilia; cardiac tox (ischemia, atrial arrhythmias); neurotox (CNS depression, somnolence, delirium, rare coma); pruritic rashes, urticaria, & erythroderma common **Interactions:** May ↑ tox *OF* cardiotox, hepatotox, myelotoxic, & nephrotoxic drugs; ↑ hypotension **W/** antihypertensive drugs; ↓ effects **W/** corticosteroids; acute Rxn **W/** iodinated contrast media up to several mo after Inf; CNS effects **W/** psychotropics **Labs:** ↓ Hgb, plt, WBC **NIPE:** Thoroughly explain serious SE of drug (hypotension, pulm edema, arrhythmias & neurotox) & that some SE are expected; ⊘ EtOH, NSAIDs, ASA

Alefacept (Amevive) [Antipsoriatic/Immunosuppressive]
Uses: *Mod/severe chronic plaque psoriasis* **Action:** Binds CD2, ↓ T lymphocyte activation **Dose:** 7.5 mg IV or 15 mg IM once/wk × 12 wk; **Caution:** [B, ?/–] PRG registry; associated w/ serious Infxn; ✓ CD4 before each dose; w/hold if < 250; D/C if < 250 × 1 mo **CI:** HIV **Disp:** 15-mg powder vial **SE:** Pharyngitis, myalgia, Inj site

Rxn, malignancy **Interactions:** ↑ Risk of immunosuppression W/ phototherapy and immunosuppressants **Labs:** ↑ LFT (monitor for liver damage); may ↑ CD4+ and CD8+, T-lymphocyte counts—Monitor; ↑ AST, ALT **NIPE:** ↑ Risk of Infxn; ∅ exposure to Infxns; Inj site inflammation; rotate sites; IV and IM different formulations; may repeat course 12 wk later if CD4 OK; immunizations up to date before use

Alemtuzumab (Campath relaunch as Lemtrada) [Monoclonal Antibody, CD52 (Recombinant, Humanized)]

WARNING: Serious, including fatal, cytopenias, Inf Rxns, and Infxns can occur; limit dose to 30 mg (single) & 90 mg (weekly), higher doses ↑ risk of pancytopenia; ↑ dose gradually & monitor during Inf, D/C for Grade 3 or 4 Inf Rxns; give prophylaxis for PCP & herpes virus Infxn **Uses:** *B-cell CLL* **Action:** CD52-directed cytolytic Ab **Dose:** *Adults.* 3 mg d 1, then ↑ dose to 30 mg/d IV 3×/wk for 12 wk (see label for escalation strategy); infuse over 2 h; premedicate w/oral antihistamine & APAP **Caution:** [C, ?/–] Do not give live vaccines; D/C for autoimmune/severe hematologic Rxns **Disp:** Inj 30 mg/mL (1 mL) **SE:** Cytopenias, Infxns, Inf Rxns, ↑/↓ BP, Inj site Rxn N/V/D, insomnia, anxiety **Interactions:** ↑ Bone marrow depression W/ antineoplastics, radiation therapy; Avoid live virus vaccines > recent therapy **Labs:** ✓ CBC & plt weekly & CD4 counts after Rx until ≥ 200 cells/mm³ **NIPE:** Instruct pt ∅ live virus vaccines o/t immunosuppression

Alendronate (Fosamax, Fosamax Plus D) [Antiosteoporotic]

Uses: *Rx & prevent osteoporosis male & postmenopausal female, Rx steroid-induced osteoporosis, Paget Dz* **Action:** ↓ Nl & abnormal bone resorption, ↓ osteoclast action **Dose:** *Osteoporosis:* Rx: 10 mg/d PO or 70 mg qwk; Fosamax plus D1 tab qwk *Steroid-induced osteoporosis:* Rx: 5 mg/d PO, 10 mg/d postmenopausal not on estrogen *Prevention:* 5 mg/d PO or 35 mg qwk *Paget Dz:* 40 mg/d PO × 6 mo; **Caution:** [C, ?] Not OK if CrCl < 35 mL/min, w/ NSAID use **CI:** Esophageal anomalies, inability to sit/stand upright for 30 min, ↓ Ca²⁺ **Disp:** Tabs 5, 10, 35, 40, 70 mg, *Fosamax Plus D:* Alendronate 70 mg w/ cholecalciferol (vit D₃) 2800 or 5600 IU **SE:** Abd pain, acid regurgitation, constipation, D/N, dyspepsia, musculoskeletal pain, jaw osteonecrosis (w/ dental procedures, chemo) **Notes:** Take 1st thing in AM w/ H₂O (8 oz) > 30 min before 1st food/ beverage of the day; do not lie down for 30 min after **Interactions:** ↓ Absorption W/ antacids, Ca supls, Fe, food; ↑ risk of upper GI bleed W/ ASA & NSAIDs **Labs:** ↓ serum Ca & phosphate **NIPE:** use Ca²⁺ & vit D supl w/ regular tab; ↑ wgt-bearing activity; ↓ smoking & EtOH use; ↑ risk of jaw fx—esp w/ dental procedures; may ↑ atypical subtrochanteric femur fxs

Alfentanil (Alfenta) [C-II] [Narcotic Analgesic]

Uses: *Adjunct in maint of anesthesia; analgesia* **Action:** Short-acting narcotic analgesic **Dose:** *Adults & Peds > 12 y.* 3–75 mcg/kg (IBW) IV Inf; total depends on duration of procedure **Caution:** [C, –] ↑ ICP, resp depression **Disp:** Inj 500 mcg/mL **SE:** ↑ HR ↓ BP arrhythmias, peripheral vasodilation, ↑ ICP, drowsiness, resp depression,

N/V/constipation, ADH release **Interactions:** ↓ Effect *W/* phenothiazines; ↑ effects *W/* BBs, CNS depressants, erythromycin **NIPE:** Monitor HR, BP, resp rate

Alfuzosin (Uroxatral) [Selective Alpha-Adrenergic Antagonist] Uses: *Symptomatic = BPH* **Action:** α-Blocker **Dose:** 10 mg PO daily stat after the same meal **Caution:** [B, ?/–] w/ any Hx ↓ BP; use w/ PDE5 inhibitors may ↓ BP; may ↑ QTC interval; IFIS during cataract surgery **CI:** w/ CYP3A4 inhib; mod–severe hepatic impair; protease inhibitors for HIV **Disp:** Tabs 10 mg ER **SE:** Postural ↓ BP, dizziness, HA, fatigue **Interactions:** ↑ Effects *W/* atenolol, azole antifungals, cimetidine, ritonavir; ↑ risk of hypotension *W/* antihypertensives, nitrates, acute ingestion of EtOH **NIPE:** Not indicated for use in women or children; take w/ food; ↑ risk of postural hypotension; ○ take other meds that prolong QT interval. Do not cut or crush

Alginic Acid + Aluminum Hydroxide & Magnesium Trisilicate (Gaviscon) [OTC] [Antacid] Uses: *Heartburn* **Action:** Protective layer blocks gastric acid **Dose:** Chew 2–4 tabs or 15–30 mL PO qid followed by H_2O **Caution:** [C, ?] Avoid w/ renal impair or Na^+-restricted diet **Disp:** Chew tabs, susp **SE:** D, constipation **Interactions:** ↓ Absorption *OF* tetracyclines

Alglucosidase Alfa (Lumizyme, Myozyme) [Recombinant Acid Alpha-Glucosidase] WARNING: Life-threatening anaphylactic Rxns seen w/ Inf; medical support measures should be immediately available; caution when ↑ CV/resp Fxn Uses: *Rx Pompe DZ* **Action:** Recombinant acid α-glucosidase; degrades glycogen in lysosomes **Dose:** *Peds 1 mo–3.5 y.* 20 mg/kg IV q2wk over 4 h (see PI) **Caution:** [B, ?/–] Illness at time of Inf may ↑ Inf Rxns **CI:** None **Disp:** Powder 50 mg/vial limited distribution **SE:** Hypersens, fever, rash, D, V, gastroenteritis, pneumonia, URI, cough, resp distress/failure, Infxns, cardiac arrhythmia, ↑/↓ HR, flushing, anemia, pain, constipation **Labs:** LFTs prior to drug initiation and then periodically; monitor for IgG antibody formation q3mo for 2 y, then annually **NIPE:** Anaphylactic Rxns commonly reported

Aliskiren (Tekturna) [Direct Renin Inhibitor] WARNING: May cause injury and death to a developing fetus; D/C stat when PRG detected Uses: *HTN* **Action:** First direct renin Inhib **Dose:** 150–300 mg/d PO **Caution:** [D, ?/–] Avoid w/ CrCl < 30 mL/min **CI:** Anuria, sulfur sensitivity **Disp:** Tabs 150, 300 mg **SE:** D, Abd pain, dyspepsia, GERD, cough, angioedema, ↓ BP, dizziness **Interactions:** ↑ Effects & levels *W/* atorvastatin, ketoconazole, & other CYP3A4 Inhibs; ↓ effects *W/* irbesartan, high-fat meal; ↓ effects *OF* furosemide plasma levels; caution w/ max doses of ACE Inhibs **Labs:** ↑ SCr, BUN, K^+, CK, uric acid **NIPE:** D/C once PRG—may cause fetal death; not recommended for < 18 y or during breast-feeding

Aliskiren & Amlodipine (Tekamlo) [Renin Inhibitor + Dihydropyridine (DHP) Calcium Channel Blocker (CCB)] WARNING: May cause fetal injury & death; D/C stat when PRG detected Uses: *HTN* **Action:** Renin Inhib w/ dihydropyridine CCB **Dose:** *Adult.* 150/5 mg PO 1 × daily; max

300/10 mg/d; max effect in 2 wk **Caution:** [D, ?/–] Do not use w/ cyclosporine/ itraconazole; avoid CrCl < 30 mL/min **Disp:** Tabs (aliskiren mg/amlodipine mg) 150/5, 150/10, 300/5, 300/10 **SE:** ↓ BP, angioedema, peripheral edema, D, dizziness, angina, MI **Interactions:** ↑ effects *W/* atorvastatin, ketoconazole; ↓ effects *W/* irbesartan; ↓ effects *OF* furosemide; Caution *W/* ACEI, K⁺ supls, K⁺-sparing diuretics, K⁺-containing salt substitutes **Labs:** ↑ SCr, BUN, K⁺, monitor lytes **NIPE:** Give consistently w/ regard to meals; absorption reduced w/ high-fat meal

Aliskiren, Amlodipine, Hydrochlorothiazide (Amturnide) [Renin Inhibitor + Dihydropyridine Calcium Channel Blocker (CCB) + Thiazide Diuretic]   **WARNING:** May cause fetal injury & death; D/C stat when PRG detected **Uses:** *HTN* **Action:** Renin Inhib, dihydropyridine CCB, & thiazide diuretic **Dose:** *Adult.* Titrate q2wk PRN to 300/10/25 mg PO max/d **Caution:** [D, ?/–] Avoid w/ CrCl < 30 mL/min; do not use w/ cyclosporine/ itraconazole; ↓ BP in salt-/volume-depleted pts; HCTZ may exacerbate/activate SLE; D/C if myopia or NAG **CI:** Anuria, sulfonamide allergy **Disp:** Tabs (aliskiren mg/amlodipine mg/HCTZ mg) 150/5/12.5, 300/5/12.5, 300/5/25, 300/10/25 **SE:** ↓ BP, hyperuricemia, angioedema, peripheral edema, D, HA, dizziness, angina, MI, nasopharyngitis **Interactions:** ↑ Effects *W/* atorvastatin, ketoconazole, EtOH; ↓ effects *W/* NSAIDs, irbesartan; ↓ effects *OF* furosemide; Caution *W/* ACEI, K⁺ supls, K⁺-sparing diuretics, K⁺-containing salt substitutes **Labs:** ↑ K⁺, monitor lytes **NIPE:** Titrate at 2-wk intervals; may need to adjust hypoglycemic agents

Aliskiren/Hydrochlorothiazide (Tekturna HCT) [Direct Renin Inhibitor with Thiazide Diuretic]   **WARNING:** May cause injury and death to a developing fetus; D/C stat when PRG detected **Uses:** *HTN* **Action:** Renin Inhib w/ thiazide diuretic **Dose:** 150 mg/12.5 mg PO qd; may ↑ after 2–4 wk up to *max* 300 mg/25 mg **Caution:** [D, –] Avoid w/ CrCl ≤ 30 mL/min **Disp:** *Tab: aliskiren mg/HCTZ mg:* 150/12.5, 150/25, 300/12.5, 300/25 **SE:** Dizziness, influenza, D, cough, vertigo, asthenia, arthralgia, angioedema **Interactions:** ↑ effects *OF* antihypertensives and possibly nondepolarizing muscle relaxants; ↑ effects *W/* ketoconazole, atorvastatin, & other CYP3A4 Inhibs as it may ↑ aliskiren levels; ↓ effects *W/* irbesartan, NSAIDs; ↓ effects *OF* furosemide; ACTH & corticosteroids ↑ the risk of hypokalemia; adjust antidiabetic drugs. Orthostatic hypotension potentiated by alcohol, CNS depressants. ↑ Risk of Li tox (avoid); ↓ BP in salt/ volume-depleted pts; in sulfonamide allergy HCTZ may exacerbate/ activate SLE **Labs:** ↑ ALT, BUN/creatinine, uric acid **NIPE:** ↓ Drug absorption w/ high-fat meal; not recommended for < 18 y or during breast-feeding; not for initial therapy

Allopurinol (Zyloprim, Aloprim) [Xanthine Oxidase Inhibitor]
Uses: *Gout, hyperuricemia of malignancy, uric acid urolithiasis* **Action:** Xanthine oxidase Inhib; ↓ uric acid production **Dose:** *Adults. PO:* Initial 100 mg/d; usual 300 mg/d; max 800 mg/d; ÷ dose if > 300 mg/d *IV:* 200–400 mg/m²/d (max 600 mg/24 h); (after meal w/ plenty of fluid) *Peds. Only for hyperuricemia of malignancy if < 10 y:*

10 mg/kg/d PO (max 800 mg) or 50–100 mg/m^2/q8h (max 300 mg/m^2/d) 200–400 mg/m^2/d IV (max 600 mg) ↓ in renal impair **Caution:** [C, M] **Disp:** Tabs 100, 300 mg; Inj 500 mg/30 mL (Aloprim) **SE:** Rash, N/V, renal impair, angioedema **Notes:** IV dose of 6 mg/mL final conc as single daily Inf or ÷ 6-, 8-, or 12-h intervals **Interactions:** ↑ Effect *OF* theophylline, oral anticoagulants; ↑ hypersensitivity Rxns *W*/ ACEIs, thiazide diuretics; ↑ risk of rash *W*/ ampicillin/ amoxicillin; ↑ BM depression *W*/ cyclophosphamide, azathioprine, mercaptopurine; ↓ effects *W*/ EtOH **Labs:** ↑ Alk phos, bilirubin, LFTs **NIPE:** ↑ Fluids to 2–3 L/d; take pc; may ↑ drowsiness; ↑ risk of acute gout attack in 1st 6 wk of Tx; Aggravates acute gout; begin after acute attack resolves

Almotriptan (Axert) [Serotonin 5-HT$_1$ Receptor Agonist] Uses: *Rx acute migraine* **Action:** Vascular serotonin receptor agonist **Dose:** *Adults. PO:* 6.25–12.5 mg PO, repeat in 2 h PRN; 2 dose/24 h max PO dose; w/ hepatic/ renal impair, w/ potent CYP3A4 6.25 mg single dose (max 12.5 mg/d) **Caution:** [C, ?/–] **CI:** Angina, ischemic heart Dz, coronary artery vasospasm, hemiplegic or basilar migraine, uncontrolled HTN, ergot use, w/ sulfonamide allergy, MAOI use w/ in 14 d **Disp:** Tabs 6.25, 12.5 mg **SE:** N, somnolence, paresthesias, HA, dry mouth, weakness, numbness, coronary vasospasm, HTN **Interactions:** ↑ Serotonin effects *OF* SSRIs, ↑ vasoactive action *OF* ergot derivatives & 5-HT agonists, ↑ effects *W*/ erythromycin, ketoconazole, itraconazole, MAOIs, ritonavir, verapamil **NIPE:** ⊘ Ergot compounds or 5-HT agonist w/in 24 h of almotriptan; ⊘ use if pregnant or breast-feeding; concurrent use w/ SSRIs may cause serotonin synd (shivering, sweating, tremors/twitching, agitation, ↑ HA); use only during migraine HA attack; avoid driving if drug causes drowsiness

Alogliptin (Nesina) [DDP-4 Inhibitor] Uses: *Monotherapy type 2 DM* **Acts:** DDP-4 inhib, ↑ insulin synth/ release **Dose:** 25 mg/d PO; if CrCl 30–60 mL/min 12.5 mg/d; CrCl < 30 mL/min 6.25 mg/d **Caution:** [B, M] 0.2% pancreatitis risk, hepatic failure, hypersens Rxn **CI:** Hypersens **Disp:** Tabs 6.25, 12.5, 25 mg **SE:** Hypoglycemia, HA, nasopharyngitis, URI **Interactions:** ↑ Effects of hypoglycemia *W*/ concurrent use of sulfonylureas or insulin **Labs:** LFTs and renal function tests prior to drug use and periodically thereafter **NIPE:** DC drug if h/o angioedema *W*/ another DDP-4, DC if s/s of pancreatitis

Alogliptin/Metformin (Kazano) [DPP-4 Inhibitor + Biguanide] **WARNING:** Lactic acidosis w/ metformin accumulation; ↑ risk w/ sepsis, vol depletion, CHF, renal/hepatic impair, excess alcohol; w/ lactic acidosis suspected D/C and hospitalize Uses: *Combo type 2 DM* **Acts:** DDP-4 inhib; ↑ insulin synth/ release w/ biguanide; ↓ hepatic glucose prod & absorption; ↑ insulin sens **Dose:** Max daily 25 mg alogliptin, 2000 mg metformin **Caution:** [B, M] May cause lactic acidosis, pancreatitis, hepatic failure, hypersens Rxn, vit B$_{12}$ def **CI:** Hx of hypersens, renal impair (♀ SCr ≥ 1.4 mg/dL or ♂ ≥ 1.5 mg/dL), metabolic acidosis **Disp:** Tabs (alogliptin mg/metformin mg): 12.5/500, 12.5/1000 **SE:** HA, nasopharyngitis, D, ↑ BP, back pain, URI **Interactions:** ↑ metformin levels *W*/

amiloride, cimetidine, digoxin, morphine, procainamide, quinine, quinidine, raniti-dine, trimeterene, trimethoprim, vancomycine, EtOH; ↑ risk of metabolic acidosis **W/** CCB, diuretics, estrogens, isoniazid, OC, phenothiazines, phenytoin, steroids, sympathomimetics, thyroid drugs, nicotine; ↑ effects of hypoglycemia **W/** concurrent use of sulfonylureas or insulin **Labs:** ↓ Glucose; LFTs and renal function tests prior to drug use and periodically thereafter; ↓ B$_{12}$ – monitor level **NIPE:** Stop drug before and for 48 h after use of intravascular iodinated contrast agents; temp D/C w/ surgery; Warn against excessive EtOH intake, may ↑ metformin lactate effect

Alogliptin/Pioglitazone (Oseni) [DPP-4 Inhibitor + Thiazolidine-dione]
WARNING: May cause/worsen CHF **Uses:** *Combo type 2 DM* **Acts:** DDP-4 inhibitor, ↑ insulin synth/release w/ thiazolidinedione; ↑ insulin sens **Dose:** 25 mg alogliptin/15 mg pioglitazone or 25 mg/30 mg/d; NYHA Class I/II, start 25 mg/15 mg **Caution:** [C, –] **CI:** CHF, NYHA Class III/IV, hx of hypersens **Disp:** Tabs (alogliptin mg/pioglitazone mg): 25/15, 25/30, 25/45, 12.5/15, 12.5/30, 12.5/45 **SE:** Back pain, nasopharyngitis, URI **Interactions:** ↑ risk of fluid retention **W/** concurrent use of insulin; ↑ effects of hypoglycemia **W/** concurrent use of sulfonylureas or insulin; ↑ effects **W/** strong CYP2C8 inhibitors (Table 10); (25 mg/15 mg max w/ strong CYP2C8 inhib); ↑ risk of CHF—monitor at start of drug and w/ drug increases; ↓ effects **W/** CYP2C8 inducers (Table 10) **Labs:** LFTs and renal function tests prior to drug use and periodically thereafter **NIPE:** May ↑ bladder CA risk (~ ↑ 3/10,000)

Alosetron (Lotronex) [Selective 5-HT$_3$ Receptor Antagonist]
WARNING: Serious GI SEs, some fatal, including ischemic colitis reported. Prescribed only through participation in the prescribing program **Uses:** *Severe D—predominant IBS in women who fail conventional Rx* **Action:** Selective 5-HT$_3$ receptor antagonist **Dose:** *Adults.* 0.5 mg PO bid; ↑ to 1 mg bid max after 4 wk; D/C after 8 wk if not controlled **Caution:** [B, ?/–] **CI:** Hx chronic/severe constipation, GI obst, strictures, toxic megacolon, GI perforation, adhesions, ischemic/UC, Crohn Dz, diverticulitis, thrombophlebitis, hypercoagulability **Disp:** Tabs 0.5, 1 mg **SE:** Constipation, Abd pain, N, fatigue, HA **Notes:** D/C stat if constipation or Sxs of ischemic colitis develop; pt must sign informed consent prior to use **Interactions:** ↑ Risk constipation **W/** other drugs that ↓ GI motility, inhibits *N*-acetyltransferase, & may influence metabolism of INH, procainamide, hydralazine **Labs:** Monitor for ↑ ALT, AST, alk phos, bilirubin **NIPE:** Administer w/o regard to food, eval effectiveness > 4 wk

Alpha-1-Protease Inhibitor (Glassia, Prolastin C) [Respiratory Agent/Alpha Protease Inhibitor Replacement]
Uses: *α$_1$-Antitrypsin deficiency* **Action:** Replace human α$_1$-protease Inhib **Dose:** 60 mg/kg IV once/wk **Caution:** [C, ?] **CI:** Selective IgA deficiencies w/ IgA antibodies **Disp:** Inj 500 mg, 1000 mg powder, 1000 mg soln vial for Inj **SE:** HA, CP, edema, MS discomfort, fever, dizziness, flu-like Sxs, allergic Rxns **Labs:** Monitor for ↑ ALT, AST **NIPE:** Inf over 30 min, ⊘ mix w/ other drugs, use w/in 3 h of reconstitution

Alprazolam (Xanax, Niravam) [C-IV] [Anxiolytic/Benzodiazepine] Uses: *Anxiety & panic disorders*, anxiety w/ depression* **Action:** Benzodiazepine; antianxiety agent **Dose:** *Anxiety:* Initial, 0.25–0.5 mg tid; ↑ to 4 mg/d max ÷ doses *Panic:* Initial, 0.5 mg tid; may gradually ↑ to response; ↓ in elderly, debilitated, & hepatic impair **Caution:** [D, –] **CI:** NAG, concomitant itra/ketoconazole **Disp:** Tabs 0.25, 0.5, 1, 2 mg *Xanax XR:* 0.5, 1, 2, 3 mg *Niravam* (ODT): 0.25, 0.5, 1, 2 mg; soln 1 mg/mL **SE:** Drowsiness, fatigue, irritability, memory impair, sexual dysfunction, paradoxical Rxns **Interactions:** ↑ CNS depression **W/** EtOH, other CNS depressants, narcotics, MAOIs, anesthetics, antihistamines, theophylline; herbs: kava kava, valerian; ↑ effect **W/** OCPs, cimetidine, INH, disulfiram, omeprazole, valproic acid, ciprofloxacin, erythromycin, clarithromycin, phenytoin, verapamil, grapefruit juice; ↑ risk **OF** ketoconazole, itraconazole, digitalis tox, ↓ effectiveness **OF** levodopa; ↓ effect **W/** carbamazepine, rifampin, rifabutin, barbiturates, cigarette smoking **Labs:** ↑ Alk phos, may cause ↓ Hct & neutropenia **NIPE:** Monitor for resp depression; avoid abrupt D/C after prolonged use

Alprostadil [Prostaglandin E₁] (Prostin VR) [Vasodilator/ Prostaglandin] **WARNING:** Apnea in up to 12% of neonates esp < 2 kg at birth **Uses:** *Conditions where ductus arteriosus blood flow must be maintained* sustain pulm/systemic circulation until OR (eg, pulm atresia/stenosis, transposition) **Action:** Vasodilator (ductus arteriosus very sensitive), plt Inhib **Dose:** 0.05–0.1 mcg/kg/min IV; ↓ to response **ECC 2010:** Maintain Ductus Patency: 0.01–0.4 mcg/kg/min **Caution:** [X, –] **CI:** Neonatal resp distress synd **Disp:** Inj 500 mcg/mL **SE:** Cutaneous vasodilation, Sz-like activity, jitteriness, ↑ temp, thrombocytopenia, ↓ BP; may cause apnea **Interactions:** ↑ Effects **OF** anticoagulants & antihypertensives, ↓ effects **OF** cyclosporine **Labs:** ↓ K+, Ca²⁺, fibrinogen **NIPE:** Dilute drug before administration, refrigerate & discard > 24 h, central line preferred, flushing indicates catheter malposition, apnea & bradycardia indicates drug OD, keep intubation kit at bedside; administered to hospitalized newborns

Alprostadil, Intracavernosal (Caverject, Edex) [GU Agent/ Prostaglandin] Uses: *ED* **Action:** Relaxes smooth muscles, dilates cavernosal arteries, ↑ lacunar spaces w/ blood entrapment **Dose:** 2.5–60 mcg intracavernosal; titrate in office **Caution:** [X, –] **CI:** ↑ Risk of priapism (eg, sickle cell); penile deformities/implants; men in whom sexual activity inadvisable **Disp:** *Caverject:* 5-, 10-, 20-, 40-mcg powder for Inj vials ± diluent syringes 10-, 20-, 40-mcg amp *Caverject Impulse:* Self-contained syringe (29 gauge) 10, 20 mcg *Edex:* 10-, 20-, 40-mcg cartridges **SE:** Local pain w/Inj **Interactions:** ↑ Effects **OF** anticoagulants & antihypertensives, ↓ effects **OF** cyclosporine **Labs:** ↓ Fibrinogen **NIPE:** Vag itching and burning in female partners, N Inj > 3x/wk or closer than 24 h/dose; counsel about priapism, penile fibrosis, hematoma risks, titrate dose in office

Alprostadil, Urethral Suppository (Muse) [GU Agent/Prostaglandin] Uses: *ED* **Action:** Urethral absorption; vasodilator, relaxes smooth muscle of corpus cavernosa **Dose:** 125–250 mcg PRN to achieve erection (max: 2 systoms/24 h);

duration is 30–60 min **Caution:** [X, –] **CI:** ↑ Priapism risk (esp sickle cell, myeloma, leukemia) penile deformities/implants; men in whom sex is inadvisable **Disp:** 125, 250, 500, 1000 mcg w/ transurethral system **SE:** ↓ BP, dizziness, syncope, penile/testicular pain, urethral burning/bleeding, priapism **Interactions:** ↑ Effects *OF* anticoagulants & antihypertensives, ↓ effects *OF* cyclosporine **Labs:** ↓ Fibrinogen **NIPE:** No more than 2 supp/24 h, counsel about priapism, urinate prior to use; titrate dose in office

Alteplase, Recombinant [tPA] (Activase) [Plasminogen Activator/Thrombolytic Enzyme]

Uses: *AMI, PE, acute ischemic stroke, & CV cath occlusion* **Action:** Thrombolytic; binds fibrin in thrombus, initiates fibrinolysis **Dose:** *ECC 2010:* STEMI 15-mg bolus; then 0.75 mg/kg over 30 min (50 mg max); then 0.50 mg/kg over next 60 min (35 mg max; max total dose 100 mg) *Acute ischemic stroke:* 0.9 mg/kg IV (max 90 mg) over 60 min; give 10% of total dose over 1 min; remaining 90% over 1 h (or 3-h Inf) PE: 100 mg over 2 h (submassive PE can administer 10-mg bolus, then 90 mg over 2 h) *Cath occlusion:* 10–29 kg 1 mg/mL; 30 kg 2 mg/2 mL **Caution:** [C, ?] **CI:** Active internal bleeding; uncontrolled HTN (SBP > 185 mm Hg/DBP > 110 mm Hg); recent (w/in 3 mo) CVA, GI bleed, trauma; intracranial or intraspinal surgery or Dzs (AVM/aneurysm/subarachnoid hemorrhage/neoplasm), prolonged cardiac massage; suspected aortic dissection, w/ anticoagulants or INR > 1.7, heparin w/in 48 h, plts <100,000, Sz at the time of stroke, significant closed head/facial trama **Disp:** Powder for Inj 2, 50, 100 mg **SE:** Bleeding, bruising (eg, venipuncture sites), ↓ BP **Interactions:** ↑ Risk of bleeding *W/* heparin, ASA, NSAIDs, abciximab, dipyridamole, eptifibatide, tirofiban; ↓ effects *W/* nitroglycerine **Labs:** ↓ Fibrinogen, monitor PT/PTT **NIPE:** Compress venipuncture site at least 30 min, bed rest during Inf; give heparin to prevent reocclusion; in AMI, doses of > 150 mg associated w/ intracranial bleeding

Altretamine (Hexalen) [Antineoplastic/Alkylating Agent]

WARNING: BM suppression, neurotox common, should be administered by experienced chemo provider **Uses:** *Palliative Rx, persistent or recurrent ovarian CA* **Action:** Unknown; ? cytotoxic/alkylating agent, ? nucleotide incorporation **Dose:** 260 mg/m²/d in 4 ÷ doses for 14–21 d of a 28-d Rx cycle; after meals & hs **Caution:** [D, ?/–] **CI:** Preexisting BM depression or neurologic tox **Disp:** Gel caps 50 mg **SE:** N/V/D, cramps; neurotox (neuropathy, CNS depression); myelosuppression, anemia **Interactions:** ↑ Effect *W/* phenobarbital, ↓ Ab response *W/* live virus vaccines, ↑ risk of tox *W/* cimetidine & hypotension *W/* MAOIs, ↑ BM depression *W/* radiation **Labs:** ↓ WBC, plt—monitor CBC, ↑ alk phos, BUN, SCr **NIPE:** Use barrier contraception, take w/ food, routine neuro exams—neurotox common

Aluminum Hydroxide (Amphojel, ALternaGEL, Dermagran) [OTC]

Uses: *Heartburn, upset or sour stomach, or acid indigestion*; supl to Rx of ↑ PO_4^{2-}; *minor cuts, burns (Dermagran)* **Action:** Neutralizes gastric acid; binds PO_4^{2-} **Dose:** *Adults.* 10–30 mL or 300–1200 mg PO q4–6h *Peds.* 5–15 mL PO q4–6h or 50–150 mg/kg/24 h PO ÷ q4–6h (hyperphosphatemia) **Caution:** [C, ?]

Disp: Tabs 300, 600 mg; susp 320, 600 mg/5 mL; oint 0.275% (*Dermagran*) **SE:** Constipation **Interactions:** ↓ Absorption & effects *OF* allopurinol, benzodiazepines, corticosteroids, chloroquine, cimetidine, digoxin, INH, phenytoin, quinolones, ranitidine, tetracycline **Labs:** ↑ Serum gastrin, ↓ serum phosphate **NIPE:** Separate other drug administration by 2 h, ↑ effectiveness of Liq form; OK in renal failure; topical ointment for cuts/burns

Aluminum Hydroxide + Alginic Acid + Magnesium Carbonate (Gaviscon Extra Strength, Liquid) [Antacid/Aluminum & Magnesium Salts] [OTC]
Uses: *Relief of heartburn, acid indigestion* **Action:** Neutralizes gastric acid **Dose:** *Adults.* 15–30 mL PO pc & hs; 2–4 chew tabs up to qid **Caution:** [C, ?] ↑ Mg^{2+}, avoid w/ renal impair **Disp:** Liq w/ AlOH 95 mg/Mg carbonate 358 mg/15 mL; Extra Strength Liq AlOH 254 mg/Mg carbonate 237 mg/15 mL; chew tabs AlOH 160 mg/Mg carbonate 105 mg **SE:** Constipation, D **Interactions:** In addition to AlOH ↓ effects *OF* histamine blockers, hydantoins, nitrofurantoin, phenothiazine, ticlopidine, ↑ effects *OF* quinidine, sulfonylureas **NIPE:** ↓ Fiber; qid doses best given pc & hs; may ↓ absorption of some drugs, take 2–3 h apart to ↓ effect

Aluminum Hydroxide + Magnesium Hydroxide (Maalox, Mylanta Ultimate Strength) [Antacid/Aluminum & Magnesium Salts] [OTC]
Uses: *Hyperacidity* (peptic ulcer, hiatal hernia, etc) **Action:** Neutralizes gastric acid **Dose:** *Adults.* 10–20 mL PO qid or PRN **Caution:** [C, ?] **Disp:** Chewtabs, susp **SE:** May ↑ Mg^{2+} w/ renal Insuff, constipation, D **Interactions:** In addition to AlOH, ↓ effects *OF* digoxin, quinolones, phenytoin, Fe supl, & ketoconazole **NIPE:** ⊘ Concurrent drug use—separate by 2h; doses qid best given pc & hs

Aluminum Hydroxide + Magnesium Hydroxide & Simethicone (Mylanta Regular Strength, Maalox Advanced) [Antacid/Aluminum & Magnesium Salts] [OTC]
Uses: *Hyperacidity w/ bloating* **Action:** Neutralizes gastric acid & defoaming **Dose:** *Adults.* 10–20 mL or 1–2 tabs PO qid or PRN, avoid in renal impair **Caution:** [C, ?] **Disp:** Tabs, susp, liq **SE:** ↑ Mg^{2+} in renal Insuff, D, constipation **Interactions:** In addition to AlOH, ↓ effects *OF* digoxin, quinolones, phenytoin, Fe supl, & ketoconazole **NIPE:** ⊘ Concurrent drug use—separate by 2 h; may affect absorption of some drugs; Mylanta II contains 2 × Al & Mg of Mylanta

Aluminum Hydroxide + Magnesium Trisilicate (Gaviscon, Regular Strength) [Antacid/Aluminum & Magnesium Salts] [OTC]
Uses: *Relief of heartburn, upset or sour stomach, or acid indigestion* **Action:** Neutralizes gastric acid **Dose:** Chew 1–2 tabs qid; avoid in renal impair **Caution:** [C, ?] **CI:** Mg^{2+}, sensitivity **Disp:** AlOH 80 mg/Mg trisilicate 20 mg/tab **SE:** ↑ Mg^{2+} in renal Insuff, constipation, D **Interactions:** In addition to Al, ↓ effects *OF* digoxin, quinolones, phenytoin, Fe supl, & ketoconazole **NIPE:** ⊘ Concurrent drug use—separate by 2 h

Alvimopan (Entereg) [Opioid Antagonist] **WARNING:** For short-term hospital use only (max 15 doses) **Uses:** *↓ Time to GI recovery w/ bowel resection and primary anastomosis* **Action:** Opioid (μ) receptor antagonist; selectively blocks GI receptors, antagonizes effects of opioids on GI motility/secretion **Dose:** 12 mg 30 min–5 h preop PO, then 12 mg bid up to 7 d; max 15 doses **Caution:** [B, ?/–] Not rec in complete bowel obstruction surgery, hepatic/renal impair **CI:** Therapeutic opioids > 7 consecutive days prior **Disp:** Caps 12 mg **SE:** Dyspepsia, urinary retention, anemia, back pain **Labs:** ↓ K+, monitor LFTs & BUN/Cr for hepatic/renal impair **NIPE:** Hospitals must be registered in Entereg Access & Support Program to use; D/C if adverse Rxns

Amantadine (Symmetrel) [Antiviral, Antiparkinsonian/ Anticholinergic-Like Medium] **Uses:** *Rx/prophylaxis influenza A (no longer recommended d/t resistance), Parkinsonism, & drug-induced EPS* **Action:** Prevents infectious viral nucleic acid release into host cell; releases dopamine & blocks reuptake of dopamine in presynaptic nerves **Dose:** *Adults. Influenza A:* 200 mg/d PO or 100 mg PO bid w/in 48 h of Sx; *EPS:* 100 mg PO bid (up to 300 mg/d ÷ doses); *Parkinsonism:* 100 mg PO daily–bid (up to 400 mg/d); *Peds 1–9 y.* 4.4–8.8 mg/kg/24 h to 150 mg/24 h max ÷ doses daily–bid *10–12 y:* 100–200 mg/d in 2 ÷ doses; ↓ in renal impair **Caution:** [C, ?/–] **Disp:** Caps 100 mg; tabs 100 mg; soln 50 mg/5 mL **SE:** Orthostatic ↓ BP, edema, insomnia, depression, irritability, hallucinations, dream abnormalities, N/D, dry mouth **Interactions:** ↑ Effects W/ HCTZ, triamterene, amiloride, pheasant's eye herb, Scopolia root, benztropine **Labs:** ↑ BUN, SCr, CPK, alk phos, bilirubin, LDH, AST, ALT **NIPE:** ⊘ D/C abruptly, take at least 4 h before sleep if insomnia occurs, eval for mental status changes, take w/ meals, ⊘ EtOH; Not for influenza use in US d/t resistance including H1N1

Ambrisentan (Letairis) [Endothelin Receptor Antagonist] **WARNING:** CIin PRG; ✓ monthly PRG tests; limited access program **Uses:** *Pulm arterial HTN* **Action:** Endothelin receptor antagonist **Dose:** *Adults.* 5 mg PO/d, max 10 mg/d; not recommended w/ hepatic impair **Caution:** [X, –] w/Cyclosporine, strong CYP3A or 2C19 inhib, inducers of P-glycoprotein, CYPs and UGTs **CI:** PRG **Disp:** Tabs 5, 10 mg **SE:** Edema, nasal congestion, sinusitis, dyspnea, flushing, constipation, HA, palpitations, hepatotoxic **Interactions:** Caution W/ cyclosporine, strong CYP3A or 2C19 Inhib, inducers of P-glycoprotein, CYPs, & UGTs **Labs:** D/CAST/ALT > 5 × ULN or bilirubin >2 × ULN or S/Sx of liver dysfunction; ↓ hct/hgb **NIPE:** Available only through the Letairis Education and Access Program (LEAP); childbearing females must use 2 methods of contraception

Amifostine (Ethyol) [Antineoplastic/Thiophosphate Cytoprotective] **Uses:** *Xerostomia prophylaxis during RT (head, neck, etc) where parotid is in radiation field; ↓ renal tox w/ repeated cisplatin* **Action:** Prodrug, dephosphorylated to active thiol metabolite; free radical scavenger binds cisplatin metabolites **Dose:** Chemo prevent: 910 mg/m^2/d 15-min IV Inf 30 min pre chemo; *Xerostomia PX:* 200 mg/m^2 over 2 min 1×/d 15 min pre-rad **Caution:** [C, ?/–] **Disp:** 500-mg vials powder, reconstitute in NS **SE:** Transient ↓ BP (> 60%), N/V, flushing w/ hot or cold chills, dizziness, somnolence, sneezing, serious skin Infxn **Interactions:** ↑ Effects *W/* antihypertensives **Labs:** ↓ Ca levels **NIPE:** Monitor BP for hypotension; ensure adequate hydration; infuse over 15 min supine; does not ↓ effectiveness of cyclophosphamide + cisplatin chemotherapy

Amikacin (Amikin) [Antibiotic/Aminoglycoside] **WARNING:** May cause nephrotoxicity, neuromuscular blockade, & respiratory paralysis **Uses:** *Serious gram(–) bacterial Infxns* & mycobacteria **Action:** Aminoglycoside; ↓ protein synth *Spectrum:* Good gram(–) bacterial coverage: *Pseudomonas* & *Mycobacterium* sp **Dose:** ***Adults &Peds.*** *Conventional:* 5–7.5 mg/kg/dose q8h; once daily: 15–20 mg/kg q24h; ↑ interval w/ renal impair *Neonates < 1200 g, 0-4 wk:* 7.5–10 mg/kg/dose q18h–24h *Age < 7 d, 1200–2000 g:* 7.5 mg/kg/dose q12h *> 2000 g:* 10 mg/kg/dose q12h *Age > 7d, 1200–2000 g:* 7.5–10 mg/kg/dose q8–12h *> 2000 g:* 7.5–10 mg/kg/dose q8h **Caution:** [O, +/–] Avoid w/ diuretics **Disp:** Inj 50 & 250 mg/mL **SE:** Renal impairment, oto **Notes:** May be effective in gram(–) resistance to gentamicin & tobramycin; follow Cr; *Levels: Peak* 30 min after Inf *Trough <* 0.5 h before next dose *Therapeutic: Peak* 20–30 mcg/mL *Trough <* 8 mcg/mL *Toxic: Peak >* 35 mcg/mL *1/2-life:* 2 h **Interactions:** ↑ Risk of ototox and nephrotox *W/* acyclovir, amphotericin B, cephalosporins, cisplatin, loop diuretics, methoxyflurane, polymyxin B, vancomycin; ↑ neuromuscular blocking effect *W/* muscle relaxants & anesthetics **Labs:** ↑ BUN, SCr, AST, ALT, serum alk phos, bilirubin, LDH **NIPE:** ↑ Fluid consumption; may cause resp depression

Amiloride (Midamor) [Potassium-Sparing Diuretic] **WARNING:** ↑ K$^+$ renal Dz, DM, elderly **Uses:** *HTN, CHF, & thiazide or loop diuretic induced* ↓ K$^+$* **Action:** K$^+$-sparing diuretic; interferes w/ K$^+$/Na$^+$ exchange in distal tubule and collecting duct **Dose:** ***Adults.*** 5–10 mg PO daily (max 20 mg/d) ***Peds.*** 0.4–0.625 mg/kg/d; ↓ w/ renal impair **Caution:** [B, ?] Avoid CrCl < 10 mL/min; **CI:** ↑ K$^+$, acute or chronic renal Dz, diabetic neuropathy, w/ other K$^+$-sparing diuretics **Disp:** Tabs 5 mg **SE:** HA, dizziness, dehydration, impotence **Interactions:** ↑ Risk of hyperkalemia *W/* ACE-I, K-sparing diuretics, NSAIDs, & K-salt substitutes; ↑ effects *OF* Li, digoxin, antihypertensives, amantadine; ↑ risk of *F* hypokalemia *W/* licorice **Labs:** ↑ K+; monitor K$^+$-monitor ECG for hyperkalemia (peaked T waves) **NIPE:** Take w/ food, I&O, daily wgt, N salt substitutes, bananas, oranges

Aminocaproic Acid (Amicar) [Antithrombotic Agent/Carboxylic Acid Derivative] **Uses:** *Excessive bleeding from systemic hyperfibrinolysis & urinary fibrinolysis* **Action:** ↓ Fibrinolysis; inhibits TPA, inhibits conversion of plasminogen to plasmin **Dose:** ***Adults.*** 4–5 g IV or PO (1st h) then 1 g/h IV or 1.25 g/h PO × 8 h or until bleeding controlled; 30 g/d max ***Peds.*** 100 mg/kg IV (1st h) then 1 g/m²/h; max 18 g/m²/d; ↓ w/ renal Insuff **Caution:** [C, ?] Not for upper urinary tract bleeding **CI:** DIC **Disp:** Tabs 500 mg, syrup 1.25 g/5 mL; Inj 250 mg/mL **SE:** ↓ BP, ↑ HR, dizziness, HA, fatigue, rash, GI disturbance, skeletal muscle weakness **Fxn Notes:** Administer × 8 h or until bleeding controlled; not for upper urinary tract bleeding **Interactions:** ↑ Coagulation *W/* estrogens & OCP **Labs:** ↓ plt, false ↑ urine amino acids **NIPE:** CK monitoring w/ long-term use, eval for thrombophlebitis & difficulty urinating

Aminoglutethimide (Cytadren) [Adrenal Steroid Inhibitor]
Uses: *Cushing synd* adrenocortical carcinoma, breast CA & PCa **Action:** ↓ Adrenal steroidogenesis & conversion of androgens to estrogens; 1st gen aromatase inhib **Dose:** Initial 250 mg PO 4 × d, titrate q1–2wk max 2 g/d; w/ hydrocortisone 20–40 mg/d; ↓ w/ renal Insuff **Caution:** [D, ?] **Disp:** Tabs 250 mg **SE:** Adrenal Insuff ("medical adrenalectomy"), hypothyroidism, masculinization, ↓ BP, N/V, rare hepatotox, rash, myalgia, fever, drowsiness, lethargy, anorexia **Interactions:** ↓ Effects *W/* dexamethasone & hydrocortisone, ↓ effects *OF* warfarin, theophylline, medroxyprogesterone **NIPE:** Masculinization reversible after D/C drug, ⊘ PRG; give q6h to ↓ N

Aminophylline (Generic) [Bronchodilator/Xanthine Derivative]
Uses: *Asthma, COPD*, & bronchospasm **Action:** Relaxes smooth muscle (bronchi, pulm vessels); stimulates diaphragm **Dose:** *Adults. Acute asthma:* Load 5.7 mg/kg IV, then 0.38–0.51 mg/kg/h (900 mg/d max) *Chronic asthma:* 380 mg/d PO ÷ q6–8h; maint ↑ 760 mg/d *Peds.* Load 5.7 mg/kg/dose IV, *1– ≤ 9 y:* 1.01 mg/kg/h; *9– ≤ 12 y:* 0.89 mg/kg/h; ↓ w/ hepatic Insuff & w/ some drugs (macrolide & quinolone antibiotics, cimetidine, propranolol) **Caution:** [C, +] Uncontrolled arrhythmias, HTN, Sz disorder, hyperthyroidism, peptic ulcers **Disp:** Tabs 100, 200 mg; PR tabs 100, 200 mg, soln 105 mg/5 mL, Inj 25 mg/mL **SE:** N/V, irritability, tachycardia, ventricular arrhythmias, Szs **Notes:** Individualize dose *Level:* 10–20 mcg/mL, toxic > 20 mcg/mL; aminophylline 85% theophylline; erratic rectal absorption **Interactions:** ↓ Effects *OF* Li, phenytoin, adenosine; ↓ effects *W/* phenobarbital, aminoglutethimide, barbiturates, rifampin, ritonavir, thyroid meds, tobacco; ↑ effects *W/* cimetidine, ciprofloxacin, erythromycin, INH, OCP, verapamil, charcoal-broiled foods, St. John's wort **Labs:** ↑ Uric acid levels, falsely ↑ levels w/ furosemide, probenecid, APAP, coffee, tea, cola, chocolate **NIPE:** ⊘ Chew or crush time-released caps & take on empty stomach, IR can be taken w/food, ↑ fluids 2 L/d, tobacco ↑ drug elimination; narrow therapeutic range

Amiodarone (Cordarone, Nexterone, Pacerone) [Ventricular Antiarrhythmic/Adrenergic Blocker]
WARNING: Liver tox, exacerbation of arrhythmias and lung damage reported **Uses:** *Recurrent VF or unstable VT*, supraventricular arrhythmias, AF **Action:** Class III antiarrhythmic inhibits alpha/beta adrenergic system (Table 9) **Dose:** *Adults. Ventricular arrhythmias: IV:* 15 mg/min × 10 min, then 1 mg/min × 6 h, maint 0.5 mg/min cont Inf or *PO:*

Load: 800–1600 mg/d PO × 1–3 wk *Maint:* 600–800 mg/d PO for 1 mo, then 200–400 mg/d *Supraventricular arrhythmias: IV:* 300 mg IV over 1 h, then 20 mg/kg for 24 h, then 600 mg PO daily for 1 wk, maint 100–400 mg daily or *PO:* Load 600–800 mg/d PO for 1–4 wk *Maint:* Slow ↓ to 100–400 mg daily *ECC 2010:* VF/VT Cardiac arrest refractory to CPR, Shock and Pressor: 300 mg IV/IO push; can give additional 150 mg IV/IO once; life-threatening arrhythmias: Max dose 2.2 g IV/24 h Rapid Inf: 150 mg IV over first 10 min (15 mg/min); can repeat 150 mg IV q10 min PRN. Slow Inf: 360 mg IV over 60 min (1 mg/min) Maint: 540 mg IV over 18 h (0.5 mg/ min) *Peds.* 10–15 mg/kg/24 h ÷ q12h PO for 7–10 d, then 5 mg/kg/24 h ÷ q12h or daily (infants require ↑ loading); *ECC 2010:* PulselessVT/refractory VF: 5mg/kg IV/IO bolus, repeat PRN to 15 mg/kg (2.2 g in adolescents)/24 h; max single dose 300 mg; perfusing SVT/ventricular arrhythmias: 5 mg/kg IV/IO load over 20–60 min; repeat PRN to 15 mg/kg (2.2 g in adolescents)/24 h **Caution:** [D, −] May require ↓ digoxin/warfarin dose, ↓ w/ liver Insuff, many drug interactions **CI:** Sinus node dysfunction, 2nd-/3rd-degree AV block, sinus brady (w/o pacemaker), iodine sensitivity **Disp:** Tabs 100, 200, 400 mg; Inj 50 mg/mL; Premixed Inf 150, 360 mg **SE:** Pulm fibrosis, exacerbation of arrhythmias, ↑ QT interval; CHF, hypo-/hyperthyroidism, liver failure, ↓ BP / ↓ HR (Inf related), dizziness, HA, corneal microdeposits, optic neuropathy/neuritis, peripheral neuropathy, photosens; blue skin **Notes:** IV conc > 2.0 mg/mL only via central line *Levels: Trough:* Just before next dose *Therapeutic:* 0.5–2.5 mcg/mL *Toxic:* > 2.5 mcg/mL *1/2-life:* 40–55 days (↓ peds) **Interactions:** ↑ Serum levels *OF* digoxin, quinidine, procainamide, flecainide, phenytoin, warfarin, theophylline, cyclosporine; ↑ levels *W/* cimetidine, indinavir, ritonavir; ↓ levels *W/* cholestyramine, rifampin, St. John's wort; ↑ cardiac effects *W/* BBs, CCB **Labs:** ↑ LFTs, ↑ T_4 & RT_3, ANA titer, ↓ T_3 **NIPE:** Monitor cardiac rhythm, BP, LFTs, thyroid Fxn, ophthalmologic exam; may cause bradycardia; ↑ photosensitivity—use sunscreen; take w/ food

Amitriptyline (Elavil) [Antidepressant/TCA]   **WARNING:** Antidepressants may ↑ suicide risk; consider risks/benefits of use. Monitor pts closely **Uses:** *Depression (not bipolar depression)* peripheral neuropathy, chronic pain, tension HA, migraine HA prophylaxis, PTSD **Action:** TCA; ↓ reuptake of serotonin & norepinephrine by presynaptic neurons **Dose:** *Adults. Initial:* 25–150 mg PO hs; may ↑ to 300 mg hs *Peds.* Not OK < 12 y unless for chronic pain *Initial:* 0.1 mg/kg PO hs, ↑ over 2–3 wk to 0.5–2 mg/kg PO hs; taper to D/C **Caution:** CV Dz, Szs [D, +/−] NAG, hepatic impair **CI:** w/ MAOIs or w/in 14 d of use, during AMI recovery **Disp:** Tabs 10, 25, 50, 75, 100, 150 mg; Inj 10 mg/mL **SE:** Strong anticholinergic SEs; OD may be fatal; urine retention, sedation, ECG changes, BM suppression, orthostatic ↓ BP, photosens **Notes:** *Levels: Therapeutic:* 100–250 ng/mL *Toxic:* > 500 ng/mL; levels may not correlate w/ effect **Interactions:** ↓ Effects *W/* carbamazepine, phenobarbital, rifampin, cholestyramine, colestipol, tobacco; ↑ effects *W/* cimetidine, quinidine, indinavir, ritonavir, CNS depressants, SSRIs, haloperidol, OCPs, BBs, phenothiazines, EtOH, evening primrose oil; ↑ effects *OF* amphetamines, anticholinergics, epinephrine, hypoglycemics, phenylephrine **Labs:** ↑ Glucose, false ↑ carbamazepine levels **NIPE:** ↑ Photosensitivity—use sunscreen; ↑ appetite & craving for sweets; ⊘ D/C abruptly; may turn urine blue-green

Amlodipine (Norvasc) [Antihypertensive, Antianginal/CCB] Uses: *HTN, stable or unstable angina* **Action:** CCB; relaxes coronary vascular smooth muscle **Dose:** 2.5–10 mg/d PO; ↓ w/ hepatic impair **Caution:** [C, ?] **Disp:** Tabs 2.5, 5, 10 mg **SE:** Edema, HA, palpitations, flushing, dizziness **Interactions:** ↑ Effect of hypotension *W/* antihypertensives, fentanyl, nitrates quinidine, EtOH, grapefruit juice; ↑ risk of neurotox *W/* Li; ↓ effects *W/* NSAIDs **NIPE:** Take w/o regard to meals; monitor for peripheral edema

Amlodipine/Atorvastatin (Caduet) [Antianginal, Antihypertensive, Antilipemic/Calcium Channel Blocker, HMG-CoA Reductase Inhibitor] Uses: *HTN, chronic stable/vasospastic angina, control cholesterol & triglycerides* **Action:** CCB & HMG-CoA reductase inhib **Dose:** Amlodipine 2.5–10 mg w/ atorvastatin 10–80 mg PO daily **Caution:** [X, –] **CI:** Active liver Dz, ↑ LFTs **Disp:** Tabs amlodipine/atorvastatin: 2.5/10, 2.5/20, 2.5/40, 5/10, 5/20, 5/40, 5/80, 10/10, 10/20, 10/40, 10/80 mg **SE:** Edema, HA, palpitations, flushing, myopathy, arthralgia, myalgia, GI upset, liver failure **Interactions:** ↑ Hypotension *W/* fentanyl, nitrates, EtOH, quinidine, other antihypertensives, grapefruit juice; ↑ effects *W/* diltiazem, erythromycin, H₂-blockers, PPI, quinidine; ↓ effects *W/* NSAIDs, barbiturates, rifampin **Labs:** Monitor LFTs & CPK **NIPE:** ⊘ D/C abruptly, ↑ photosensitivity—use sunscreen; rare risk of rhabdomyolysis; instruct pt to report muscle pain/ weakness

Amlodipine/Olmesartan (Azor) [Calcium Channel Blocker + Angiotensin II Receptor Blocker] **WARNING:** Use of renin-angiotensin agents in PRG can cause injury and death to fetus, D/C stat when PRG detected Uses: *Hypertension* **Action:** CCB w/ angiotensin II receptor blocker **Dose:** *Adults.* Initial 5 mg/20 mg, max 10 mg/40 mg qd **Caution:** [C (1st tri), D (2nd, 3rd tri), –] w/K⁺ supl or K⁺-sparing diuretics, renal impair, RAS, severe CAD, AS **CI:** PRG **Disp:** Tab amlodipine/olmesartan 5 mg/20 mg, 10/20, 5/40, 10/40 **SE:** Edema, vertigo, dizziness, ↓ BP **Labs:** ↓ Hgb & Hct; monitor LFTs & BUN/Cr **NIPE:** May need ↓ dose in elderly; not recommended in children

Amlodipine/Valsartan (HA Exforge) [Calcium Channel Blocker (Dihydropyridine) + Angiotensin II Receptor Blocker] **WARNING:** Use of renin-angiotensin agents in PRG can cause fetal injury and death, D/C immediately when PRG detected Uses: *HTN* **Action:** CCB w/ angiotensin II receptor blocker **Dose:** *Adults.* Initial 5 mg/160 mg, may ↑ after 1–2 wk, max 320 mg/320 mg qd, start elderly at ½ initial dose **Caution:** [C (1st tri), D (2nd, 3rd tri),–] w/K⁺ supl or K⁺-sparing diuretics, renal impair, RAS, severe CAD **CI:** PRG **Disp:** Tabs amlodipine/valsartan: 5/160, 10/160, 5/320, 10 mg/320 mg **SE:** Edema, vertigo, nasopharyngitis, URI, dizziness, ↓ BP **Interactions:** ↑ Risk of hyperkalemia *W/* concomitant K⁺

supls, K+-sparing diuretics, K+-containing salt substitutes; ↑ SCr in HF **NIPE:** ⊘ PRG or breast-feeding; max effects w/in 2 wk after dose change

Amlodipine/Valsartan/HCTZ (Exforge Hct) [Calcium Channel Blocker + Angiotensin Receptor Blocker + Diuretic] WARNING: Use of renin-angiotensin agents in PRG can cause fetal injury and death, D/C immediately when PRG detected **Uses:** *HTN* (not initial Rx) **Action:** CCB, angiotensin II receptor blocker, & thiazide diuretic **Dose:** 5–10/160–320/12.5–25 mg, 1 tab × 1 d, may ↑ dose after 2 wk; max dose 10/320/25 mg **Caution:** [D, –] w/ Severe hepaticorenal impair **CI:** Anuria, sulfonamide allergy **Disp:** Tabs amlodipine/valsartan/HCTZ: 5/160/12.5, 10/160/12.5, 5/160/25, 10/160/25, 10/320/25 **SE:** Edema, dizziness, HA, fatigue, nasopharyngitis, dyspepsia, N, back pain, muscle spasm, ↓ BP **Interactions:** ↑ Risk of hypotension *W/* diuretics, antihypertensives **Labs:** ↑/↓ K+, ↑ BUN, ↑ SCr **NIPE:** Monitor BP for hypotension; ⊘ PRG or breast-feeding; ↑ risk of hyperkalemia w/ concomitant K+ supls, K+-sparing diuretics, K+-containing salt substitutes; ↑ SCr in HF

Ammonium Aluminum Sulfate [Alum] [GU Astringent] [OTC] **Uses:** *Hemorrhagic cystitis when saline bladder irrigation fails* **Action:** Astringent **Dose:** 1–2% soln w/ constant NS bladder irrigation **Caution:** [+/–] **Disp:** Powder for recons **SE:** Encephalopathy possible; can precipitate & occlude catheters **Labs:** Monitor Al levels, especially w/ renal Insuff **NIPE:** Safe to use w/o anesthesia & w/ vesicoureteral reflux

Amoxicillin (Amoxil Moxatag) [Antibiotic/Aminopenicillin] **Uses:** *Ear, nose, & throat, lower resp, skin, urirnary tract Infxns from susceptible gram(+) bacteria* endocarditis prophylaxis, *H pylori* eradication w/ other agents (gastric ulcers) **Action:** β-Lactam antibiotic; ↓ cell wall synth *Spectrum:* Gram(+) (*Streptococcus* sp, *Enterococcus* sp); some gram(–) (*H influenzae, E coli, N gonorrhoeae, H pylori, & P mirabilis*) **Dose: *Adults.*** 250–500 mg PO tid or 500–875 mg bid ER: 775 mg, 1 × d; *Peds.* 25–100 mg/kg/24 h PO ÷ q8h; ↓ in renal impair **Caution:** [B, +] **Disp:** Caps 250, 500 mg; chewtabs 125, 200, 250, 400 mg; susp 50, 125, 200, 250 mg/mL, & 400 mg/5 mL; tabs 500, 875 mg; ER: 775 mg **SE:** D; rash **Interactions:** ↑ Effects *OF* warfarin, ↑ effects *W/* probenecid, disulfiram, ↑ risk of rash *W/* allopurinol, ↓ effects *OF* OCP, ↓ effects *W/* tetracyclines, chloramphenicol **Labs:** ↑ Serum alk phos, LDH, LFTs, false(+) direct Coombs test **NIPE:** Space med over 24 h; eval for super Infxn; use barrier contraception; cross hypersensitivity w/PCN; many *E coli* strains resistant; chewtabs contain phenylalanine

Amoxicillin & Clavulanic Acid (Augmentin, Augmentin 600 ES, Augmentin XR) [Antibiotic/Aminopenicillin, Beta-Lactamase Inhibitor] **Uses:** *Ear, lower resp, sinus, urinary tract, skin Infxns caused by β-lactamase-producing H influenzae, S aureus, & E coli* **Action:** β-lactam antibiotic w/ β-lactamase Inhib *Spectrum:* Gram(+) same as amoxicillin alone, MSSA; gram(–) as w/ amoxicillinalone, β-lactamase-producing *H influenzae, Klebsiella* sp, *M catarrhalis Dose: Adults.* 250–500 mg PO q8h or 875 mg q12h; XR 2000 mg PO q12h *Peds.* 20–40 mg/kg/d as amoxicillin PO ÷ q8h or 45–90 mg/kg/d ÷ q12h; ↓ in renal impair; take w/ food **Caution:** [B, enters breast milk] **Disp:** Supplied (as amoxicillin/ clavulanic): Tabs 250/125, 500/125, 875/125 mg; chewtabs 125/31.25, 200/28.5, 250/62.5, 400/57 mg; susp 125/31.25, 250/62.5, 200/28.5, 400/57 mg/5 mL; susp: ES 600/42.9 mg/5 mL; XR tab 1000/62.5 mg **SE:** Abd discomfort, N/V/D, allergic Rxn, vaginitis **Interactions:** ↑ Effects *OF* warfarin, methotrexate, ↑ effects *W/* probenecid, disulfiram, ↑ risk of rash *W/* allopurinol, ↓ effects *OF* OCP, ↓ effects *W/* tetracyclines, chloramphenicol **Labs:** ↑ Serum alk phos, LDH, LFTs, false(+) direct Coombs test **NIPE:** Space med over 24 h, eval for super Infxn, use barrier contraception; do not substitute two 250-mg tabs for one 500-mg tab (possible OD of clavulanic acid); max clavulanic acid 125 mg/dose

Amphotericin B (Fungizone) [Antifungal/Polyene Macrolide]

Uses: *Severe systemic fungal Infxns; oral & cutaneous candidiasis* **Action:** Binds ergosterol in the cell membrane to alter permeability **Dose:** *Adults & Peds.* 0.25–1.5 mg/kg/24 h IV over 2–6 h (25–50 mg/d or qod). Total varies w/ indication ↑ PR, N/V **Caution:** [B, ?] **Disp:** Powder (Inj) 50 mg/vial **SE:** ↓ anaphylaxis, HA, fever, chills, nephrotox, ↓ BP, anemia, rigors **SE Interactions:** ↑ Nephrotoxic effects *W/* antineoplastics, cyclosporine, furosemide, vancomycin, aminoglycosides, ↑ hypokalemia *W/* corticosteroids, skeletal muscle relaxants **Labs:** ↓ K+, Mg2+ from renal wasting; monitor Cr/LFTs/K/Mg; ↑ serum bilirubin, serum cholesterol **NIPE:** Monitor CNS effects & ⊘ take hs; ↓ in renal impair; pretreatment w/ APAP & diphenhydramine ± hydrocortisone; ↓ SE

Amphotericin B Cholesteryl (Amphotec) [Antifungal/Polyene Macrolide]

Uses: *Aspergillosis if intolerant/refractory to conventional amphotericin B*, systemic candidiasis **Action:** Binds ergosterol in fungal membrane, alters permeability **Dose:** *Adults & Peds.* 3–4 mg/kg/d; 1 mg/kg/h Inf, 7.5 mg/kg/d max; ↓ w/ renal Insuff **Caution:** [B, ?] **Disp:** Powder for Inj 50, 100 mg/vial **SE:** Anaphylaxis; fever, chills, HA, N/V, ↑ HR; nephrotox, ↓ BP, infusion Rxns, anemia **Interactions:** See Amphotericin B **Labs:** Monitor LFTs, lytes; ↓ platelets, ↓ K+, ↓ Mg2+ **NIPE:** Do not use in-line filter

Amphotericin B Lipid Complex (Abelcet) [Antifungal/Polyene Macrolide]

Uses: *Refractory invasive fungal Infxn in pts intolerant to conventional amphotericin B* **Action:** Binds ergosterol in fungal membrane, alters permeability **Dose:** *Adults &Peds.* 2.5–5 mg/kg/d IV × 1 daily **Caution:** [B, ?] **Disp:** Inj 5 mg/mL **SE:** Anaphylaxis; fever, chills, HA, nephrotox, ↓ BP, anemia **Interactions:** See Amphotericin B **Labs:** ↑ SCr, ↓ K+, ↓ Mg2+ **NIPE:** Filter w/ 5-mcm needle; do not mix in lyte-containing solns; if Inf > 2 h, manually mix bag

Amphotericin B Liposomal (AmBisome) [Antifungal/Polyene Macrolide]

Uses: *Refractory invasive fungal Infxn w/ intolerance to conventional amphotericin B; cryptococcal meningitis in HIV; empiric for febrile neutropenia; visceral leishmaniasis* **Action:** Binds ergosterol in fungal membrane, alters membrane permeability **Dose:** *Adults & Peds.* 3–6 mcg/kg/d, Inf 60–120 min; varies by indication; ↓ in renal Insuff **Caution:** [B, ?] **Disp:** Powder Inj 50 mg **SE:** Anaphylaxis, fever, chills, HA, ↓ K+, ↓ Mg2+, nephrotox, ↓ BP, anemia **Interactions:** See amphotericin B **Labs:** ↑ LFTs, ↓ K+, ↓ Mg2+ **NIPE:** Do not use < 1-mcg filter

Ampicillin [Antibiotic/Aminopenicillin]   **Uses:** *Resp, GU, or GI tract Infxns, meningitis d/t gram(−) & (+) bacteria; SBE prophylaxis* **Action:** β-Lactam antibiotic; ↓ cell wall synth **Spectrum:** Gram(+) (*Streptococcus* sp, *Staphylococcus* sp, *Listeria*); gram(−) (*Klebsiella* sp, *E coli, H influenzae, P mirabilis, Shigella* sp, *Salmonella* sp) **Dose:** *Adults.* 1000 mg–2 g IM or IV q4–6h or 250–500 mg PO q6h; varies by indication *Peds Neonates. <7d:* 50–100 mg/kg/24 h IV ÷ q8h *Term infants:* 75–150 mg/kg/24 h ÷ q6–8h IV or PO *Children >1 mo:* 200 mg/kg/24 h ÷ q6h IM or IV; 50–100 mg/kg/24 h ÷q6h PO up to 250 mg/dose *Meningitis:* 200–400 mg/kg/24 h ÷ q6h IV; ↓ w/ renal impair; take on empty stomach **Caution:** [B, M] Cross-hypersens w/PCN **Disp:** Caps 250, 500 mg; susp 125 mg/5 mL, 250 mg/5 mg/mL; powder (Inj) 125, 250, 500 mg, 1, 2, 10 g/vial **SE:** D, rash, allergic Rxn **Notes:** Many *E coli* resistant **Interactions:** ↓ Effects *OF* OCP & atenolol, ↓ effects *W/* chloramphenicol, erythromycin, tetracycline, & food; ↑ effects *OF* anticoagulants & MTX; ↑ risk of rash *W/* allopurinol; ↑ effects *W/* probenecid & disulfiram **Labs:** ↑ LFTs, serum protein, serum theophylline, serum uric acid; ↓ serum estrogen, serum cholesterol, serum folate; false(+) direct Coombs test, urine glucose, & urine amino acids **NIPE:** Take on empty stomach & around the clock; may cause candidal vaginitis; use barrier contraception

Ampicillin-Sulbactam (Unasyn) [Antibiotic/Aminopenicillin & Beta-Lactamase Inhibitor] **Uses:** *Gynecologic, intra-Abd, skin Infxns d/t β-lactamase-producing S aureus, Enterococcus, H influenzae, P mirabilis, & Bacteroide ssp* **Action:** β-Lactam antibiotic & β-lactamase inhib **Spectrum:** Gram(+) & (−) as for amp alone; also *Enterobacter, Acinetobacter, Bacteroides* **Dose:** *Adults.* 1.5–3 g IM or IV q6h *Peds.* 100–400 mg ampicillin/kg/d (150–300 mg Unasyn) q6h; ↓ w/ renal Insuff **Caution:** [B, M] **Disp:** Powder for Inj 1.5, 3 g/vial,15 g bulk package **SE:** Allergic Rxns, rash, D, Inj site pain **Notes:** A 2:1 ratio ampicillin:sulbactam **Interactions:** ↓ Effects *OF* OCP & atenolol, ↓ effects *W/* chloramphenicol, erythromycin, tetracycline, & food; ↑ effects *OF* anticoagulants & MTX; ↑ risk of rash *W/* allopurinol; ↑ effects *W/* probenecid & disulfiram **Labs:** ↑ LFTs, serum protein, serum theophylline, serum uric acid; ↓ serum estrogen, serum cholesterol, serum folate; false(+) direct Coombs test, urine glucose, & urine amino acids **NIPE:** Take around the clock; may cause candidal vaginitis; use barrier contraception

Anakinra   (Kineret)   [Antirheumatic/Immunomodulator]   **Uses:** *Reduce S/Sxs of mod-severe active RA, failed 1 or more DMARD* **Action:** Human

IL-1 receptor antagonist **Dose:** 100 mg SQ daily; w/ CrCl < 30 mL/min, qod **Caution:** [B, ?] Only >1% y, avoid in active Inf **CI:** *E coli*–derived proteins allergy **Disp:** 100-mg prefilled syringes; 100 mg (0.67 mL/vial) **SE:** ↓ WBC esp w/TNF-blockers, Inj site Rxn (may last up to 28 d), Infxn, N/D, Abd pain, flu-like sx, HA **Interactions:** ↓ Effects *OF* immunizations; ↑ risk of Infxns if combined *W/* TNF-blocking drugs **Labs:** ↓WBCs, plts, ANC **NIPE:** ✓ Immunizations up-to-date prior to starting Rx; Store drug in refrigerator; ⊘ light exposure, & discard unused portion; ⊘ use soln if discolored or has particulate matter

Anastrozole (Arimidex) [Antineoplastic/Nonsteroidal Aromatase Inhibitor] Uses: *Breast CA: postmenopausal w/ metastatic breast CA, adjuvant Rx postmenopausal early hormone-receptor (+) breast CA* Action: Selective nonsteroidal aromatase Inhib, ↓ circulatory estradiol Dose: 1 mg/d Caution: [X, ?/–] CI: PRG Disp: Tabs 1 mg SE: N/V/D, HTN, flushing, ↑ bone/ tumor pain, HA, somnolence, mood disturbance, depression, rash, fatigue, weakness; Interactions: None noted Labs: ↑ GTT, LFTs, alk phos, total & LDL cholesterol; no effect on adrenal steroids or aldosterone NIPE: May ↓ fertility & cause fetal damage; eval for pain & administer adequate analgesia; may cause Vag bleeding 1st few wk

Anidulafungin (Eraxis) [Antifungal/Echinocandin] Uses: *Candidemia, esophageal candidiasis, other *Candida* Infxn (peritonitis, intra-Abd abscess)* Action: Echinocandin; ↓ cell wall synth Spectrum: *C albicans, C glabrata, C parapsilosis, C Tropicalis* Dose: *Candidemia, others:* 200 mg IV × 1, then 100 mg IV daily [Tx ≥ 14 d after last (+) culture]; *Esophageal candidiasis:*100 mg IV × 1, then 50 mg IV daily (Tx > 14 d and 7 d after resolution of Sx); 1.1 mg/min max Inf rate Caution: [B, ?/–] CI: Echinocandin hypersens Disp: Powder 50, 100 mg/vial SE: Histamine-mediated Inf Rxns (urticaria, flushing, ↓ BP, dyspnea, etc), fever, N/V/D, HA, hep, worsening hepatic failure Labs: ↑ LFTs, ↓ K⁺ NIPE: ↓ Inf rate to < 1.1 mg/min w/ Inf Rxns; monitor ECG for hypokalemia (flattened T waves)

Anthralin (Dritho, Zithranol, Zithranol-RR) [Keratolytic Dermatologic Agent] Uses: *Psoriasis* Action: Keratolytic Dose: Apply daily Caution: [C, ?] CI: Acutely inflamed psoriatic eruptions, erythroderma Disp: Cream, 0.5, 1, 1.2%; shampoo SE: Irritation; hair/fingernails/skin discoloration, erythema Interactions: ↑ Tox if used stat after long-term topical corticosteroid therapy NIPE: May stain fabric; external use only; ⊘ sunlight-mechanical areas

Antihemophilic Factor [AHF, Factor VIII) (Monoclate) [Antihemophilic] Uses: *Classic hemophilia A* Action: Provides factor VIII needed to convert prothrombin to thrombin Dose: *Adults & Peds.* 1 AHF unit/kg ↑ factor VIII level by 2 IU/dL; units required = (wgt in kg)(desired factor VIII ↑ as % nl) × (0.5); minor hemorrhage = 20–40% nl; mod hemorrhage/minor surgery = 30–50% nl; major surgery, life-threatening hemorrhage = 80–100% nl Caution: [C, ?] Disp: ✓ each vial for units contained, powder for recons SE: Rash, fever, HA, chills, N/V

Notes: Determine % nl factor VIII before dosing **Interactions:** None **Labs:** Monitor CBC & direct Coombs test **NIPE:** ⊘ ASA; immunize against hep B; D/C if tachycardic

Antihemophilic Factor (Recombinant) (Advate, Helixate FS, Kogenate FS Recombinate, Xyntha) [Clotting Factor] Uses: *Control/ prevent bleeding & surgical prophylaxis in hemophilia A* **Action:** ↑ Levels of factor VIII **Dose:** *Adults.* Required units = body wgt (kg) × desired factor VIII rise (IU/dL or % of nl) × 0.5 (IU/kg per IU/dL); frequency/duration determined by type of bleed (see PI) **Caution:** [C, ?/–] Severe hypersens Rxn possible **CI:** None **Disp:** ✓ Each vial for units contained, powder for recons **SE:** HA, fever, N/V/D, weakness, allergic Rxn **NIPE:** Monitor for the development of factor VIII neutralizing antibodies

Antithrombin, Recombinant (Atryn) [Antithrombin] Uses: *Prevent peri-op/peri-partum thromboembolic events w/ hereditary antithrombin (AT) deficiency* **Action:** Inhibits thrombin and factor Xa **Dose:** *Adults.* Based on pre-Rx AT level, BW (kg) and drug monitoring; see package. Goal AT levels 0.8–1.2 IU/mL **Caution:** [C+, /–] Hypersens Rxns; ↑ effect of heparin/LMWH **CI:** Hypersens to goat/ goat milk proteins **Disp:** Powder 1750 IU/vial **SE:** Bleeding, infusion site Rxn **Interactions:** ↑ Effects *OF* heparin, LMW heparins **Labs:** ✓ aPTT and antifactor Xa **NIPE:** Monitor for bleeding or thrombosis

Antithymocyte Globulin (See Lymphocyte Immune Globulin) [Immunosuppressive Agent]

Apixaban (Eliquis) [Factor Xa Inhibitor] **WARNING:** ↑ Risk of spinal/ epidural hematoma w/ paralysis & ↑ thrombotic events w/ D/C in afib pts; monitor closely Uses: *Prevent CVA/TE in nonvalvular afib* **Acts:** Factor Xa inhib **Dose:** 5 mg bid; 2.5 mg w/2 of the following: > 80 y, wgt < 60 kg, SCr ≥ 1.5; 2.5 mg w/ strong dual inhib of CYP3A4 and P-glycoprotein; if on 2.5 mg do **NOT** use w/ strong dual inhib of CYP3A4 and P-glycoprotein **Caution:** [B, –] Do not use w/ prosthetic valves **CI:** Pathological bleeding & apixaban hypersens **Disp:** Tabs 2.5, 5 mg **SE:** Bleeding **Interactions:** ↑ Effects *W/* dual inhibitors of CYP3A4 (Table 10); ↑ risk of bleeding *W/* ASA, antiplatelets, fibrinolytics, anticoagulants, heparin, thrombolytics, SSRIs, SNRIs, NSAID; ↓ effects *W/* CYP3A4 inducers such as carbamazepine, phenytoin, rifampin, St. John's wort **NIPE:** If missed dose, do **NOT** double next dose; no antidote to reverse; anticoagulant effect can last 24 h after dose

Apomorphine (Apokyn) [Antiparkinsonian/Dopamine Agonist] Uses: *Acute, intermittent hypomobility ("off") episodes of Parkinson Dz* **Action:** Dopamine agonist **Dose:** *Adults.* 0.2 mL SQ supervised test dose; if BP OK, initial 0.2 mL (2 mg) SQ during "off" periods; only 1 dose per "off" period; titrate dose; 0.6 mL (6 mg) max single doses; use w/ antiemetic; ↓ in renal impair **Caution:** [C, ?] Avoid EtOH; antihypertensives, vasodilators, cardio- or cerebrovascular Dz, hepatic impair **CI:** IV administration, 5-HT₃ antagonists, sulfite allergy **Disp:** Inj

10 mg/mL, 3-mL pen cartridges **SE:** Emesis, syncope, ↑ QT, orthostatic ↓ BP, somnolence, ischemia, Inj site Rxn, edema, N/V, hallucination, abuse potential, dyskinesia, fibrotic conditions, priapism, CP/angina, yawning, rhinorrhea **Interactions:** ↑ Risk of hypotension **W/** alosetron, dolasetron, granisetron, ondansetron, palonosetron **Labs:** ECG—monitor for prolongation of QT interval **NIPE:** Daytime somnolence may limit activities; trimethobenzamide 300 mg tid PO orotherron–5-HT₃ antagonist antiemetic given 3 d prior to & up to 2 mo following initiation

Apraclonidine (Iopidine) [Glaucoma Agent/Alpha-Adrenergic Agonist] Uses:* Control post-op intraocular pressure, HTN* **Action:** α_2-Adrenergic agonist **Dose:** 1–2 gtt of 0.5% tid; 1 gtt of 1% before and after surgical procedure **Caution:** [C, ?] **CI:** w/in 14 d of or w/ MAOI **Disp:** 0.5%, 1% soln **SE:** Ocular irritation, lethargy, xerostomia, blurred vision **Interactions:** ↑ HTN crisis **W/** MAOIs; ↑ risk of hypotension **W/** antihypertensives, cardiac glycosides, neuroleptics; ↑ effects **OF** CNS depressants, EtOH; ↓ IOP **W/** pilocarpine or topical BBs **NIPE:** Monitor CV status of pts w/ CAD; potential for dizziness

Apremilast (Otezla) Uses: *Tx psoriatic arthritis * **Action:** PDE4 inhib **Dose:** *Adults.* Titrate to 30 mg 2×/d (day 1: 10 mg AM, day 2: 10 mg AM & PM, day 3: 10 mg AM & 20 mg AM, day 4: 20 mg AM & PM, day 5: 20 mg AM & 30 mg PM, day 6 and after: 30 mg bid); CrCl < 30 mL/min: ↓ to 30 mg daily **W/P:** [C, ?/–] May cause/worsen depression or ↓ wgt (monitor wgt); ↓ effect w/ strong CYP450 enzyme inducers (eg, rifampin, phenobarbital, carbamazepine, phenytoin) **CI:** Apremilast/component hypersens **Disp:** Tabs 10, 20, 30 mg **SE:** N/V/D, HA, wgt loss, URI **NIPE:** Take w/o regard to food; swallow whole; ⊘ crush, break, or chew before swallowing; observe for ↑ depression s/sx

Aprepitant (Emend, Oral) [Centrally Acting Antiemetic] Uses: *Prevents N/V associated w/ emetogenic CA chemotherapy (eg, cisplatin) (use in combo w/ other antiemetics)*, post-op N/V* **Action:** Substance P/neurokinin 1 (NK₁) receptor antagonist **Dose:** 125 mg PO day 1, 1 h before chemotherapy, then 80 mg PO q AM days 2 & 3; post-op N/V: 40 mg PO w/in 3 h of induction **Caution:** [B, ?/–] substrate & mod CYP3A4 inhib; CYP2C9 inducer (Table 10); Effect OCP and warfarin **CI:** Use w/ pimozide or cisapride **Disp:** Caps 40, 80, 125 mg **SE:** Fatigue, asthenia, hiccups **Interactions:** ↑ Effects **W/** clarithromycin, diltiazem, itraconazole, ketoconazole, nefazodone, nelfinavir, ritonavir, troleandomycin; ↑ effects **OF** alprazolam, astemizole, cisapride, dexamethasone, methylprednisolone, midazolam, pimozide, terfenadine, triazolam, & chemotherapeutic agents, eg docetaxel, etoposide, ifosfamide, imatinib, irinotecan, paclitaxel, vinblastine, vincristine, vinorelbine; ↓ effects **W/** paroxetine, rifampin; ↓ effects **OF** OCPs, paroxetine, phenytoin, tolbutamide, warfarin **Labs:** ↑ ALT, AST, BUN, alk phos, leukocytes **NIPE:** Use barrier contraception; take w/o regard to food; see also Fosaprepitant (Emend, Inj)

Arformoterol (Brovana) [Long-Acting Beta-2 Agonist] WARNING: Long-acting β_2-adrenergic agonists may increase the risk of asthma-related death.

Use only for pts not adequately controlled on other asthma-controller meds; safety + efficacy in asthma not established in COPD* **Action:** Selective LA β₂-adrenergic agonist **Dose:** *Adults.* 15 mcg bid nebulization **Caution:** [C, ?] **CI:** Hypersens **Disp:** Soln: 15 mcg/2 mL **SE:** Pain, back pain, CP, D, sinusitis, nervousness, palpitations, allergic Rxn, peripheral edema, rash, leg cramps **Interactions:** ↑ Risk of prolonged QT interval *W/* MAOIs, TCAs; ↑ risk of hypokalemia *W/* steroids; ↓ effects *W/* aminophylline, BBs, K⁺-depleting diuretics, theophylline **Labs:** Monitor K⁺ **NIPE:** Not for acute bronchospasm; refrigerate, use stat after opening

Argatroban (Generic) [Anticoagulant/Thrombin Inhibitor]
Uses: *Prevent/Tx thrombosis in HIT, PCI in pts w/ HIT risk* **Action:** Anticoagulant, direct thrombin inhib **Dose:** 2 mcg/kg/min IV; adjust until a PTT 1.5–3 × baseline not to exceed 100 s; 10 mcg/kg/min max; ↓ w/ hepatic impair **Caution:** [B, ?] Avoid PO anticoagulants, ↑ bleeding risk; avoid use w/ thrombolytics in critically ill pts **CI:** Overt major bleed **Disp:** Inj 100 mg/mL; premixed Inf 50, 125 mg **SE:** AF, cardiac arrest, cerebrovascular disorder, ↓ BP, VT, N/V/D, sepsis, cough, renal tox **Interactions:** ↑ Risk of bleeding *W/* anticoagulants, feverfew, garlic, ginger, ginkgo, ↑ risk of intracranial bleed *W/* thrombolytics **Labs:** ↑ aPTT, PT, INR, ACT, thrombin time; ↓ Hgb; ✓ aPTT w/ Inf start and after each dose change **NIPE:** Report ↑ bruising & bleeding; ⊘ breast feeding; steady state in 1–3 h

Aripiprazole (Abilify, Abilify Discmelt) [Antipsychotic/Psychotropic] **WARNING:** Increased mortality in elderly w/ dementia-related psychosis; ↑ suicidal thinking in children, adolescents, and young adults w/ MDD **Uses:** *Schizophrenia adults & peds 13–17 y, mania or mixed episodes associated w/ bipolar disorder, MDD in adults, agitation w/ schizophrenia* **Action:** Dopamine & serotonin antagonist **Dose:** *Adults. Schizophrenia:* 10–15 mg PO/d *Acute agitation:* 9.75 mg/1.3 mL IM *Bipolar:* 15 mg/d *MDD adjunct* w/ other antidepressants initial 2 mg/d *Peds. Schizophrenia: 13–17 y:* Start 2 mg/d, usual 10 mg/d; max 30 mg/d for all adult and peds uses; ↓ dose w/ CYP3A4/CYP2D6 inhib (Table 10); ↑ dose w/ CYP3A4 inducer **Caution:** [C, −] w/Low WBC, CV Dz **Disp:** Tabs 2, 5, 10, 15, 20, 30 mg; Discmelt (disintegrating tabs 10, 15 mg) soln 1 mg/mL; Inj 7.5 mg/mL **SE:** Neuroleptic malignant synd, tardive dyskinesia, orthostatic ↓ BP, cognitive & motor impair **Interactions:** ↑ Effects *W/* ketoconazole, quinidine, fluoxetine, paroxetine, ↓ effects*W/* carbamazepine **Labs:** ↑ Glucose, monitor CBC, monitor for leukopenia, neutropenia, & agranulocytosis **NIPE:** ⊘ Breast-feed, consume EtOH, or use during PRG; use barrier contraception; ↑ fluid intake; Discmelt contains phenylalanine

Armodafinil (Nuvigil) [Binds Dopamine Receptor] **Uses:** *Narcolepsy, SWSD, and OSAHS* **Action:** ?; binds DA receptor, ↓ DA reuptake **Dose:** *Adults. OSAHS/narcolepsy:* 150 or 250 mg PO daily in AM *SWSD:* 150 mg PO qd 1 h prior to start of shift; ↓ w/ hepatic impair; monitor for interactions w/ substrates

CYP3A4/5, CYP7C19 **Caution:** [C, ?] **CI:** Hypersensitivity to modafinil/armodafinil **Disp:** Tabs 50, 150, 250 mg **SE:** HA, N, dizziness, insomnia, xerostomia, rash including SJS, angioedema, anaphylactoid Rxns, multiorgan hypersensitivity Rxns **Interactions:** *Avoid:* May significantly ↑ effects W/ fosamprenavir, itraconazole, ketoconazole, lopinavir, nelfinavir, ritonavir, telithromycin, tipranavir; ↑ effects W/ chloramphenicol, clarithromycin, conivaptan, erythromycin, fluvoxamine, imatinib, nefazodone, posaconazole, voriconazole; ↑ effects OF carisoprodol, clomipramine, desipramine, diazepam, doxepin, ifosfamide, imipramine, propranolol, phenytoins, pentamidine, tiagabine, warfarin, caffeine; ↑ effects of CV &/or CNS stimulation W/ caffeine, ergotamine, stimulants/anorexiants; ↑ effects of HTN crisis W/ linezolid, MAOIs; ↓ effects W/ barbiturates, carbamazepine, nevirapine, phenytoin, rifampin, rifapentine, warfarin, St. John's wort *Avoid:* May significantly ↓ effects OF atazanavir, clopidogrel, OC, darunavir, dasatinib, delavirdine, dronedarone, erlotinib, everolimus, indinavir, irinotecan, itraconazole, ixabepilone, ketoconazole, lapatinib, lopinavir, nelfinavir, nilotinib, pazopanib, ritonavir, saquinavir, sunitinib, telithromycin, temsirolimus, tipranavir, tolvaptan; ↓ effects OF alfentanil, amiodarone, aprepitant, aripiprazole, bexarotene, bortezomib, bosentan, buprenorphine, buspirone, carbamazepine, CCBs, cinacalcet, cisapride, clozapine, colchicine, conivaptan, corticosteroids, cyclosporine, dapsone, darifenacin, disopyramide, docetaxel, doxorubicins, efavirenz, eplerenone, ethosuximide, fentanyl, gefitinib, maraviroc, meperidine, methadone, nevirapine, quinidine, paclitaxel, pimozide, proguanil, propoxyphene, repaglinide, risperidone, sildenafil, sirolimus, statins, sufentanil, tacrolimus, tandalafil, theophylline, tramadol, trazadone, zaleplon, ziprasidone, zonisamide **Labs:** ↑ GGT, alk phos **NIPE:** Monitor BP, ↑ risk for psychosis, suicidal ideation, mania; may cause dependency; lower doses in elderly

Artemether & Lumefantrine (Coartem) [Antiprotozolal/Antimalarial]
Uses: *Acute, uncomplicated malaria (P falciparum)* **Action:** Antiprotozoal/antimalarial **Dose:** *Adults > 16 y.* 25–< 35 kg: 3 tabs hour 0 & 8 day 1, then 3 tabs bid day 2&3 (18 tabs/course) ≥35 kg: 4 tabs hour 0 & 8 day 1, then 4 tabs bid day 2 & 3 (24 tabs/course) *Peds 2 mo–< 16 y.* 5–<15 kg: 1 tab at hour 0 & 8 day 1, then 1 tab bid day 2 & 3 (6 tabs/course) 15–<25 kg: 2 tabs at hour 0 & 8 day 1, then 2 tabs bid day 2 & 3 (12 tabs/course) 25–<35 kg: 3 tabs at hour 0 & 8 day 1, then 3 tabs bid on day 2 & 3 (18 tabs/course) ≥ 35 kg: See Adult dose **Caution:** [C, ?] ↑ QT, hepatic/renal impair, CYP3A4 inhib/substrate/inducers, CYP2D6 substrates **CI:** Component hypersens **Disp:** Tabs artemether 20 mg/lumefantrine 120 mg **SE:** Palp, HA, dizziness, chills, sleep disturb, fatigue, anorexia, N/V/D, Abd pain, weakness, arthralgia, myalgia, cough, splenomegaly, fever, anemia hepatomegaly **Interactions:** ↑ risk of prolonged QT w/ antifungals, amiodarone, disopyramide, fluroquinolones, macrolides, procainamide, quinidine, sotalol, antiarrhythmics, antipsychotics, antihistamines; ↓ effects OF/ OCP; **Labs:** ↑ AST, ↑ QT **NIPE:** Not recommended w/ other agents that ↑ QT—monitor ECG

Artificial Tears (Tears Naturale) [Ocular Lubricant] [OTC] Uses: *Dry eyes* Action: Ocular lubricant Dose: 1–2 gtt prn Disp: OTC soln SE: Mild stinging, temperature, blurred vision

Asenapine Maleate (Saphris) [Atypical Antipsychotic (Dibenzo-Oxepino Pyrrole)] WARNING: ↑ Mortality in elderly w/ dementia-related psychosis Uses: *Schizophrenia; manic/mixed bipolar disorder* Action: DA/serotonin antagonist Dose: *Adults. Schizophrenia:* 5 mg bid; max 20 mg/d *Bipolar disorder:* 5–10 mg bid Caution: [C, ?/–] Disp: SL tabs 5, 10 mg SE: Dizziness, insomnia, edema, ↑/↓ BP, somnolence, akathisia, oral hypoesthesia, EPS, ↑ wgt, ↑ QT interval, hyperprolactinemia, neuroleptic malignant syndrome, severe allergic Rxns Interactions: Avoid drugs that ↑ QT interval (eg, Class Ia or Class III antiarrhythmics, ziprasidone, chlorpromazine, thioridazine, moxifloxacin, alcohol), ↑ effects *OF* antihypertensives; ↓ effects *W/* fluvoxamine Labs: ↑ Glucose, ↑ TG, ↓ WBC NIPE: Do not swallow/crush/chew tab; avoid eating/drinking 10 min after dose

L-Asparaginase (Elspar) [Antineoplastic/Protein Synthesis Inhibitor] Uses: *ALL* (in combo w/ other agents) Action: Protein synth inhib Dose: Unit/m^2/dose based on protocol Caution: [C, ?] CI: Active/ Hx pancreatitis; Hx of allergic Rxn, thrombosis or hemorrhagic event w/prior Rx w/ asparaginase Disp: Powder (Inj) 10,000 units/vial SE: Allergy 15–35% (urticarial to anaphylaxis): fever, chills, N/V, anorexia, coma, azotemia, Abd cramps, depression, agitation, Sz, pancreatitis, coagulopathy Interactions: ↑ Effects *W/* prednisone, vincristine; ↓ effects *OF* MTX, sulfonylureas, insulin Labs: ✓ Glucose, coagulation studies, LFTs; ↓ T$_4$- & T$_3$-binding globulin, serum albumin, total cholesterol, plasma fibrinogen; ↑ BUN, glucose, uric acid, LFTs, alk phos NIPE: ⊘ Fluid intake; monitor for bleeding; monitor I&O & wgt; ⊘ EtOH or ASA; test dose OK

Aspirin (Bayer, Ecotrin, St. Joseph's) [Antipyretic, Analgesic/Salicylate] [OTC] Uses: *CABG, PTCA, carotid endarterectomy, ischemic stroke, TIA, ACS/MI, arthritis, pain, HA, fever, inflammation*, Kawasaki Dz Action: Prostaglandin inhib by COX-2 inhib Dose: *Adults. Pain, fever:* 325–650 mg q4–6h PO or PR (4 g/d max) *Plt Inhib:* 81–325 mg PO daily; *Prevent MI:* 81 (preferred)–325 mg PO daily *ECC 2010:* ACS: 160–325 mg non-enteric coated PO ASAP (chewing preferred at ACS onset) *Peds. Antipyretic:* 10–15 mg/kg/dose PO or PR q4–6h; *Kawasaki Dz:* 80–100 mg/kg/d ÷ q6h, then 3–5 mg/kg/d after fever resolves for at least 48 h or total 14 d; for all uses < 10 mg/kg/d max; avoid w/ CrCl < 10 mL/min, severe liver Dz Caution: [C, M] Linked to Reye synd; avoid w/viral illness in peds < 16 y CI: Allergy to ASA, chickenpox/flu Sxs, synd of nasal polyps, angioedema, & bronchospasm to NSAIDs, bleeding disorders Disp: Tabs 325, 500 mg; chewtabs 81 mg; EC tabs 81, 162, 325, 500 mg; effervescent tabs 500 mg; sup 300, 600 mg; caplet 81, 375, 500 mg SE: GI upset, erosion, & bleeding Notes: Salicylate levels: *Therapeutic:* 100–250 mcg/mL *Toxic:* > 300 mcg/mL Interactions: ↑ Effects *W/* anticoagulants, ammonium chloride, antibiotics, ascorbic acid, furosemide, methionine, nizatidine, NSAIDs, verapamil, EtOH, feverfew, garlic, ginkgo, horse chestnut, kelpware (black-tang), prickly ash, red clover; ↓ effects **W/** antacids, activated charcoal, corticosteroids, griseofulvin, NaHCO₃, ginseng, food; ↑ effects **OF** ACEI, hypoglycemics, insulin, Li, MTX, phenytoin, sulfonamides, valproic acid; ↓ effects **OF** BBs, probenecid, spironolactone, sulfinpyrazone **Labs:** False(−) of urinary glucose & urinary ketone tests, serum albumin, total serum phenytoin, T₃, & T₄ **NIPE:** D/C 1 wk prior to surgery; avoid/ limit EtOH; chronic ASA use may result in ↓ folic acid, Fe-deficiency anemia, & hypernatremia; ⊘ foods ↑ salicylate (eg, curry powder, paprika, licorice, prunes, raisins, tea; take ASA w/ food or milk); report S/Sxs bleeding/GI pain/ringing in ears

Aspirin, Butalbital, & Caffeine Compound (Fiorinal) [C-III] [Analgesic & Barbiturate] Uses: *Tension HA*, pain **Action:** Barbiturate w/ analgesic **Dose:** 1–2 PO q4h PRN, max 6 tabs/d; dose in renal/hepatic Dz **Caution:** [C (D w/ prolonged use or high doses at term)] **CI:** ASA allergy, GI ulceration, bleeding disorder, porphyria, synd of nasal polyps, angioedema, & bronchospasm to NSAIDs **Disp:** Caps/tabs ASA 325 mg/butalbital 50 mg/caffeine 40 mg **SE:** Drowsiness, dizziness, GI upset, ulceration, bleeding, lightheadedness, heartburn, confusion, HA **Interactions:** ↑ Effect **OF** benzodiazepines, CNS depressants, chloramphenicol, methylphenidate, propoxyphene, valproic acid; ↓ effects **OF** BBs, corticosteroids, chloramphenicol, cyclosporines, doxycycline, griseofulvin, haloperidol, OCPs, phenothiazines, quinidine, TCAs, theophylline, warfarin **NIPE:** Butalbital habit-forming; D/C 1 wk prior to surgery; use barrier contraception, avoid or limit EtOH

Aspirin + Butalbital, Caffeine, & Codeine (Fiorinal + Codeine) [C-III] [Analgesic & Barbiturate & Narcotic] Uses: *Complex tension HA* **Action:** Sedative and narcotic analgesic **Dose:** 1–2 tabs/ caps PO q4h PRN max 6/d **Caution:** [C, −] CI: Allergy to ASA and codeine; synd of nasal polyps, angioedema, & bronchospasm to NSAIDs, bleeding diathesis, peptic ulcer or sig GI lesions, porphyria **Disp:** Caps contain 325 mg ASA, 40 mg caffeine, 50 mg butalbital, 30 mg codeine **SE:** Drowsiness, dizziness, GI upset, ulceration, bleeding **Interactions:** ↑ Effects **W/** narcotic analgesics, MAOIs, neuromuscular blockers; ↑ effects **W/** tobacco smoking; ↑ effects **OF** digitoxin, phenytoin, rifampin; ↓ resp & CNS depression **W/** cimetidine **Labs:** ↑ Plasma amylase & lipase **NIPE:** D/C 1 wk prior to surgery, avoid/ limit EtOH; may cause constipation, ↑ fluids & fiber; take w/ milk to ↓ GI distress

Atazanavir (Reyataz) [Antiretroviral/HIV-1 Protease Inhibitor] Uses: *HIV-1 Infxn* **Action:** Protease inhib **Dose:** Antiretroviral naïve 300 mg PO daily w/ ritonavir 100 mg or 400 mg PO daily; experienced pts 300 mg w/ ritonavir 100 mg; when given w/ efavirenz 600 mg, administer atazanavir 400 mg + ritonavir 100 mg once/d; separate doses from didanosine; ↓ w/ hepatic impair **Caution:** [B,−]; ↑ Levels of statins sildenafil, antiarrhythmics, warfarin, cyclosporine, TCAs; ↓ w/ St. John's wort, PPIs, H₂-receptor antagonists; do not use w/ salmeterol, colchicine (w/ renal/hepatic failure); adjust dose w/ bosentan, tadalafil for PAH **CI:** w/ Midazolam, triazolam, ergots, pimozide, simvastatin, lovastatin, cisapride, etravirine, indinavir, rifampin, alpha 1-adrenoreceptor antagonist (alfuzosin), PDE5 inhibitor sildenafil **Disp:** Caps 100, 150, 200, 300 mg **SE:** HA, N/V/D, rash, Abd pain, DM, photosens, ↑ PR interval **Interactions:** May have less adverse effect on cholesterol; if given w/ H₂-blocker, administer with food and separate by 10 h; if given w/ PPI, separate by 12 h; concurrent use not recommended inexperienced pts; ↑ effects W/ amprenavir, clarithromycin, indinavir, lamivudine, lopinavir, ritonavir, saquinavir, stavudine, tenofovir, zalcitabine, zidovudine; ↑ effects OF amiodarone, atorvastatin, CCBs, clarithromycin, cyclosporine, diltiazem, irinotecan, lidocaine, lovastatin, OCPs, rifabutin, quinidine, saquinavir, sildenafil, simvastatin, sirolimus, tacrolimus, TCAs, warfarin; ↓ effects W/ antacids, antimycobacterials, efavirenz, esomeprazole, H₂-receptor antagonists, lansoprazole, omeprazole, rifampin, St. John's wort **Labs:** ↑ ALT, AST, total bilirubin, amylase, lipase, serum glucose, ↓ Hgb, neutrophils **NIPE:** CDC rec HIV-infected mothers not to breast-feed; take w/ food; will not cure HIV or ↓ risk of transmission; use barrier contraception; ↑ risk of skin and/or scleral yellowing; administer with food

Atenolol (Tenormin) [Antihypertensive, Antianginal/Beta-Blocker]

WARNING: Avoid abrupt withdrawl (esp CAD pts), gradual taper to ↓ acute ↑ HR, HTN, +/- ischemia **Uses:** *HTN, angina, post-MI* **Action:** Selective β-adrenergic receptor blocker **Dose:** *HTN & angina:* 25–100 mg/d PO *ECC 2010:* AMI: 5 mg IV over 5 min; in 10 min, 5 mg slow IV; if tolerated in 10 min, start 50 mg PO, titrate; ↓ in renal impair **Caution:** [D, M] DM, bronchospasm; abrupt D/C can exacerbate angina & ↑ MI risk **CI:** ↓ HR, cardiogenic shock, cardiac failure, 2nd-/3rd-degree AV block, sinus node dysfunction, pulm edema **Disp:** Tabs 25, 50, 100 mg **SE:** ↓ HR, ↓ BP, 2nd-/3rd-degree AV block, dizziness, fatigue **Interactions:** ↑ Effects W/ other antihypertensives esp diltiazem & verapamil, nitrates, EtOH; ↑ bradycardia W/ adenosine, digitalis glycosides, dipyridamole, physostigmine, tacrine; ↓ effects W/ ampicillin, antacids, NSAIDs, salicylates; ↑ effects OF lidocaine; ↓ effects OF DA, glucagons, insulin, sulfonylureas **Labs:** ↑ ANA titers, BUN, glucose, serum lipoprotein, K⁺, triglyceride, uric acid levels; ↓ HDL **NIPE:** May mask S/Sxs hypoglycemia; may ↑ sensitivity to cold; may ↑ depression, wheezing, orthostatic hypotension

Atenolol & Chlorthalidone (Tenoretic [Antihypertensive, Antianginal/Beta-Blocker & Diuretic]

Uses: *HTN* **Action:** β-Adrenergic blockade w/ diuretic **Dose:** 50–100 mg/d PO based on atenolol; ↓ dose w/ CrCl < 35 mL/min **Caution:** [D, ?/–] DM, bronchospasm **CI:** See atenolol; anuria, sulfonamide cross-sensitivity **Disp:** Atenolol 50 mg/chlorthalidone 25 mg; atenolol 100 mg/chlorthalidone 25 mg **SE:** ↓ HR, ↓ BP, 2nd-/3rd-degree AV block, dizziness, fatigue; photosens **Interactions:** ↑ Effects W/ other antihypertensives; ↓ effects W/ cholestyramine, NSAIDs; ↑ effects OF Li, digoxin, ↓ effects of sulfonylureas **Labs:** ↑ CPK, serum ammonia, amylase, Ca²⁺, cholesterol, glucose;

↓ serum Cl⁻, Mg²⁺, K⁺, Na⁻ **NIPE:** Take in AM to prevent nocturia, use sunblock > SPF 15, photosensitivity, monitor S/Sxs gout

Atomoxetine (Strattera) [ADHD/Selective Norepinephrine Reuptake Inhibitor] WARNING: ↑ Frequency of suicidal thinking; monitor closely especially in peds pts. **Uses:** *ADHD* **Action:** Selective norepinephrinere uptake inhib **Dose:** *Adults & children > 70 kg.* 40 mg PO/d, after 3 d minimum, ↑ to 80–100 mg ÷ daily–bid *Peds < 70 kg.* 0.5 mg/kg ×3 d, then ↑ 1.2 mg/kg daily or bid (max 1.4 mg/kg or 100 mg); ↓ dose w/ hepatic Insuff or in combo w/ CYP2D6 inhib (Table 10) **Caution:** [C, ?/–] Known structural cardiac anomalies, cardiac Hx hepatotoxicity **CI:** NAG, w/ or w/in 2 wk of D/C an MAOI **Disp:** Caps 10, 18, 25, 40, 60, 80, 100 mg **SE:** HA, insomnia, dry mouth, Abd pain, N/V, anorexia, ↑ BP, tachycardia, wgt loss, somnolence, sexual dysfunction, jaundice **Labs:** ↑ LFTs **NIPE:** AHA rec: all children receiving stimulants for ADHD receive CV assessment before therapy initiated; D/C immediately w/ jaundice

Atorvastatin (Lipitor) [Antilipemic/HMG-CoA Reductase Inhibitor] Uses: Dyslipidemia, primary prevention CVD Dz **Action:** HMG-CoA reductase inhib **Dose:** Initial 10–20 mg/d, may ↑ to 80 mg/d **Caution:** [X, –] **CI:** Active liver Dz **Disp:** Tabs 10, 20, 40, 80 mg **SE:** Myopathy, HA, arthralgia, myalgia, GI upset, CP, edema, insomnia, dizziness, liver failure **Interactions:** ↑ Effects *W/* azole antifungals, erythromycin, nefazodone, protease Inhibs, grapefruit juice; ↓ effects *W/* antacids, bile acid sequestrants; ↑ effects *OF* digoxin, levothyroxine, OCPs **Labs:** Monitor LFTs; ↑ LFTs, CPK; ↓ lipid levels **NIPE:** Instruct pt to report unusual muscle pain or weakness; ⊘ EtOH, breast-feeding, or while PRG

Atovaquone (Mepron) [Antiprotozoal] Uses: *Rx & prevention PCP & *Toxoplasma gondii* encephalitis, babesiosis (w/ azithromycin) **Action:** ↓ Nucleic acid & ATP synth **Dose:** *Rx:* 750 mg PO bid for 21 d *Prevention:* 1500 mg PO once/d (w/ meals) **Caution:** [C, ?] **Disp:** Susp 750 mg/5 mL **SE:** Fever, HA, anxiety, insomnia, rash, N/V, cough, pruritis, weakness **Interactions:** ↓ Effects *W/* metoclopramide, rifabutin, rifampin, tetracycline **Labs:** Monitor LFTs w/ long-term use **NIPE:** ↑ Absorption w/ meal esp high-fat meal

Atovaquone/Proguanil (Malarone) [Antimalarial] Uses: *Prevention or Rx *P falciparum* malaria* **Action:** Antimalarial **Dose:** *Adults: Prevention:* 1 tab PO 1–2 d before, during, & 7 d after leaving endemic region; *Rx:* 4 tabs PO single dose daily ×3 d *Peds.* See PI **Caution:** [C, ?] **CI:** Prophylactic use when CrCl < 30 mL/ min **Disp:** Tabs atovaquone 250 mg/proguanil 100 mg; peds 62.5 mg/25 mg **SE:** HA, fever, myalgia, Abd pain, dizziness, weakness, N/V **Interactions:** ↓ Effects *W/* metoclopramide, rifabutin, rifampin, tetracycline **Labs:** ↑ LFTs, monitor LFTs w/ long-term use **NIPE:** ↑ Absorption w/ meal esp high-fat meal

Atracurium (Tracrium) [Skeletal Muscle Relaxant/Neuromuscular Blocker] Uses: *Anesthesia adjunct to facilitate ET intubation, facilitate ventilation in ICU pts* **Action:** Nondepolarizing neuromuscular blocker **Dose:** *Adults*

& Peds > 2 y. 0.4–0.5 mg/kg IV bolus, then 0.08–0.1 mg/kg q20–45min PRN; ICU: 0.4–0.5 mg/kg/min titrated **Caution:** [C, ?] **Disp:** Inj 10 mg/mL **SE:** Flushing **Interactions:** ↑ Effects *W/* general anesthetics, aminoglycosides, bacitracin, BBs, β-agonists, clindamycin, CCBs, diuretics, lidocaine, Li, MgSO₄, narcotic analgesics, procainamide, quinidine, succinylcholine, trimethaphan, verapamil; ↓ effects *W/* Ca, carbamazepine, phenytoin, theophylline, caffeine **Labs:** Monitor BUN, Cr, LFTs **NIPE:** Drug does not affect consciousness or pain; inability to speak until drug wears off; pt must be intubated & on controlled ventilation; use adequate amounts of sedation & analgesia

Atropine, Ophthalmic (Isopto Atropine, Generic) [Antiarrhythmic/Anticholinergic] **Uses:** *Mydriasis, cycloplegia, uveitis* **Action:** Antimuscarinic; cycloplegic, dilates pupils **Dose:** *Adults. Refr Action:* 1–2 gtt 1 h before *Uveitis:* 1–2 gtt daily–qid **CI:** NAG, adhesions between iris and lens **Disp:** 1% ophthal soln, 1% oint **SE:** Local irritation, burning, blurred vision, light sensitivity **Interactions:** ↑ Effects *W/* amantadine, antihistamines, disopyramide, procainamide, quinidine, TCA, thiazides, betel palm, squaw vine; ↓ effects *W/* antacids, levodopa; ↓ effects *OF* phenothiazines **NIPE:** Compress lacrimal sac 2–3 min after instillation; effects can last 1–2 wk; ↑ risk of photophobia

Atropine, Systemic (AtroPen Auto-Injector) [Antiarrhythmic/Anticholinergic] **Uses:** *Preanesthetic; symptomatic ↓ HR & asystole, AV block, organophosphate (insecticide) and acetylcholinesterase (nerve gas) inhib antidote; cycloplegic* **Action:** Antimuscarinic; blocks acetylcholine at parasympathetic sites, cycloplegic **Dose:** *Adults. ECC 2010:* **Asystole or PEA:** Routine use for asystole or PEA no longer recommended. *Bradycardia:* 0.5 mg IV q3–5 min as needed; max 3 mg or 0.04 mg/kg; *Preanesthetic:* 0.4–0.6 mg IM/IV *Poisoning:* 1–2 mg IV bolus, repeat q3–5min PRN to reverse effects *Peds. ECC 2010:* **Symptomatic bradycardia:** 0.02 mg/kg IV/IO (min dose 0.1 mg, max single dose 0.5 mg); repeat PRN × 1; max total dose 1 mg or 0.04 mg/kg child, 3 mg adolescent **Caution:** B/[C, +] **CI:** NAG, adhesions between iris and lens, pyloric stenosis, prostatic hypertrophy **Disp:** Inj 0.05, 0.1, 0.4, 1 mg/mL; *AtroPen Auto-Injector:* 0.25, 0.5, 1, 2 mg/dose **SE:** Flushing, mydriasis, tachycardia, dry mouth & nose, blurred vision, urinary retention, constipation, psychosis **Notes:** SLUDGE (Salivation, Lacrimation, Urination, Diaphoresis, Gastrointestinal motility, Emesis) are Sx of organophosphate poisoning; Auto-Injector limited distribution; see also Atropine Opthalmic **Interactions:** ↑ Effects *W/* amantadine, antihistamines, disopyramide, procainamide, quinidine, TCA, thiazides, betel palm, squaw vine; ↓ effects *W/* antacids, levodopa; ↓ effects *OF* phenothiazines **Labs:** ↓ Gastric motility & emptying may affect results of upper GI series **NIPE:** Monitor I&O, ↑ fluids & oral hygiene, wear dark glasses to ↓ photophobia

Atropine/Pralidoxime (DuoDote) [Antiarrhythmic/Anticholinergic/Antidote] **WARNING:** For use by personnel w/ appropriate training; wear protective garments; do not rely solely on medication, evacuation & decontamination

ASAP Uses: *Nerve agent (tabun, sarin, others) or organophosphate insecticide poisoning* Action: Atropine blocks effects of excess acetylcholine; pralidoxime reactivates acetylcholinesterase inactivated by poisoning Dose: 1 Inj in midlateral thigh; wait 10–15 min for effect; w/ severe Sx give 2 additional Inj; if alert/oriented no more doses Caution: [C, ?] Disp: Auto-injector 2.1 mg atropine/600 mg pralidoxime SE: Dry mouth, blurred vision, dry eyes, photophobia, confusion, HA, tachycardia, ↑ BP, flushing, urinary retention, constipation, Abd pain, N, V, emesis Interactions: ↑ Effects W/ amantadine, antihistamines, disopyramide, procainamide, quinidine, TCA, thiazides, betel palm, squaw vine; ↑ effects OF barbiturates; ↓ effects W/ antacids, levodopa; ↓ effects OF phenothiazines Labs: ↑ ALT, AST, Cr NIPE: Severe Sx of poisoning: confusion, dyspnea w/ copious secretions, weakness, twitching, involuntary urination & defecation, convulsions, unconsciousness; limited distribution. For use by personnel w/ appropriate training; wear protective garments; do not rely solely on medication; evacuation and decontamination ASAP.

Avanafil (Stendra) [Phosphodiesterase Type 5 Inhibitor] Uses:
ED Acts: ↓ Phosphodiesterase type 5 (PDE5) (responsible for cGMP breakdown); ↑ cGMP activity to relax smooth muscles to ↑ flow to corpus cavernosum Dose: (men only) 100 mg PO 30 min before sex activity, no more than 1/d; ↑/↓ dose 50–200 mg based on effect; do not use w/ strong CYP3A4 inhib; use 50 mg w/ mod CYP3A4 inhib; w/ or w/o food Caution: [C, ?] Priapism risk; hypotension w/ BP meds or substantial alcohol; seek immediate attention w/ hearing loss or acute vision loss (may be NIAON); w/ CYP3A4 inhib (eg, ketoconazole, ritonavir, erythromycin) ↑ effects; do not use w/ severe renal/hepatic impair CI: w/ Nitrates or if sex not advised Disp: Tabs 50, 100, 200 mg SE: HA, flushing, nasal congestion, nasopharyngitis, back pain Interactions: ↑ risk of hypotension W/ alpha-blockers, antihypertensives, nitrates, EtOH NIPE: More rapid onset than sildenafil (15–30 min)

Axitinib (Inlyta) [Kinase Inhibitor] Uses: *Advanced RCC* Acts: TKI
inhibitor Dose: Adults. 5 mg PO q12h; if tolerated > 2 wks, ↑ to 7 mg q12h, then 10 mg q12h; w or w/o food; swallow whole; ↓ dose by ½ w/ moderate hepatic impair; avoid w/or ↓ dose by ½ if used w/ strong CYP3A4/5 inhib Caution: [D, ?] w/ brain mets, recent GI bleed Disp: Tabs 1, 5 mg SE: N/V/D/C, HTN, fatigue, asthenia, ↓ appetite, ↓ wgt, hand-foot synd, venous/arterial thrombosis; hemorrhage, GI perf/fistula, proteinuria, hypertensive crisis, impaired wound healing, reversible posterior leukoencephalopathy synd Labs: ↑ LFTs, ↓ thyroid levels; monitor thyroid function, LFTs, proteinuria NIPE: Hold 24 h prior to surgery; use adequate contraception during therapy

Azathioprine (Imuran, Azasan) [Immunosuppressant/ Purine
Antagonist] WARNING: May ↑ neoplasia w/ chronic use; mutagenic and hematologic tox possible Uses: *Adjunct to prevent renal transplant rejection, RA*, SLE, Crohn Dz, UC Action: Immunosuppressive; antagonizes purine metabolism Dose: Adults: Crohn and UC: Start 50 mg/d, ↑ 25 mg/d q1–2wk, target dose

2–3 mg/kg/d *Adults & Peds. Renal transplant:* 3–5 mg/kg/d IV/PO single daily dose, then 1–3 mg/kg/d, maint; RA 1 mg/kg/d once daily or ÷ div × 6–8 wk, ↑ 0.5 mg/kg/d q4wk to 2.5 mg/kg/d; ↓ w/ renal Insuff **Caution:** [D, ?/–] **CI:** PRG **Disp:** Tabs, 50, 75, 100 mg; powder for Inj 100 mg **SE:** GI intolerance, fever, chills, leukopenia, ↑ risk Infxns, thrombocytopenia **Interactions:** ↑ Effects *W/* allopurinol; ↓ effects *OF* antineoplastic drugs, cyclosporine, myelosuppressive drugs, MTX; ↑ risk of severe leucopenia *W/* ACEI; ↓ effects *OF* nondepolarizing neuromuscular blocking drugs, warfarin **Labs:** ↑ LFTs, bilirubin; monitor CBC, LFTs during therapy **NIPE:** Handle Inj w/ cytotoxic precautions; do not administer live vaccines on drug; dose per local transplant protocol, usually start 1–3 d pretransplant; ⊘ PRG, breast-feeding; ↑ risk of infection.

Azelastine (Astelin, Astepro, Optivar) [Antihistamine/H₁-Receptor Antagonist]

Uses: *Allergic rhinitis (rhinorrhea, sneezing, nasal pruritus); vasomotor rhinitis; allergic conjunctivitis* **Action:** Histamine H₁-receptor antagonist **Dose:** *Adults & Peds > 12 y.* Nasal: 1–2 sprays/nostril bid Ophthal: 1 gtt in each affected eye bid *Peds 5–11 y.* 1 spray/nostril 1× d **Caution:** [C, ?/–] **CI:** Component sensitivity **Disp:** Nasal 137 mcg/spray; ophthal soln 0.05% **SE:** Somnolence, bitter taste, HA, cold Sx (rhinitis, cough) **Interactions:** ↑ Effects *W/* cimetidine; ↑ effects *OF* EtOH, CNS depressants **Labs:** ↑ AST, ↓ skin Rxns to antigen skin tests **NIPE:** Systemically absorbed; clear nares before administration; prime pump before use

Azilsartan (Edarbi) [Angiotensin II Receptor Blocker]

WARNING: Use in 2nd/3rd trimester can cause fetal injury and death; D/C when PRG detected **Uses:** *HTN* **Action:** ARB **Dose:** *Adults.* 80 mg PO 1 × d; consider 40 mg PO 1 × dif on high dose diuretic **Caution:** [D, ?] Correct vol/salt depletion before **Disp:** Tabs 40 mg, 80 mg **SE:** D, ↓ BP, N, asthenia, fatigue, dizziness, cough **Interactions:** ↑ Risk of renal toxicity *W/* NSAIDs, COX-2 inhibitors **Labs:** Monitor SCr esp in elderly and volume depleted pts **NIPE:** If pt salt/volume depleted, correct before starting drug; may be used alone or in combination with other antihypertensives

Azilsartan & Chlorthalidone (Edarbyclor) [ARB & Diuretic]

WARNING: Use in 2nd/3rd trimester can cause fetal injury and death; D/C when PRG detected *Uses:* *HTN* **Acts:** ARB w/ thiazide diuretic **Dose:** *Adults.* 40/12.5 mg–40/25 mg PO 1 × d **Caution:** [D, ?/–] Correct vol/salt depletion prior to use **CI:** Anuria **Disp:** Tabs (azilsartan/chlorthalidone) 40/12.5, 40/25 mg **SE:** N/D, ↓ BP, asthenia, fatigue, dizziness, cough, hyperuricemia, photosens **Interactions:** ↑ Risk of hypotension & hyperkalemia *W/* ACEIs, ARBs; ↑ risk of renal impairment *W/* NSAIDs; ↑ effects *OF* Li **Labs:** ↑ Glucose, ↓ K+

Azithromycin (Zithromax) [Antibiotic/Macrolide]

Uses: *Community-acquired pneumonia, pharyngitis, otitis media, skin Infxns, nongonococcal (chlamydial) urethritis, chancroid & PID; Rx & prevention of MAC in HIV* **Action:** Macrolide antibiotic; bacteriostatic; ↓ protein synth *Spectrum:*

Chlamydia, H ducreyi, H influenzae, Legionella, M catarrhalis, M pneumoniae, M hominis, N gonorrhoeae, S aureus, S agalactiae, S pneumoniae, S pyogenes **Dose: Adults.** *Resp tract Infxns: PO:* Caps 500 mg/d 1, then 250 mg/d PO × 4 d; *Sinusitis* 500 mg/d PO × 3 d; *IV:* 500 mg × 2 d, then 500 mg PO × 7–10 d *Nongonococcal urethritis:* 1 g PO × 1 *Gonorrhea, uncomplicated:* 2 g PO × 1 *Prevent MAC:* 1200 mg PO once/wk *Otitis media:* 10 mg/kg PO day 1, then 5 mg/kg/d days 2–5 *Pharyngitis* (≥ 2 y): 12 mg/kg/d PO × 5 d; take susp on empty stomach; tabs OK w/ or w/o food; ↓ w/ CrCl < 10 mL/min **Caution:** [B, +] May ↑ QTc w/ arrhythmias **Disp:** Tabs 250, 500, 600 mg; Z-Pack (5-d, 250 mg); Tri-Pak (500-mg tabs × 3); susp 2 g; single-dose packet (ZMAX) ER susp (2 g) susp 100, 200 mg/5 mL; Inj powder 500 mg; 2.5 mL **SE:** GI upset, metallic taste **Interactions:** ↓ Effects *W/* Al- & Mg-containing antacids, atovaquone, food (suspension); ↑ effects *OF* alfentanil, barbiturates, bromocriptine, carbamazepine, cyclosporine, digoxin, disopyramide, ergot alkaloids, phenytoin, pimozide, terfenadine, theophylline, triazolam, warfarin; ↓ effects *OF* penicillins **Labs:** May ↑ serum bilirubin, alkphos, BUN, Cr, CPK, glucose, K⁺, LFTs, LDH, PT; may ↓ WBC, plt count, serum folate **NIPE:** Monitor S/Sxs super Infxns; use sunscreen & protective clothing

Azithromycin Ophthalmic 1% (AzaSite) [Antibiotic/Macrolide]
Uses: *Bacterial conjunctivitis* **Dose: Adults & Peds > 1 year.** 1 gtt bid, q8–12h × 2 d, then 1 gtt q day × 5d. **Caution:** [↑B, ?] **CI:** None **Disp:** 1% in 2.5 mL bottle **SE:** Irritation, burning, stinging, contact dermatitis, corneal erosion, dry eye, dysgeusia, nasal congestion, sinusitis, ocular discharge, keratitis **NIPE:** Avoid contact w/ use

Aztreonam (Azactam) [Antibiotic/Monobactam]
Uses: *Aerobic gram(−) UTIs, lower resp, intra-Abd, skin, gynecologic Infxns & septicemia* **Action:** Monobactam, ↓ cell wall synth. *Spectrum:* Gram(−) (*Pseudomonas, E coli, Klebsiella, H influenzae, Serratia, Proteus, Enterobacter, Citrobacter*) **Dose: Adults.** 1–2 g IV/IM q6–12h *UTI:* 500 mg–1 g IV q8–12h *Meningitis:* 2 g IV q6–8h *Peds.* 90–120 mg/kg/d ÷ q6–8h; ↓ in renal impair **Caution:** [B, +] **Disp:** Inj (soln), 1 g, 2g/50 mL Inj powder for recons 1 g, 2 g **SE:** N/V/D, rash, pain at Inj site **Interactions:** ↑ Effects *W/* probenecid, aminoglycosides, β-lactam antibiotics; ↓ effects *W/* cefoxitin, chloramphenicol, imipenem **Labs:** ↑ LFTs, alk phos, SCr, PT, PTT, & (+) direct Coombs test **NIPE:** No gram(+) or anaerobic activity; OK in PCN-allergic pts; monitor S/Sxs super Infxn; taste changes w/ IV administration

Aztreonam, Inhaled (Cayston) [Monobactam]
Uses: *Improve respiratory Sx in CF pts w/ P aeruginosa* **Action:** Monobactam: ↓ cell wall synth **Dose: Adults & Peds ≥ 7 y.** One dose × 28 d (space doses q4h) **Caution:** [B, +] w/ β-lactam allergy **CI:** Allergy to aztreonam **Disp:** Lyophilized **SE:** Allergic Rxn, bronchospasm, cough, nasal congestion, wheezing, pharyngolaryngeal pain, V, Abd pain, chest discomfort, pyrexia, rash **NIPE:** Use immediately after reconstitution, use only w/Altera Nebulizer System; bronchodilator prior to use

Bacitracin & Polymyxin B, Ophthalmic (AK-Poly-Bac Ophthalmic, Polysporin Ophthalmic); Bacitracin, Neomycin, & Polymyxin B, Ophthalmic (Neo-Polycin, Neosporin Ophthalmic); Bacitracin, Neomycin, Polymyxin B, & Hydrocortisone, Ophthalmic (Neo-Polycin HC, Cortisporin Ophthalmic) [Antibiotic/ Anti-Inflammatory] Uses: *Steroid-responsive inflammatory ocular conditions* **Action:** Topical antibiotic w/ anti-inflammatory **Dose:** Apply q3–4h into conjunctival sac **Caution:** [C, ?] **CI:** Viral, mycobacterial, fungal eye Infxn **Disp:** See Bacitracin, topical equivalents, next listing **Interactions:** ↑ Effects W/ neuromuscular blocking agents, anesthetics, nephrotoxic drugs **NIPE:** May cause blurred vision

Bacitracin, Topical (Baciguent); Bacitracin & Polymyxin B, Topical (Polysporin); Bacitracin, Neomycin, & Polymyxin B, Topical (Neosporin); Bacitracin, Neomycin, Polymyxin B, & Hydrocortisone, Topical (Cortisporin); [Antibiotic/Anti-Inflammatory/Analgesic] Uses: Prevent/Rx of *minor skin Infxns* **Action:** Topical antibiotic w/ added components (anti-inflammatory & analgesic) **Dose:** Apply sparingly bid–qid **Caution:** [C, ?] Not for deep wounds, puncture, or animal bites **Disp:** Bacitracin 500 units/g oint & powder; bacitracin 500 units/polymyxin B sulfate 10,000 units/g oint & powder; bacitracin 400 units/neomycin 3.5 mg/polymyxin B 5000 units/g oint; bacitracin 400 units/neomycin 3.5 mg/polymyxin B 5000 units/hydrocortisone 10 mg/g oint; bacitracin 500 units/neomycin 3.5 mg/polymyxin B 5000 units/lidocaine 40 mg/g oint **NIPE:** Ophthal, systemic, & irrigation forms available, not generally used d/t potential tox

Baclofen (Lioresal Intrathecal, Gablofen) [Antispasmodic/ Skeletal Muscle Relaxant] **WARNING:** Abrupt discontinuation, especially of IT use, can lead to organ failure, rhabdomyolysis, and death **Uses:** *Spasticity d/t severe chronic disorders (eg, MS, amyotrophic lateral sclerosis, or spinal cord lesions)*, trigeminal neuralgia, intractable hiccups **Action:** Centrally acting skeletal muscle relaxant; ↓ transmission of monosynaptic & polysynaptic cord reflexes **Dose:** *Adults.* Initial, 5 mg PO tid; ↑ q3d to effect; max 80 mg/d. *IT:* Via implantable pump (see PI) *Peds 2–7 y.* 20–30 mg ÷ q8h (max 60 mg); *> 8 y.* max 120 mg/d; *IT:* Via implantable pump (see PI); ↓ in renal impair; take w/ food or milk **Caution:** [C, +] Epilepsy, neuropsychological disturbances **Disp:** Tabs 10, 20 mg; IT Inj 50, 500, 1000, 2000 mcg/mL **SE:** Dizziness, drowsiness, insomnia, rash, fatigue, ataxia, weakness, ↓ BP **Interactions:** ↑ CNS depression W/ CNS depressants, MAOIs, EtOH, antihistamines, opioid analgesics, sedatives, hypnotics; ↑ effects *OF* antihypertensives, clindamycin, guanabenz; ↑ risk of resp paralysis & renal failure W/ aminoglycosides **Labs:** ↑ Serum glucose, AST, ammonia, alk phos **NIPE:** Take oral meds w/ food to ↓ GI distress; ⊘ EtOH

Balsalazide (Colazal) [Anti-Inflammatory/GI Drug] Uses: *Ulcerative colitis* Action: 5-ASA derivative, anti-inflammatory Dose: 2.25 g (3 caps) tid × 8–12 wk Caution: [B, ?/–] Severe renal failure CI: Mesalamine or salicylate hypersens Disp: Caps 750 mg SE: Dizziness, HA, N, Abd pain, agranulocytosis, renal impair, allergic Rxns Notes: Daily dose of 6.75 g = 2.4 g mesalamine Interactions: Oral antibiotics may interfere W/ mesalamine release in the colon Labs: ↑ Bilirubin, CPK, LFTs, LDH NIPE: ✓ If ASA allergy; take w/ food & swallow caps whole; ulcerative colitis exacerbation upon initiation of Rx.

Basiliximab (Simulect) [Immunosuppressant/Monoclonal Antibody] WARNING: Use only under the supervision of a physician experienced in immunosuppression therapy in an appropriate facility Uses: *Prevent acute transplant rejection* Action: IL-2 receptor antagonists Dose: *Adults & Peds > 35 kg.* 20 mg IV 2 h before transplant, then 20 mg IV 4 d post transplant. *Peds < 35 kg.* 10 mg 2 h prior to transplant; same dose IV 4 d post transplant Caution: [B, ?/–] CI: Hypersensitivity to murine proteins Disp: Inj powder 10, 20 mg SE: Edema, ↑ BP, HTN, HA, dizziness, fever, pain, Infxn, GI effects, electrolyte disturbances Notes: A murine/human MoAb Interactions: May ↑ immunosuppression W/ other immunosuppressive drugs; use W/ echinacea & melatonin may interfere with immunosuppression Labs: ↑ Cholesterol, BUN, Cr, lipids, uric acid; ↓ serum Mg phosphate, plts, Hgb, Hct, Ca²⁺, ↑ or ↓ glucose, K⁺ NIPE: Monitor for Infxns—hypersensitivity Rxns—can occur up to 24 h following administration, IV dose over 20–30 min

BCG [Bacillus Calmette-Guérin] (TheraCys, Tice BCG) [Antineoplastic, Antituberculotic] WARNING: Contains live, attenuated mycobacteria; transmission risk; handle as biohazard; nosocomial & disseminated Infxns reported in immunosuppressed Uses: *Bladder CA (superficial)*, TB prophylaxis Action: Attenuated live BCG culture, immunomodulator Dose: *Bladder CA:* 1 vial prepared & instilled in bladder for 2 h; repeat once/wk × 6 wk; then 1 Tx at 3, 6, 12, 18, & 24 mo after Caution: [C, ?] Asthma w/ TB immunization CI: Immunosuppresion, PRG, steroid use, febrile illness, UTI, gross hematuria, w/ traumatic catheterization Disp: Powder 81 mg (TheraCys), 50 mg (Tice BCG) SE: *Intravesical:* Hematuria, urinary frequency, dysuria, bacterial UTI, rare BCG sepsis, malaise, fever, chills, pain, N/V, anorexia, anemia Interactions: ↓ Effects W/ antimicrobials, immunosuppressives, radiation Labs: Prior BCG may cause false(+) PPD NIPE: PPD is not contraindicated in BCG vaccinated persons; monitor for S/Sxs systemic Infxn, report persistent pain on urination or blood in urine; routine US adult BCG immunization not recommended. Use for children who are PPD(–) & continually exposed to untreated/ineffectively treated adults or whose TB strain is INH/rifampin resistant. Used for healthcare workers in high-risk environments; intravesical use, dispose/void in toilet w/ chlorine bleach

Becaplermin (Regranex Gel) [Growth Factor] **WARNING:** ↑ Mortality d/t malignancy reported; use w/ caution in known malignancy **Uses:** Local wound care adjunct w/ *diabetic foot ulcers* **Action:** Recombinant PDGF, enhances granulation tissue **Dose:** *Adults.* Based on lesion: calculate the length of gel, measure the greatest length of ulcer by the greatest width; tube size and measured result determine the formula used in the calculation. Recalculate q1–2wk based on change in lesion size *15-g tube:* (length × width) × 0.6 = length of gel (in inches) or for *2-g tube:* (length × width) × 1.3 = length of gel (in inches) *Peds.* See package insert **Caution:** [C, ?] **CI:** Neoplasmatic site **Disp:** 0.01% gel in 2-, 15-g tubes **SE:** Rash **Interactions:** None known **NIPE:** Dosage recalculated q1–2wk; use w/ good wound care; wound must be vascularized; reassess after 10 wk if ulcer not ↓ by 30% or not healed by 20 wk

Beclomethasone (QVAR) [Antiasthmatic/Synthetic Corticosteroid] **Uses:** Chronic *asthma* **Action:** Inhaled corticosteroid **Dose:** *Adults & Peds 5–11 y.* 40–160 mcg 1–4 Inh bid; initial 40–80 mcg Inh bid if on bronchodilators alone; 40–160 mcg bid w/ other inhaled steroids; 320 mcg bid max; taper to lowest effective dose bid; rinse mouth/throat after **Caution:** [C, ?] **CI:** Acute asthma **Disp:** PO metered-dose inhaler; 40, 80 mcg/Inh **SE:** HA, cough, hoarseness, oral candidiasis **Interactions:** None noted **NIPE:** Use inhaled bronchodilator prior to inhaled steroid, rinse mouth after inhaled steroid; not effective for acute asthma; effect in 1–2 d or as long as 2 wk

Beclomethasone Nasal (Beconase AQ) [Anti-Inflammatory/Corticosteroid] **Uses:** *Allergic rhinitis, nasal polyps* **Action:** Inhaled steroid **Dose:** *Adults & Peds. Aqueous inhaler:* 1–2 sprays/nostril bid **Caution:** [C, ?] **Disp:** Nasal metered-dose inhaler 42 mcg/spray **SE:** Local irritation, burning, epistaxis **Interactions:** None noted **NIPE:** Prior use of decongestant nasal gtt if edema or secretions, may take several days for full steroid effect

Bedaquiline Fumarate (Sirturo) [Diarylquinoline/Antimycobacterial] **WARNING:** ↑ QT can occur and may be additive w/ other QT-prolonging drugs; ↑ risk of death vs placebo, only use when an effective TB regimen cannot be provided **Uses:** *Tx of MDR TB* **Acts:** Diarylquinoline antimycobacterial **Dose:** 400 mg/d 2/wk, then 200 mg 3/wk for 22 wk **Caution:** [B, –] ↑ QT, ECG freq; D/C if ventricular arrhythmias or QTc > 500 ms; hepatic Rxn **CI:** w/ Drugs that ↑ QTc **Disp:** Tabs 100 mg **SE:** HA, N, arthralgias, hemoptysis, CP; **Interactions:** ↑ risk of QT prolongation W/ fluoroquinolones, macrolides, clofazimine; ↑ effects *W/* strong Inhib of CYP3A4 such as: ketoconazole, amiodarone, norfloxacin, verapamil, grapefruit (Table 10); avoid w/in < 14 d use of CYP3A4 Inhib; ↓ effects *W/* strong CYP3A4 inducers such as: carbamazepine, glucocorticoids, phenytoin, phenobarbital, rifampin, St John's wort (Table 10) **Labs:** Frequent ECG for QT prolongation; LFTs, D/C w/ AST/ALT > 8 × ULN, T bili > 2 × ULN or LFT elevations persist > 2 wk; D/C w/ renal failure **NIPE:** ✓ ECG if pt c/o dizziness; swallow drug whole w/ H_2O; take w/ food to ↓ GI distress

Belatacept (Nulojix) [Selective T-Cell Costimulation Blocker]
WARNING: May ↑ risk of posttransplant lymphoproliferative disorder (PTLD) mostly CNS; ↑ risk of Infxn; for use by physicians experienced in immunosuppressive therapy; ↑ risk of malignancies; not for liver transplant **Uses:** *Prevent rejection in EBVpositive kidney transplant recipients* **Action:** T-cell costimulation blocker **Dose:** *Day 1* (transplant day, pre-op) & *Day 5* 10 mg/kg; end of wk 2, wk 4, wk 8, wk 12 after transplant 10 mg/kg; *Maint:* End of wk 16 after transplant 4 wk 5 mg/kg **Caution:** [C, –] w/ CYP3A4 Inhib/inducers, other anticoagulants or plt Inhib **CI:** EBV seronegative or unknown EBV status **Disp:** 250 mg Inj **SE:** Anemia, N/V/D, UTI edema, constipation, ↑ BP, pyrexia, graft dysfunction, cough, HA; **Interactions:** ⊘ W/ Live-virus vaccines **Labs:** ↑/↓ K⁺, ↓ WBC **NIPE:** REMS; use in combo w/ basiliximab, mycophenolatemofetil (MMF), & steroids; PML with excess belatacept dosing

Belimumab (Benlysta) **Uses:** *SLE* **Acts:** B-lymphocyte Inhib **Dose:** *Adults.* 10 mg/kg IV q2wk × 3 doses, then q4wk; Inf over 1 h; premed against Inf & hypersensitivity Rxns **Caution:** [C, ?/–] h/o active or chronic Infxns; possible ↑ mortality **CI:** Live vaccines, hypersens **Disp:** Inj powder 120, 400 mg/vial **SE:** N/D, bronchitis, nasopharyngitis, pharyngitis, insomnia, extremity pain, pyrexia, depression, migraine, serious/fatal hypersensitivity, anaphylaxis **Interactions:** ⊘ Use W/ live-virus vaccines; ⊘ use W/ other biological drugs **Labs:** ↓ Leukocyte count **NIPE:** Not for severe active lupus nephritis or CNS lupus or w/ other biologics or IV cyclophosphamide

Belladonna & Opium Suppositories (Generic) [C-II] [Antispasmodic, Analgesic] **Uses:** *Mod–severe pain associated w/ bladder spasms* **Action:** Antispasmodic, analgesic **Dose:** 1 supp PR 1–2/d (up to 4 doses/d) **Caution:** [C, ?] **CI:** Glaucoma, resp depression, severe renal or hepatic Dz, convulsive disorder, acute alcoholism **Disp:** 30 mg opium/16.2 mg belladonna extract; 60 mg opium/16.2 mg belladonna extract **SE:** Anticholinergic (eg, sedation, urinary retention, constipation) **Interactions:** ↑ Effects W/ CNS depressants, TCAs; ↓ effects W/ phenothiazine **Labs:** ↑ LFTs **NIPE:** ⊘ Refrigerate; moisten finger & supp before insertion; may cause blurred vision

Benazepril (Lotensin) [Antihypertensive/ACEI] **WARNING:** PRG avoid use **Uses:** *HTN* **Action:** ACE Inhib **Dose:** 10–80 mg/d PO **Caution:** [D, –] **CI:** Angioedema **Disp:** Tabs 5, 10, 20, 40 mg **SE:** Symptomatic ↓ BP w/ diuretics; dizziness, HA, nonproductive cough **Interactions:** ↑ Effects W/ α-blockers, diuretics, capsaicin; ↓ effects W/ NSAIDs, ASA; ↑ effects OF insulin, Li; ↑ risk of hyperkalemia W/ TMP & K⁺-sparing diuretics **Labs:** ↑ BUN, SCr, K⁺; ↓ Hgb; monitor ECG for signs of hyperkalemia (peaked T waves) **NIPE:** Persistent cough and/or taste changes may develop; ⊘ PRG, D/C if angioedema

Bendamustine (Treanda) [Alkylating Agent] **Uses:** *CLL, B-cell NHL* **Action:** Mechlorethamine derivative; alkylating agent **Dose:** *Adults.* 100

mg/m^2 IV over 30 min on days 1 & 2 of 28-d cycle, up to 6 cycles (w/tox see package insert for dose changes); NHL: 120 mg/m^2 IV over 30 min d 1 & 2 of 21-d tx cycle up to 8 cycles; do not use w/ CrCl < 40 mL/min, severe hepatic impair) **Caution:** [D, ?/–] Do not use w/ CrCl < 40 mL/min, severe hepatic impair **CI:** Hypersensitivity to bendamustine or mannitol **Disp:** Inj powder 25 mg, 100 mg **SE:** Pyrexia, N/V, dry mouth, fatigue, cough, stomatitis, rash, myelosuppression, Infxns, Inf Rxns & anaphylaxis, tumor lysis synd, skin Rxns, extravasation **Interactions:** ↑ Effects **W/** CYP1A2 Inhibs (Table 10); ↓ effects **W/** CYP1A2 inducers **Labs:** ↑ LFTs **NIPE:** Consider use of allopurinol to prevent tumor lysis synd; ⊘ PRG or breast-feeding

Benzocaine (Americaine, Hurricaine, Lanacane, Various) [OTC Topical Anesthetic]   Uses: *Topical anesthetic, lubricant on ET tubes, catheters, etc; pain relief in external otitis, cerumen removal, skin conditions, sunburn, insect bites, mouth and gum irritation, hemorrhoids* **Action:** Topical local anesthetic **Dose:** *Adults & Peds > 1 y. Anesthetic lubricant:* Apply evenly to tube/instrument; other uses per manufacturer instructions **Caution:** [C, –] Do not use on broken skin; see provider if condition does not respond; avoid in infants and those w/ pulmonary Dzs **Disp:** Many site-specific OTC forms creams, gels, liquids, sprays, 2–20% **SE:** Itching, irritation, burning, edema, erythema, pruritus, rash, stinging, tenderness, urticaria; methemoglobinemia (infants or in COPD) **NIPE:** Use minimum amount to obtain effect; methemoglobinemia S/Sxs: HA, lightheadedness, SOB, anxiety, fatigue, pale, gray or blue-colored skin, & tachycardia; S/Sxs may appear w/ in minutes to 1–2 h after use of benzocaine; treat w/ IV methylene blue

Benzocaine & Antipyrine (Auralgan) [Otic Anesthetic]   Uses: *Analgesia in severe otitis media* **Action:** Anesthetic w/local decongestant **Dose:** Fill ear & insert a moist cotton plug; repeat 1–2 h PRN **Caution:** [C, ?] **CI:** w/ Perforated eardrum **Disp:** Soln 5.4% antipyrine, 1.4% benzocaine **SE:** Local irritation, methemoglobimemia, ear discharge **Interactions:** May ↓ effects **OF** sulfonamides

Benzonatate (Tessalon, Zonatuss) [Antitussive]   Uses: Symptomatic relief of *nonproductive cough* **Action:** Anesthetizes the stretch receptors in the resp passages **Dose:** *Adults & Peds > 10y.* 100 mg PO tid (max 600 mg/d) **Caution:** [C, ?] **Disp:** Caps 100, 150, 200 mg **SE:** Sedation, dizziness, GI upset **Interactions:** ↑ CNS depression **W/** antihistamines, EtOH, hypnotics, opioids, sedatives **NIPE:** ↑ Fluid intake to liquefy secretions; do not chew or puncture the caps; deaths reported in peds < 10 y w/ ingestion

Benztropine   (Cogentin)   [Antiparkinsonian/Anticholinergic]   Uses: *Parkinsonism & drug-induced extrapyramidal disorders* **Action:** Anticholinergic & antihistaminic effects **Dose:** *Adults. Parkinsonism:* initial 0.5–1 mg PO/IM/IV qhs, ↑ q5–6d PRN by 0.5 mg, usual dose 1–2 mg, 6 mg/d max *Extrapyramidal:* 1–4 mg PO/IV/IM qd–bid *Peds > 3 y.* 0.02–0.05 mg/kg/dose 1–2/d **Caution:** [C, ?] w/ urinary Sxs, NAG, hot environments, CNS or mental disorders, other phenothiazines or TCA **CI:** < 3 y, pyloric/duodenal obstruction, myasthenia gravis; **Disp:** Tabs 0.5, 1, 2 mg; Inj 1 mg/mL **SE:** Anticholinergic (tachycardia, ileus, N/V, etc), anhidrosis, heat stroke **Interactions:** ↑ Sedation & depressant effects *W/* EtOH & CNS depressants; ↑ anticholinergic effects *W/* antihistamine phenothiazine, quinidine, disopyramide, TCAs, MAOIs; ↑ effect *OF* digoxin; ↓ effect *OF* levodopa; ↓ effects *W/* antacids & antidiarrheal drugs **NIPE:** May ↑ susceptibility to heat stroke, take w/ meals to avoid GI upset

Benzyl Alcohol (Ulesfia) [Pediculicide] Uses: *Head lice* Action: Pediculicide **Dose:** Apply volume for hair length to dry hair; saturate the scalp; leave on 10 min; rinse w/ water; repeat in 7 d *Hair length 0–2 in:* 4–6 oz *2–4 in:* 6–8 oz *4–8 in:* 8–12 oz *8–16 in:* 12–24 oz *16–22 in:* 24–32 oz *> 22 in:* 32–48 oz **Caution:** [B, ?] Avoid eyes **Contra:** None **Disp:** 5% lotion 4, 8 oz bottles **SE:** Pruritus, erythema, irritation (local, eyes) **NIPE:** Use fine-tooth/nit comb to remove nits & dead lice; avoid contact w/ eyes; wash hands after application; does not have ovicidal activity

Bepotastine Besilate (Bepreve) [Antihistamine/Mast Cell Stabilizer] Uses: *Allergic conjunctivitis* Action: H_1-receptor antagonist **Dose:** *Adults.* 1 gtt into affected eye(s) bid **Caution:** [C, ?/–] **Disp:** Soln 1.5% **SE:** Mild taste, eye irritation, HA, nasopharyngitis **NIPE:** Do not use while wearing contacts, reinsert 10 min > dosing if eye not red

Beractant (Survanta) [Lung Surfactant] Uses: *Prevention & Rx RDS in premature infants* Action: Replaces pulm surfactant **Dose:** 100 mg/kg via ET tube; repeat q6h PRN; max 4 doses **Disp:** Susp 25 mg of phospholipid/mL **SE:** Transient ↓ HR, desaturation, apnea **Interactions:** None noted **NIPE:** ↑ Risk of nosocomial sepsis after Rx w/ this drug

Besifloxacin (Besivance) [Antibiotic/Quinolone] Uses: *Bacterial conjunctivitis* Action: Inhibits DNA gyrase & topoisomerase IV **Dose:** *Adults & Peds > 1 y.* 1 gtt into eye(s) tid 4–12 h apart × 7 d **Caution:** [C, ?] Remove contacts during Tx **Contra:** None **Disp:** 0.6% susp **SE:** HA, redness, blurred vision, irritation **NIPE:** ⊘ Wear contact lenses during Tx or if symptomatic

Betaxolol (Kerlone) [Antihypertensive/Beta-Blocker] Uses: *HTN* **Action:** Competitively blocks β-adrenergic receptors, $β_1$ **Caution:** [C ?/–] **CI:** Sinus ↓ HR, AV conduction abnormalities, uncompensated cardiac failure **Dose:** 5–20 mg/d **Disp:** Tabs 10, 20 mg **SE:** Dizziness, HA, ↓ HR, edema, CHF, fatigue, lethargy **Interactions:** ↑ Effects *W/* anticholinergics, verapamil, general anesthetics; ↓ effects *W/* thyroid drugs, amphetamine, cocaine, ephedrine, epinephrine, norepinephrine, phenylephrine, pseudoephedrine, NSAIDs; ↑ effects *OF* insulin, digitalis glycosides; ↓ effects *OF* theophylline, DA, glucagon **Labs:** ↑ BUN, serum lipoprotein, glucose, K^+, triglyceride, uric acid, ANA titers **NIPE:** May ↑ sensitivity to cold, ⊘ D/C abruptly

Betaxolol, Ophthalmic (Betoptic) [Beta-Blocker] Uses: Open-angle glaucoma **Action:** Competitively blocks β-adrenergic receptors **Dose:** 1–2 gtt bid

Caution: [C, ?/–] **Disp:** Soln 0.5%; susp 0.25% **SE:** Local irritation photophobia
Additional NIPE: Use sunglasses to ↓ exposure; may cause photophobia, review instillation procedures

Bethanechol (Urecholine) [Urinary Tract Stimulant/Cholinergic Agonist] **Uses:** *Acute post-op/postpartum nonobstructive urinary retention; neurogenic bladder w/ retention* **Action:** Stimulates cholinergic smooth muscle in bladder & GI tract **Dose:** *Adults.* Initial 5–10 mg PO, then repeat qh until response or 50 mg, typical 10–50 mg tid–qid, 200 mg/d max tid–qid; 2.5–5 mg SQ tid–qid & PRN *Peds.* 0.3–0.6 mg/kg/24 h PO ÷ tid–qid; take on empty stomach **Caution:** [C, –] **CI:** BOO, PUD, epilepsy, hyperthyroidism, ↓ HR, COPD, AV conduction defects, Parkinsonism, ↓ BP, vasomotor instability **Disp:** Tabs 5, 10, 25, 50 mg **SE:** Abd cramps, D, salivation, ↓ BP **Interactions:** ↑ Effects *W/* BBs, tacrine, cholinesterase Inhibs; ↓ effects *W/* atropine, anticholinergic drugs, procainamide, quinidine, epinephrine **Labs:** ↑ In serum AST, ALT, amylase, lipase, bilirubin **NIPE:** Do not use IM/IV; may cause blurred vision; monitor I&O; take on an empty stomach

Bevacizumab (Avastin) [Antineoplastic/Monoclonal Antibody] **WARNING:** Associated w/GI perforation, wound dehiscence, & fatal hemoptysis **Uses:** *Met colorectal CA w/ 5-FU, NSCLC w/ paclitaxel and carboplatin; glioblastoma; metastatic RCC w/ IFN-α* **Action:** Vascular endothelial GF inhibitor **Dose:** *Adults. Colon:* 5 mg/kg or 10 mg/kg IV q14d *NSCLC:* 15 mg/kg q21d; 1st dose over 90 min; 2nd over 60 min, 3rd over 30 min if tolerated; *RCC:* 10 mg/kg IV q2wk w/ IFN-α **Caution:** [C, –] Do not use w/in 28 d of surgery if time for separation of drug & anticipated surgical procedures is unknown; D/C w/ serious adverse effects **CI:** None **Disp:** 100 mg/4 mL, 400 mg/16 mL vials **SE:** Wound dehiscence, GI perforation, tracheoesophageal fistula, arterial thrombosis, hemoptysis, hemorrhage, HTN, proteinuria, CHF, Inf Rxns, D, leukopenia **Labs:** Monitor for ↑ proteinuria **NIPE:** Monitor for ↑ BP q2–3wk during Tx

Bicalutamide (Casodex) [Antineoplastic/Nonsteroidal Antiandrogen] **Uses:** *Advanced PCa w/ GnRH agonists (eg, leuprolide, goserelin)* **Action:** Nonsteroidal antiandrogen **Dose:** 50 mg/d **Caution:** [X, ?] **CI:** Women **Disp:** Caps 50 mg **SE:** Hot flashes, ↓ loss of libido, impotence, edema, pain, D/N/V, gynecomastia **Interactions:** ↑ Effects *OF* anticoagulants, TCAs, phenothiazines; ↓ effects *OF* antipsychotic drugs **Labs:** ↑ LFTs **NIPE:** Monitor PSA, may experience hair loss

Bicarbonate (See Sodium Bicarbonate)

Bisacodyl (Dulcolax) [OTC] [Stimulant Laxative] **Uses:** *Constipation; pre-op bowel prep* **Action:** Stimulates peristalsis **Dose:** *Adults.* 5–15 mg PO or 10 mg PR PRN *Peds < 2 y.* 5 mg PR PRN *> 2 y.* 5 mg PO or 10 mg PR PRN (do not chew tabs or give w/in 1 h of antacids or milk) **Caution:** [C, ?] **CI:** Abd pain or obstruction; N/V **Disp:** EC tabs 55, 10 mg supp 10 mg, enema soln 10 mg/30 mL **SE:** Abd cramps, proctitis, & inflammation w/ suppositories **Interactions:**

Antacids & milk ↑ dissolution of EC causing Abd irritation **Labs:** ↑ Phosphate, Na; ↓ Ca, Mg, K⁺ **NIPE:** ↑ Fluid intake & high-fiber foods, ⊘ take w/ milk or antacids

Bismuth Subcitrate/Metronidazole/Tetracycline (Pylera) [Antibacterial/Antiprotozoal] **Uses:** *H pylori* Infxn w/ omeprazole* **Action:** Eradicates *H pylori*, see agents **Dose:** 3 caps qid w/ omeprazole 20 mg bid for × 10 d **Caution:** [D, –] **CI:** PRG, peds < 8 y (tetracycline during tooth development causes teeth discoloration), w/ renal/hepatic impair, component hypersensitivity **Disp:** Caps w/ 140 mg bismuth subcitrate potassium, 125 mg metronidazole, & 125 mg tetracycline hydrochloride **SE:** Stool abnormality, N, anorexia, D, dyspepsia, Abd pain, HA, flu-like synd, taste perversion, vaginitis, dizziness **Interactions:** See multiple drug interactions for each component **Labs:** ↓ Neutrophils, WBC **NIPE:** EtOH use may cause disulfiram-like Rxn; possible occurrence of metallic taste & reddish-brown urine; take w/ food; see SE for each component; [metronidazole carcinogenic in animals.]

Bismuth Subsalicylate (Pepto-Bismol) [Antidiarrheal/Adsorbent] [OTC] **Uses:** Indigestion, N, & *D*; combo for Rx of *H pylori* Infxn* **Action:** Antisecretory & anti-inflammatory **Dose:** **Adults.** 2 tabs or 30 mL PO PRN (max 8 doses/ 24 h) **Peds** (For all max 8 doses/24 h) *3–6 y.* 1/3 tabs or 5 mL PO PRN *6–9 y.* 2/3 tabs or 10 mL PO PRN *9–12 y.* 1 tab or 15 mL PO PRN **Caution:** [C, D (3rd tri), –] Avoid w/renal failure; Hx severe GI bleed, influenza or chickenpox (↑ risk of Reye synd) **CI:** h/o Severe GI bleeding or coagulopathy, ASA allergy **Disp:** Chew tabs; caplets 262 mg; Liq 262, 525 mg/15 mL; susp 262 mg/15 mL **SE:** May turn tongue & stools black **Interactions:** ↑ Effects *OF* ASA, MTX, valproic acid; ↓ effects *OF* tetracyclines; ↑ effects *W/* corticosteroids, probenecid **Labs:** ↑ Lipid levels; may interfere w/ GI tract x-rays **NIPE:** Chew tabs, ⊘ swallow whole; may darken tongue & stool to black

Bisoprolol (Zebeta) [Antihypertensive/Beta-Blocker] **Uses:** *HTN* **Action:** Competitively blocks β₁-adrenergic receptors **Dose:** 2.5–10 mg/d (max dose 20 mg/d); ↓ w/ renal impair **Caution:** [C ?/ –] **CI:** Sinus bradycardia, AV conduction abnormalities, uncompensated cardiac failure **Disp:** Tabs 5, 10 mg **SE:** Fatigue, lethargy, HA, ↓ HR, edema, CHF **Notes:** Not dialyzed **Interactions:** ↑ Bradycardia *W/* adenosine, amiodarone, digoxin, dipyridamole, neostigmine, physostigmine, tacrine; ↑ effects *W/* cimetidine, fluoxetine, prazosin; ↓ effects *W/* NSAIDs, rifampin; ↓ effects *OF* theophylline, glucagon **Labs:** ↑Alk phos, BUN, cholesterol, glucose, K⁺, triglycerides, uric acid **NIPE:** ⊘ D/C abruptly, may mask S/Sxs hypoglycemia, take w/o regard to food

Bivalirudin (Angiomax) [Anticoagulant/Direct Thrombin Inhibitor] 0020aa **Uses:** *Anticoagulant w/ ASA in unstable angina undergoing PTCA, PCI, or in pts undergoing PCI w/or at risk of HIT/HITTS* **Action:** Anticoagulant, thrombin Inhib **Dose:** 0.75 mg/kg IV bolus, then 1.75 mg/kg/h for duration of procedure and up to 4 h post procedure; ✓ ACT 5 min after bolus, may repeat 0.3 mg/ kg bolus if necessary (give w/ aspirin ASA 300–325 mg/d; start pre-PTCA)

Caution: [B, ?] **CI:** Major bleeding **Disp:** Powder 250 mg for Inj **SE:** ↓ BP, bleeding, back pain, N, HA **Interactions:** ↑ Risk of bleeding *W/* heparin, warfarin, oral anticoagulants **Labs:** ↑ PT, PTT **NIPE:** Monitor venipuncture site for bleeding; instruct pt to watch for bleeding, bruising, or tarry stool

Bleomycin Sulfate (Generic) [Antineoplastic/Antibiotic]
WARNING: Idiopathic Rxn (↓ BP, fever, chills, wheezing) in lymphoma pts; pulm fibrosis; should be administered by chemo experienced provider **Uses:** *Testis CA; Hodgkin Dz & NHLs; cutaneous lymphomas; & squamous cell CA (head & neck, larynx, cervix, skin, penis); malignant pleural effusion sclerosing agent* **Action:** Induces DNA breakage (scission) **Dose:** (per protocols): **Caution:** [D, ?] **CI:** w/ Hypersens, idiosyncratic Rxn **Disp:** Powder (Inj) 15, 30 units **SE:** Hyperpigmentation & allergy (rash to anaphylaxis); fever in 50%; lung tox (idiosyncratic & dose related); pneumonitis w/ fibrosis; Raynaud phenomenon, N/V **Notes:** Test dose 1 unit, esp in lymphoma pts; lung tox w/ total dose > 400 units or single dose > 30 units; avoid high Fio_2 in general anesthesia to ↓ tox **Interactions:** ↑ Effects *W/* cisplatin & other antineoplastic drugs; ↓ effects *OF* digoxin & phenytoin **Labs:** ↑ Uric acid, WBC; monitor BUN, Cr, pulm Fxn tests **NIPE:** Eval lungs for adventitious sounds; transient hair loss; ⊘ immunizations, breast-feeding; use contraception method

Boceprevir (Victrelis) [HCVNS3/4A Protease Inhibitor/Hep C Antiviral] **Uses:** *Chronic hep C genotype 1, w/ compensated liver Dz, including naïve to Tx or failed Tx w/ peginterferon & ribavirin* **Action:** Hep C antiviral **Dose:** *Adults.* After 4 wk of peginterferon & ribavirin, then 800 mg tid w/ food for 44 wks w/ peginterferon & ribavirin; must be used w/ peginterferon and ribavirin **Caution:** [B, X w/ peginterferon and ribavirin, –] (X because must be used w/ peginterferon and ribavirin, class B by itself) **CI:** All CIs to peginterferon and ribavirin; men if PRG female partner; drugs highly dependent on CYP3A4/5 including alfuzosin, sildenafil, tadalafil, lovastatin, simvastatin, ergotamines, cisapride, triazolam, midazolam, rifampin, St. John's wort, phenytoin, carbamazepine, phenobarbital, drosperinone **Disp:** caps 200 mg **SE:** Anemia, ↓ WBCs, neutrophils, fatigue, insomnia, HA, anorexia, N/V/D, dysgeusia, alopecia **Interactions:** ↑ Effects *OF* CYP3A4/5 substrates (eg, including alfuzosin, sildenafil, tadalafil, lovastatin, simvastatin, ergotamines, cisapride, triazolam, midazolam, rifampin, St. John's wort, phenytoin, carbamazepine, phenobarbital, drosperinone) ↓ effect *OF* ethinylestradiol; strong Inhib CYP3A4/5 ↓ effects *W/* CYP3A4/5 Inhibs **Labs:** ↓ Hct/ WBC/neutrophils—monitor **NIPE:** Not a monotherapy; PRG test before; take w/ food; ✓ HCV-RNA levels wks 4, 8, 12, 24, end of Tx; ✓ WBC w/ diff at wks 4, 8, 12

Bortezomib (Velcade) [Antineoplastic/Proteosome Inhibitor]
Uses: *Rx multiple myeloma or mantel cell lymphoma w/ one failed previous Rx* **Action:** Proteasome Inhib **Dose:** Per protocol or PI; ↓ dose w/ hematologic tox, neuropathy **Caution:** [D, ?/–] w/ Drugs CYP450 metabolized (Table 10) **Disp:** 3.5 mg

vial Inj powder **SE:** Asthenia, GI upset, anorexia, dyspnea, HA, orthostatic ↓ BP, edema, insomnia, dizziness, rash, pyrexia, arthralgia, neuropathy **Interactions:** ↑ Risk of peripheral neuropathy *W/* amiodarone, antivirals, INH, nitrofurantoin, statins; ↑ risk hypotension *W/* antihypertensives; ↑ effects *W/* cimetidine, clarithromycin, diltiazem, disulfiram, erythromycin, fluoxetine, propoxyphene, verapamil, zafirlukast; ↓ effects *W/* amiodarone, carbamazepine, phenobarbital, phenytoin, rifampin **Labs:** ↓ Hgb, Hct, neutrophils, plts **NIPE:** ⊘ PRG or breast-feeding; use contraception; caution w/ driving d/t fatigue/dizziness; ↑ fluids if c/o N/V; may worsen neuropathy

Bosutinib Monohydrate (Bosulif) [Tyrosine Kinase Inhibitor]

Uses: *Ph₊ CML intolerant/resistant to prior Tx* **Acts:** TKI **Dose:** 500 mg/d, ↑ dose to 600 mg/d by wk 8 w/ incomplete reponse, or by wk 12 w/ cytogenetic incomplete response and no grade 3/greater adverse Rxn; w/ hepatic impair 200 mg/d **Caution:** [D, –] GI toxicity; ↓ BM, fluid retention; hold/ ↓ dose or D/C w/ toxicity **CI:** Hypersens **Disp:** Tabs 100, 500 mg **SE:** N, V, D, Abd pain, fever, rash, fatigue, anemia **Interactions:** ↑ Effects *W/* concomitant use of strong or moderate CYP3A and/or P-gp inhibitors (eg, ritonavir, indinavir, nelfinavir, saquinavir, ketoconazole, boceprevir, telaprevir, itraconazole, voriconazole, posaconazole, clarithromycin, telithromycin, nefazodone, conivaptan, fluconazole, darunavir, erythromycin, diltiazem, atazanavir, aprepitant, amprenavir, fosamprenavir, crizotinib, imatinib, verapamil, grapefruit products, ciprofloxacin); ↑ effects OF/ digoxin; ↓ effects *W/* concomitant use of strong or moderate CYP3A inducers (eg, rifampin, phenytoin, carbamazepine, St. John's wort, rifabutin, phenobarbital, bosentan, nafcillin, efavirenz, modafinil ethavirine); ↓ effects *W/* proton pump inhibitors **Labs:** ↓ Plts; ✓ CBC/ LFTs q mo **NIPE:** Avoid w/ mod/strong CYP3A Inhib & inducers; avoid use of PPIs—use short-acting antacids or H2 blockers & separate dosing by 2 h or more

Botulinum Toxin Type A [AbobotulinumtoxinA] (Dysport) [Neuromuscular Blocker/Neurotoxin]

WARNING: Effects may spread beyond Tx area leading to swallowing and breathing difficulties (may be fatal); Sxs may occur hours to weeks after Inj **Uses:** *Cervical dystonia (adults), glabellar lines (cosmetic)* **Action:** Neurotoxin, ↓ ACH release from nerve endings, ↓ neuromuscular transmission **Dose:** *Cervical dystonia:* 500 units IM ÷ units into muscles; re-treat no less than 12–16 wk PRN dose range 250–100 units based on response. *Glabellar lines:* 50 units ÷ in 10 units/Inj into muscles, do not administer at intervals < q3mo, repeat no less than q3mo **Caution:** [C, ?] Sedentary pt to resume activity slowly after Inj; aminoglycosides and nondepolarizing muscle blockers may ↑ effects; do not exceed dosing **CI:** Hypersens to components (cow milk), Infxn at Inj site **Disp:** 300, 500 units, 60 Inj **SE:** Anaphylaxis, erythema multiforme, dysphagia, dyspnea, syncope, HA, NAG **Interactions:** ↑ Effects *W/* aminoglycosides, other botulinum toxin products **NIPE:** Botulinum toxin products not interchangeable; Inj site pain

Botulinum Toxin Type A [IncobotulinumtoxinA] (Xeomin) [Neuro-muscular Blocker/Neurotoxin]   WARNING: Effects may spread beyond Tx area leading to swallowing and breathing difficulties (may be fatal); Sxs may occur hours to weeks after Inj Uses: *Cervical dystonia (adults), glabellar lines* **Action:** Neurotoxin, ↓ ACH release from nerve endings, ↓ neuromuscular transmission **Dose:** *Cervical dystonia:* 120 units IM ÷ dose into muscles; *Glabellar lines:* 4 units into each of the 5 sites (total = 20 units), do not administer at intervals < q3mo **Caution:** [C, ?] Sedentary pt to resume activity slowly after Inj; aminoglycosides and nondepolarizing muscle blockers may ↑ effects; do not exceed dosing **CI:** Hypersensitivity to components (cow milk), Infxn at Inj site **Disp:** 50, 100 units, Inj **SE:** Dysphagia, neck/ musculoskeletal pain, muscle weakness **Interactions:** ↑ Effects *W/* aminoglycosides, other botulinum toxin products **NIPE:** Effect 12–16 wk w/ 5000–10,000 units; botulinum toxin products not interchangeable; Inj site pain

Botulinum Toxin Type A [AnabotulinumtoxinA] (Botox, Botox Cosmetic) [Neuromuscular Blocker/Neurotoxin]   WARNING: Effects may spread beyond Tx area leading to swallowing/breathing difficulties (may be fatal); Sxs may occur hours to weeks after Inj Uses: *Glabellar lines (cosmetic) < 65 y, blepharospasm, cervical dystonia, axillary hyperhidrosis, strabismus, chronic migraine, upper limb spasticity, incontinence in OAB due to neurologic Dz* **Action:** Neurotoxin, ↓ ACH release from nerve endings; denervates sweat glands/muscles **Dose:** *Adults. Glabellar lines (cosmetic):* 0.1 mL IM × 5 sites q3–4mo *Blepharospasm:* 1.25–2.5 units IM/ site q3mo; max 200 units/30 d total *Cervical dystonia:* 198–300 units IM ÷ < 100 units into muscle *Hyperhidrosis:* 50 units intradermal/each axilla *Strabismus:* 1.25–2.5 units IM/ site q3mo; inject eye muscles w/ EMG guidance *Chronic migraine:* 155 units total, 0.1 mL (5 unit) Inj ÷ into 7 head/neck muscles *Upper limb spasticity:* Dose based on Hx use EMG guidance **Caution:** [C, ?] w/ Neurologic Dz; do not exceed doses; sedentary pt to resume activity slowly after Inj; aminoglycosides and nondepolarizing muscle blockers may ↑ effects; do not exceed dosing **CI:** Hypersensitivity to components, Infxn at Inj site **Disp:** Inj powder, single-use vial (dilute w/NS); (*Botox cosmetic*) 50, 100 units (*Botox*) 100, 200 unit vials; store 2–8°C **SE:** Anaphylaxis, erythema multiforme, dysphagia, dyspnea, syncope, HA, NAG **Interactions:** ↑ Effects *W/* aminoglycosides, other botulinum toxin products **NIPE:** Effect 12–16 wk w/ 5000–10,000 units; botulinum toxin products not interchangeable; Inj site pain; do not exceed total dose of 360 units q12–16wk

Botulinum Toxin Type B [RimabotulinumtoxinB] (Myobloc) [Neuromuscular Blocker/Neurotoxin]   WARNING: Effects may spread beyond Tx area leading to swallowing and breathing difficulties (may be fatal); Sxs may occur hours to weeks after Inj Uses: *Cervical dystonia (adults)* **Action:** Neurotoxin, ↓ ACH release from nerve endings, ↓ neuromuscular transmission **Dose:** *Cervical dystonia:* 2500–5000 units IM ÷ dose units into muscles; lower dose if näive Caution: [C, ?] Sedentary pt to resume activity slowly after Inj; aminoglycosides and nondepolarizing muscle blockers may ↑↑ effects; do not exceed dosing CI: Hypersensitivity to components, Infxn at Inj site Dose: Inj 5000 units/mL SE: Anaphylaxis, erythema multiforme, dysphagia, dyspnea, syncope, HA, NAG Interactions: ↑ Effects W/ aminoglycosides, other botulinum toxin products NIPE: Effect 12–16 wk w/ 5000–10,000 units; botulinum toxin products not interchangeable; Inj site pain out

Brentuximab Vedotin (Adcetris) [CD30-Directed Antibody-Drug Conjugate]
WARNING: JC virus Infxn leading to PML and death may occur Uses: * Hodgkin lymphoma, systemic anaplastic large cell lymphoma* Action: CD30-directed antibody-drug conjugate Dose: Adult. 1.8 mg/kg IV over 30 min q3wk; max 16 cycles; pts > 100 kg, dose based on wgt of 100 kg; ↓ dose w/ periph neuropathy & neutropenia (see label) Caution: [D, ?/–] CI: w/ Bleomycin Disp: Inj (powder) 50 mg/vial SE: Periph neuropathy, N/V/D, HA, dizziness, pain, arthralgia, myalgia, insomnia, anxiety, alopecia, night sweats, URI, fatigue, pyrexia, rash, cough, dyspnea, Inf Rxns, tumor lysis synd, PML, SJS, pulmonary tox Interactions: ↑ Effects W/ strong CYP3A4 Inhibitors such as amiodarone, ciprofloxacin, clarithromycin, diltiazem, ketoconazole, verapamil, grapefruit (Table 10); ↓ effects W/ strong CYP3A4 inducers such as carbamazepine, glucocorticoids, phenytoin, rifampin, St. John's wort (Table 10) Labs: ↓ WBC, Hgb, plt NIPE: Monitor for neuropathy; give by IV infusion over 30 min

Brimonidine (Alphagan P) [Alpha Agonist/Glaucoma Agent]
Uses: *Open-angle glaucoma, ocular HTN* Action: α_2-Adrenergic agonist Dose: 1gtt in eye(s) tid (wait 15 min to insert contacts) Caution: [B, ?] CI: MAOI Rx Disp: 0.15, 0.1, 0.2%, soln SE: Local irritation, HA, fatigue Interactions: ↑ Effects OF antihypertensives, BBs, cardiac glycosides, CNS depressants; ↓ effects W/ TCAs NIPE: ⊘ EtOH, insert soft contact lenses 15+ min after drug use

Brimonidine, Topical (Mirvaso) [Alpha Agonist]
Uses: *Tx of rosacea* Action: α2-Adrenergic agonist Dose: Adults. Apply pea-size quantity to forehead, chin, nose, & cheeks 1 ×/ d Caution: [B, ?/–] w/ h/o depression, orthostatic ↓ BP, severe CV Dz, cerebral or coronary Insuff, scleroderma, thromboangiitis obliterans, Sjögren synd, Raynaud (may potentiate vascular insufficiency) Disp: Gel 0.33% CI: None SE: Flushing, erythema, skin burning sensation, contact dermatitis, acne, HA, nasopharyngitis, ↑ IOP Notes: Do not apply to eyes/lips NIPE: Wash hands after applying; avoid use during PRG/breast-feeding

Brimonidine/Timolol (Combigan) [Alpha-2 Agonist + Noncardioselective Beta-Blocker]
Uses: *↓ IOP in glaucoma or ocular HTN* Action: Selective α_2-adrenergic agonist and nonselective β-adrenergic antagonist Dose: Adults & Peds ≥ 2 y. 1 gtt bid Caution: [C, –] CI: Asthma, severe COPD, sinus bradycardia, 2nd-/3rd-degree AV block, CHF cardiac failure, cardiogenic shock, component hypersens Disp: Soln: (2 mg/mL brimonidine, 5 mg/mL timolol) 5, 10, 15 mL SE: Allergic conjunctivitis, conjunctival folliculosis, conjunctival

hyperemia, eye pruritus, ocular burning & stinging **Interactions:** ↑ Risk of conduction defects *W/* digoxin, CCBs; ↓ effects *OF* epinephrine; may ↑ or ↓ effects *W/* other CNS depressants, systemic BB, reserpine, quinidine, SSRIs, other CYP2D6 Inhibs (Table 10) **NIPE:** Instill other ophthal products 5 min apart

Brinzolamide (Azopt) [Carbonic Anhydrase Inhibitor/Glaucoma Agent] **Uses:** *Open-angle glaucoma, ocular HTN* **Action:** Carbonic anhydrase Inhib **Dose:** 1 gtt in eye(s) tid **Caution:** [C, ?/–] **CI:** Sulfonamide allergy **Disp:** 1% susp **SE:** Blurred vision, dry eye, blepharitis, taste disturbance, HA **Interactions:** ↑ Effects *W/* oral carbonic anhydrase Inhibs **Labs:** Check LFTs, BUN, Cr **NIPE:** ⊘ Use drug if ↓ renal & hepatic studies or allergies to sulfonamides; shake well before use; insert soft contact lenses 15+ min after drug use; wait 10 min before use of other topical ophthal drugs; may cause blurred vision or taste changes

Brinzolamide/Brimonidine (Simbrinza) **Uses:** *↓ IOP in open-angle glaucoma or ocular HTN* **Action:** Carbonic anhydrase Inhib and α₂-adrenergic agonist **Dose:** *Adults.* 1 gtt in eye(s) tid **Caution:** [C, ?/–] sulfonamide hypersensitivity Rxn (brinzolamide); corneal endothelium cell loss; not rec if CrCl < 30 mL/min **CI:** Component hypersensitivity **Disp:** Ophthal susp (brinzolamide/ brimonidine): 10/2 mg/mL **SE:** Eye irritation/allergy, blurred vision, dysgeusia, dry mouth, HA, fatigue **NIPE:** Shake well before use; remove contacts during admin, reinsert after 15 min; separate other topical eye meds drugs by 5 min

Bromfenac (Prolensa) **Uses:** *↓ Inflame & ocular pain post cataract surgery* **Action:** NSAID **Dose:** *Adults.* 1 gtt in eye(s) 1 d prior & 14 d post-surgery **Caution:** [C, ?/–] Sulfite hypersensitivity; may delay healing, keratitis, ↑ bleeding time **CI:** None **Disp:** Ophthal soln: 0.07% **SE:** Eye pain, blurred vision, photophobia, anterior chamber inflammation, foreign body sensation **NIPE:** Shake well before use; remove contacts during admin, reinsert after 10 min; separate other topical eye meds drugs by 10 min

Bromocriptine (Parlodel) [Antiparkinson/Dopamine Receptor Agonist] **Uses:** *Parkinson Dz, hyperprolactinemia, acromegaly, pituitary tumors* **Action:** Agonist to striatal dopamine receptors; ↓ prolactin secretion **Dose:** Initial, 1.25 mg PO bid; titrate to effect, w/food **Caution:** [B, –] **CI:** uncontrolled HTN, PRG, severe CAD or CV Dz **Disp:** Tabs 2.5 mg; caps 5 mg **SE:** ↓ BP, Raynaud phenomenon, dizziness, N, GI upset, hallucinations **Interactions:** ↑ Effects *W/* erythromycin, fluvoxamine, nefazodone, sympathomimetics; ↓ effects *W/* phenothiazines, antipsychotics **Labs:** ↑ BUN, AST, ALT, CPK, alk phos, uric acid **NIPE:** ⊘ Breast-feeding, PRG, OCPs; drug may cause intolerance to EtOH, return of menses & suppression of galactorrhea may take 6–8 wk; take drug w/ meals

Bromocriptine Mesylate (Cycloset) [Dopamine Receptor Agonist] **Uses:** *Improve glycemic control in adults w/ type 2 DM* **Action:** Dopamine receptor agonist; ? DM mechanism **Dose:** *Initial:* 0.8 mg PO daily, ↑ weekly by 1 tab; usual dose 1.6–4.8 mg 1 × d; w/in 2 h after waking w/ food **Caution:** [B, –] May cause orthostatic ↓ BP, psychotic disorders; not for type 1 DM or DKA; avoid w/ dopamine antagonists/receptor agonists **CI:** Hypersensitivity to ergots drugs, w/ syncopal migraine, nursing mothers **Disp:** Tabs 0.8 mg **SE:** N/V, fatigue, HA, dizziness, somnolence **Interactions:** ↑ Effects *OF* antihypertensives, levodopa, triptans; strong CYP3A4 inhibitors/inducers many ↑ or ↓ levels of cycloset; ↓ effects *W/* amitriptyline, haloperidol, imipramine, loxapine, MAO inhibitors, methyldopa, phenothiazines, reserpine **Labs:** ↑ Alk phos, ALT, AST, BUN, CK, uric acid **NIPE:** ↑ Risk of syncope; ↑ risk of HTN; may restore fertility

Budesonide (Rhinocort Aqua, Pulmicort) [Anti-Inflammatory/ Glucocorticoid] Uses: *Allergic & nonallergic rhinitis, asthma* **Action:** Steroid **Dose:** *Adults.* *Rhinocort Aqua:* 1 spray/each nostril/d *Pulmicort Flexhaler:* 1–2 Inh bid *Pulmicort Aqua intranasal:* 1 spray/each nostril/d; *Pulmicort flexhaler:* 1–2 Inh bid *Respules:* 0.25–0.5 mg daily or bid (rinse mouth after PO use) **Caution:** [B, ?/–] **CI:** w/ Acute asthma **Disp:** *Flexhaler,* 90, 180 mcg/Inh; *Respules,* 0.25, 0.5, 1 mg/2 mL; *Rhinocort Aqua,* 32 mcg/spray **SE:** HA, N, cough, hoarseness, *Candida* Infxn, epistaxis **Interactions:** ↑ Effects *W/* ketoconazole, itraconazole, ritonavir, indinavir, saquinavir, erythromycin, & grapefruit juice **NIPE:** Shake inhaler well before use, rinse mouth & wash inhaler after use, swallow caps whole, ⊘ exposure chickenpox or measles

Budesonide, Oral (Entocort EC) [Anti-Inflammatory, Corticosteroid] Uses: *Mild–mod Crohn Dz* **Action:** Steroid, anti-inflammatory **Dose:** *Adults.* Initial, 9 mg PO qAM to 8 wk max: maint 6 mg PO qAM taper by 3 mo; avoid grapefruit juice **CI:** Hypersensitivity **Caution:** [C, ?/–] DM, glaucoma, cataracts, HTN, CHF **Disp:** Caps 3 mg ER **SE:** HA, N, ↑ wgt, mood change, *Candida* Infxn, epistaxis **Interactions:** ↑ Effects *W/* erythromycin, indinavir, itraconazole, ketoconazole, ritonavir, grapefruit **Labs:** ↑ Alk phos, C-reactive protein, ESR, WBC; ↓ Hgb, Hct **NIPE:** Do not cut/crush/chew caps; taper on D/C

Budesonide/Formoterol (Symbicort) [Anti-Inflammatory, Bronchodilator/Beta-2 Agonist] **WARNING:** Long-acting β_2-adrenergic agonists may ↑ risk of asthma-related death. Use only for pts not adequately controlled on other meds **Uses:** *Rx of asthma, main in COPD (chronic bronchitis and emphysema)* **Action:** Steroid w/ LA selective β_2-adrenergic agonist **Dose:** *Adults & Peds > 12 y.* 2 Inh bid (use lowest effective dose), 640 mcg/18 mcg/d max **Caution:** [C, ?/–] **CI:** Status asthmaticus/acute episodes **Disp:** Inh (budesonide formoterol) 80/4.5 mcg, 160/4.5 mcg **SE:** HA, GI discomfort, nasopharyngitis, palpitations, tremor, nervousness, URI, paradoxical bronchospasm, hypokalemia, cataracts, glaucoma **Interactions:** ↑ Effects *W/* adrenergics; ↑ hypokalemic effects *W/* cardiac glycosides, diuretics, steroids; ↑ risk of ventricular arrhythmias *W/* MAOIs, TCA, quinidine, phenothiazines; ↓ effects W/ BBs **Labs:** ↑ Serum glucose; ↓ K⁺ **NIPE:** ⊘ EtOH; not for acute bronchospasm; not for transferring pt from chronic systemic steroids; rinse & spit w/ H₂O after each dose

Bumetanide (Bumex) [Diuretic/Loop]   **WARNING:** Potent diuretic, may result in profound fluid & electrolyte loss   **Uses:** *Edema from CHF, hepatic cirrhosis, & renal Dz* **Action:** Loop diuretic; ↓ reabsorption of Na⁺ & Cl⁻, in ascending loop of Henle & the distal tubule **Dose:** *Adults.* 0.5–2 mg/d PO; 0.5–1 mg IV/IM q8–24h (max 10 mg/d) *Peds.* 0.015–0.1 mg/kg PO q6–24h (max 10 mg/d) **Caution:** [C, ?/–] **CI:** Anuria, hepatic coma, severe electrolyte depletion **Disp:** Tabs 0.5, 1, 2 mg; Inj 0.25 mg/mL **SE:** Dizziness, ototox **Interactions:** ↑ Effects W/ antihypertensives, thiazides, nitrates, EtOH, clofibrate; ↑ effects OF Li, warfarin, thrombolytic drugs, anticoagulants; ↑K⁺ loss W/ carbenoxolone, corticosteroids, terbutaline; ↑ ototox W/ aminoglycosides, cisplatin; ↓ effects W/ cholestyramine, colestipol, NSAIDs, probenecid, barbiturates, phenytoin **Labs:** ↑ Cr, uric acid; ↓ serum K⁺, Ca²⁺, Na⁺, Mg⁺ **NIPE:** Take drug w/food, take early to prevent nocturia, daily wgt; monitor fluid & lytes; monitor ECG for hypokalemia (flattened T waves)

Bupivacaine (Marcaine) [Anesthetic]   **WARNING:** Avoid 0.75% for OB anesthesia d/t reports of cardiac arrest and death **Uses:** *Local, regional, & spinal anesthesia, obstetrical procedures* local & regional analgesia **Action:** Local anesthetic **Dose:** *Adults & Peds.* Dose dependent on procedure (tissue vascularity, depth of anesthesia, etc) (Table 1) **Caution:** [C, –]. Severe bleeding, ↓ BP, shock & arrhythmias, local Infxns at site, septicemia **CI:** Obstetrical paracervical block anesthesia **Disp:** Inj 0.25%, 0.5%, 0.75% **SE:** ↓ BP, ↓ HR, dizziness, anxiety **Interactions:** ↑ Effects W/ BBs, hyaluronidase, ergot-type oxytocics, MAOI, TCAs, phenothiazines, vasopressors, CNS depressants; ↓ effects W/ chloroprocaine **NIPE:** Anesthetized area has temporary loss of sensation & Fxn

Buprenorphine (Buprenex) [C-III] [Analgesic/Opioid Agonist-Antagonist]   **Uses:** *Mod/severe pain* **Action:** Opiate agonist–antagonist **Dose:** 0.3–0.6 mg IM or slow IV push q6h PRN **Caution:** [C, –] **Disp:** 0.3 mg/mL **SE:** Sedation, ↓ BP, resp depression **Notes:** Withdrawal if opioid-dependent **Interactions:** ↑ Effects of resp & CNS depression W/ EtOH, opiates, benzodiazepines, TCAs, MAOIs, other CNS depressants **Labs:** ↓ Alk phos, Hgb, Hct, erythrocyte count **NIPE:** ⊘ EtOH & other CNS depressants

Buprenorphine, Transdermal (Butrans) [C-III] [Opioid Analgesic]   **WARNING:** Limit use to severe around the clock chronic pain; assess for opioid abuse/addiction before use; 20 mcg/h max d/t ↑ QTc; avoid heat on patch, may result in OD **Uses:** *Mod/severe chronic pain requiring around the clock opioid analgesic* **Action:** Opiate agonist–antagonist **Dose:** Wear patch × 7 d; if opioid naïve start 5 mcg/h; see label for conversion from opioid; wait 72 h before Δ dose; wait 3 wk before using same application site **Caution:** [C, –] **CI:** Resp depression, severe asthma, ileus, component hypersensitivity, short-term opioid need, post-op/mild/intermittent pain **Disp:** Transdermal patch 5, 10, 20 mcg/h **SE:**

N/V, HA, site Rxns pruritus, dizziness, constipation, somnolence, dry mouth **Interactions:** ↑ Effects W/ CNS & resp depressants (eg, benzodiazepines, muscle relaxants, tricyclics, phenothiazines), EtOH; do not give w/in 14 d of MAOIs; ↑ risk of cardiac effects W/ Class Ia (eg, quinidine, procainamide, disopyramide) or Class III antiarrhythmics (eg, sotalol, amiodarone, dofetilide) **NIPE:** Taper on D/C

Buprenorphine & Naloxone (Suboxone) [C-III] [Opioid (Partial Agonist–Antagonist) + Opioid Antagonist] Uses: *Maint opioid withdrawal* **Action:** Opioid agonist–antagonist + opioid antagonist **Dose:** Usual: 4–24 mg/d SL ↑/↓ by 2/0.5 mg or 4/1 mg to effect of S/Sxs **Caution:** [C, +/–] **CI:** Hypersensitivity **Disp:** SL film *Buprenorphine/naloxone:* 2/0.5, 8/2 mg **SE:** Oral hypoparesthesia, HA, V, pain, constipation, diaphoresis **Interactions:** ↑ Effects W/ CYP3A4 Inhibs (eg, azole antifungals, macrolides, HIV protease Inhibs) **NIPE:** Not for analgesia; dissolve under tongue, do not swallow tabs or film

Bupropion (Aplenzin XR, Wellbutrin, Wellbutrin SR, Wellbutrin XL Zyban) [Aminoketone] **WARNING:** All pts being treated w/bupropion for smoking cessation Tx should be observed for neuropsychiatric S/Sxs (hostility, agitation, depressed mood, and suicide-related events; most during/after; *Zyban;* Sxs may persist following D/C; closely monitor for worsening depression or emergence of suicidality, increased suicidal behavior in young adults Uses: *Depression, smoking cessation adjunct*, ADHD, not for peds use **Action:** Weak Inhib of neuronal uptake of serotonin & norepinephrine; ↓ neuronal dopamine reuptake **Dose:** *Depression:* 100–450 mg/d ÷ bid–tid; SR 150–200 mg bid; XL 150–450 mg daily *Smoking cessation (Zyban, Wellbutrin XR):* 150 mg/d × 3 d, then 150 mg bid × 8–12 wk, last dose before 6 PM; ↓ dose w/ renal/hepatic impair **Caution:** [C, ?/–] **CI:** Sz disorder, Hx anorexia nervosa or bulimia, MAOI, w/in 14 d, abrupt D/C of EtOH or sedatives; inhibitors/inducers of CYP2B6 (Table 10) **Disp:** Tabs 75, 100 mg; SR tabs 100, 150, 200 mg; XL tabs 150, 300 mg; Zyban 150 mg tabs, Aplenzin XR tabs: 175, 348, 522 mg **SE:** Xerostomia, dizziness, Szs, agitation, insomnia, HA, tachycardia, ↓ wgt **Interactions:** ↑ Effects W/ cimetidine, levodopa, MAOIs; ↑ risk of Szs W/ EtOH, phenothiazines, antidepressants, theophylline, TCAs, or abrupt withdrawal of corticosteroids, benzodiazepines **Labs:** ↓ Prolactin level **NIPE:** Drug may ↑ adverse events including Szs; take 3–4 wk for full effect; ⊘ EtOH or CNS depressants; ⊘ abrupt D/C; SR & XR do not cut/chew/crush

Buspirone [Anxiolytic] Uses: *Generalized anxiety disorder* **Action:** Antianxiety; antagonizes CNS serotonin & dopamine receptors **Dose:** *Initial:* 7.5 mg PO bid; ↑ by 5 mg q2–3d to effect; usual 20–30 mg/d; max 60 mg/d **CI:** Hypersensitivity **Caution:** [B, ?/–] Avoid w/ severe hepatic/renal Insuff, w/ MAOI **Disp:** Tabs 5, 7.5, 10, 15, 30 mg **SE:** Drowsiness, dizziness, HA, N, EPS, serotonin synd, hostility, depression **Interactions:** ↑ Effects W/ erythromycin, clarithromycin, itraconazole, ketoconazole, diltiazem, verapamil, grapefruit juice; ↓ effects W/ carbamazepine, rifampin, phenytoin, dexamethasone, phenobarbital, fluoxetine **Labs:** ↑

Glucose; ↓ WBC, plts **NIPE:** ↑ Sedation w/ EtOH, therapeutic effects may take up to 4 wk; no abuse potential or physical/ psychologic dependence

Busulfan (Myleran, Busulfex) [Antineoplastic/Alkylating Drug]

WARNING: Can cause severe bone marrow suppresion, should be administered by an experienced provider **Uses:** *CML*, preparative regimens for allogeneic & ABMT in high doses **Action:** Alkylating agent **Dose:** (per protocol) **Caution:** [D, ?] **Disp:** Tabs 2 mg, Inj 60 mg/10 mL **SE:** Bone marrow suppression, ↑ BP, pulm fibrosis, N (w/ high-dose), gynecomastia, adrenal Insuff, skin hyperpigmentation, ↑ HR, rash, weakness, Sz **Interactions:** ↑ Effects *W/* APAP; ↑ BM suppression *W/* antineoplastic drugs w/ radiation therapy; ↑ uric acid levels *W/* probenecid & sulfinpyrazone; ↓ effects *W/* itraconazole, phenytoin **Labs:** ↑ Glucose, ALT, bilirubin, BUN, Cr, uric acid; monitor CBC, LFTs **NIPE:** ⊘ Immunizations, PRG, breast-feeding; ↑ fluids; use barrier contraception; ↑ risk of hair loss, rash, darkened skin pigment; ↑ susceptibility to Infxn

Butabarbital, Hyoscyamine Hydrobromide, Phenazopyridine (Pyridium Plus) [Urinary Tract Analgesic & Sedative]

Uses: *Relieve urinary tract pain w/ UTI, procedures, trauma* **Action:** Phenazopyridine (topical anesthetic), hyoscyamine (parasympatholytic, ↓ spasm) & butabarbital (sedative) **Dose:** 1 PO qid, pc, & hs; w/ antibiotic for UTI, 2 d max **Caution:** [C, ?] **Disp:** Tabs butabarbital/hyoscyamine/phenazopyridine 15 mg/0.3 mg/150 mg **SE:** HA, rash, itching, GI distress, methemoglobinemia, hemolytic anemia, anaphylactoid-like Rxns, dry mouth, dizziness, drowsiness, blurred vision **Labs:** Effects urine test results **NIPE:** Colors urine orange, may tint skin, sclera; stains clothing/contacts

Butorphanol (Stadol) [C-IV] [Analgesic/Opiate Agonist–Antagonist]

Uses: *Anesthesia adjunct, pain & migraine HA* **Action:** Opiate agonist–antagonist w/ central analgesic actions **Dose:** 0.5-4 mg IM or IV q3–4h PRN *Migraine:* 1 spray in 1 nostril, repeat × 1, 60–90 min, then q3–4h in renal impair **Caution:** [C, +] **Disp:** Inj 1, 2 mg/mL; nasal 1 mg/spray (10 mg/mL) **SE:** Drowsiness, dizziness, nasal congestion **Interactions:** ↑ Effects *W/* EtOH, antihistamines, cimetidine, CNS depressants, phenothiazines, barbiturates, skeletal-muscle relaxants, MAOIs; ↓ effects *OF* opiates **Labs:** ↑ Serum amylase & lipase **NIPE:** ⊘ EtOH or other CNS depressants; may induce withdrawal in opioid dependency

C1 Esterase Inhibitor [Human] (Berinert, Cinryze) [C1 Inhibitor]

Uses: *Berinert:* Rx acute Abd or facial attacks of HAE*, *Cinryze:* Prophylaxis of HAE* **Action:** ↓ complement system by ↑ Factor XIIa & kallikrein activation **Dose:** *Adults & Adolescents. Berinert:* 20 units/kg IV × 1; *Cinryze:* 1000 units IV q3–4d **Caution:** [C, ?/–] Hypersens Rxns, monitor for thrombotic events, may contain infectious agents **CI:** Hypersens Rxns to C1 esterase inhibitor preparations **Disp:** 500 units/vial **SE:** HA, Abd pain, N/V/D, muscle spasms, pain, subsequent HAE attack, anaphylaxis, thromboembolism **NIPE:** Contains human plasma, monitor for possible Infxn transmission; use dedicated IV line to administer; provide pt w/ instructions/training for self-admin & recognition of S/Sx HAE

Cabazitaxel (Jevtana) [Taxane Antimicrotubule] **WARNING:** Neutropenic deaths reported; ✓ CBCs, CI w/ ANC ≤ 1500 cells/mm³; severe hypersens (rash/erythema, ↓ BP, bronchospasm) may occur, D/C drug & Tx; CI w/ Hx of hypersens to cabazitaxel or others formulated w/ polysorbate 80 **Uses:** *Hormone refractory metastatic PCa after taxotere* **Action:** Microtubule inhib **Dose:** 25 mg/m² IV Inf (over 1 h) q3wk w/ prednisone 10 mg PO daily; premed w/ antihistamine, corticosteroid, H₂ antagonist; do not use w/ bilirubin ≥ ULN, AST/ALT ≥ 1.5 × ULN **Caution:** [D, ?/–] w/ CYP3A inhib/inducers **CI:** See Warning **Disp:** 40 mg/mL Inj **SE:** ↓ WBC, ↓ Hgb, ↓ plt, sepsis, N/V/D, constipation, Abd/back/Jt pain, dysgeusia, fatigue, hematuria, neuropathy, anorexia, cough, dyspnea, alopecia, pyrexia, hypersens Rxn, renal failure **Interactions:** ↑ Effects *OF* CYP3A4 Inhibs (eg, ketoconazole, clarithromycin, atazanavir, nefazodone, nelfinavir, ritonavir, saquinavir, voriconazole); ↓ effects *OF* CYP3A4 inducers (eg, phenytoin, carbamazepine, rifampin, phenobarbital) (may antagonize cabazitaxel), St. John's wort **Labs:** ↓ WBC, ↓ Hgb, ↓ plt **NIPE:** Follow presmedication protocol—severe hypersensitivity Rxn can occur; monitor closely pts > 65 y; maintain adeq hydration

Cabozanitinib (Cometriq) **WARNING:** GI perf/fistulas, severe and sometimes fatal hemorrhage (3%) including GI bleed/hemoptysis **Uses:** *Metastatic medullary thyroid CA* **Acts:** Multi TKI **Dose:** 140 mg/d, do NOT eat 2 h ac or 1 h pc **Caution:** [D, –] D/C w/ arterial thromboembolic events; dehiscence; ↑ BP, ONJ; palmar-plantar erythrodysesthesia synd; proteinuria; reversible posterior leukoencephalopathy **CI:** w/ Severe bleed **Disp:** Caps 20, 80 mg **SE:** N, V, Abd pain, constipation, stomatitis, oral pain, dysgeusia, fatigue, ↓ wgt, anorexia, ↑ BP, ↑ AST/ALT, ↑ alk phos, ↑ bili, ↓ Ca, ↓ PO₄, ↓ plts, ↓ lymphocytes, ↓ neutrophils **Notes:** A CYP3A4 subs, w/ strong CYP3A4 induc ↓ cabozantinib exposure; w/ strong CYP3A4 inhib ↑ cabozantinib exposure; ✓ for hemorrhage. **NIPE:** ⊘ PRG; use effective contraception during Tx & × 4 mo after Tx completion; ⊘ grapefruit products; ⊘ food intake 2 h before or 1 h after taking

Calcipotriene (Dovonex) [Keratolytic] **Uses:** *Plaque psoriasis* **Action:** Synthetic vitamin D₃ analog **Dose:** Apply bid **Caution:** [C, ?] **CI:** ↑ Ca²⁺; vit D tox; do not apply to face **Disp:** Cream; foam oint; soln 0.005% **SE:** Skin irritation, dermatitis **Interactions:** None noted **Labs:** Monitor serum Ca **NIPE:** Wash hands after application or wear gloves to apply, D/C drug if ↑ Ca; ⊘ excessive sun or artifical light exposure

Calcitonin (Fortical, Miacalcin) [Hypocalcemic, Bone Resorption Inhibitor/Thyroid Hormone] **Uses:** *Miacalcin:* *Paget Dz, emergent Rx hypercalcemia, postmenopausal osteoporosis* *Fortical:* *Postmenopausal osteoporosis*; osteogenesis imperfecta **Action:** Polypeptide hormone (salmon derived), inhibits osteoclasts **Dose:** *Paget Dz:* 100 units/d IM/SQ initial, 50 units/d or 50–100 units q1–3d maint *Hypercalcemia:* 4 units/kg IM/SQ q12h; ↑ to 8 units/kg q12h, max q6h *Osteoporosis:* 100 units/qod IM/SQ; intranasal 200 units = 1 nasal spray/d **Caution:**

[C, ?] **Disp:** *Fortical, Miacalcin* nasal spray 200 IU/activation; **Inj,** *Miacalcin* 200 units/mL (2 mL) **SE:** Facial flushing, N, Inj site edema, nasal irritation, polyuria, may ↑ granular casts in urine **Notes:** *Fortical* is rDNA derived from salmon **Interactions:** Prior Tx w/ alendronate, risedronate, etidronate or pamidronate may ↓ effects *OF* calcitonin **Labs:** May ↑ granular casts in urine; ↓ serum Li; monitor serum Ca & alkphos **NIPE:** Allergy skin test prior to use; take hs to < N/V; flushing > Inj is transient; N > Inj will < w/ continued Tx; for nasal spray alternate nostrils daily; ensure adequate Ca & vit D intake

Calcitriol (Rocaltrol, Calcijex) [Antihypocalcemic/Vitamin D Analog] **Uses:** *Predialysis reduction of ↑ PTH levels to treat bone Dz; ↑ Ca²⁺ on dialysis* **Action:** 1,25-Dihydroxycholecalciferol (vit D analog); ↑ Ca²⁺ & phosphorus absorption; ↑ bone mineralization **Dose:** *Adults. Renal failure:* 0.25 mcg/d PO, ↑ 0.25 mcg/d q4–8wk PRN; 0.5–4 mcg 3×/wk IV, ↑ PRN *Hypoparathyroidism:* 0.5–2 mcg/d **Peds.** *Renal failure:* 15 ng/kg/d, ↑ PRN; maint 30–60 ng/kg/d *Hypoparathyroidism: < 5 y:* 0.25–0.75 mcg/d *> 6 y:* 0.5–2 mcg/d **Caution:** [C, ?] ↑ Mg²⁺ possible w/ antacids **CI:** ↑ Ca²⁺; vit D tox **Disp:** Inj 1 mcg/mL (in 1 mL); caps 0.25, 0.5 mcg; soln 1 mcg/mL **SE:** ↑ Ca²⁺ possible **Interactions:** ↑ Effect *W/* thiazide diuretics; ↓ effect *W/* cholestyramine, colestipol, ketoconazole **Labs:** Monitor for ↑ Ca²⁺, cholesterol, BUN, AST, ALT; ↓ alk phos **NIPE:** ⊘ Mg-containing antacids or supls; use non-aluminum phosphate binders & low-phosphate diet to control serum phosphate; maintain adeq fluid intake

Calcitriol, Ointment (Vectical) [Vitamin D₃ Derivative] **Uses:** *Mild/mod plaque psoriasis* **Action:** Vit D₃ analog **Dose:** *Adults.* Apply to area bid; max 200 g/wk **Caution:** [C, ?/–] Avoid excess sunlight **CI:** None **Disp:** Oint 3 mcg/g (5-, 100-g tube) **SE:** Hypercalcemia, hypercalciuria, nephrolithiasis, worsening psoriasis, pruritus, skin discomfort **Interactions:** ↑ Risk of hypercalcemia *W/* thiazide diuretics, calcium supls or high doses of vit D **Labs:** Monitor for hypercalcemia **NIPE:** ↑ Absorption may occur w/ occlusive dressing; D/C Tx until normocalcemia returns; ⊘ apply to eyes, lips, facial skin; avoid excessive sunlight or artificial light

Calcium Acetate (PhosLo) [Calcium Supplement, Antiarrhythmic/Mineral, Electrolyte] **Uses:** *ESRD-associated hyperphosphatemia* **Action:** Ca²⁺ supl w/o aluminum to ↓ PO₄²⁻ absorption **Dose:** 2–4 tabs PO w/meals **Caution:** [C, +] **CI:** ↑ Ca²⁺ renal calculi **Disp:** GelCap 667 mg **SE:** Can ↑ Ca²⁺, hypophosphatemia, constipation **Interactions:** ↑ Effects *OF* quinidine; ↓ effects *W/* large intake of dietary fiber, spinach, rhubarb; ↓ effects *OF* atenolol, CCB, etidronate, tetracyclines, fluoroquinolones, phenytoin, Fe salts, thyroid hormones **Labs:** Monitor for ↑ Ca²⁺; ↓ Mg²⁺ **NIPE:** ⊘ EtOH, caffeine, tobacco; separate Ca supls & other meds by 1–2 h; adeq w/fluids during meals for ↑ effectiveness

Calcium Carbonate (Tums, Alka-Mints) [Antacid, Calcium Supplement/Mineral, Electrolyte] [OTC] **Uses:** *Hyperacidity associated w/ peptic ulcer Dz, hiatal hernia, etc* **Action:** Neutralizes gastric acid **Dose:**

500 mg–2 g PO PRN, 7 g/d max; ↓ w/ renal impair **Caution:** [C, ?] **CI:** ↑ CA, ↓ phos, renal calculi, suspected digoxin tox **Disp:** Chewtabs 350, 420, 500, 550, 750, 850 mg; susp **SE:** ↑ Ca²⁺, ↓ PO⁴⁻, constipation **Interactions:** ↓ Effect *OF* tetracyclines, fluoroquinolones, Fe salts, & ASA; ↓ Ca absorption *W/* high intake of dietary fiber **Labs:** Monitor for ↑ Ca²⁺, ↓ Phos, & Mg²⁺ **NIPE:** ↑ Fluids; drug may cause constipation; ⊘ EtOH, caffeine, tobacco; separate Ca supls & other meds & fiber-containing foods by 1–2 h, chew tabs well; take w/ or immediately after meals w/ ↑H₂O

Calcium Glubionate (Calcionate) [Calcium Supplement Antiarrhythmic/Mineral, Electrolyte] [OTC]
Uses: *Rx & prevent calcium deficiency* **Action:** Ca²⁺ supl **Dose:** *Adults.* 1000–1200 mg/d ÷ doses **Peds.** 200–1300 mg/d mg/kg/d **Caution:** [C, ?] **CI:** ↑ Ca²⁺ **Disp:** OTC syrup 1.8 g/5 mL = elemental Ca 115 mg/5 mL **SE:** ↑ Ca²⁺, ↓ PO⁴⁻, constipation **Interactions:** ↑ Effects *OF* quinidine; ↓ effect *OF* tetracyclines; ↓ Ca absorption *W/* high intake of dietary fiber **Labs:** ↑Ca²⁺, ↓ Mg²⁺, ↓ PO⁴⁻ **NIPE:** ⊘ EtOH, caffeine, tobacco, separate Ca supls & other meds & fiber-containing foods by 1–2 h; give on empty stomach for Tx of ↑ phosphatemia

Calcium Salts (Chloride, Gluconate, Gluceptate) [Calcium Supplement, Antiarrhythmic/Mineral, Electrolyte]
Uses: *Ca²⁺ replacement*, VF, Ca²⁺ blocker tox (CCB), *severe ↑ Mg²⁺ tetany*, hyperphosphatemia in ESRD* **Action:** Ca²⁺ supl/replacement **Dose:** *Adults.* *Replacement:* 1–2 g/d PO. *Tetany:* 1 g CaCl over 10–30 min; repeat in 6 h PRN *ECC 2010: Hyperkalemia/hypermagnesemia/CCB OD:* 500–1000 mg (5–10 mL of 10% soln) IV; repeat PRN; comparable dose of 10% calcium gluconate is 15–30 mL *Peds. Tetany:* 10 mg/kg CaCl over 5–10 min; repeat in 6–8 h or use Inf (200 mg/kg/d max). *ECC 2010: Hypocalcemia/hyperkalemia/hypermagnesemia/CCB OD:* Calcium chloride or gluconate 20 mg/kg (0.2 mL/kg) slow IV/IO, repeat PRN; central venous route preferred *Adults &Peds.* ↓ Ca²⁺ d/t citrated blood Inf: 0.45 mEq Ca/100 mL citrated blood Inf (↓ in renal impair) **Caution:** [C, ?] **CI:** ↑ Ca²⁺, suspected digoxin tox **Disp:** CaCl Inj 10% = 100 mg/mL = Ca 27.2 mg/mL = 10-mL amp; Ca gluconate Inj 10% = 100 mg/mL = Ca 9 mg/mL; tabs 500 mg = 45-mg Ca, 650 mg = 58.5 mg Ca, 975 mg = 87.75-mg Ca, 1 g = 90 mg Ca; Ca gluceptate Inj 220 mg/mL = 18 mg/mL Ca **SE:** ↓ HR, cardiac arrhythmias, ↑ Ca²⁺, constipation **Notes:** CaCl 270 mg (13.6 mEq) elemental Ca/g, & calcium gluconate 90 mg (4.5 mEq) Ca/g. RDA for Ca: *Peds < 6 mo:* 210 mg/d; *6 mo–1 y:* 270 mg/d; *1–3 y:* 500 mg/d; *4–9 y:* 800 mg/d; *10–18 y:* 1200 mg/d. *Adults.* 1000 mg/d; *> 50 y:* 1200 mg/d **Interactions:** ↑ Effects *OF* quinidine & digitalis; ↓ effects *OF* tetracyclines, quinolones, verapamil, CCBs, Fe salts, ASA, atenolol; ↓ Ca absorption *W/* high intake of dietary fiber **Labs:** Monitor for ↑ Ca²⁺, ↓ Mg²⁺ **NIPE:** ⊘ EtOH, caffeine, tobacco; separate Ca supls & other meds/fiber-containing foods by 1–2 h

Calfactant (Infasurf) [RDS Agent/Surfactant]
Uses: *Prevention & Rx of RDS in infants* **Action:** Exogenous pulm surfactant **Dose:** 3 mL/kg instilled into lungs. Can repeat 3 total doses given 12 h apart **Caution:** [?, ?] **Disp:** Intratracheal

susp 35 mg/mL **SE:** Monitor for cyanosis, airway obst, ↓ HR during administration **Interactions:** None noted **NIPE:** Only for intratracheal use; ⊘ reconstitute, dilute, or shake vial; refrigerate & keep away from light; no need to warm soln prior to use; ✓ freq ABGs; ✓ lungs for adventitious breath sounds (crackles, rales, rhonchi)

Canagliflozin (Invokana) **Uses:** *Type 2 DM* **Acts:** Sodium-glucose co-transporter 2 (SGLT2) inhib **Dose:** *Adults.* Start 100 mg/d; ↑ to 300 mg PRN w/ GFR > 60 mL/min **Caution:** [C, −] ↓ BP from ↓ vol from glucosuria; ↑ K+; ↑ Cr, ✓ renal Fxn; genital mycotic infections; hypoglycemia lower risk than insulin & sulfonylureas; hypersens **CI:** Hypersens reaction, severe renal impairment (GFR < 45 mL/min) **Disp:** Tabs 100, 300 mg **SE:** UTI, genital mycotic infections (3–15%) less likely to occur in circumcised males, polyuria, ↑ K+, ↑ PO_4^{3-}, ↑ Mg^{2+}, ↑ creat, ↑ LDL-chol **Notes:** First in class w/ FDA approval; may ↑ CV morbidity in first 30 d of Tx; CrCl 45–60 mL/min 100 mg/d max, do NOT use w/ CrCl < 45 mL/min; wgt loss likely; do not use w/ severe liver Dz; ↑ adverse events in geriatric pop; metabolized by UDP-glucuronosyl transferase 1A9 & 2B4, concomitant rifampin, phenytoin, or ritonavir use reduces exposure, may need to ↑ dose; may need to ↓ digoxin dose. **NIPE:** Give before 1st meal of the day; change position slowly; ✓ for orthostatic BP

Candesartan (Atacand) [Antihypertensive/ARB] **WARNING:** w/ PRG D/C immediately **Uses:** *HTN, CHF*, **Action:** Angiotensin II receptor antagonist **Dose:** 4–32 mg/d (usual 16 mg/d) **Caution:** [C (1st tri), D (2nd tri), ?/−] w/ renal disease **CI:** Component hypersens **Disp:** Tabs 4, 8, 16, 32 mg **SE:** Dizziness, HA, flushing, angioedema; ↑ K+, ↑ SCr **Interactions:** ↑ Effects *W*/ cimetidine; ↑ risk of hyperkalemia *W*/ amiloride, spironolactone, triamterene, K+ supls, TMP; ↑ effects *OF* Li; ↓ effects *W*/ phenobarbital, rifampin **Labs:** ↑ SCr, ↑ K+, monitor for albuminuria, hyperglycemia, triglyceridemia, uricemia **NIPE:** ⊘ Breast-feeding or PRG, use barrier contraception, may take 4–6 wk for full effect, adequate fluid intake, take w/o regard to food

Capsaicin (Capsin, Zostrix, Others) [Topical Anesthetic/Analgesic] [OTC] **Uses:** Pain d/t *postherpetic neuralgia*, *arthritis, diabetic neuropathy*, *minor pain of muscles & joints*; **Action:** Topical analgesic **Dose:** Apply tid–qid **Caution:** [B, ?] **Disp:** OTC creams; gel; lotions; roll-ons **SE:** Local irritation, neurotox, cough **Interactions:** May ↑ cough *W*/ ACEIs **NIPE:** External use only; wk to onset of action; ⊘ contact w/eyes or broken/ irritated skin; apply w/ gloves; transient stinging/ burning; ⊘ bandage or wrap treated area

Captopril (Capoten, Others) [Antihypertensive/ACEI] **Uses:** *HTN, CHF, MI*, LVD, diabetic neuropathy **Action:** ACE Inhib **Dose:** *Adults. HTN:* Initial, 25 mg PO bid–tid; ↑ to maint q1–2wk by 25-mg increments/dose (max 450 mg/d) to effect *CHF:* Initial, 6.25–12.5 mg PO tid; titrate PRN *LVD:* 50 mg PO tid. *DN:* 25 mg PO tid **Peds.** Infants 0.15–0.3 mg/kg/dose PO ÷ 1–4 doses **Children:** Initial, 0.3–0.5 mg/kg/dose PO; ↑ to 6 mg/kg/d max in 2–4 ÷ doses; 1 h ac; ↓ dose renal impairment **Caution:** [D, −] **CI:** Hx angioedema **Disp:** Tabs 12.5, 25, 50, 100 mg **SE:** Rash, proteinuria, cough, ↑ K⁺ **Interactions:** ↑ Effects W/ antihypertensives, diuretics, nitrates, probenecid, black catechu; ↓ effects W/ antacids, ASA, NSAIDs, food; ↑ effects OF digoxin, insulin, oral hypoglycemics, Li **Labs:** False (+) urine acetone; ↑ K⁺; may ↓ glucose, Hgb, Hct, RBC, WBC, plt **NIPE:** ⊘ PRG, breast-feeding, K⁺-sparing diuretics; take w/o food, give 1 h < meals; may take 2 wk for full therapeutic effect; ⊘ skip or reduce dose (↑ risk of rebound HTN)

Carbamazepine (Tegretol XR, Carbatrol, Epitol, Equetro) [Anticonvulsant/Analgesic]

WARNING: Aplastic anemia & agranulocytosis have been reported w/ carbamazepine; pts w/ Asian ancestry should be tested to determine potential for skin Rxns **Uses:** *Epilepsy, trigeminal neuralgia, acute mania w/ bipolar disorder (Equetro)* EtOH withdrawal **Action:** Anticonvulsant **Dose:** **Adults.** *Initial:* 200 mg PO bid or 100 mg 4 ×/d as susp; ↑ by 200 mg/d; usual 800–1200 mg/d ÷ doses *Acute Mania (Equetro):* 400 mg/d, adjust by 200 mg/d to response 1600 mg/d max **Peds < 6 y.** 10–20 mg/kg ÷ bid-tid or qid (susp) **6–12 y.** *Initial:* 200 mg/d bid (tab) or qid (susp), ↑ 100 mg/d, usual: 400–800 mg/d, max 1000 mg/d; ↓ in renal impair; take w/ food **Caution:** [D, M] **CI:** w/in 14 d, w/ nefazodone, MAOI use, Hx BM suppression **Disp:** Tabs 200 mg; chewtabs 100 mg; XR tabs 100, 200, 400 mg; *Equetro* Caps ER 100, 200, 300 mg; susp 100 mg/5 mL **SE:** Drowsiness, dizziness, blurred vision, N/V, rash, SJS/toxic epidermal necrolysis (TEN), ↓ Na⁺, leukopenia, agranulocytosis **Notes:** *Trough:* Just before next dose *Therapeutic peak:* 8–12 mcg/mL (monotherapy), 4–8 mcg/mL (polytherapy) *Toxic trough:* > 15 mcg/mL; *half-life:* 15–20 h; generic products not interchangeable, many drug interactions, administer susp in 3–4 ÷ doses daily; skin txn (SJS/TEN) ↑ w/ HLA-B* 1502 allele **Interactions:** ↑ Effects W/ cimetidine, clarithromycin, danazol, diltiazem, felbamate, fluconazole, fluoxetine, fluvoxamine, INH, itraconazole, ketoconazole, macrolides, metronidazole, propoxyphene, protease Inhibs, valproic acid, verapamil, grapefruit juice; ↑ effects OF Li, MAOIs; ↓ effects W/ phenobarbital, phenytoin, primidone, plantain; ↓ effects OF benzodiazepines, corticosteroids, cyclosporine, doxycycline, felbamate, haloperidol, OCPs, phenytoin, theophylline, thyroid hormones, TCAs, warfarin **Labs:** ↑ Na+, monitor CBC & drug levels; ↑ eosinophil count; ↓ Hgb, Hct, WBC, plts; ↓ LFTs, thyroid hormones; ↑ BUN **NIPE:** Take w/ food; ⊘ grapefruit products; ⊘ EtOH; may cause photosensitivity—use sunscreen; use barrier contraception; abrupt withdrawal may cause Sz; ⊘ breast-feeding or PRG; monitor bld levels/ CBC freq during 1st 3 mo of Tx & qm × 2–3 y thereafter

Carbidopa/Levodopa (Sinemet, Parcopa) [Antiparkinsonian/Dopamine Agonist]

Uses: *Parkinson Dz* **Action:** ↑ CNS dopamine levels **Dose:** 25/100 mg tid, ↑ as needed (max 200/2000 mg/d) **Caution:** [C, ?] **CI:** NAG, suspicious skin lesion (may activate melanoma), melanoma, MAOI use (w/in 14 d) **Disp:** Tabs (mg carbidopa/mg levodopa) 10/100, 25/100, 25/250; tabs SR (mg carbidopa/mg levodopa) 25/100, 50/200; ODT 10/100, 25/100, 25/250 **SE:** Psych disturbances, orthostatic ↓ BP, dyskinesias, cardiac arrhythmias **Interactions:** ↑ Risk of hypotension W/ antihypertensives; ↑ risk of HTN W/ MAOIs; ↑ effects W/ antacids; ↓ effects W/ anticholinergics, anticonvulsants, benzodiazepines, haloperidol, Fe, methionine, papaverine, phenothiazines, phenytoin, pyridoxine, reserpine, spiramycin, tacrine, thioxanthenes, high-protein food **Labs:** ↑ Alk phos, AST, bilirubin, BUN, uric acid, ↓ Hgb, plts, WBCs **NIPE:** Darkened urine & sweat may result; ⊘ crush or chew SR tabs; space doses evenly while awake; take w/o food; muscle or eyelid twitching may suggest tox

Carboplatin (Paraplatin) [Antineoplastic/Alkylating Agent]

WARNING: Administration only by physician experienced in CA chemotherapy; ↓ PLT, anemia, ↑ Infxn; BM suppression possible; anaphylaxis and V may occur **Uses:** *Ovarian*, lung, head & neck, testicular, urothelial, & brain CA, NHL & allogeneic & ABMT in high doses **Action:** DNA cross-linker; forms DNA-platinum adducts **Dose:** Per protocols based on target (Calvert formula: mg = AUC × [25 + calculated GFR]); adjust based on plt count, CrCl, & BSA (Egorin formula); up to 1500 mg/m² used in ABMT setting (per protocols) **Caution:** [D, ?] severe hepatic tox **CI:** Severe BM suppression, excessive bleeding **Disp:** Inj 50-, 150-, 450-, 650-mg vial (10 mg/mL) **SE:** Pain, ↓ Na⁺/Mg²⁺/Ca²⁺/K⁺, anaphylaxis, ↓ BM, N/V/D, nephrotox, hematuria, neurotox, ↑ LFTs **Notes:** Physiologic dosing based on Culvert or Egorin formula allows ↑ doses w/ ↓ tox **Interactions:** ↑ Myelosuppression W/ myelosuppressive drugs; ↑ hematologic effects W/ BM suppressants; ↑ bleeding W/ ASA; ↑ nephrotox W/ nephrotoxic drugs; ↓ effects OF phenytoin **Labs:** Monitor for ↑ LFTs, BUN, Cr; ↓ Mg²⁺, Na, Ca, K, CBC levels **NIPE:** ⊘ U sew/Al needles or IV administration sets, PRG, breast-feeding; antiemetics prior to administration may prevent N/V, maint adequate food & fluid intake; ⊘ immunizations w/o MD approval

Carfilzomib (Kyprolis)

Uses: *Multiple myeloma w/ > 2 prior therapies and prog w/in 60 d* **Acts:** Proteasome inhib **Dose:** 20 mg/m₂/d, if tolerated ↑ to 27 mg/m²/d; IV over 2–10 min; cycle = 2 consecutive d/wk × 3 wk, then 12-d rest; hydrate before and after admin, premedicate w/ dexamethasone first cycle, dose escalation or if infusion reactions **Caution:** [D, –] CHF, cardiac ischemia; pulm HTN, dyspnea; tumor lysis synd; ↓ plts, ↓ plts, ✓ plts; hepatic toxicity, ✓ LFTs **CI:** None **Disp:** Vial, 60 mg powder **SE:** N, D, fever, fatigue, dyspnea, ARF, anemia, ↓ plts, ↓ lymphocytes, ↑ LFTs, peripheral neuropathy **NIPE:** Avoid dehydration; ⊘ PRG; use effective contraception during Tx; ✓ for SOB—usually occurs w/in 1 day of dosing

Carisoprodol (Soma)

Uses: *Acute (limit 2–3 wk) painful musculoskeletal conditions* **Acts:** Centrally acting muscle relaxant **Dose:** 250–350 mg PO tid-qid **Caution:** [C, M] Tolerance may result; w/ renal/hepatic impair, w/ CYP219 poor metabolizers **CI:** Allergy to meprobamate; acute intermittent porphyria **Disp:** Tabs 250, 350 mg **SE:** CNS depression, drowsiness, dizziness, HA, tachycardia, weakness, rare Sz **Notes:** Avoid EtOH & other CNS depressants; avoid abrupt D/C; available in combo w/ ASA or codeine. **NIPE:** Avoid EtOH & other CNS depressants;

avoid abrupt D/C (withdrawal); available incombo w/ ASA or codeine; ⊘ breast-feeding; take w/food if GI upset; for short-term use (2–3 wk)

Carmustine [BCNU] (BiCNU, Gliadel) [Antineoplastic, Alkylating Agent] WARNING: BM suppression, dose-related pulm tox possible; administer under direct supervision of experienced physician Uses: *Primary or adjunct brain tumors, multiple myeloma, Hodgkin & non-Hodgkin lymphoma*, induction for autologous stem cell or BMT (off-label) surgery & RT adjunct high-grade glioma and recurrent glioblastoma (*Gliadel* implant) Action: Alkylating agent; nitrosourea forms DNA cross-links to inhibit DNA Dose: 150–200 mg/m² q6–8wk single or ÷ dose daily Inj over 2 d; 20–65 mg/m² q4–6wk; 300–600 mg/m² in BMT (per protocols); up to 8 implants in CNS op site; ↓ w/ hepatic & renal impair Caution: [D,?/–] ↓ WBC, RBC, plt counts, renal/hepatic impair CI: ↓ BM, PRG Disp: Inj 100 mg/vial *Gliadel* wafer: 7.7 mg SE: Inf Rxn, ↓ BP, N/V, ↓WBC & plt, phlebitis, facial flushing, hepatic/ renal dysfunction, pulm fibrosis (may occur years after), optic neuroretinitis; heme tox may persist 4–6 wk after dose Notes: Do not give course more frequently than q6wk (cumulative tox) Interactions: ↑ Bleeding W/ ASA, anticoagulants, NSAIDs; ↑ hepatic dysfunction W/ etoposide; ↑ suppression of BM W/ cimetidine, radiation or additional antineoplastics; ↓ effects OF phenytoin, digoxin; ↓ pulm Fxn Labs: ↑ AST, alk phos, bilirubin; ↓ Hgb, Hct, WBC, RBC, plt counts; monitor PFTs NIPE: ⊘ PRG, breast-feeding, exposure to Infxns, ASA products; obtain baseline PFTs w/ freq ✓ PFTs during Tx, monitor pulm status

Carteolol Ophthalmic (Generic) [Beta-Blocker/Glaucoma Agent] Uses: *↑ IOP pressure, chronic open-angle glaucoma* Action: Blocks β-adrenergic receptors (β₁, β₂), mild ISA Dose: Ophthal 1 gtt in eye(s) bid Caution: [C, ?/–] Cardiac failure, asthma CI: Sinus bradycardia; heart block > 1st degree; bronchospasm Disp: Ophthal soln 1% SE: conjunctival hyperemia, anisocoria, keratitis, eye pain NIPE: Ophthal drug may cause photophobia & risk of burning; may ↑ cold sensitivity, mental confusion; no value in CHF; oral forms no longer available in US

Carvedilol (Coreg, Coreg CR) [Antihypertensive/Alpha-1 & Beta-Blocker] Uses: *HTN, mild–severe CHF, LVD post-MI* Action: Blocks adrenergic receptors, β₁, β₂, α₁ Dose: *HTN:* 6.25–12.5 mg bid or CR 20–80 mg PO daily. *CHF:* 3.125–25 mg bid; w/ food to minimize orthostatic ↓ BP Caution: [C, ?/–] Asthma, DM CI: Decompensated CHF, 2nd-/3rd-degree heart block, SSS, severe ↓ HR w/o pacemaker, acute asthma, severe hepatic impair Disp: Tabs 3.125, 6.25, 12.5, 25 mg; CR tabs 10, 20, 40, 80 mg SE: Dizziness, fatigue, hyperglycemia, may mask/potentiate hypoglycemia, bradycardia, edema, hypercholesterolemia Interactions: ↑ Effects W/ cimetidine, clonidine, MAOIs, reserpine, verapamil, fluoxetine, paroxetine, EtOH; ↑ effects OF digoxin, hypoglycemics, cyclosporine, CCBs; ↓ effects W/ rifampin, NSAIDs Labs: ↑ Digoxin levels; ↑ LFTs, K⁺, triglycerides, uric acid, BUN, Cr, alk phos, glucose; ↓ pt, INR, plts

NIPE: Do not D/C abruptly; food slows absorption but reduces risk of dizziness; ✓ BP standing 1 h after dose; may cause dry eyes w/ contact lenses; takes 1–2 wk for full effect

Caspofungin (Cancidas) [Antifungal/Echinocandin] Uses: *Invasive aspergillosis refractory/intolerant to standard Rx, candidemia & other candida Inf*, empiric Rx in febrile neutropenia w/ presumed fungal Infxn **Action:** Echinocandin; ↓ fungal cell wall synth; highest activity in regions of active cell growth **Dose:** 70 mg IV load day 1, 50 mg/d IV; slow Inf over 1 h; ↓ in hepatic impair **Caution:** [C, ?/−] Do not use w/ cyclosporine **CI:** Allergy to any component **Disp:** Inj 50, 70 mg powder for recons **SE:** Fever, N/V, thrombophlebitis at site, ↑ LFTs, ↓ BP, edema, ↑ HR, rash, ↓ K, D, Inf Rxn **Interactions:** ↑ Effects W/ cyclosporine; ↓ effects W/ carbamazepine, dexamethasone, efavirenz, nelfinavir, nevirapine, phenytoin, rifampin; ↓ effect OF tacrolimus **Labs:** ↑ LFTs, serum alk phos; ↓ K+, Hgb, Hct **NIPE:** Monitor during Inf; infuse slowly over 1 h & ⊘ mix w/ other drugs; limited experience beyond 2 wk of Rx; ↓ BP, edema; ↑ HR, rash; ✓ S/Sx hepatic dysfunction

Cefaclor (Ceclor, Raniclor) [Antibiotic/Cephalosporin-2nd Generation] Uses: *Bacterial Infxns of the upper & lower resp tract, skin, bone, urinary tract* **Action:** 2nd-gen cephalosporin; ↓ cell wall synth. *Spectrum:* More gram(−) activity than 1st-gen cephalosporins; effective against gram(+) (*Streptococcus* sp, *S aureus*); good gram(−) against *H influenza, E coli, Klebsiella, Proteus* **Dose:** *Adults.* 250–500 mg PO > q8h. *Peds.* 20–40 mg/kg/d PO ÷ 8–12 h; ↓ renal impair **Caution:** [B, M] **CI:** Cephalosporin/PCN allergy **Disp:** Caps 250, 500 mg; tabs ER 500 mg; susp 125, 250, 375 mg/5 mL **SE:** Rash, eosinophilia, ↑ LFTs, HA, rhinitis, vaginitis **Interactions:** ↑ Bleeding W/ anticoagulants; ↑ nephrotox W/ aminoglycosides, loop diuretics; ↑ effects W/ probenecid; ↓ effects W/ antacids, chloramphenicol **Labs:** ↑ LFTs, eosinophilia; ↓ Hgb, Hct, plts, WBC; false(+) direct Coombs test **NIPE:** Take w/food to < GI upset; monitor for super Infxn, ⊘ antacids w/in 2 h of XR tabs; chewable tabs must be chewed; space doses evenly

Cefadroxil (Duricef) [Antibiotic/Cephalosporin-1st Generation] Uses: *Infxns skin, bone, upper & lower resp tract, urinary tract* **Action:** 1st-gen cephalosporin; ↓ cell wall synth. *Spectrum:* Good gram(+) (group A β-hemolytic *Streptococcus, Staphylococcus*); gram(−) (*E coli, Proteus, Klebsiella*) **Dose:** *Adults.* 1–2 g/d PO, 2 ÷ doses *Peds.* 30 mg/kg/d ÷ bid; ↓ in renal impair **Caution:** [B, M] **CI:** Cephalosporin/PCN allergy **Disp:** Caps 500 mg; tabs 1 g; susp, 250, 500 mg/5 mL **SE:** N/V/D, rash, eosinophilia, ↑ LFTs **Interactions:** ↑ Nephrotox W/ aminoglycosides, loop diuretics; ↑ effects W/ probenecid **Labs:** ↑ LFTs, eosinophilia, BUN, Cr; ↓ Hgb, Hct, plts, WBC false(+) direct Coombs test **NIPE:** Take w/ food to < GI upset; monitor for super Infxn; space doses evenly; refrigerate oral suspension

Cefazolin (Ancef, Kefzol) [Antibiotic/Cephalosporin-1st Generation] Uses: *Infxns of skin, bone, upper & lower resp tract, urinary tract*

Action: 1st-gen cephalosporin; β-lactam ↓ cell wall synth *Spectrum:* Good gram(+) bacilli & cocci, (*Streptococcus, Staphylococcus* [except *Enterococcus*]); some gram(−) (*E coli, Proteus, Klebsiella*) **Dose:** *Adults.* 1–2 g IV q8h **Peds.** 25–100 mg/kg/d IV ÷ q6–8h; ↓ in renal impair **Caution:** [B, M] **CI:** Cephalosporin/PCN allergy **Disp:** Inj **SE:** D, rash, eosinophilia, ↑ LFTs, Inj site pain **Notes:** Widely used for surgical prophylaxis **Interactions:** ↑ Bleeding *W/* anticoagulants; ↑ nephrotox *W/* aminoglycosides, loop diuretics; ↑ effects *W/* probenecid; ↓ effects *W/* antacids, chloramphenicol **Labs:** ↑ LFTs, eosinophils; false(+) direct Coombs test, Clinitest; monitor PT in pts w/ hepatic/renal impair, long-term use, or on anticoagulant therapy **NIPE:** Take w/ food to < GI upset; monitor for super Infxn; monitor renal Fxn; complete full Tx course

Cefdinir (Omnicef) [Antibiotic/Cephalosporin-3rd Generation]

Uses: *Infxns of the resp tract, skin, and skin structure* **Action:** 3rd-gen cephalosporin; ↓ cell wall synth *Spectrum:* Many gram(+) & (−) organisms; more active than cefaclor & cephalexin against *Streptococcus, Staphylococcus*; some anaerobes **Dose:** *Adults.* 300 mg PO bid or 600 mg/d PO **Peds.** 7 mg/kG PO bid or 14 mg/kg/d PO; ↓ in renal impair **Caution:** [B, M] w/ PCN-sensitive pts, serum sickness-like Rxns reported **CI:** Hypersens to cephalosporins **Disp:** Caps 300 mg; susp 125, 250 mg/5 mL **SE:** Anaphylaxis, D, rare pseudomembranous colitis, HA **Interactions:** ↑ Bleeding *W/* anticoagulants; ↑ nephrotox *W/* aminoglycosides, loop diuretics; ↑ effects *W/* probenecid; ↓ effects *W/* antacids, chloramphenicol; ↓ effects *W/* Fe supls **Labs:** ↑ LFTs, eosinophils; false(+) direct Coombs test & Clinitest **NIPE:** Take w/food to < GI upset; monitor for super Infxn; stools may initially turn red in color; instruct pt to report persistent D; ⊘ antacids w/in 2 h of this drug; space doses evenly; suspension contains sugar

Cefditoren (Spectracef) [Antibiotic/Cephalosporin-3rd Generation]

Uses: *Acute exacerbations of chronic bronchitis, pharyngitis, tonsillitis; skin Infxns* **Action:** 3rd-gen cephalosporin; ↓ cell wall synth *Spectrum:* Good gram(+) (*Streptococcus & Staphylococcus*); gram(−) (*H influenzae & M catarrhalis*) **Dose:** *Adults & Peds > 12 y. Skin also pharyngitis, tonsillitis:* 200 mg PO bid × 10 d *Chronic bronchitis:* 400 mg PO bid × 10 d; avoid antacids w/in 2 h; take w/meals; ↓ in renal impair **Caution:** [B, ?] Renal/hepatic impair **CI:** Cephalosporin/PCN allergy, milk protein, or carnitine deficiency **Disp:** Tabs 200, 400 mg **SE:** HA, N/V/D, colitis, nephrotox, hepatic dysfunction, SJS, toxic epidermal necrolysis, allergic Rxns **Notes:** Causes renal excretion of carnitine; tabs contain milk protein **Interactions:** ↑ Bleeding *W/* anticoagulants; ↑nephrotox *W/* aminoglycosides, loop diuretics; ↑ effects *W/* probenecid; ↓ effects *W/* antacids, chloramphenicol **Labs:** ↑ LFTs; ↓ PT, monitor PT in renal or hepatic impair or poor nutritional state; false(+) direct Coombs test & Clinitest **NIPE:** High-fat meal will ↑ bioavailability; monitor for super Infxn; report persistent D; ⊘ antacids w/in 2 h of this drug; causes renal excretion of carnitine; tabs contain milk protein

Cefepime (Maxipime) [Antibiotic/Cephalosporin-4th Generation]
Uses: *Comp/uncomp UTI, pneumonia, empiric febrile neutropenia, skin/soft tissue Infxns, comp intra-Abd Infxns* **Action:** 4th-gen cephalosporin; ↓ cell wall synth *Spectrum:* Gram(+) *S pneumoniae, S aureus,* gram(−) *K pneumoniae, E coli, P aeruginosa,* & *Enterobacter* sp **Dose: Adults.** 1–2 g IV q8–12h **Peds.** 50 mg/kg q8h for febrile neutropenia; 50 mg/kg bid for skin/soft-tissue Infxns; ↓ in renal impair **Caution:** [B, +]; Sz risk w/ CrCl < 60 mL/min; adjust dose w/ renal Insuff **CI:** Cephalosporin/ PCN allergy **Disp:** Inj 500 mg, 1, 2 g **SE:** Rash, pruritus, N/V/D, fever, HA **Interactions:** ↑ Nephrotox *W/* aminoglycosides, loop diuretics; ↑ effects *W/* probenecid **Labs:** ↑ LFTs; ↓ Hgb, Hct, PT; (+) Coombs test w/o hemolysis **NIPE:** Monitor for super Infxn; report persistent D; monitor Inf site for inflammation; can give IM or IV; ✓ ↑ risk of neurotoxicity in pts w/ renal impairment (confusion, hallucinations, stupor, coma, seizures)

Cefixime (Suprax) [Antibiotic/Cephalosporin-3rd Generation]
Uses: *Resp tract, skin, bone, & urinary tract Infxns* **Action:** 3rd-gen cephalosporin; ↓ cell wall synth *Spectrum: S pneumoniae, S pyogenes, H influenzae,* & enterobacteria **Dose: Adults.** 400 mg PO ÷ daily–bid **Peds.** 8 mg/kg/d PO ÷ daily–bid; ↓ w/ renal impair **Caution:** [B, ?] **CI:** Cephalosporin/ PCN allergy **Disp:** Tabs 400 mg, 100, 200 mg chew tab, susp 100, 200 mg/5 mL **SE:** N/V/D, flatulence, & Abd pain **Interactions:** ↑ Nephrotox *W/* aminoglycosides, loop diuretics; ↑ effects *W/* nifedipine, probenecid **Labs:** ↑ LFTs, eosinophils, BUN, Cr monitor renal & hepatic Fxn; WBC; false(+) direct Coombs test **NIPE:** Monitor for super Infxn; after mixing susp it is stable for 14 d w/o refrigeration; use susp for otitis media; take w/o regard to food; ✓ for S/Sx thrush; space doses evenly

Cefotaxime (Claforan) [Antibiotic/Cephalosporin-3rd Generation]
Uses: *Infxns of lower resp tract, skin, bone & jt, urinary tract, meningitis, sepsis, PID, GC* **Action:** 3rd-gen cephalosporin; ↓ cell wall synth *Spectrum:* Most gram(−) (not *Pseudomonas*), some gram(+) cocci *S pneumoniae, S aureus* (penicillinase/nonpenicillinase producing), *H influenzae* (including ampicillin-resistant), not *Enterococcus*; many PCN-resistant pneumococci **Dose: Adults.** *Uncomplicated Infxn:* 1 g IV/IM q12h; *Mod–severe Infxn* 1–2 g IV/IM q 8–12 h; Severe/septicemia 2 g IV/IM q4–8h; *GC urethritis, cervicitis, rectal in female:* 0.5 g IM × 1; rectal GC men 1 g IM × 1; **Peds.** 50–200 mg/kg/d IV ÷ q6–8h; ↓ w/ renal/hepatic impair **Caution:** [B, +] Arrhythmia w/ rapid Inj; w/ colitis **CI:** Cephalosporin/PCN allergy **Disp:** Powder for Inj 500 mg, 1, 2, 10 g, premixed Inf 20 mg/mL, 40 mg/mL **SE:** D, rash, pruritus, colitis, eosinophilia, ↑ transaminases **Interactions:** ↑ Nephrotox *W/* aminoglycosides, loop diuretics; ↑ effects *W/* probenecid **Labs:** ↑LFTs, eosinophils, transaminases, BUN, Cr; ↓ Hgb, Hct, plts, WBC **NIPE:** Monitor for super Infxn; IM Inj deep into large muscle mass; rotate Inf sites; ✓ for S/Sx thrush; space doses evenly

Cefotetan (Cefotan) [Antibiotic/Cephalosporin-2nd Generation]

Uses: *Infns of the upper & lower resp tract, skin, bone, urinary tract, Abd, & gynecologic system* **Action:** 2nd-gen cephalosporin; ↓ cell wall synth *Spectrum:* Less active against gram(+) anaerobes including *B fragilis*; gram(−), including *E coli, Klebsiella,* & *Proteus* **Dose: Adults.** 1–3 g IV q12h **Peds.** 20–40 mg/kg/d IV ÷ q12h (6 g/d max) ↓ w/ renal impair **Caution:** [B, +] May ↑ bleeding risk; w/ Hx of PCN allergies, w/other nephrotoxic drugs **CI:** Cephalosporin/PCN allergy **Disp:** Powder for Inj 1, 2, 10 g **SE:** D, rash, eosinophilia, ↑ transaminases, hypoprothrombinemia, & bleeding (d/t MTT side chain) **Interactions:** ↑ Bleeding *W/* anticoagulants; ↑ nephrotox *W/* aminoglycosides, loop diuretics **Labs:** ↑ LFTs, eosinophils; ↓ Hgb, Hct, plts **NIPE:** Monitor for super Infxn; rotate Inf sites; may interfere w/ warfarin; ⊘ ETOH

Cefoxitin (Mefoxin) [Antibiotic/Cephalosporin-2nd Generation]

Uses: *Infns of the upper & lower resp tract, skin, bone, urinary tract, Abd, & gynecologic system* **Action:** 2nd-gen cephalosporin; ↓ cell wall synth *Spectrum:* Good gram(−) against enteric bacilli (ie, *E coli, Klebsiella,* & *Proteus*); anaerobic: *B fragilis* **Dose: Adults.** 1–2 g IV q6–8h **Peds.** 80–160 mg/kg/d ÷ q4–6h (12 g/d max); ↓ w/ renal impair **Caution:** [B, M] **CI:** Cephalosporin/PCN allergy **Disp:** Powder for Inj 1, 2, 10 g **SE:** D, rash, eosinophilia, ↑ transaminases **Interactions:** ↑ Nephrotox *W/* aminoglycosides, loop diuretics; ↑effects *W/* probenecid **Labs:** ↑ LFTs, eosinophils, transaminases, BUN, Cr; ↓ Hgb, Hct, plts **NIPE:** Monitor for super Infxn, report persistent D

Cefpodoxime (Vantin) [Antibiotic/Cephalosporin-3rd Generation]

Uses: *Rx resp, skin, & urinary tract Infxns* **Action:** 3rd-gen cephalosporin; ↓ cell wall synth *Spectrum: S pneumonia* or non-β-lactamase-producing *H influenzae*; acute uncomplicated *N gonorrhoeae*; some uncomplicated gram(−) (*E coli, Klebsiella, Proteus*) **Dose: Adults.** 100–400 mg PO q12h **Peds.** 10 mg/kg/d PO ÷ bid; ↓ in renal impair, w/ food **Caution:** [B, M] **CI:** Cephalosporin/PCN allergy **Disp:** Tabs 100, 200 mg; susp 50, 100 mg/5 mL **SE:** D, rash, HA, eosinophilia, ↑ transaminases **Interactions:** Drug interactions w/ agents that ↑ gastric pH; ↑ nephrotox *W/* aminoglycosides, loop diuretics; ↑ effects *W/* probenecid; ↓ effects *W/* antacids, chloramphenicol **Labs:** ↑ LFTs, eosinophils, transaminases, BUN, Cr; ↓ Hgb, Hct, plts; (+) Coombs test **NIPE:** Food will ↑ absorption & < GI upset; monitor for super Infxn; take w/in 2 h of antacids; evenly space doses

Cefprozil (Cefzil) [Antibiotic/Cephalosporin-2nd Generation]

Uses: *Rx resp tract, skin, & urinary tract Infxns* **Action:** 2nd-gen cephalosporin; ↓ cell wall synth *Spectrum:* Active against MSSA, *Streptococcus,* & gram(−) bacilli (*E coli, Klebsiella, P mirabilis, H influenzae, Moraxella*) **Dose: Adults.** 250–500 mg PO daily–bid **Peds.** 7.5–15 mg/kg/d PO ÷ bid; ↓ in renal impair **Caution:** [B, M] **CI:** Cephalosporin/PCN allergy **Disp:** Tabs 250, 500 mg; susp 125, 250 mg/5 mL **SE:** D, dizziness, rash, eosinophilia, ↑ transaminases **Interactions:** ↑ Nephrotox

W/ aminoglycosides, loop diuretics; ↑ effects *W/* probenecid; ↓ effects *W/* antacids, chloramphenicol **Labs:** ↑ LFTs, eosinophils, transaminases; ↓ Hgb, Hct, plts **NIPE:** Food will ↑ absorption & < GI upset, monitor for super Infxn; ⊘ take w/in 2 h of antacids; stable after reconstition for 14 d—keep refrigerated; use higher doses for otitis & pneumonia; evenly space doses

Ceftaroline (Teflaro) [Cephalosporin] Uses: *Tx skin/skin structure Infxn & CAP* **Action:** Unclassified ("5th-gen") cephalosporin; ↓ cell wall synthesis *Spectrum:* Gram(+) *Staph aureus* (MSSA/MRSA), *Strep pyogenes, Strep agalactiae, Strep pneumoniae*; gram(−) *E coli, K pneumoniae, K oxytoca, H influenzae* **Dose: Adults.** 600 mg IV q12h; CrCl 30–50 mL/min: 400 mg IV q12h; CrCl 15–29 mL/min: 300 mg IV q12h; CrCl < 15 mL/min, 200 mg IV q12h; Inf over 1 h **Caution:** [B. ?/−] Monitor for *C difficile*–associated D **CI:** Cephalsporin sensitivity **Disp:** Inj 600 mg **SE:** Hypersens Rxn, D/N, rash, constipation, ↓ K⁺ phlebitis, ↑ LFTs **Labs:** ↑ LFTs, (+) Coombs test; ↓ K⁺ **NIPE:** ✓ Suprainfxn; ✓ S/Sx thrush; space doses evenly

Ceftazidime (Fortaz, Tazicef) [Antibiotic/Cephalosporin-3rd Generation] Uses: *Rx resp tract, skin, bone, urinary tract Infxns, meningitis, & septicemia* **Action:** 3rd-gen cephalosporin; ↓ cell wall synth *Spectrum: P aeruginosa* sp, good gram(−) activity **Dose: Adults.** 500–2 g IV/IM q8–12h **Peds.** 30–50 mg/ kg/dose IV q8h 6g/d max; ↓ in renal impair **Caution:** [B,+] PCN sensitivity **CI:** Cephalosporin/PCN allergy **Disp:** Powder for Inj 500 mg, 1, 2, 6 g **SE:** D, rash, eosinophilia, ↑ transaminases **Interactions:** ↑ Nephrotox *W/* aminoglycosides, loop diuretics; ↑ effects *W/* probenecid; ↓ effects *W/* antacids, chloramphenicol **Labs:** ↑ LFTs, eosinophils, transaminases; ↓ Hgb, Hct, plts **NIPE:** Food will ↑ absorption & < GI upset, monitor for super Infxn; ⊘ take w/in 2 h of antacids; stable after reconstition for 14 d—keep refrigerated; use only for proven or strongly suspected Infxn to ↓ development of drug resistance; ✓ S/Sx thrush

Ceftibuten (Cedax) [Antibiotic/Cephalosporin-3rd Generation] Uses: *Rx resp tract, skin, urinary tract Infxns, & otitis media* **Action:** 3rd-gen cephalosporin; ↓ cell wall synth. *Spectrum: H influenzae & M catarrhalis*; weak against *S pneumoniae* **Dose: Adults.** 400 mg/d PO **Peds.** 9 mg/kg/d PO; ↓ in renal impair; take on empty stomach (susp) **Caution:** [B, +/−] **CI:** Cephalosporin/ PCN allergy **Disp:** Caps 400 mg; susp 90 mg/5 mL **SE:** D, rash **Interactions:** ↑ Nephrotox *W/* aminoglycosides, loop diuretics; ↑ effects *W/* probenecid; ↓ effects *W/* antacids, chloramphenicol **Labs:** ↑ LFTs, eosinophils, transaminases; ↓ Hgb, Hct, plts **NIPE:** Take oral suspension 1 h < or 2 h > a meal; monitor for super Infxn; stable after reconstition for 14 d—keep refrigerated; ✓ S/S × thrush; report persistant D

Ceftriaxone (Rocephin) [Antibiotic/Cephalosporin-3rd Generation] WARNING: Avoid in hyperbilirubinemic neonates or co-infusion *w/* calcium-containing products **Uses:** *Resp tract (pneumonia), skin, bone, Abd & urinary tract

Infxns, meningitis, septicemia, GC, PID, perioperative* **Action:** 3rd-gen cephalosporin; ↓ cell wall synth *Spectrum:* Mod gram(+); excellent β-lactamase producers **Dose:** *Adults.* 1–2 g IV/IM q12–24h *Peds.* 50–100 mg/kg/d IV/IM ÷ q12–24h **Caution:** [B, +] **CI:** Cephalosporin allergy; hyperbilirubinemic neonates **Disp:** Powder for Inj 250 mg, 500 mg, 1, 2, 10 g; premixed 20, 40 mg/mL **SE:** D, rash, ↑ WBC, thrombocytosis, eosinophilia, ↑ LFTs **Interactions:** ↑ Nephrotox *W/* aminoglycosides, loop diuretics; ↑ effects *W/* probenecid **Labs:** ↑ LFTs, eosinophils, BUN, Cr; ↓ Hgb, Hct, plts **NIPE:** ✓ for super Infxn; solns are stable for 24 h at room temperature after dilution; IM Inj deep into large muscle mass; ✓ S/Sx thrush

Cefuroxime (Ceftin [PO], Zinacef [Parenteral]) [Antibiotic/ Cephalosporin-2nd Generation]
Uses: *Upper & lower resp tract, skin, bone, urinary tract, Abd, gynecologic Infxns* **Action:** 2nd-gen cephalosporin; ↓ cell wall synth *Spectrum:* Staphylococci, group B streptococci, *H influenzae, E coli, Enterobacter, Salmonella,* & *Klebsiella* **Dose:** *Adults.* 750 mg–1.5 g IV q6h or 250–500 mg PO bid *Peds.* 75–150 mg/kg/d IV ÷ q8h or 20–30 mg/kg/d PO ÷ bid; ↓ w/renal impair; take PO w/food **Caution:** [B, +] **CI:** Cephalosporin/ PCN allergy **Disp:** Tabs 250, 500 mg; susp 125, 250 mg/5 mL; powder for Inj 750 mg, 1.5, 7.5 g **SE:** D, rash, eosinophilia, ↑ LFTs **Notes:** Cefuroxime film-coated tabs & susp not bioequivalent; do not substitute on a mg/mg basis; IV crosses blood–brain barrier **Interactions:** ↑ Nephrotox *W/* aminoglycosides, loop diuretics; ↑ effects *W/* probenecid; ↑ effects *W/* Al & Mg antacids **Labs:** ↑ LFTs, eosinophils, BUN, Cr; ↓ Hgb, Hct, plts **NIPE:** ✓ For super Infxn; high-fat meals ↑ drug bioavailability; give suspension w/ food; IM Inj deep into large muscle mass; avoid crushing tab due to bitter taste

Celecoxib (Celebrex) [Anti-Inflammatory/COX-2 Inhibitor]
WARNING: ↑ Risk of serious CV thrombotic events, MI, & stroke; can be fatal; ↑ risk of serious GI adverse events including bleeding, ulceration, & perforation of the stomach or intestines; can be fatal **Uses:** *OA, RA, ankylosing spondylitis, acute pain, primary dysmenorrhea, preventive in FAP* **Action:** NSAID; ↓ COX-2 pathway **Dose:** 100–200 mg/d or bid; FAP: 400 mg PO bid; ↓ w/ hepatic impair; take w/ food/milk **Caution:** [C/D (3rd tri), ?] w/ Renal impair **CI:** Sulfonamide allergy, perioperative CABG **Disp:** Caps 50, 100, 200, 400 mg **SE:** See Warning; GI upset, HTN, edema, renal failure, HA **Interactions:** ↑ Effects *W/* fluconazole; ↑ effects *OF* Li; ↑ risks of GI upset and/or bleeding *W/* ASA, NSAIDs, warfarin, EtOH; ↓ effects *W/* Al- & Mg-containing antacids, ↓ effects *OF* thiazidediuretics, loop diuretics, ACEIs **Labs:** ↑ LFTs, BUN, Cr, CPK, alk phos; monitor for hypercholesterolemia, hyperglycemia, hypokalemia, hypophosphatemia, albuminuria, hematuria **NIPE:** Take w/ food if GI distress; watch for Sxs of GI bleed; no effect on plt/bleeding time; can affect drugs metabolized by P450 pathway; ⊘ antacids

Centruroides (Scorpion) Immune F(ab')₂ (Anascorp)
Uses: *Antivenom for scorpion envenomation w/ symptoms* **Acts:** IgG, bind/neutralize

Centruroides sculpturatus toxin **Dose: *Adult/Peds*.** 3 vials, recons w/ 5 mL NS, combine all 3, dilute to 50 mL, Inf IV over 10 min; 1 vial q 30–60 min PRN Sx **W/P:** [C, M] hypersens, especially w/ Hx equine protein Rxn **CI:** None **Disp:** Vial **SE:** Fever, N, V, pruritus, rash, myalgias, serum sickness **Notes:** Use only w/ important symptoms (loss of muscle control, abn eye movements, slurred speech, resp distress, salivation, vomiting); may contain infectious agents. **NIPE:** ✓ Pt closely during and for up to 60 min following infusion completion for resolution of clinical signs of envenomation (loss of muscle control, abnl eye movements, slurred speech, resp distress, excessive salivation, frothing at mouth, V)

Cephalexin (Keflex, Generic) [Antibiotic/Cephalosporin-1st Generation]

Uses: *Skin, bone, upper/lower resp tract (streptococcal pharyngitis), otitis media, uncomp cystitis Infxns* **Action:** 1st-gen cephalosporin; ↓ cell wall synth *Spectrum: Streptococcus* (including β-hemolytic), *Staphylococcus, E coli, Proteus,* & *Klebsiella* **Dose: *Adults & Peds > 15 y.*** 250–1000 mg PO qid; Rx cystitis 7–14 d (4 g/d max) ***Peds < 15 y.*** 25–100 mg/kg/d PO ÷ bid–qid; ↓ in renal impair; w/ or w/o food **Caution:** [B, +] **CI:** Cephalosporin/ PCN allergy **Disp:** Caps 250, 500 mg; susp, 125, 250 mg; susp 250 mg/5 **SE:** D, rash, eosinophilia, gastritis, dyspepsia. ↑ LFTs, *C difficile* colitis, vaginitis **Interactions:** ↑ Nephrotox **W/** aminoglycosides, loop diuretics; ↑ effects **W/** probenecid **Labs:** ↑ LFTs, eosinophils, alkphos, bilirubin, LDH; ↓ Hgb, Hct, plts **NIPE:** Food will ↑ absorption & < GI upset; monitor for super Infxns; oral susp stable for 14 d after reconstitution if refrigerated

Certolizumab Pegol (Cimzia) [Tumor Necrosis Factor Blocker]

WARNING: Serious Infxns (bacterial, fungal, TB, opportunistic) possible. D/C w/ severe Infxn/sepsis, test and monitor for TB w/ Tx; lymphoma/ other CA possible in children/adolescents **Uses:** *Crohn Dz w/ inadequate response to conventional Tx; mod–severe RA* **Action:** TNF-α blocker **Dose:** *Crohn: Initial:* 400 mg SQ, repeat 2 & 4 wk after; *Maint:* 400 mg SQ q4wk *RA: Initial:* 400 mg SQ, repeat 2 & 4 wk after; *Maint:* 200 mg SQ qowk or 400 mg SQ q4wk **Caution:** [B, ?] Infxn, TB, autoimmune Dz, demyelinating CNS Dz, hep B reactivation **CI:** None **Disp:** Inj. powder for reconstitution 200 mg; Inj. soln: 200 mg/mL (1 mL) **SE:** HA, N, URI, serious Infxns, TB, opportunistic Infxns, malignancies, demyelinating Dz, CHF, pancytopenia, lupus-like synd, new onset psoriasis **Interactions:** ↑ Risk of Infxn **W/** immunosuppressants **Labs:** May interfere w/ coagulation tests such as PTT **NIPE:** Do not give live/attenuated vaccines during therapy; avoid use w/ anakinra; 400 mg dose is 2 Inj of 200 mg each; monitor for Infxn

Cetirizine (Zyrtec, Zyrtec D) [Allergy/Antihistamine] [OTC]

Uses: *Allergic rhinitis & other allergic Sxs including urticaria* **Action:** Nonsedating antihistamine; *Zyrtec D* contains decongestant **Dose: *Adults & Children > 6 y.*** 5–10 mg/d. *Zyrtec D:* 5/120 mg PO bid whole ***Peds 6–11 mo.*** 2.5 mg daily. ***12 mo–5 y.*** 2.5 mg daily–bid; ↓ to qd in renal/hepatic impair **Caution:** [C, ?/–] w/ HTN, BPH, rare CNS stimulation, DM, heart Dz **CI:** Allergy to cetirizine, hydroxyzine **Disp:** Tabs 5, 10 mg; chew tabs 5, 10 mg; syrup 5 mg/5 mL; *Zyrtec D:*

Tabs 5/120 mg (cetirizine/pseudoephedrine) **SE:** HA, drowsiness, xerostomia **Interactions:** ↑ Effects *W/* anticholinergics, CNS depressants, theophylline, EtOH **Labs:** May cause false(−) w/allergy skin tests **NIPE:** ⊘ Take w/EtOH or CNS depressants can potentiate sedation; sun exposure can cause photosensitivity; swallow ER tabs whole

Cetuximab (Erbitux) [Antineoplastic/Recombinant Monoclonal Antibody] WARNING: Severe Inf Rxns including rapid onset of airway obst (bronchospasm, stridor, hoarseness), urticaria, & ↓ BP; permanent D/C required; ↑ risk sudden death & cardiopulmonary arrest **Uses:** *EGFR + metastatic colorectal CA w/ or w/o irinotecan, unresectable head/neck small cell CA w/ RT; monotherapy in metastatic head/neck CA* **Action:** Human/mouse recombinant MoAb; binds EGFR, ↓ tumor cell growth **Dose:** Per protocol; load 400 mg/m² IV over 2 h; 250 mg/m² given over 1 h weekly **Caution:** [C,−] **Disp:** Inj 100 mg/50 mL **SE:** Acneiform rash, asthenia/malaise, N/V/D, Abd pain, alopecia, Inf Rxn, derm tox, interstitial lung Dz, fever, sepsis, dehydration, kidney failure, PE **Notes:** Assess tumor for EGFR before Rx; pretreatment w/ diphenhydramine **Interactions:** N Topical steroids; ↑ possibility of cardiotox *W/* radiation & cisplatin **Labs:** Monitor lytes, Mg²⁺, Ca during & after drug therapy **NIPE:** ⊘ PRG; monitor for Inf Rxns for 1 h after Inf; during 1st 2 wk observe for skin tox; w/ mild SE ↓ Inf rate by 50%; limit sun exposure & UV light; use sunscreen; ⊘ immunizations w/o MD approval

Charcoal, Activated (Superchar, Actidose, Liqui-Char) [Adsorbent] Uses: *Emergency poisoning by most drugs & chemicals (see CI)* **Action:** Adsorbent detoxicant **Dose:** Give w/ 70% sorbitol (2 mL/kg); repeated use of sorbitol not OK *Adults. Acute intoxication:* 25–100 g/dose *GI dialysis:* 20–50 g q6h for 1–2 d *Peds 1–12 y. Acute intoxication:* 1–2g/kg/dose *GI dialysis:* 5–10g/dose q4–8h **Caution:** [C, ?] May cause V (hazardous w/ petroleum & caustic ingestions); do not mix w/ dairy **CI:** Not effective for cyanide, mineral acids, caustic alkalis, organic solvents, Fe, EtOH, methanol poisoning, Li; do not use sorbitol in pts w/ fructose intolerance, intestinal obst, non intact GI tracts **Disp:** Powder, liq, caps, tabs **SE:** Some Liq dosage forms in sorbitol base (acathartic); V/D, black stools, constipation **Notes:** Charcoal w/sorbitol not OK in children < 1 y; protect airway in lethargic/comatose pts **Interactions:** ↓ Effects if taken w/ ice cream, milk, sherbet; ↓ effects *OF* digoxin & absorption of other oral meds, ↓ effects *OF* syrup of ipecac **Labs:** Monitor for ↓ K⁺ & Mg²⁺ **NIPE:** Most effective if given w/in 30 min of acute poisoning; only give to conscious pts; ⊘ use w/ intestinal obstruction

Chloral Hydrate (Aquachloral, Supprettes) [Sedative/Hypnotic/ CNS Depressant] [C-IV] Uses: *Short-term nocturnal & pre-op sedation* **Action:** Sedative hypnotic; active metabolite trichloroethanol **Dose:** *Adults. Hypnotic:* 500 mg–1 g PO or PR 30 min hs or before procedure *Sedative:* 250 mg PO or PR tid *Peds. Hypnotic:* 20–50 mg/kg/24 h PO or PR 30 min hs or before procedure

Sedative: 5–15 mg/kg/dose q8h; avoid w/CrCl < 50 mL/min or severe hepatic impair **Caution:** [C, +] Porphyria & in neonates, long-term care facility residents **CI:** Allergy to components; severe renal, hepatic, or cardiac Dz **Disp:** Caps 500 mg; syrup 500 mg/5 mL; supp 325, 500 mg **SE:** GI irritation, drowsiness, ataxia, dizziness, nightmares, rash **Interactions:** ↑ Effects W/ antihistamines, barbiturates, paralde-hyde, CNS depressants, opiate analgesics, EtOH; ↑ effects OF anticoagulants **Labs:** ↑ Eosinophils, BUN; ↓ WBCs **NIPE:** ⊘ Take w/ EtOH, CNS depressants; ⊘ chew or crush caps; may accumulate; tolerance may develop > 2 wk; taper dose; mix syrup in H$_2$O or fruit juice; ⊘ use w/ severe liver or renal Dz

Chlorambucil (Leukeran) [Antineoplastic/Alkylating Agent]   WARN-ING: Myelosuppressive, carcinogenic, teratogenic, associated w/ infertility Uses: *CLL, Hodgkin Dz*, Waldenström macroglobulinemia **Action:** Alkylating agent (nitrogen mustard) **Dose:** (per protocol) 0.1–0.2 mg/kg/d for 3–6 wk or 0.4 mg/kg/dose q2wk; ↓w/ renal impair **Caution:** [D, ?] Sz disorder & BM suppression; affects human fertility **CI:** Previous resistance; alkylating agent allergy; w/ live vaccines **Disp:** Tabs 2 mg **SE:** ↓ BM, CNS stimulation, N/V, drug fever, rash, sec-ondary leukemias, alveolar dysplasia, pulm fibrosis, hepatotoxic **Interactions:** ↑ BM suppression W/ antineoplastic drugs & immunosuppressants; ↑ risk of bleed-ing W/ ASA, anticoagulants **Labs:** ↑ Urine & serum uric acid, ALT, alk phos; ↓ Hgb, Hct, neutrophil, plts, RBCs, WBCs; monitor LFTs, CBC, plts, serum uric acid **NIPE:** ⊘ PRG, breast-feeding, Infxn; ↑ fluids to 2–3 L/d; monitor lab work periodically & CBC w/ differential weekly during drug use; may cause hair loss; ↓ dose if pt has received radiation; ⊘ take w/ acidic foods, hot foods, spicy food, take 30–60 min before food; ⊘ immunizations; avoid contact w/ recent recipients of live vaccines

Chlordiazepoxide (Librium, Mitran, Libritabs) [Anxiolytic, Seda-tive/Hypnotic/Benzodiazepine] [C-IV]   Uses: *Anxiety, tension, EtOH withdrawal*, & pre-op apprehension **Action:** Benzodiazepine; antianxiety agent **Dose:** *Adults. Mild anxiety:* 5–10 mg PO tid–qid or PRN *Severe anxiety:* 25–50 mg PO q6–8h or PRN *Peds > 6 y.* 5 mg PO q6–8h; ↓ in renal impair, elderly **Caution:** [D, ?] Resp depression, CNS impair, Hx of drug dependence; avoid in hepatic impair **CI:** Preexisting CNS depression, NAG **Disp:** Caps 5, 10, 25 mg **SE:** Drows-iness, CP, rash, fatigue, memory impair, xerostomia, wgt gain **Interactions:** ↑ Effects W/ antidepressants, antihistamines, anticonvulsants, barbiturates, general anesthetics, MAOIs, narcotics, phenothiazine, cimetidine, disulfiram, fluconazole, itraconazole, ketoconazole, OCPs, INH, metoprolol, propoxyphene, propranolol, valproic acid, EtOH, grapefruit juice, kava kava, valerian; ↑ effects OF digoxin, phenytoin; ↓ effects W/ aminophylline, antacids, carbamazepine, theophylline, rifampin, rifabutin, tobacco; ↓ effects OF levodopa **Labs:** ↑ LFTs, alk phos, biliru-bin, triglycerides; ↓ granulocytes **NIPE:** ⊘ EtOH, PRG, breast-feeding; risk of photosensitivity—use sunscreen, orthostatic hypotension, tachycardia; erratic IM absorption; smoking ↓ effectiveness

Chlorothiazide (Diuril) [Antihypertensive/Thiazide Diuretic] Uses: *HTN, edema* **Action:** Thiazide diuretic **Dose:** *Adults.* 500 mg–1g PO daily–bid; 500–1000 mg/24 h PO (for edema only) *Peds > 6 mo.* 10–20 mg/kg/24 h PO ÷ bid; 4 mg/kg ÷ daily bid IV; OK w/ food **Caution:** [C, +] **CI:** Sensitivity to thiazides/sulfonamides, anuria **Disp:** Tabs 250, 500 mg; susp 250 mg/5 mL; Inj 500 mg/vial **SE:** ↓ K+, Na+, dizziness, hyperglycemia, hyperuricemia, hyperlipidemia, photosens **Interactions:** ↑ Effects *W/* ACEI, amphotericin B, corticosteroids; ↑ effects *OF* diazoxide, Li, MTX; ↓ effects *W/* colestipol, cholestyramine, NSAIDs; ↓ effects *OF* hypoglycemics **Labs:** ↓ K+, Na+; ↑ CPK, cholesterol, glucose, lytes, uric acid; monitor electrolytes **NIPE:** ⊘ Use IM/SQ; take early in the day to avoid nocturia; monitor for gout, hyperglycemia, photosensitivity—use sunblock, I&O, wgt

Chlorpheniramine (Chlor-Trimeton, Others) [OTC] [Antihistamine/Propylamine] <mark>**WARNING:** OTC meds w/ chlorpheniramine should not be used in peds < 2 y</mark> **Uses:** *Allergic rhinitis*, common cold **Action:** Antihistamine **Dose:** *Adults.* 4 mg PO q4–6h or 8–12 mg PO bid of SR 24 mg/d *Peds.* 0.35 mg/kg/24 h PO ÷ q4–6h or 0.2 mg/kg/24 h SR **Caution:** [C, ?/−] BOO; NAG; hepatic Insuff **CI:** Allergy **Disp:** Tabs 4 mg; SR tabs 12 mg **SE:** Anticholinergic SE & sedation common, postural ↓ BP, QT changes, extrapyramidal Rxns, photosens **Interactions:** ↑ Effects *W/* other CNS depressants, EtOH, opioids, sedatives, MAOIs, atropine, haloperidol, phenothiazine, quinidine, disopyramide; ↑ effects *OF* epinephrine; ↓ effects *OF* heparin, sulfonureas **Labs:** False(−) w/ allergy testing **NIPE:** D/C drug 4 d prior to allergy testing; take w/ food if GI distress; ⊘ cut/crush/chew ER forms; do not take > 7 days in a row; not for use in children under 2 y of age

Chlorpromazine (Thorazine) [Antipsychotic, Antiemetic/ Phenothiazine] Uses: *Psychotic disorders, N/V*, apprehension, intractable hiccups **Action:** Phenothiazine antipsychotic; antiemetic **Dose:** *Adults. Psychosis:* 30–800 mg/d in 1–4 ÷ doses, start low dose, ↑ PRN; typical 200–600 mg/d; 1–2 g/d may be needed in some cases. *Severe Sxs:* 25 mg IM/IV initial; may repeat in 1–4 h; then 25–50 mg PO or PR tid. *Hiccups:* 25–50 mg PO tid–qid *Children > 6 mo. Psychosis & N/V:* 0.5–1 mg/kg/dose PO q4–6h or IM/ IV q6–8h **Caution:** [C, ?/−] Safety inchildren < 6 mo not established; Szs, avoid w/ hepatic impair, BM suppression **CI:** Sensitivity w/ phenothiazines; NAG **Disp:** Tabs 10, 25, 50, 100, 200 mg; Inj 25 mg/mL **SE:** Extrapyramidal SE & sedation α-adrenergic blocking properties; ↓ BP; ↑ QT interval **Interactions:** ↑ Effects *W/* amodiaquine, chloroquine, sulfadoxine–pyrimethamine, antidepressants, narcotic analgesics, propranolol, quinidine, BBs, MAOIs, TCAs, EtOH, kava kava; ↑ effects *OF* anticholinergics, centrally acting antihypertensives, propranolol, valproic acid; ↓ effects *W/* antacids, antidiarrheals, barbiturates, Li, tobacco; ↓ effects *OF* anticonvulsants, guanethidine, levodopa, Li, warfarin **Labs:** False(+) urine bilirubin; false(+) or (−) PRG test; ↑ alk phos, bilirubin, CK, GGT, eosinophil count; ↓ Hgb, Hct, granulocytes, plts, WBC **NIPE:** ⊘ D/C abruptly; dilute

PO conc in 2–4 oz of Liq; risk of photosensitivity—use sunscreen; risk of tardive dyskinesia; take w/ food if GI upset; may darken urine; full effect may take up to 6 wks

Chlorpropamide (Diabinese) [Hypoglycemic/Sulfonylurea]
Uses: *Type 2 DM* **Action:** Sulfonylurea; ↑ pancreatic insulin release; ↑ peripheral insulin sensitivity; ↓ hepatic glucose output **Dose:** 100–500 mg/d; w/ food, ↓ hepatic impair **Caution:** [C,?/–] CrCl < 50 mL/min; ↓ in hepatic impair **CI:** Cross-sensitivity w/ sulfonamides **Disp:** Tabs 100, 250 mg **SE:** HA, dizziness, rash, photosens, hypoglycemia, SIADH **Interactions:** ↑ Effects **W/** ASA, NSAIDs, anticoagulants, BBs, chloramphenicol, guanethidine, insulin, MAOIs, rifampin, sulfonamides, EtOH, juniper berries, ginseng, garlic, fenugreek, coriander, dandelion root, celery, bitter melon, ginkgo; ↓ effects **W/** diazoxide, thiazide diuretics **Labs:** ↑Alk phos, bilirubin, BUN, Cr, cholesterol; ↓ glucose Hgb, Hct, plts, WBC **NIPE:** ⊘ EtOH (disulfiram-like Rxn); ⊘ PRG, breast-feeding

Chlorthalidone [Antihypertensive/Thiazide Diuretic] **Uses:** *HTN* **Action:** Thiazidediuretic **Dose:** *Adults.* 25–100 mg PO daily **Peds.** (Not approved) 2 mg/kg/dose PO 3×/wk or 1–2 mg/kg/d PO; ↓ in renal impair; OK w/ food, milk **Caution:** [B, +] **CI:** Cross-sensitivity w/ thiazides or sulfonamides; anuria **Disp:** Tabs 25, 50, mg **SE:** Dizziness, photosensitivity, hyperglycemia, hyperuricemia, sexual dysfunction **Interactions:** ↑ Effects **W/** ACEIs, diazoxide; ↑ effects **OF** digoxin, Li, MTX; ↓ effects **W/** cholestyramine, colestipol, NSAIDs; ↓ effects **OF** hypoglycemics; ↓ K+ **W/** amphotericin B, carbenoxolone, corticosteroids **Labs:** ↑ Bilirubin, Ca2+, Cr, uric acid; ↑ glucose in DM; ↓ Mg2+, K+, Na+ **NIPE:** May take w/food & milk, take early in day, use sunblock; ↑ K+-rich foods in diet; avoid ETOH

Chlorzoxazone (Parafon Forte DSC, Others) [Skeletal Muscle Relaxant/ANS Drug] **Uses:** *Adjunct to rest & physical therapy Rx to relieve discomfort associated w/ acute, painful musculoskeletal conditions* **Action:** Centrally acting skeletal muscle relaxant **Dose:** *Adults.* 500–750 mg PO tid–qid **Peds.** 20 mg/kg/d in 3–4 ÷ doses **Caution:** [C, ?] Avoid EtOH & CNS depressants **CI:** Severe liver Dz **Disp:** Tabs 250, 500, 750 mg **SE:** Drowsiness, tachycardia, dizziness, hepatotox, angioedema **Interactions:** ↑ Effects **W/** antihistamines, CNS depressants, MAOIs, TCAs, opiates, EtOH, watercress **Labs:** ↑ Alk phos, bilirubin; monitor LFTs **NIPE:** Urine may turn reddish purple or orange; reduce dose as improvement occurs

Cholecalciferol [Vitamin D₃] (Delta D) [Vitamin/Dietary Supplement] **Uses:** Dietary supl to Rx vit D deficiency **Action:** ↑ Intestinal Ca2+ absorption **Dose:** 400–1000 IU/d PO **Caution:** [A(D doses above the RDA), +] **CI:** ↑ Ca2+, hypervitaminosis, allergy **Disp:** Tabs 400, 1000 IU **SE:** Vit D tox (renal failure, HTN, psychosis) **Notes:** 1 mg cholecalciferol = 40,000 IU vit D activity **Interactions:** ↑ Risk of arrhythmias **W/** cardiac glycosides; ↓ effects **W/** cholestyramine, colestipol, mineral oil, orlistat, phenobarbital, phenytoin **Labs:** ↑ BUN, Ca, cholesterol, Cr, LFTs, urine urea **NIPE:** Vit D is fat-soluble; mineral oil interferes w/ vit D absorption; vit D is needed for Ca absorption

Cholestyramine (Questran, Questran Light, Prevalite) [Antilipemic, Bile Acid Sequestrant]
Uses: *Hypercholesterolemia; hyperlipidemia, pruritus associated w/ partial biliary obst;* hyperlipidemia, pruritus associated w/ partial biliary obst* *pseudomembranous colitis, dig tox, hyperoxaluria **Action:** Binds intestinal bile acids, forms insoluble complexes **Dose:** *Adults.* Titrate: 4 g/d–bid ↑ to max 24 g/d ÷ 1–6 doses/d *Peds.* 240 mg/kg/d in 2–3 ÷ doses max 8 g/d **Caution:** [C, ?] Constipation, phenylketonuria, may interfere w/other drug absorption; consider supl w/ fat-soluble vits **CI:** Complete biliary or bowel obst; w/ mycophenolate hyperlipoproteinemia types III, IV, V **Disp:** *(Questran)* 4 g cholestyramine resin/9 g powder; *(Prevalite)* w/aspartame: 4 g resin/5.5 g powder; *(Questran Light):* 4 g resin/5 g powder **SE:** Constipation, Abd pain, bloating, HA, rash, vit K deficiency **Interactions:** ↓ Effects *OF* APAP, amiodarone, anticoagulants, ASA, cardiac glycosides, clindamycin, corticosteroids, diclofenac, fat-soluble vits, gemfibrozil, glipizide, Fe salts, MTX, methyldopa, nicotinic acid, PCNs, phenobarbital, phenytoin, propranolol, thiazide diuretics, tetracyclines, thyroid drugs, troglitazone, warfarin if given w/ this drug **Labs:** ↑ Alk phos, PT; ↓ cholesterol, folic acid, vit A, D, K, ✓ Fluids, take other drugs 1–2 h before or 6 h after; OD may cause GI obst; mix 4 g in 2–6 oz of noncarbonated beverage; take w/ meals

Ciclesonide, Inhalation (Alvesco) [Corticosteroid]
Uses: *Asthma maint* **Action:** Inhaled steroid **Dose:** *Adults & Peds > 12 y. On bronchodilators alone:* 80 mcg bid (320 mcg/d max). *Inhaled corticosteroids:* 80 mcg bid (640 mcg/d max) *On oral corticosteroids:* 320 mcg bid (640 mcg/d max) **Caution:** [C, ?] **CI:** Status asthmaticus or other acute episodes of asthma, hypersens **Disp:** Inh 80, 160 mcg/actuation 60 doses **SE:** HA, nasopharyngitis, sinusitis, pharyngolaryngeal pain, URI, arthralgia, nasal congestion **Labs:** Monitor for ↓ BMD **NIPE:** Oral *Candida* risk, rinse mouth & spit after; taper systemic steroids slowly when transferring to ciclesonide; monitor growth in pediatric pts; counsel on use of device, clean mouthpiece weekly; monitor for changes in vision, ↑ IOP, cataracts

Ciclesonide, Nasal (Omnaris) [Corticosteroid]
Uses: Allergic rhinitis **Action:** Nasal corticosteroid **Dose:** *Adults/Peds > 12 y. Omnaris* 2 sprays, *Zettona* 1 spray each nostril 1×/d **Caution:** [C, ?/–] w/ ketoconazole; monitor peds for growth ↓ **CI:** Component allergy **Disp:** Intranasal spray, *Omnaris,* 50 mcg/spray (120 doses); *Zettona* 37 mcg/spray (60 doses) **SE:** Adrenal suppression, delayed nasal wound healing, URI, HA, ear pain, epistaxis ↑ risk viral Dz (eg, chickenpox), delayed growth in children **Interactions:** ↑ Effects *W/* ketoconazole **NIPE:** ↑ Risk viral Dz (eg, chickenpox), delayed growth in children; monitor for vision changes; full effect may take 1–2 wks for allergic rhinitis

Ciclopirox (Ciclodan, CNL8, Loprox, Pedipirox-4 Nail Kit, Penlac) [Antifungal/Antibiotic]
Uses: *Tinea pedis, tinea cruris, tinea corporis, cutaneous candidiasis, tinea versicolor, tinea rubrum* **Action:** Antifungal antibiotic;

cellular depletion of essential substrates &/or ions **Dose: *Adults & Peds > 10 y.*** Massage into affected area bid *Onychomycosis:* Apply to nails daily, w/removal q7d **Caution:** [B, ?] **CI:** Component sensitivity **Disp:** Cream 0.77%, gel 0.77%, topicals usp 0.77%, shampoo 1%, nail lacquer 8% **SE:** Pruritus, local irritation, burning **Interactions:** None noted **NIPE:** Nail lacquer may take 6 mo to see improvement; cream/gel/lotion see improvement by 4 wk; D/C w/ irritation; avoid dressings; gel best for athlete's foot

Cidofovir (Vistide) [Antiviral/Inhibits DNA Synthesis] WARNING: Renal impair is the major tox. Neutropenia possible, ✓ CBC before dose. Follow administration instructions. Possible carcinogenic, teratogenic Uses:
CMV retinitis w/ HIV **Action:** Selective inhib viral DNA synth **Dose:** *Rx:* 5 mg/kg IV over 1 h once/wk for 2 wk w/ probenecid. *Maint:* 5 mg/kg IV once/2 wk w/ probenecid (2 g PO 3 h prior to cidofovir, then 1 g PO at 2 h & 8 h after cidofovir); ↓ in renal impair **Caution:** [C, −] SCr > 1.5 mg/dL or CrCl < 55 mL/min or urine protein ≥ 100 mg/dL; w/ other nephrotoxic drugs **CI:** Probenecid/sulfa allergy **Disp:** Inj 75 mg/mL **SE:** Renal tox, chills, fever, HA, N/V/D, ↓ plt, ↓ WBC **Interactions:** ↑ Nephrotox *W/* aminoglycosides, amphotericin B, foscarnet, IV pentamidine, NSAIDs, vancomycin; ↑ effects *W/* zidovudine **Labs:** ↑ SCr, BUN, alkphos, LFTs, urine protein; ↓ Ca, Hgb, Hct, neutrophils, plts; monitor for hematuria, glycosuria, hypocalcemia, hyperglycemia, hypokalemia, hyperlipidemia **NIPE:** Coadminister oral probenecid w/ each dose to < GI upset; possible hair loss; hydrate w/ NS prior to each Inf; use effective contraception during & 1 mo after therapy; men should use barrier contraception during & 3 mo after therapy; ⊘ PRG, breast-feeding.

Cilostazol (Pletal) [Antiplatelet, Arterial Vasodilator/Phosphodiesterase Inhibitor] WARNING: PDE III inhib have ↓ survival w/ class III/IV heart failure Uses:
↓ Sxs of intermittent claudication **Action:** Phosphodiesterase III inhib; ↑ cAMP in plts & blood vessels, vasodilation & inhibit plt aggregation **Dose:** 100 mg PO bid, 1/2 h before or 2 h after breakfast & dinner **Caution:** [C, ?] ↓ Dose w/ drugs that inhibit CYP3A4 & CYP2C19 (Table 10) **CI:** CHF, hemostatic disorders, active bleeding **Disp:** Tabs 50, 100 mg **SE:** HA, palpitation, D **Interactions:** ↑ Effects *W/* diltiazem, macrolides, omeprazole, fluconazole, itraconazole, ketoconazole, sertraline, grapefruit juice; ↑ effects *OF* ASA; ↓ effects *W/* cigarette smoking **Labs:** ↑ HDL; ↓ triglycerides **NIPE:** Take on empty stomach; ⊘ grapefruit products; may take up to12 wk to ↓ cramping pain; may cause dizziness

Cimetidine (Tagamet, Tagamet HB 200 [OTC]) [Antiulcerative/ H₂-Receptor Antagonist] Uses:
Duodenal ulcer; ulcer prophylaxis in hypersecretory states (eg, trauma, burns); & GERD **Action:** H₂-receptor antagonist **Dose: Adults.** *Active ulcer:* 2400 mg/d IV cont Inf or 300 mg IV q6h; 400 mg PO bid or 800 mg hs; *Maint:* 400 mg PO hs *GERD:* 300–600 mg PO q6h; maint 800 mg PO hs **Peds. Infants.** 10–20 mg/kg/24 h PO or IV ÷ q6–12h **Children.**

20–40 mg/kg/24 h PO or IV ÷ q6h; ↓ w/ renal Insuff & in elderly **Caution:** [B, +] Many drug interactions (P-450 system); do not use w/ clopidogrel (↓ effect) **CI:** Component sensitivity **Disp:** Tabs 200 (OTC), 300, 400, 800 mg; liq 300 mg/5 mL; Inj 300 mg/2 mL **SE:** Dizziness, HA, agitation, ↓ plt, gynecomastia **Interactions:** ↑ Effects *OF* benzodiazepines, disulfram, flecainide, INH, lidocaine, OCPs, sulfonylureas, warfarin, theophylline, phenytoin, metronidazole, triamterene, procainamide, quinidine, propranolol, diazepam, nifedipine, TCAs, procainamide, tacrine, carbamazepine, valproic acid, xanthines; ↓ effects *W/* antacids, tobacco; ↓ effects *OF* digoxin, ketoconazole, cefpodoxime, indomethacin, tetracyclines **Labs:** ↑ Cr, LFTs; ↓ Hgb, Hct, neutrophils, plt counts **NIPE:** Take w/ meals; monitor for gynecomastia, breast pain, impotence; take 1 h before or 2 h after antacids; ⊘ EtOH

Cinacalcet (Sensipar) [Hyperparathyroidism Agent/Calcimimetic]
Uses: *Secondary hyperparathyroidism in CRF; ↑ Ca²⁺ in parathyroid CA* **Action:** ↓ PTH by ↑ calcium-sensing receptor sensitivity **Dose:** *Secondary hyperparathyroidism:* 30 mg PO daily *Parathyroid carcinoma:* 30 mg PO bid; titrate q2–4wk based on calcium & PTH levels; swallow whole; take w/ food **Caution:** [C, ?/–] w/ Szs, adjust w/ CYP3A4 inhib (Table 10) **Disp:** Tabs 30, 60, 90 mg **SE:** N/V/D, myalgia, dizziness, ↓ Ca²⁺ **Interactions:** ↑ Effects *W/* CYP3A4 Inhibs such as ketoconazole, itraconazole, erythromycin; ↑ effects *OF* drugs metabolized at CYP2D6 such as TCA, thioridazine, flecainide, vinblastine **Labs:** ↓ Ca²⁺; monitor Ca²⁺, PO₄, PTH **NIPE:** Must take drug w/ vit D and/or phosphate binders; ↑ conc of drug if taken w/ food; ⊘ break, crush, chew coated tabs

Ciprofloxacin (Cipro, Cipro XR) [Antibiotic/Fluoroquinolone]
WARNING: ↑ Risk of tendonitis & tendon rupture; ↑ risk w/ age > 60, transplant pts may worsen MG Sxs **Uses:** *Rx lower resp tract, sinuses, skin & skin structure, bone/joints, complex intra-Abd Infxn (w/ metronidazole), typhoid, infectious D, uncomp GC, inhal anthrax UT Infxns, including prostatitis* **Action:** Quinolone antibiotic; ↓ DNA gyrase *Spectrum:* Broad gram(+) & (–) aerobics; little *Streptococcus*; good *Pseudomonas, E coli, B fragilis, P mirabilis, K pneumoniae, C jejuni,* or *Shigella* **Dose:** *Adults.* 250–750 mg PO q12h; XR 500–1000 mg PO q24h; or 200–400 mg IV q12h; ↓ in renal impair **Caution:** [C, ?/–] Children < 18 y; avoid in MG **CI:** Component sensitivity; w/ tizanidine **Disp:** Tabs 100, 250, 500, 750 mg; tabs XR 500, 1000 mg; susp 5 g/100 mL, 10 g/100 mL; Inj 200, 400 mg; premixed piggyback 200, 400 mg/100 mL **SE:** Restlessness, N/V/D, rash, ruptured tendons, ↑ LFTs, peripheral neuropathy risk **Interactions:** ↑ Effects *W/* probenecid; ↑ effects *OF* diazepam, theophylline, caffeine, metoprolol, propranolol, phenytoin, warfarin; ↓ effects *W/* antacids, didanosine, Fe salts, Mg, sucralfate, NaHCO₃, zinc **Labs:** ↑ LFTs, alk phos, serum bilirubin, LDH, BUN, SCr, K⁺, PT, triglycerides; ↓ plts, WBC **NIPE:** ⊘ Give to children < 18 y; ↑ fluids to 2–3 L/d, may cause photosensitivity—use sunblock; avoid antacids; reduce/restrict caffeine intake; most tendon problems in Achilles, rare shoulder & hand

Ciprofloxacin, Ophthalmic (Ciloxan) [Antibiotic/Fluoroquinolone Opthalmic Agent] Uses: *Rx & prevention of ocular Infxns (conjunctivitis, blepharitis, corneal abrasions)* **Action:** Quinolone antibiotic; ↓ DNA gyrase **Dose:** 1–2 gtt in eye(s) q2h while awake for 2 d, then 1–2 gtt q4h while awake for 5 d, oint 1/2-in ribbon in eye tid × 2d, then bid × 5d **Caution:** [C, ?/–] **CI:** Component sensitivity **Disp:** Soln 3.5 mg/mL; oint 0.3%, 3.5 g **SE:** Local irritation **Interactions:** ↑ Theophylline levels; ↑ effects *OF* oral anticoagulants; ↑ renal tox **W/** cyclosporine **NIPE:** Limited systemic absorption

Ciprofloxacin, Otic (Cetraxal) [Antibiotic/Quinolone Otic Agent] Uses: *Otitis externa* **Action:** Quinolone antibiotic; ↓ DNA gyrase *Spectrum: P aeruginosa, S aureus* **Dose:** *Adults & Peds > 1 y.* 0.25 mL in ear(s) q12h × 7 d **Caution:** [C, ?/–] **CI:** Component sensitivity **Disp:** Soln 0.2% **SE:** Hypersens Rxn, ear pruritus/pain, HA, fungal super Infxn **NIPE:** Limited systemic absorption; instruct pt on proper instillation technique

Ciprofloxacin & Dexamethasone, Otic (Ciprodex Otic) [Antibiotic/Fluoroquinolone Otic Agent] Uses: *Otitis externa, otitis media peds* **Action:** Quinolone antibiotic; ↓ DNA gyrase; w/ steroid **Dose:** *Adults.* 4 gtt in ear(s) bid × 7 d. *Peds > 6 mo.* 4 gtt in ear(s) bid for 7 d **Caution:** [C, ?/–] **CI:** Viral ear Infxns **Disp:** Susp ciprofloxacin 0.3% & dexamethasone 1% **SE:** Ear discomfort **NIPE:** OK w/ tympanostomy tubes; D/C if super Infxn or hypersensitivity; limited systemic absorption; shake immediately before use; protect drug from light

Ciprofloxacin & Hydrocortisone, Otic (Cipro HC Otic) [Antibiotic/Fluoroquinolone Otic Agent] Uses: *Otitis externa* **Action:** Quinolone antibiotic; ↓ DNA gyrase; w/ steroid **Dose:** *Adults & Peds > 1 y.* 3 gtt in ear(s) bid × 7 d **Caution:** [C, ?/–] **CI:** Perforated tympanic membrane, viral Infxns of the external canal **Disp:** Susp ciprofloxacin 0.2% & hydrocortisone 1% **SE:** HA, pruritus **NIPE:** D/C if hypersensitive Rxn; hold bottle in hand 1–2 min before use to warm susp & minimize dizziness; ⊘ use w/ perforated tympanic membrane

Cisplatin (Platinol, Platinol AQ) [Antineoplastic/Alkylating Agent] WARNING: Anaphylactic-like Rxn, ototox, cumulative renal tox; doses > 100 mg/m² q3–4 wk rarely used, do not confuse w/carboplatin Uses: *Testicular, bladder, ovarian*, SCLC, NSCLC, breast, head & neck, & penile CAs; osteosarcoma; peds brain tumors **Action:** DNA-binding; denatures double helix; intrastrand cross-linking **Dose:** 10–20 mg/m²/d for 5 d q3wk; 50–120 mg/m² q3–4wk (per protocols); ↓ w/ renal impair **Caution:** [D, –] Cumulative renal tox may be severe; ↓ BM, hearing impair, preexisting renal Insuff **CI:** w/Anthrax or live vaccines, platinum-containing compound allergy; w/ cidofovir **Disp:** Inj 1 mg/mL **SE:** Allergic Rxns, N/V, nephrotox (↑ w/ administration of other nephrotoxic drugs; minimize w/ NS Inf & mannitol diuresis, high-frequency hearing loss in 30%, peripheral "stocking glove"-type neuropathy, cardiotox (ST-, T-wave changes), ↓ Mg²⁺, mild ↓ BM, hepatotox; renal impair dose-related & cumulative **Notes:** Give taxanes before platinum derivatives

Interactions: ↑ Effects *OF* antineoplastic drugs & radiation therapy; ↑ ototox *W/* loop diuretics; ↑ nephrotox *W/* aminoglycosides, amphotericin B, vancomycin; ↓ effects *W/* Nathiosulfate; ↓ effects *OF* phenytoin **Labs:** ✓ Mg²⁺, lytes before & w/in 48 h after cisplatin; ↑ BUN, Cr, serum bilirubin, AST, uric acid; ↓ Ca²⁺, Mg²⁺, phosphate, Na⁺, K⁺, RBC, WBC, plts **NIPE:** May cause infertility, ⊘ immunizations or products w/ ASA; instruct pt to report signs of Infxn; ✓ for ototoxicity (tinnitus; ↓ hrg) wear protective gloves & handle drug w/ extreme care; ⊘ PRG

Citalopram (Celexa) [Antidepressant/SSRI] **WARNING:** Closely monitor for worsening depression or emergence of suicidality, particularly in pts < 24 y; not for peds **Uses:** *Depression* **Action:** SSRI **Dose:** Initial 20 mg/d, may ↑ to 40 mg/d max dose; ↓ 20 mg/d max > 60 y, w/ cimetidine, or hepatic/renal Insuff **Caution:** [C, +/−] Hx of mania, Szs & pts at risk for suicide, ↑ risk serotonin synd w/ triptans, linezolid, lithium, tramadol, St. John's wort; use w/ other SSRIs, SNRIs, or tryptophan not rec **CI:** MAOI or w/in 14 d of MAOI use **Disp:** Tabs 10, 20, 40 mg; soln 10 mg/5 mL **SE:** Somnolence, insomnia, anxiety, xerostomia, N, diaphoresis, sexual dysfunction; may ↑ Qt interval and cause arrhythmias; ↓ Na⁺/SIADH **Interactions:** ↑ Effects *W/* azole antifungals, cimetidine, Li, macrolides, EtOH; ↑ effects *OF* BBs, carbamazepine, CNS drugs, warfarin; ↓ effects *W/* carbamazepine; ↓ effects *OF* phenytoin; may cause fatal Rxn *W/* MAOIs **Labs:** ↑ LFTs; May cause ↓ Na⁺/SIADH **NIPE:** ⊘ PRG, breast-feeding, use barrier contraception; ⊘ ETOH; report ↑ depression, suicidal ideation immediately

Citric Acid/Magnesium Oxide/Sodium Picosulfate (Prepopik) **Uses:** *Colonoscopy colon prep* **Acts:** Stimulant/osmotic laxative **Dose:** Powder recons w/ 5-oz cold water; "Split Dose": 1st dose night before and 2nd dose morning of procedure; OR "Day Before": 1st dose afternoon/early eve day before and 2nd dose later evening; clear liquids after dose **W/P:** [B, ?] Fluid/electrolyte abnormalities, arrhythmias, seizures; ↑ risk in renal Insuff or w/ nephrotox drugs; mucosal ulcerations; aspiration risk **CI:** CrCl < 30 mL/min; GI perf/obstr/ileus/gastric retention/toxic colitis/megacolon **Disp:** Packets, 16.1 g powder (10 mg sodium picosulfate, 3.5 g mag oxide, 12 g anhyd citric acid) w/ dosing cup **SE:** N,V, D, HA, Abd pain, cramping, bloating **Notes:** Meds taken 1 h w/in dose might not be absorbed. **NIPE:** ⊘ Use other laxatives while using Prepopik; if severe bloating, distention, or abd pain occur w/1st packet, delay 2nd administration until Sx resolve; dissolve in 5 oz cold H₂O

Cladribine (Leustatin) [Antineoplastic Agent/Purine Nucleoside Analog] **WARNING:** Dose-dependent reversible myelosuppression; neurotox, nephrotox, administer by physician w/ experience in chemotherapy regimens **Uses:** *HCL, CLL, NHLs, progressive MS* **Action:** Induces DNA strand breakage; interferes w/ DNA repair/synth; purine nucleoside analog **Dose:** 0.09–0.1 mg/kg/d cont IV Inf for 1–7 d (per protocols); ↓ w/renal impair **Caution:** [D, ?/−] Causes neutropenia & Infxn **CI:** Component sensitivity **Disp:** Inj 1 mg/mL **SE:** ↓ BM, T-lymphocyte ↓ may be prolonged (26–34 wk), fever in 46%, tumor lysis synd, Infxns (especially lung & IV sites), rash (50%), HA, fatigue, N/V **Interactions:** ↑ Risk of bleeding *W/* anticoagulants, NSAIDs, salicylates, ↑ risk of nephrotox *W/* amphotericin B **Labs:** Monitor CBC, LFTs, SCr **NIPE:** ⊘ PRG, breast-feeding; consider prophylactic allopurinol; ⊘ immunizations or contact w/ recent recipients of live virus vaccine; avoid those w/ active infections

Clarithromycin (Biaxin, Biaxin XL) [Antibiotic/Macrolide] Uses: *Upper/lower resp tract, skin/skin structure Infxns, *H pylori* Infxns, & Infxns caused by nontuberculosis (atypical) *Mycobacterium*; prevention of MAC Infxns in HIV Infxn* **Action:** Macrolide antibiotic, ↓ protein synth *Spectrum:* H influenzae, M catarrhalis, S pneumoniae, M pneumoniae, & H pylori Dose: **Adults.** 250–500 mg PO bid or 1000 mg (2 × 500 mg XL tab)/d *Mycobacterium:* 500 mg PO bid **Peds > 6 mo.** 7.5 mg/kg/dose PO bid; ↓ w/ renal impair **Caution:** [C, ?] Antibiotic-associated colitis; rare ↑ QT & ventricular arrhythmias; not rec w/ PDE5 inhib **CI:** Macrolide allergy; w/ Hx jaundice w/ Biaxin; w/ cisaride, pimozide, astemizole, terfenadine, ergotamines; w/ colchicine & renal impair; w/ statins; w/ ↑ QT or ventricular arrhythmias **Disp:** Tabs 250, 500 mg; susp 125, 250 mg/5 mL; 500 mg XL tab SE: ↑ QT interval, causes metallic taste, N/D, Abd pain, HA, rash **Interactions:** ↑ Effects *W/* amprenavir, indinavir, nelfinavir, ritonavir; ↑ effects *OF* atorvastatin, buspirone, clozapine, colchicine, diazepam, felodipine, itraconazole, lovastatin, simvastatin, methylprednisolone, theophylline, phenytoin, quinidine, digoxin, carbamazepine, triazolam, warfarin, ergotamine, alprazolam, valproic acid; ↓ effects *W/* EtOH; ↓ effects *OF* PCN, zafirlukast **Labs:** ↑ Serum AST, ALT, GTT, alk phos, LDH, total bilirubin, BUN, Cr, PT, INR; ↓ WBC **NIPE:** May take w/o regard to food; do not refrigerate susp & discard > 14 d; space doses evenly

Clemastine Fumarate (Tavist, Dayhist, Antihist-1) [OTC] [Antihistamine] Uses: *Allergic rhinitis & Sxs of urticaria* **Action:** Antihistamine Dose: **Adults & Peds >12 y.** 1.34 mg bid–2.68 mg tid; max 8.04 mg/d; **6–12 y.** 0.67–1.34 mg bid (max 4.02/d) < 6 y: 0.335–0.67 mg/d ÷ into 2–3 doses (max 1.34 mg/d) **Caution:** [B, M] BOO: ⊘ Do not take w/ MAOI **CI:** NAG **Disp:** Tabs 1.34, 2.68 mg; syrup 0.67 mg/5 mL SE: Drowsiness, dyscoordination, epigastric distress, urinary retention **Interactions:** ↑ Effects *W/* CNS depressants, MAOIs, EtOH; ↓ effects *OF* heparin, sulfonylureas **NIPE:** ⊘ EtOH, sedatives; ↑ excitability (particularly in children)

Clevidipine (Cleviprex) [Antihypertension/Calcium Channel Blocker] Uses: *HTN when PO not available/desirable* **Action:** Dihydropyridine CCB, potent arterial vasodilator Dose: 1–2 mg/h IV then maint 4–6 mg/h; 21 mg/h max **Caution:** [C, ?] ↓ BP, syncope, rebound HTN, reflex tachycardia, CHF Contra: Hypersens: component or formulation (soy, egg products); impaired lipid metabolism; severe aortic stenosis **Disp:** Inj 0.5 mg/mL (50 mL, 100 mL) SE: AF, fever, insomnia, N/V, HA, renal impair **Interactions:** ↑ Risk of reflex tachycardia w/ BB **NIPE:** Monitor BP & pulse during Inf & until stabilized; monitor for rebound HTN at least 8 h after Inf ends

Clindamycin (Cleocin, Cleocin-T, Others) [Antibiotic/Lincomycin Derivative] WARNING: Pseudomembranous colitis may range from mild to life-threatening

Uses: *Rx aerobic & anaerobic Infxns; topical for severe acne & Vag Infxns* **Action:** Bacteriostatic; interferes w/ protein synth *Spectrum:* Streptococci (eg, pneumococci), staphylococci, & gram(+) & (−) anaerobes; no activity against gram(−) aerobes **Dose:** *Adults. PO:* 150–450 mg PO q6–8h. *IV:* 300–600 mg IV q6h or 900 mg IV q8h *Vag cream:* 1 applicator hs × 7 d. *Vag supp:* Insert 1 qhs × 3 d *Topical:* Apply 1% gel, lotion, or soln bid *Peds. Neonates.* (Avoid use; contains benzyl alcohol) 10–15 mg/kg/24 h ÷ q8–12h *Children >1 mo.* 10–30 mg/kg/24 h ÷ q6–8h, to a max of 1.8 g/d PO or 4.8 g/d IV *Topical:* Apply 1%, gel, lotion, or soln bid; ↓ in severe hepatic impair **Caution:** [B, +] Can cause fatal colitis **CI:** Hx pseudomembranous colitis **Disp:** Caps 75, 150, 300 mg; susp 75 mg/5 mL; Inj 300 mg/2 mL; Vag cream 2%, topical soln 1%, gel 1%, lotion 1%, Vag sup 100 mg **SE:** D may be *C difficile* pseudomembranous colitis, rash, ↑ LFTs **Interactions:** ↑ Effects of neuromuscular blockage *W/* tubocurarine, pancuronium; ↓ effects *W/* erythromycin, kaolin, foods *W/* Na cyclamate **Labs:** ↑ LFTs; monitor CBC, LFTs, BUN, Cr; ↓ WBC, plts **NIPE:** D/C drug w/ D, eval for *C difficile;* ⊘ intercourse, tampons, douches while using Vag cream; take oral meds w/ 8 oz H₂O; space doses evenly

Clindamycin/Benzoyl Peroxide (Benzaclin)

Uses: *Topical for acne vulgaris* **Action:** Bacteriostatic antibiotic w/ keratolytic **Dose:** Apply bid (AM & PM) **Caution:** [C, ?] Pseudomembranous colitis reported **CI:** Component sensitivity, Hx UC/antibiotic-associated colitis **Disp:** Gel 10 mg (clindamycin [1%] and benzoyl peroxide [5%]) **SE:** Dry skin, pruritus, peeling, erythema, sunburn, allergic Rxns **Notes:** May bleach hair/fabrics; not approved in peds. **NIPE:** D/C w/ D, eval for *C difficile;* ⊘ exposure to natural or artificial sunlight, use sunscreen/protective clothing

Clindamycin & Tretinoin (Veltin Gel, Ziana) [Lincosamide + Retinoid]

Uses: *Acne vulgaris* **Action:** Lincosamide abx (↓ protein synthesis) w/a retinoid; *Spectrum: P acnes* **Dose:** *Adults (> 12 y).* Apply pea-size amount to area qd **Caution:** [C, ?/−] Do not use w/ erythromycin products **CI:** Hx regional enteritis/UC/abx-assoc colitis **Disp:** TopGel (clindamycin 1.2%/tretinoin 0.025%) **SE:** Dryness, irritation, erythema, pruritis, exfoliation, dermatitis, sunburn **Interaction:** May ↑ neuromuscular blockers **NIPE:** Avoid eyes, lips, mucous membranes; avoid erythromycin or additive irritation w/ topical products (eg, alcohol, drying agents); avoid sun & UV light; D/C w/D, eval for *C difficile*

Clobazam (Onfi) [C-IV]

Uses: *Szs assoc w/ Lennox-Gastaut synd* **Action:** Potentiates GABA neurotransmission; binds to benzodiazepine GABAₐ receptor **Dose:** *Adults & Peds.* ≥ 2 y. ≤ 30 kg: 5 mg PO/d, titrate weekly 20 mg/d max; *> 30 kg:*

10 mg daily, titrate weekly 40 mg/d max; divide dose bid if > 5 mg/d; may crush & mix w/ applesauce; ↓ dose in geriatric pts, CYP2C19 poor metabolizers, & mild–moderate hepatic impair; ↓ dose weekly by 5–10 mg/d w/ D/C **Caution:** [C, ±] physical/psychological dependence & suicidal ideation/behavior; withdrawal Sxs w/ rapid dose ↓; alcohol ↑ clobazam levels by 50%; adjust w/ CYP2C19 Inhib, ↓ dose of drugs metabolized by CYP2D6; may ↓ contraceptive effect **Disp:** Tabs 5, 10, 20 mg **SE:** Somnolence, sedation, cough, V, constipation, drooling, UTI, aggression, dysarthria, fatigue, insomnia, ataxia, pyrexia, lethargy, ↑/↓ appetite. **NIPE:** ⊘ abruptly D/C; ⊘ ETOH; ✓ report depression, suicidal ideation, aggressive behaviors; give w/o regard to food

Clofarabine (Clolar) [Antineoplastic; Purine Nucleoside Antimetabolite]   **Uses:** Rx relapsed/refractoryALL after at least 2 regimens in children 1–21 y **Action:** Antimetabolite; ↓ ribonucleotide reductase w/ false nucleotide base-inhibiting DNA synth **Dose:** 52 mg/m² IV over 2 h daily × 5 d (repeat q2–6wk); per protocol; ↓ w/ renal impair **Caution:** [D, –] **Disp:** Inj 20 mg/20 mL **SE:** N/V/D, anemia, leukopenia, thrombocytopenia, neutropenia, Infxn, ↑ AST/ALT **Interactions:** ↑ Additive risk w/ hepatotoxic or nephrotoxic drugs **Labs:** ↑ AST, ALT, Cr, Hgb, Hct; monitor serum uric acid, phosphate, Ca & Cr bid for 2–3 d after starting chemotherapy **NIPE:** Monitor for tumor lysis synd & systemic inflammatory response synd (SIRS)/capillary leak synd; hydrate well; ⊘ immunizations; ⊘ exposure to those w/ active infections or recent recipients of live virus vaccines; ⊘ PRG

Clomiphene (Clomid, Serophene) [Ovulatory Stimulant]   **Uses:** *Tx ovulatory dysfunction in women desiring PRG* **Action:** Nonsteroidal ovulatory stimulant; estrogen antagonist **Dose:** 50 mg × 5 d; if no ovulation ↑ to 100 mg × 5 d @ 30 d later; ovulation usually 5–10 d post-course, time coitus w/ expected ovulation time **Caution:** [X; ?/–] r/o PRG & ovarian enlargement **CI:** Hypersens, uterine bleed, PRG, ovarian cysts (not due to olycystic ovary synd), liver Dz, thyroid/adrenal dysfunction **Disp:** Tabs 50 mg **SE:** Ovarian enlargement, vasomotor flushes **NIPE:** D/C with visual changes. ⊘ Use if PRG

Clomipramine (Anafranil) [Tricyclic]   **WARNING:** Closely monitor for suicidal ideation or unusual behavior changes **Uses:** *OCD, *depression, chronic pain, panic attacks **Action:** TCA; ↑ synaptic serotonin & norepinephrine **Dose:** *Adults.* Initial 25 mg/d PO in ÷ doses; ↑ over few wk 250 mg/d max QHS *Peds > 10 y.* Initial 25 mg/d PO in ÷ doses; ↑over few wk 200 mg/d or 3 mg/kg/d max given hs **Caution:** [C; +/–] **CI:** w/ MAOI, linezolid, IV methylene blue (risk serotonin synd), TCA allergy, during AMI recovery **Disp:** Caps 25, 50, 75 mg **SE:** Anticholinergic (xerostomia, urinary retention, constipation), somnolence **Interactions:** ↑ Effects *OF* other CNS depressants, anticholinergics, sympathomimetics, other protein-bound drugs, EtOH; ↑ effects *W/* CYP2D6 and/or CYP1A2 Inhibs; ↓ effects *W/* barbiturates, carbamazepine, phenytoin, other CYP450 inducers; blocks guanethidine, clonidine **Labs:** Monitor plasma levels with cimetidine, SSRIs, phenothiazines

NIPE: Take with food; do not take w/in 14 d of MAOI, ⊘ abruptly D/C; ⊘ ETOH; maximum effect may take 2–4 wk

Clonazepam (Klonopin) [C-IV] [Anticonvulsant/Benzodiazepine]

Uses: *Lennox-Gastaut synd, akinetic & myoclonic Szs, absence Szs, panic attacks*, RLS, neuralgia, parkinsonian dysarthria, bipolar disorder **Action:** Benzodiazepine; anticonvulsant **Dose:** *Adults.* 1.5 mg/d PO in 3 ÷ doses; ↑ by 0.5–1 mg/d q3d PRN up to 20 mg/d *Peds.* 0.01–0.03 mg/kg/24 h PO ÷ tid; ↑ to 0.1–0.2 mg/kg/24 h ÷ tid; 0.2 mg/kg/d max; avoid abrupt D/C **Caution:** [D, M] Elderly pts, resp Dz, CNS depression, severe hepatic impair, NAG **CI:** Severe liver Dz, acute NAG **Disp:** Tabs 0.5, 1, 2 mg, oral disintegrating tabs 0.125, 0.25, 0.5, 1, 2 mg **SE:** CNS (drowsiness, dizziness, ataxia, memory impair) **Interactions:** ↑ CNS depression W/ antidepressants, antihistamines, opiates, benzodiazepines; ↑ effects W/ cimetidine, disulfiram, fluoxetine, INH, itraconazole, ketoconazole, metoprolol, valproic acid, EtOH, kava kava, valerian; ↓ effects W/ phenytoin **Labs:** ↑ LFTs, ↓ WBC, plts **NIPE:** ⊘ D/C abruptly; can cause retrograde amnesia; a CYP3A4 substrate; ⊘ ETOH

Clonidine, Epidural (Duraclon)

WARNING: Dilute 500 mcg/mL before use; not rec for OB, postpartum or periop pain management due to ↓ BP/HR **Uses:** *w/ Opiates for severe pain in cancer patients uncontrolled by opiates alone* **Action:** Centrally acting analgesic **Dose:** 30 mcg/h by epidural Inf **Caution:** [C, ?/M] May ↓ HR/resp CI: See Warning; clonidine sens, Inj site Infxn, anticoagulants, bleed diathesis, use above C4 dermatome **Disp:** 500 mcg/mL; dilute to 100 mcg/mL w/ NS (preservative free) **SE:** ↓ BP, dry mouth, N/V, somnolence, dizziness, confusion, sweating, hallucinations, tinnitus **Notes:** Avoid abrupt D/C; may cause nervousness, rebound ↑ BP **NIPE:** ⊘ Use in severe CV Dz; needs CV assessment before starting epidural clonidine (Duraclon) used for chronic CA pain; ✓ S/ Sx ↑ depression; ✓ VS freq 1st few days following Tx

Clonidine, Oral (Catapres) [Antihypertensive/Centrally Acting Sympatholytic]

Uses: *HTN*, opioid, EtOH, & tobacco withdrawal, ADHD **Action:** Centrally acting α-adrenergic stimulant **Dose:** *Adults.* 0.1 mg PO bid, adjust daily by 0.1–0.2-mg increments (max 2.4 mg/d) *Peds.* 5–10 mcg/kg/d ÷ q8–12 h (max 0.9 mg/d); ↓ in renal impair **Caution:** [C, +/−] Avoid w/ β-blocker, elderly, severe CV Dz, renal impair; use w/ agents that affect sinus node may cause severe ↓ HR **CI:** Component sensitivity **Disp:** Tabs 0.1, 0.2, 0.3 mg **SE:** drowsiness, orthostatic ↓ BP, xerostomia, constipation, ↓ HR, dizziness **Interactions:** ↑ Sedation W/ CNS depressants; ↓ antihypertensive effects W/ amphetamines, BB, MAOIs TCA **Labs:** ↑ Glucose **NIPE:** More effective for HTN if combined w/ diuretics; withdraw slowly, rebound HTN w/ abrupt D/C of doses > 0.2 mg bid; ADHD use in peds; change position slowly

Clonidine, Oral, Extended Release (Kapvay) [Antihypertensive/Centrally Acting Sympatholytic]

Uses: *ADHD alone or as adjunct* **Action:** Central α-adrenergic stimulant **Dose:** *Adults, Peds > 6y.* Initial 0.1 mg

Total Daily Dose	Morning Dose	Bedtime Dose
0.1 mg/d	N/A	0.1 mg
0.2 mg/d	0.1 mg	0.1 mg
0.3 mg/d	0.2 mg	0.2 mg
0.4 mg/d	0.1 mg	0.2 mg

qhs, then adjust weekly to bid; split dose based on table; do not crush/chew; do not substitute other products as mg dosing differs; > 0.4 mg/d not rec **Caution:** [C, +/−] May cause severe ↓ HR & ↓ BP; w/ BP meds **CI:** Component sensitivity **Disp:** Tabs ER 0.1, 0.2 mg **SE:** Somnolence, fatigue, URI, irritability, sore throat, insomnia, nightmares, emotional disorder, constipation, congestion, ↑ temperature, dry mouth, ear pain **Interactions:** ↑ Effects *OF* other CNS depressants, antihypertensives, EtOH; ↑ cardiac Sx (AV block, bradycardia) *W/* digitalis, CCB, BB **NIPE:** On D/C, ↓ no more than 0.1 mg q3–7d; swallow whole; titrate by response

Clonidine, Transdermal (Catapres TTS) [Antihypertensive/ Centrally Acting Sympatholytic] Uses: *HTN* **Action:** Centrally acting α-adrenergic stimulant **Dose:** 1 patch q7d to hairless area (upper arm/torso); titrate to effect; ↓ w/ severe renal impair **Caution:** [C,+/−] Avoid w/ β-blocker, withdraw slowly, in elderly, severe CV Dz and w/ renal impair; use w/ agents that affect sinus node may cause severe ↓ HR **CI:** Component sensitivity **Disp:** TTS-1, TTS-2, TTS-3 (delivers 0.1, 0.2, 0.3 mg, respectively, of clonidine/d for 1 wk) **SE:** Drowsiness, orthostatic ↓ BP, xerostomia, constipation, ↓ HR **Interactions:** ↑ Sedation *W/* CNS depressants; ↓ antihypertensive effects *W/* amphetamines, BB, MAOIs TCA **Labs:** ↑ Glucose, CK **NIPE:** Do not D/C abruptly (rebound HTN) doses > 2 TTS-3 usually not associated w/ ↑ efficacy; steady state in 2–3 d; ⊘ cut patch to adjust dose

Clopidogrel (Plavix, Generics) [Antiplatelet/Platelet Aggregation Inhibitor] Uses: *Reduce atherosclerotic events*, administer ASAP in ECC setting w/ high-risk ST depressior T-wave inversion **Action:** ↓ Plt aggregation **Dose:** 75 mg/d *ECC 2010:* ACS: 300–600 mg PO loading dose, then 75 mg/d PO; full effects take several days. **Caution:** [B, ?] Active bleeding; risk of bleeding from trauma & other; TTP; liver Dz; other CYP2C19 (eg, fluconazole); OK w/ ranitidine, famotidine **CI:** Coagulation disorders, active/intracranial bleeding; CABG planned w/in 5–7 d **Disp:** Tabs 75, 300 mg **SE:** ↑ bleeding time, GI intolerance, HA, dizziness, rash, thrombocytopenia, ↓ WBC **Interactions:** Do not use with PPI or other CYP2C19 (eg, fluconazole); OK with ranitidine, famotidine; ↑ risk of GI bleed *W/* ASA, NSAIDs, heparin, warfarin, feverfew, garlic, ginger, ginkgo; ↑ effects **OF** phenytoin, tamoxifen, tolbutamide **Labs:** ↑ LFTs; ↓ plts, WBC **NIPE:** plt aggregation to baseline 5 d after D/C; plt transfusion to reverse acutely; take w/o regard to food; ✓ for bleeding; notify DDS/MD of med use before surgery or procedures

Clorazepate (Tranxene) [Anxiolytic, Anticonvulsant, Sedative/ Hypnotic/Benzodiazepine] [C-IV] Uses: *Acute anxiety disorders, acute EtOH withdrawal Sxs, adjunctive therapy in partial Szs* **Action:** Benzodiazepine; antianxiety agent **Dose:** *Adults.* 15–60 mg/d PO single or ÷ doses *Elderly & debilitated pts.* Initial 7.5–15 mg/d in ÷ doses *EtOH withdrawal: Day 1:* Initial 30 mg; then 30–60 mg ÷ doses *Day 2:* 45–90 mg ÷ doses *Day 3:* 22.5–45 mg ÷ doses *Day 4:* 15–30 mg ÷ doses; after Day 4, 15–30 mg ÷ doses, then 7.5–15 mg/d ÷ doses *Peds.* 3.75–7.5 mg/dose bid to 60 mg/d max ÷ bid–tid **Caution:** [D, ?/–] Elderly; Hx depression **CI:** NAG; Not OK < 9 y of age **Disp:** Tabs 3.75, 7.5, 15 mg **SE:** CNS depressant effects (drowsiness, dizziness, ataxia, memory impair), ↓ BP **Interactions:** ↑ Effects **W/** antidepressants, antihistamines, barbiturates, MAOIs, opiates, phenothiazines, cimetidine, disulfiram, EtOH; ↑ effects **OF** levodopa; ↓ effects **W/** rifampin, ginkgo, tobacco **Labs:** ↑ Alk phos; monitor pts w/ renal/hepatic impair (drug may accumulate) **NIPE:** ⊘ D/C abruptly; may cause dependence; ⊘ ETOH; ✓ for ↑ depression, suicidal ideation, ↓ Sz control

Clotrimazole (Lotrimin, Mycelex, Others) [Antifungal] [OTC] Uses: *Candidiasis & tinea Infxns* **Action:** Antifungal; alters cell wall permeability *Spectrum:* Oropharyngeal candidiasis, dermatophytoses, superficial mycoses, cutaneous candidiasis, & vulvovaginal candidiasis **Dose:** *PO: Prophylaxis:* One troche dissolved in mouth tid *Rx:* 1 troche dissolved in mouth 5 ×/d for 14 d. *Vag 1% cream:* 1 applicator-full hs for 7 d. *2% cream:* 1 applicator-full hs for 3 d. *Tabs:* 100 mg vaginally hs for 7 d or 200 mg (2 tabs) vaginally hs for 3 d or 500-mg tabs vaginally hs once *Topical:* Apply bid 10–14 d **Caution:** [B (C if PO), ?] Not for systemic fungal Infxn; safety in children < 3 y not established **CI:** Component allergy **Disp:** 1% cream; soln; troche 10 mg; vag cream 1%, 2% **SE:** *Topical:* Local irritation; *PO:* N/V, ↑ LFTs **Interactions:** ↑ Effects **OF** cyclosporine, tacrolimus; ↓ effects **OF** spermicides **Labs:** ↑ LFTs **NIPE:** PO prophylaxis immunosuppressed pts; wash hands before/after applying

Clotrimazole & Betamethasone (Lotrisone) [Antifungal, Anti- Inflammatory] Uses: *Fungal skin Infxns* **Action:** Imidazole antifungal & anti-inflammatory. *Spectrum:* Tinea pedis, cruris, & corporis **Dose:** Children ≥ 17 y. Apply & massage into area bid for 2–4 wk **Caution:** [C, ?] Varicella Infxn **CI: Children** < 12 y **Disp:** Cream 1% & 0.05% 15, 45 g; lotion 1% & 0.05%; 30 mL **SE:** Local irritation, rash **NIPE:** Not for diaper dermatitis or under occlusive dressings

Clozapine (Clozaril, FazaClo, Versacloz) [Antipsychotic/Dibenzo- diazepine Derivative] **WARNING:** Myocarditis, agranulocytosis, Szs, & orthostatic ↓ BP associated w/ clozapine; ↑ mortality in elderly w/ dementia-related psychosis **Uses:** *Refractory severe schizophrenia*; childhood psychosis; obsessive-compulsive disorder (OCD), bipolar disorder **Action:** "Atypical" TCA **Dose:** 1 2 . 5 mg daily or bid initial; ↑ to 300–450 mg/d over 2 wk; maintain lowest dose possible; do not D/C abruptly **Caution:** [B, +/–] Monitor for psychosis & cholinergic rebound **CI:** Uncontrolled epilepsy; comatose state; WBC < 3500 cells/mm³ & ANC < 2000 cells/mm³ before Rx or < 3000 cells/mm³ during Rx; Eos > 4000/mm³ **Disp:** Orally disintegrating tabs (ODTs) 12.5, 25, 100, 150, 20 mg; tabs 25, 100 mg; susp 50 mg/mL **SE:** Sialorrhea, tachycardia, drowsiness, ↑ wgt, constipation, incontinence, rash, Szs, CNS stimulation, hyperglycemia **Interactions:** ↑ Effects *W/* clarithromycin, cimetidine, erythromycin, fluoxetine, paroxetine, quinidine, sertraline; ↑ depressant effects *W/* CNS depressants, EtOH; ↑ effects *OF* digoxin, warfarin; ↓ effects *W/* carbamazepine, phenytoin, primidone, phenobarbital, valproic acid, St. John's wort, nutmeg, caffeine; ↓ effects *OF* phenytoin **Labs:** Monitor WBCs; weekly CBC mandatory 1st 6 mo, then qowk **NIPE:** ↑ Risk of developing agranulocytosis; ◌ abrupt D/C; ◌ ETOH, caffeine, ✓ fever, flu-like symptoms; give w/o regard to food

Cocaine [C-II] [Narcotic Analgesic] Uses: *Topical anesthetic for mucous membranes* **Action:** Narcotic analgesic, local vasoconstrictor **Dose:** Lowest topical amount that provides relief; 3 mg/kg max **Caution:** [C, ?] **CI:** PRG, ocular anesthesia **Disp:** Topical soln & viscous preparations 4–10%; powder **SE:** CNS stimulation, nervousness, loss of taste/smell, chronic rhinitis, CV tox, abuse potential **Interactions:** ↑ Effects *W/* MAOIs, ↑ risk of HTN & arrhythmias *W/* epinephrine **NIPE:** Use only on PO, laryngeal, & nasal mucosa; do not use on extensive areas of broken skin

Codeine [C-II] [Analgesic, Antitussive/Opioid] Uses: *Mild–mod pain; symptomatic relief of cough* **Action:** Narcotic analgesic; ↓ cough reflex **Dose:** *Adults.* *Analgesic:* 15–60 mg PO or IM q4h PRN; 360 mg max/24 h *Antitussive:* 10–20 mg PO q4h PRN; max 120 mg/d *Peds.* *Analgesic:* 0.5–1 mg/kg/dose PO q4–6h PRN *Antitussive:* 1–1.5 mg/kg/24 h PO ÷ q4h; max 30 mg/24 h; ↓ in renal/hepatic impair **Caution:** [C (D if prolonged use or high dose at term), +] Hx drug abuse, severe hepatic impair **CI:** Component sensitivity **Disp:** Tabs 15, 30, 60 mg; soln 30 mg/5 mL; Inj 15, 30 mg/mL **SE:** Drowsiness, constipation, ↓ BP **Interactions:** ↑ CNS depression *W/* CNS depressants, antidepressants, MAOIs, TCAs, barbiturates, benzodiazepines, muscle relaxants, phenothiazines, cimetidine, antihistamines, sedatives, EtOH; ↑ effects *OF* digitoxin, phenytoin, rifampin; ↓ effects *W/* nalbuphine, pentazocine, tobacco **Labs:** ↑ Amylase, lipase, ↑ urine morphine **NIPE:** Usually combined w/ APAP for pain or w/ agents (eg, terpin-hydrate) as an antitussive; 120 mg IM = 10 mg IM morphine; give w/ food to ↓ GI distress; ◌ EtOH

Colchicine (Colcrys) [Antigout Agent/Colchicum Alkaloid] Uses: *Acute gouty arthritis & prevention of recurrences; familial Mediterranean fever*; primary biliary cirrhosis **Action:** ↓ Migration of leukocytes; ↓ leukocyte lactic acid production Dose: *Acute gout:* 1.2 mg load, 0.6 mg 1 h later, then prophylactic 0.6 mg/qd-bid *FMF: Adult* 1.2–2.4 mg/d *Peds* > *4 y see label* Caution: [C, +] w/ P-glycoprotein or CYP3A4 inhib in pt w/ renal or hepatic impair; ↓ dose or avoid in elderly or w/ indinavir CI: Serious renal, GI, hepatic, or cardiac disorders; blood dyscrasias Disp: Tabs 0.6 mg SE: N/V/D, Abd pain, BM suppression, hepatotox Notes: IV no longer available Interactions: ↑ Risk of leukopenia W/ phenylbutazone; ↓ effects W/ loop diuretics; ↓ effects *OF* vit B₁₂ Labs: ↑ Alk phos, ALT, AST; ↓ cholesterol, Hgb, Hct, plts; false(+) urine Hgb & RBCs NIPE: ⊘ EtOH; give w/ adeq H₂O; maintain hydration (8–10 8-oz glasses); ⊘ grapefruit products; D/C when gout pain is resolved or w/ N, V, D

Colesevelam (WelChol) [Antilipemic/Bile Acid Sequestrant] Uses: *↓↓ LDL & total cholesterol alone or in combo w/ an HMG-CoA reductase inhib, improve glycemic control in type 2 DM* Action: Bile acid sequestrant Dose: 3 tabs PO bid or 6 tabs daily w/meals Caution: [B, ?] Severe GI motility disorders; in pts w/ triglycerides > 300 mg/dL (may ↑ levels); use not established in peds CI: Bowel obst, serum triglycerides > 500; Hx hypertriglyceridemia-pancreatitis Disp: Tabs 625 mg; oral susp 1.875, 3.75 g SE: Constipation, dyspepsia, myalgia, weakness Interactions: ↓ Vit absorption Labs: Monitor lipids NIPE: Take w/ food & Liq; may ↓ absorption of fat-soluble vits; ✓ lipids, HbA1c, BG to assess therapeutic effect

Colestipol (Colestid) [Antilipemic/Bile Acid Sequestrant] Uses:* Adjunct to ↓ serum cholesterol in primary hypercholesterolemia, relieve pruritus associated w/ ↑ bile acids* Action: Binds intestinal bile acids to form insoluble complex Dose: *Granules:* 5–30 g/d ÷ 2–4 doses; tabs: 2–16 g/d ÷ daily–bid Caution: [C, ?] Avoid w/ high triglycerides, GI dysfunction Disp: Bowel obst Disp: Tabs 1 g; granules 5 g/pack or scoop SE: Constipation, Abd pain, bloating, HA, GI irritation & bleeding Interactions: ↓ Absorption *OF* numerous drugs esp anticoagulants, cardiac glycosides, digitoxin, digoxin, phenobarbital, PCN G, tetracycline, thiazide diuretics, thyroid drugs Labs: ↑ Alk phos; PT prolonged NIPE: Take other meds 1 h before or 4 h after colestipol; do not use dry powder; mix w/ beverages, cereals, etc; may ↓ absorption of other medications & fat-soluble vits

Conivaptan HCL (Vaprisol) [Hyponatremic Agent/Vasopressin Receptor Antagonist] Uses: Euvolemic & hypervolemic hyponatremia Action: Dual arginine vasopressin V_{1A}/V_2 receptor antagonist Dose: 20 mg IV × 1 over 30 min, then 20 mg cont IV Inf over 24 h; 20 mg/d cont IV Inf for 1–3 more d; may ↑ to 40 mg/dif Na⁺ not responding; 4 d max use; use large vein, change site q24h Caution: [C, ?/–] Rapid ↑ Na⁺ (> 12 mEq/L/24 h) may cause osmotic demyelination syndj impaired renal/hepatic Fxn; may ↑ digoxin levels; CYP3A4 inhib (Table 10) CI: Hypovolemic hyponatremia; w/ CYP3A4 inhib; anuria Disp: Inj 20 mg/100 mL SE: Inf site Rxns, HA, N/V/D, constipation, orthostatic ↓ BP, thirst, dry mouth, pyrexia, pollakiuria, polyuria, Infxn Interactions: ↑ Effects *OF* amlodipine, digoxin, midazolam, simvastatin, & CYP3A4 Inhibs such as clarithromycin, itraconazole, ketoconazole, ritonavir **Labs:** May ↑ digoxin level; ↓ K⁺, Na⁺, Mg²⁺; monitor Na⁺; D/C w/ very rapid ↑ Na⁺ **NIPE:** Mix only w/ 5% dextrose; D/C w/ very rapid ↑ Na⁺; monitor Na⁺, vol, & neurologic status; change position slowly

Conjugated Estrogens/Bazedoxifene (Duavee) **WARNING:** Do not use w/ additional estrogen; ↑ risk endometrial CA; do not use to prevent CV Dz or dementia; ↑ risk of stroke & DVT in postmenopausal (50–79 y); ↑ dementia risk in postmenopausal (> 65 y) **Uses:** *Tx mod/severe menopausal vasomotor Sx; Px postmenopausal osteoporosis* **Action:** Conj estrogens w/ estrogen agonist/antagonist **Dose:** Adults. One tab PO daily **Caution:** [X, –] w/ CYP3A4 inhib may ↑ exposure; do not use w/progestins, other estrogens; w/ Hx of CV Dz; ↑ risk gallbladder Dz; D/C w/vision loss, severe ↑ TG, jaundice; monitor thyroid function if on thyroid Rx **CI:** Hepatic impair; deficiency of protein C or S, antithrombin, other thrombophilic Dz; AUB; Hx breast CA; estrogen-dependent neoplasia; Hx of TE; PRG, child-bearing potential, nursing mothers; component hypersens **Disp:** Tab (conj estrogens/bazedoxifene): 0.45/20 mg **SE:** N/D, dyspepsia, abd pain, oropharyngeal/neck pain, dizziness, muscle spasms, hot flush **Notes:** Use for shortest duration for benefit; not rec > 75 y. **NIPE:** Take same time of day; take w/food if nausea occurs; ⊘ smoking; ⊘ grapefruit products; ✓ and teach pt S/Sx of DVT; D/C w/ PRG

Copper IUD Contraceptive (ParaGard T380A) [Contraceptive] **Uses:** *Contraception, long-term (up to 10 y)* **Action:** ?, interfere w/ sperm survival/transport **Dose:** Insert any time during menstrual cycle; replace at 10 y max **Caution:** [C,?] Remove w/ intrauterine PRG, increased risk of comps w/ PRG & device in place **CI:** Acute PID or in high-risk behavior, postpartum endometritis, cervicitis **Disp:** 309 mg IUD **SE:** PRG, ectopic PRG, pelvic Infxn w/ or w/o immunocompromised, embedment, perforation, expulsion, Wilson Dz, fainting w/ insert, Vag bleeding, expulsion **NIPE:** Counsel pt does not protect against STD/HIV; see package insert for detailed instructions; 99% effective

Cortisone, Systemic & Topical See Steroids and Tables 2 & 3

Crizotinib (Xalkori) **Uses:** *Locally advanced/metastatic NSCLC anaplastic lymphoma kinase (ALK)-positive* **Acts:** TKI **Dose:** Adult. 250 mg PO bid; swallow whole; see label for tox adjustments **W/P:** [D, ?/–] w/ Hepatic impair & CrCl < 30 mL/min; may cause ↑ QT (monitor); ↓ dose w/ CYP3A substrates; avoid w/ strong CYP3A inducers/inhib & CYP3A substrates w/ narrow therapeutic index **Disp:** Caps 200, 250 mg **SE:** N/V/D, constipation, Abd pain, stomatitis, edema, vision disorder, hepatotox, pneumonitis, pneumonia, PE, neutropenia, thrombocytopenia, lymphopenia, HA, dizziness, fatigue, cough, dyspnea, URI, fever, arthralgia, ↓ appetite, rash, neuropathy **Notes:** ✓ CBC & LFTs monthly. **NIPE:** Take w/o regard to food; ⊘ grapefruit products; ⊘ crush or cut; use effective contraception during Tx & 3 mos after Tx; ⊘ ETOH

Crofelemer (Fulyzaq) **Uses:** *Noninfectious diarrhea w/ HIV on antiretrovirals* **Acts:** Inhibits cAMP-stimulated CF transmembrane conductance regulator

Cl⁻ channel and Ca-activated Cl⁻ channels of intestinal epithelial cells, controls Cl⁻ and fluid secretion **Dose:** 125 mg bid **W/P:** [C, –] **CI:** None **Disp:** Tab 125 mg DR **SE:** Flatulence, cough, bronchitis, URI, ↑ bili **Notes:** R/O infectious D before; do not crush/chew tabs; minimal absorb, drug interact unlikely. **NIPE:** R/O infectious etiologies for D before starting crofelemer; ⊘ PRG; can take w/o regard to food; ⊘ crush or chew; swallow tablet whole

Cromolyn Sodium (Intal, NasalCrom, Opticrom, Others) [Anti-asthmatic/Mast Cell Stabilizer]

Uses: *Adjunct to the Rx of asthma; prevent exercise-induced asthma; allergic rhinitis; ophthal allergic manifestations*; food allergy, systemic mastocytosis, IBD **Action:** Antiasthmatic; mast cell stabilizer **Dose:** *Adults & Children > 12 y.* **Inh:** 20 mg (as powder in caps) inhaled qid *PO:* 200 mg qid 15–20 min ac, up to 400 mg qid *Nasal instillation:* Spray once in each nostril 2–6 ×/d *Ophthal:* 1–2 gtt in each eye 4–6 ×d **Peds.** **Inh:** 2 puffs qid of metered-dose inhaler *PO: Infants < 2 y.* (not OK) 20 mg/kg/d in 4 ÷ doses *2–12 y.* 100 mg qid ac **Caution:** [B, ?] w/ Renal/hepatic impair **CI:** Acute asthmatic attacks **Disp:** PO conc 100 mg/5 mL; soln for nebulizer 20 mg/2 mL; nasal soln 40 mg/mL; ophthal soln 4% **SE:** Unpleasant taste, hoarseness, coughing **Interactions:** None noted **Labs:** Monitor pulm Fxn tests **NIPE:** No benefit in acute Rx; 2–4 wk for max effect in perennial allergic disorders; for ophthalmic use: ⊘ contact lenses; ⊘ use with other ocular drugs

Cyanocobalamin [Vitamin B₁₂] (Nascobal) [Vitamin B/Dietary Supplement]

Uses: *Pernicious anemia & other vit B₁₂ deficiency states; ↑ requirements d/t PRG; thyrotoxicosis; liver or kidney Dz* **Action:** Dietary vit B₁₂ supl **Dose:** *Adults.* 30 mcg/d × 5–10 d intranasal: 500 mcg once/wk for pts in remission, then 100 mcg IM or SQ daily for 5–10 d, then 100 mcg IM 2 ×/wk for 1 mo, then 100 mcg IM monthly. *Peds.* Use 0.2 mcg/kg × 2 d test dose; if OK 30–50 mcg/d for 2 or more wk (total 1000 mcg) then maint: 100 mg/mo **Caution:** [A (C if dose exceeds RDA), +] **CI:** Allergy to cobalt; hereditary optic nerve atrophy; Leber Dz **Disp:** Tabs 50, 100, 250, 500, 1000, 2500, 5000 mcg; Inj 1000 mcg/mL; intranasal (Nascobal) gel 500 mcg/0.1 mL **SE:** Itching, D, HA, anxiety **Interactions:** ↓ Effects d/t malabsorption of B₁₂ *W/* aminosalicylic acid, aminoglycosides, chloramphenicol, EtOH **Labs:** ↓ K⁺ levels **NIPE:** PO absorption erratic & not recommended; OK for use w/ hyperalimentation; use nasal preparation 1 h before or 1 h after intake of hot foods/liquids

Cyclobenzaprine (Flexeril) [Skeletal Muscle Relaxant/ANS Agent]

Uses: *Relief of muscle spasm* **Action:** Centrally acting skeletal muscle relaxant; reduces tonic somatic motor activity **Dose:** 5–10 mg PO bid–qid (2–3 wk max) **Caution:** [B, ?] Shares the toxic potential of the TCAs; urinary hesitancy, NAG **CI:** Do not use concomitantly or w/in 14 d of MAOIs; hyperthyroidism; heart failure; arrhythmias **Disp:** Tabs 5, 10 mg **SE:** Sedation & anticholinergic effects **Interactions:** ↑ Effects of CNS depression *W/* CNS depressants, TCAs, barbiturates, EtOH; ↑ risk of HTN & convulsions *W/* MAOIs **NIPE:** ↑ Fluids &

fiber for constipation; may inhibit mental alertness or physical coordination; ⊘ ETOH

Cyclobenzaprine, Extended Release (Amrix) [Skeletal Muscle Relaxant/ANS Agent] **Uses:** *Muscle spasm* **Action:** ? Centrally acting long-term muscle relaxant **Dose:** 15–30 mg PO daily 2–3 wk; 30 mg/d max **Caution:** [B, ?/–] w/ Urinary retention, NAG, w/ EtOH/CNS depressant **CI:** MAOI w/in 14 d, elderly, arrhythmias, heartblock, CHF, MI recovery phase, ↑ thyroid **Disp:** Caps ER 15, 30 mg **SE:** Dry mouth, drowsiness, dizziness, HA, N, blurred vision, dysgeusia **Interactions:** ↑ Effects of CNS depression *W/* CNS depressants, TCAs, barbiturates, EtOH; ↑ risk of HTN & convulsions *W/* MAOIs **NIPE:** ↑ Fluids & fiber constipation; may inhibit mental alertness or physical coordination; avoid abrupt D/C w/ long-term use; take same time daily; avoid use in elderly, hepatic impairment

Cyclopentolate Ophthalmic (Cyclogyl, Cylate) [Anticholinergic/ Cycloplegic Mydriatic Agent] **Uses:** *Cycloplegia, mydriasis* **Action:** Cycloplegic mydriatic, anticholinergic inhibits iris sphincter and ciliary body **Dose:** *Adults.* 1 gtt in eye 40–50 min pre-procedure, may repeat × 1 in 5–10 min *Peds.* As adult, children 0.5%; infants use 0.5% **Caution:** [C (may cause late-term fetal anoxia/↓ HR), +/–], w/ premature infants, HTN, Down synd, elderly **CI:** NAG **Disp:** Ophthal soln 0.5, 1, 2% **SE:** Tearing, HA, irritation, eye pain, photophobia, arrhythmia, tremor, ↑ IOP, confusion **Interactions:** ↓ Effects *OF* carbachol, cholinesterase Inhibs, pilocarpine **NIPE:** Burning sensation when instilled; compress lacrimal sac for several min after dose; heavily pigmented irises may require ↑ strength; peak 25–75 min, cycloplegia 6–24 h, mydrias is up to 24 h; 2% soln may result in psychotic Rxns & behavioral disturbances in peds; ↑ sensitivity to light, protect eyes in bright light during dilation; avoid driving while pupils are dilated

Cyclopentolate with Phenylephrine (Cyclomydril) [Anticholinergic/ Cycloplegic Mydriatic, Alpha-Adrenergic Agonist] **Uses:** *Mydriasis greater than cyclopentolate alone* **Action:** Cycloplegic mydriatic, α-adrenergic agonist w/ anticholinergic to inhibit iris sphincter **Dose:** 1 gtt in eye q5–10 min (max 3 doses) 40–50 min pre-procedure **Caution:** (C [may cause late-term fetal anoxia/ ↓ HR, +/–] HTN, or elderly w/ CAD **CI:** NAG **Disp:** Ophthal soln cyclopentolate 0.2%/phenylephrine 1% (2, 5 mL) SE: Tearing, HA, irritation, eye pain, photophobia, arrhythmia, tremor **NIPE:** Compress lacrimal sac for several min after dose; heavily pigmented irises may require ↑ strength; peak 25–75 min, cycloplegia 6–24 h, mydriasis up to 24 h; ↑ sensitivity to light, protect eyes in bright light during dilation; avoid driving while pupils are dilated

Cyclosporine (Gengraf, Neoral, Sandimmune) [Immunosuppressant/ Polypeptide Antibiotic] **WARNING:** ↑ risk neoplasm, ↑ risk skin malignancies, ↑ risk HTN & nephrotox **Uses:** *Organ rejection in kidney, liver, heart, & BMT w/ steroids; RA; psoriasis* **Action:** Immunosuppressant; reversible inhibition of immunocompetent lymphocytes **Dose:** *Adults & Peds. PO:* 15 mg/kg/12 h pretransplant; after 2 wk, taper by 5 mg/wk to 5–10 mg/kg/d. *IV:* If NPO, give 1/3 PO dose IV; ↓ in renal/hepatic impair **Caution:** [C, –] Dose-related risk of nephrotox/hepatotox/serious fatal Infxns; live, attenuated vaccines may be less effective; may induce fatal malignancy; many drug interactions; ↑ risk of Infxns after D/C **CI:** Renal impair; uncontrolled HTN; w/ lovastatin, simvastatin **Disp:** Caps 25, 100 mg; PO soln 100 mg/mL; Inj 50 mg/mL **SE:** May ↑ BUN & Cr & mimic transplant rejection; HTN; HA; hirsutism **Notes:** Levels: *Trough:* Just before next dose *Therapeutic:* Variable 150–300 ng/mL RIA **Interactions:** ↑ Effects W/ azole antifungals, allopurinol, amiodarone, anabolic steroids, CCBs, cimetidine, chloroquine, clarithromycin, clonidine, diltiazem, macrolides, metoclopramide, nicardipine, NSAIDs, OCPs, ticlopidine, grapefruit juice; ↑ nephrotox W/ aminoglycosides, amphotericin B, acyclovir, colchicine, enalapril, ranitidine, sulfonamides; ↑ risk of digoxin tox; ↑ risk of hyperkalemia W/ diuretics, ACEIs; ↓ effects W/ barbiturates, carbamazepine, INH, nafcillin, pyrazinamide, phenytoin, rifampin, sulfonamides, St. John's wort, alfalfa sprouts, astragalus, echinacea, licorice; ↓ effects *OF* immunizations **Labs:** ↑ SCr, BUN, LFTs, LDL, glucose; ↓ Hgb, plts, WBCs; monitor Cr, CBC, LFTs **NIPE:** Monitor BP & ✓ for hyperglycemia, hyperkalemia, hyperuricemia; risk of photosensitivity—use sunscreen; administer in glass container; Neoral & Sandimmune not interchangeable; take same time of day; ⊘ grapefruit products

Cyclosporine Ophthalmic (Restasis) [Immunosuppressant/Anti-Inflammatory] Uses: *↑ Tear production suppressed d/t ocular inflammation* **Action:** Immune modulator, anti-inflammatory **Dose:** 1 gtt bid each eye 12 h apart; OK w/ artificial tears, allow 15 min between **Caution:** [C, –] **CI:** Ocular Infxn, component allergy **Disp:** Single-use vial 0.05% **SE:** Ocular burning/ hyperemia **NIPE:** ⊘ Children < 16 y; may insert contact lenses 15 min after instillation; mix vial well

Cyproheptadine (Periactin) [Antihistamine, Antipruritic] Uses: *Allergic Rxns; itching* **Action:** Phenothiazine antihistamine; serotonin antagonist **Dose:** *Adults.* 4–20 mg PO ÷ q8h; max 0.5 mg/kg/d *Peds 2–6 y.* 2 mg bid–tid (max 12 mg/24 h) *7–14 y.* 4 mg bid–tid; ↓ in hepatic impair **Caution:** [B, ?] Elderly, CV Dz, asthma, thyroid Dz, BPH **CI:** Neonates or < 2 y; NAG; BOO; acute asthma; GI obst; w/MAOI **Disp:** Tabs 4 mg; syrup 2 mg/5 mL **SE:** Anticholinergic, drowsiness **Interactions:** ↑ Effects W/ CNS depressants, MAOIs, EtOH; ↓ effects *OF* epinephrine, fluoxetine **Labs:** False(–) allergy skin testing **NIPE:** ↑ Risk photosensitivity—use sunscreen, take w/ food if GI distress; may stimulate appetite; ⊘ breast-feeding

Cytarabine [ARA-C] (Cytosar-U) [Antineoplastic/Antimetabolite] **WARNING:** Administration by experienced physician in properly equipped facility; potent myelosuppressive agent **Uses:** *Acute leukemias, CML, NHL; IT for leukemic meningitis or prophylaxis* **Action:** Antimetabolite; interferes w/ DNA synth **Dose:** 100–150 mg/m²/d for 5–10 d (low dose); 3 g/m² q12h for 6–12 doses (high dose); 1 mg/kg 1–2/wk (SQ maint); 5–75 mg/m² up to 3/wk IT (per protocols); ↓ in renal/ hepatic impair **Caution:** [D, ?] In elderly, w/ marked BM suppression, ↓ dosage by ↓ the number of days of administration **CI:** Component sensitivity **Disp:** Inj 100, 500, 1, 2 g, also 20, 100 mg/mL **SE:** ↓ BM, N/V/D, stomatitis, flu-like synd, rash on palms/soles, hepatic/cerebellar dysfunction w/high doses, noncardiogenic pulm edema, neuropathy, fever **Interactions:** ↓ Effects *OF* digoxin, flucytosine **Labs:** ↓ Uric acid, ↓ Hgb, Hct, plts, RBCs, WBCs **NIPE:** ⊘ EtOH, NSAIDs, ASA, PRG, breast-feeding, immunizations; little use in solid tumors; high-dose tox limited by corticosteroid ophth soln; ↑ fluid intake; ✓ for infxn

Cytarabine Liposome (DepoCyt) [Antineoplastic/Antimetabolite]
WARNING: Can cause chemical arachnoiditis (N/V/HA, fever) ↓ severity w/ dexamethasone. Administer by experienced physician in properly equipped facility **Uses:** *Lymphomatous meningitis* **Action:** Antimetabolite; interferes w/DNA synth **Dose:** 50 mg IT q14d for 5 doses, then 50 mg IT q28d × 4 doses; use dexamethasone prophylaxis **Caution:** [D, ?] May cause neurotox; blockage to CSF flow may ↑ the risk of neurotox; use in peds not established **CI:** Active meningeal Infxn **Disp:** IT Inj 50 mg/5 mL **SE:** Neck pain/rigidity, HA, confusion, somnolence, fever, back pain, N/V, edema, neutropenia, ↓ plt, anemia **Interactions:** ↓ Effects *OF* digoxin, flucytosine **Labs:** ↑ Uric acid, ↓ Hgb, Hct, plts, RBCs, WBCs **NIPE:** EtOH, NSAIDs, ASA, PRG, breast-feeding, immunizations; cytarabine liposomes are similar in microscopic appearance to WBCs; caution in interpreting CSF studies; ✓ & educate for S/Sx of neurotoxicity; Tx concurrently w/ dexamethasone

Cytomegalovirus Immune Globulin [CMV-IGIV] (CytoGam) [Immune Globulin] **Uses:** *Prophylaxis/attenuation CMV Dz w/ transplantation* **Action:** IgG antibodies to CMV **Dose:** 150 mg/kg/dose w/in 72 h of transplant & wk 2, 4, 6, 8; 100–150 mg/kg/dose wk 12, 16 post transplant; 50–100 mg/kg/dose **Caution:** [C, ?] Anaphylactic Rxns; renal dysfunction **CI:** Allergy to immunoglobulins; IgA deficiency **Disp:** Inj 50 mg/mL **SE:** Flushing, N/V, muscle cramps, wheezing, HA, fever, noncardiogenic pulm edema, renal Insuff, aseptic meningitis **Interactions:** ↓ Effects *OF* live virus vaccines **NIPE:** IV only; administer by separate line; do not shake; ✓ VS continuously during infusion; ✓ S/Sx infection, receive prompt Tx

Dabigatran (Pradaxa) [Direct Thrombin Inhibitor] **WARNING:** Pradaxa D/C w/o adequate anticoagulation ↑ stroke risk **Uses:** *↓ Risk stroke/ systemic embolism w/ non-valvular AF* **Action:** Thrombin Inhib **Dose:** CrCl > 30 mL/min: 150 mg PO bid; CrCl 15–30 mL/min: 75 mg PO bid **Caution:** [C, ?/–] Avoid w/ P-glycoprotein inducers (eg, rifampin) **CI:** Active bleeding; prosthetic valve **Disp:** Caps 75, 150 mg **SE:** Bleeding, gastritis, dyspepsia **Interactions:** ↑ Effects *W/* ketoconazole, amiodarone, quinidine, clopidogrel, verapamil; ↑ risk of bleeding *W/* fibrinolytics, heparin, NSAIDs, plt Inhibs; ↓ effects *W/* rifampin

Labs: Monitor aPTT **NIPE:** Do not chew/break/open caps; see label to convert between anticoagulants; do not undergo surgery or dental procedures while using dabigatran—D/C 1–5 days prior to invasive/surgical procedures

Dabrafenib (Tafinlar) Uses: *Met melanoma (single agent) w/BRAF V600E mut; combo w/ trametinib w/BRAF V600E or V600K mut* **Action:** TKI **Dose:** *Adults.* *As single agent:* 150 mg PO bid; *Combo:* 150 mg PO bid + trametinib 2 mg PO 1 x/d; 1 h ac or 2 h pc; see label dosage mods w/tox **Caution:** [D, –] embryo-fetal tox; may cause new malignancies, tumor promotion in BRAF wild-type melanoma, ↑ bleeding risk, cardiomyopathy, VTE, ocular tox, skin tox, ↑ glucose, febrile Rxn; risk of hemolytic anemia w/ G6PD def; avoid w/ strong Inhib/inducers CYP3A4 & CYP2C8; use w/ substrates of CYP3A4, CYP2C8, CYP2C9, CYP2C19, or CYP2B6 may ↓ efficacy of these agents **CI:** None **Disp:** Caps 50, 75 mg **SE:** See Caution; single agent: hyperkeratosis, pyrexia, arthralgia, papilloma, alopecia, HA, palmar-plantar erythrodysesthesia synd; w/trametinib: N/V/D, constipation, abd pain, pyrexia, chills, fatigue, rash, edema, cough, HA, arthralgia, night sweats, ↓ appetite, myalgia **NIPE:** Take w/o food ≥ 1 h ac or ≥ 2 h pc; swallow whole - ⊘ chew/crush/split; withhold if temp > 101.3°F; use nonhormonal contraception w/Tx and for 2 wk after D/C of single therapy or 4 mo after D/C w/ trametinib; may ↓ spermatogenesis

Dacarbazine (DTIC) [Antineoplastic/Alkylating Agent] WARNING: Causes hematopoietic depression, hepatic necrosis, may be carcinogenic, teratogenic Uses: *Melanoma, Hodgkin Dz, sarcoma* **Action:** Alkylating agent; antimetabolite as a purine precursor; ↓ protein synth, RNA, & especially DNA **Dose:** 2–4.5 mg/kg/d for 10 consecutive d or 250 mg/m²/d for 5 d (per protocols); ↓ in renal impair **Caution:** [C, –] In BM suppression; renal/hepatic impair **CI:** Component sensitivity **Disp:** Inj 100, 200 mg **SE:** ↓ BM, N/V, hepatotox, flu-like synd, ↓ BP, photosens, alopecia, facial flushing, facial paresthesias, urticaria, phlebitis at Inj site **Interactions:** ↑ Risk of bleeding *W/* anticoagulants, ASA; ↓ effects *W/* phenobarbital, phenytoin **Labs:** ↑ AST, ALT; ↓ plts, RBCs, WBCs; monitor CBC, plt **NIPE:** Risk of photosensitivity—use sunscreen; hair loss; Infxn; avoid extrav; to ↓ pain/burning at injection site may increase diluent, reduce infusion rate & apply cold compresses

Daclizumab (Zenapax) [Immunosuppressant/Immunomodulator] WARNING: Administration under skilled supervision in properly equipped facility Uses: *Prevent acute organ rejection* **Action:** IL-2 receptor antagonist **Dose:** 1 mg/kg/dose IV; 1st dose pretransplant, then 1 mg/kg q14d × 4 doses **Caution:** [C, ?] **CI:** Component sensitivity **Disp:** Inj 5 mg/mL **SE:** Hyperglycemia, edema, HTN, ↓ BP, constipation, HA, dizziness, anxiety, nephrotox, pulm edema, pain, anaphylaxis/hypersensitivity **Interactions:** ↑ Risk of mortality *W/* corticosteroids, cyclosporine, mycophenolate mofetil **NIPE:** Immunizations; Infxns; ↑ fluid intake; administration w/in 4 h of prep

Dactinomycin (Cosmegen) [Antineoplastic/Antibiotic] **WARNING:** Administration under skilled supervision in properly equipped facility; powder & soln toxic, corrosive, mutagenic, carcinogenic, & teratogenic; avoid exposure and use precautions **Uses:** *Choriocarcinoma, Wilms tumor, Kaposi and Ewing sarcomas, rhabdomyosarcoma, uterine and testicular CA* **Action:** DNA-intercalating agent **Dose:** *Adults.* 15 mcg/kg/d for 5 d q3–6 wk or 400–600 mcg/m^2 for 5 d q3–6wk *Peds. Sarcoma* (per protocols); ↓ in renal impair **Caution:** [D, ?] **CI:** Concurrent/recent chickenpox or herpes zoster; infants < 6 mo **Disp:** Inj 0.5 mg **SE:** Myelo-/immunosuppression, severe N/V/D, alopecia, acne, hyperpigmentation, radiation recall phenomenon, tissue damage w/ extrav, hepatotox **Interactions:** ↑ Effects *OF* BM suppressants, radiation therapy; ↓ effects *OF* vit K **Labs:** Monitor CBC; ↓ Hgb, Hct, plts, RBCs, WBCs **NIPE:** ⊘ PRG, breast-feeding; risk of irreversible infertility; reversible hair loss; ↑ fluids to 2–3; use sunscreen L/d; classified as antibiotic but not used as antimicrobial

Dalfampridine (Ampyra) [Potassium Channel Blocker] **Uses:** *Improve walking w/ MS* **Action:** K$^+$ channel blocker **Dose:** 10 mg PO q12h max dose/d 20 mg; **Caution:** [C, ?/–] Not w/ other 4-aminopyridines **CI:** Hx Sz; w/ CrCl ≤ 50 mL/min **Disp:** Tab ER 10 mg **SE:** HA, N, constipation, dyspepsia, dizziness, insomnia, UTI, nasopharyngitis, back pain, pharyngolaryngeal pain, asthenia, balance disorder, MS relapse, paresthesia, Sz **NIPE:** Do not cut/chew/crush/dissolve tab; take w/o regard to food; may cause dizziness—caution driving

Dalteparin (Fragmin) [Anticoagulant/Low-Molecular-Weight Heparin] **WARNING:** ↑ Risk of spinal/epidural hematoma w/ LP **Uses:** *Unstable angina, non-Q-wave MI, prevent & Rx DVT following surgery (hip, Abd), pt w/ restricted mobility, extended therapy Rx for PE DVT in CA pt* **Action:** LMW heparin **Dose:** *Angina/MI:* 120 units/kg (max 10,000 units) SQ q12h w/ ASA. *DVT prophylaxis:* 2500–5000 units SQ 1–2 h pre-op, then daily for 5–10 d *Systemic anticoagulation:* 200 units/kg/d SQ or 100 units/kg bid SQ *CA:* 200 IU/kg (max 18,000 IU) SQ q24h × 30 d, mo 2–6 150 IU/kg SQ q24h (max 18,000 IU) **Caution:** [B, ?] In renal/hepatic impair, active hemorrhage, cerebrovascular Dz, cerebral aneurysm, severe HTN **CI:** HIT; pork product allergy; w/ mifepristone **Disp:** Inj multiple ranging from 2500 units (16 mg/0.2 mL) to 25,000 units/mL (3.8 mL) *prefilled vials* **SE:** Bleeding, pain at site, ↓ plt **Interactions:** ↑ Bleeding *W/* oral anticoagulants, plt Inhibs, warfarin, garlic, ginger, ginkgo, ginseng, chamomile **Labs:** ↑ AST, ALT; monitor CBC & plts **NIPE:** ⊘ Give IM or IV; administration SQ route only; limit alcohol; bleeding precautions

Dantrolene (Dantrium, Revonto) [Skeletal Muscle Relaxant/ Hydantoin Derivative] **WARNING:** Hepatotox reported; D/C after 45 d if no benefit observed **Uses:** *Rx spasticity d/t upper motor neuron disorders (eg, spinal cord injuries, stroke, CP, MS); malignant hyperthermia* **Action:** Skeletal muscle relaxant **Dose:** *Adults. Spasticity:* 25 mg PO daily; ↑ 25 mg to effect to 100 mg PO q8h (400 mg/d max) *Peds.* 0.5 mg/kg/dose/d; ↑ by 0.5

mg/kg dose tid to 2 mg/kg dose tid (max 400 mg/d) *Adults & Peds. Malignant hyperthermia: Rx:* Cont rapid IV, start 1 mg/kg until Sxs subside or 10 mg/kg is reached *Postcrisis follow-up:* 4–8 mg/kg/d in 3–4 ÷ doses for 1–3 d to prevent recurrence **Caution:** [C, ?] Impaired cardiac/pulm/hepatic Fxn **CI:** Active hepatic Dz; where spasticity needed to maintain posture or balance **Disp:** Caps 25, 50, 100 mg; powder for Inj 20 mg/vial **SE:** Hepatotox, ↑ LFTs, drowsiness, dizziness, rash, muscle weakness, D/N/V, pleural effusion w/ pericarditis, blurred vision, hep, photosens **Interactions:** ↑ Effects *W/* CNS depressants, antihistamines, opiates, EtOH; ↑ risk of hepatotox *W/* estrogens; ↑ risk of CV collapse & VF *W/* CCBs; ↓ plasma protein binding *W/* clofibrate, warfarin **Labs:** ↑ LFTs—monitor **NIPE:** ↑ Risk of photosensitivity—use sunblock; ⊘ EtOH, CNS depressants, sunlight

Dapagliflozin (Farxiga) **Uses:** * Type 2 DM * **Acts:** SGLT2 Inhib **Dose:** 5–10 mg PO q AM; do not use if GFR < 60 mL/min **Caution:** [C, –] ↓ BP due to ↓ intravascular vol; ↑ Cr, check renal fxn; ↓ BS risk w/ insulin/insulin secretagogue; ↑ LDL; bladder CA **CI:** Hypersens rxn; severe renal impair (< 30 mL/min), end-stage renal Dz, dialysis **Disp:** Tabs 5, 10 mg **SE:** UTI, female genital mycotic Infxn, nasopharyngitis, see Caution **Notes:** No clinical trials to date to show ↓ in macrovascular complications **NIPE:** Maintain adequate hydration to ↓ risk of hypotension; okay to take w/ or w/o food—but consistency in how taken is advised; monitor BS

Dapsone, Oral [Antileprotic, Antimalarial] **Uses:** *Rx & prevent PCP; toxoplasmosis prophylaxis; leprosy* **Action:** Unknown; bactericidal **Dose:** *Adults.* PCP prophylaxis 50–100 mg/d PO; Rx PCP 100 mg/d PO w/ TMP 15–20 mg/kg/d for 21 d *Peds. PCP prophylaxis alternated* **Dose:** (> 1 mo) 4 mg/kg/dose once/wk (max 200 mg); Rx PCP: 1–2 mg/kg/24 h PO daily; max 100 mg/d **Caution:** [C, +] G6PD deficiency; severe anemia **CI:** Component sensitivis; rash, cholestatic jaundice **Disp:** Tabs 25, 100 mg **SE:** Hemolysis, methemoglobinemia, agranulocytosis, rash, cholestatic jaundice **Interactions:** ↑ Effects *W/* probenecid, TMP; ↓ effects *W/* activated charcoal, rifampin **Labs:** Monitor CBC, LFTs **NIPE:** ↑ Risk of photosensitivity—use sunblock; absorption ↑ by an acidic environment; take w/o regard to food; wait ≥ 2 h before taking antacids; for leprosy, combine w/ rifampin & other agents

Dapsone, Topical (Aczone) [Antileprotic, Antimalarial] **Uses:** *Topical for acne vulgaris* **Action:** Unknown; bactericidal **Dose:** Apply pea-size amount and rub into areas bid; wash hands after **Caution:** [C, +] G6PD deficiency; severe anemia **CI:** Component sensitivity **Disp:** 5% gel **SE:** Skin oiliness/peeling, dryness, erythema **Labs:** Check G6PD levels before use; follow CBC if G6PD deficient **NIPE:** Not for oral, ophthalmic, or intravag use

Daptomycin (Cubicin) [Antibiotic/Cyclic Lipopeptide Antibacterial] **Uses:** *Complicated skin/skin structure Infxns d/t gram(+) organisms* *S aureus,* bacteremia, MRSA endocarditis **Action:** Cyclic lipopeptide; rapid membrane depolarization & bacterial death. *Spectrum: S aureus* (including MRSA), *S pyogenes, S agalactiae, S dysgalactiae* subsp *Equisimilis,* & *E faecalis* (vancomycin-susceptible strains only) **Dose:** *Skin:* 4 mg/kg IV daily × 7–14 d (over 2 min) *Bacteremia & Endocarditis:* 6 mg/kg q24h; ↓ w/ CrCl < 30 mL/min or dialysis: q48h **Caution:** [B, ?] w/ HMG-CoA Inhib **Disp:** Inj 500 mg/10 mL **SE:** Anemia, constipation, N/V/D, HA, rash, site Rxn, muscle pain/weakness, edema, cellulitis, hypo-/hyper-glycemia, ↑ alkaline phosphatase, cough, back pain, Abd pain, ↓ K⁺, anxiety, CP, sore throat, cardiac failure, confusion, *Candida* Infxns **Interactions:** ↓ Effects *OF* anticoagulants; ↓ effects *OF* tobramycin; ↓ effects *W/* tobramycin **Labs:** Monitor CPK baseline & weekly, LFTs, PT, INR; ↑ alk phos, CPK, LFTs; ↓ Hgb, Hct, K⁺ **NIPE:** Safety & efficacy not established in pts < 18 y; consider D/C HMG-CoA reductase Inhibits to ↓ myopathy risk limit EtOH; may cause dizziness—caution driving; not for Rx PNA

Darbepoetin Alfa (Aranesp) [Antianemic/Hematopoietic]
WARNING: Associated w/ ↑ CV, thromboembolic events and/or mortality; D/C if Hgb > 12 g/dL; may increase tumor progression and death in CA pts **Uses:** *Anemia associated w/ CRF*, anemia in nonmyeloid malignancy w/ concurrent chemotherapy **Action:** ↑ Erythropoiesis, recombinant erythropoietin variant **Dose:** 0.45 mcg/kg single IV or SQ qwk; titrate, do not exceed target Hgb of 12 g/dL; use lowest doses possible, see PI to convert from Epogen **Caution:** [C, ?] May ↑ risk of CV &/or neurologic SE in renal failure; HTN; w/ Hx Szs **CI:** Uncontrolled HTN, component allergy **Disp:** 25, 40, 60, 100, 200, 300 mcg/mL, 150 mcg/0.075 mL in polysorbate or albumin excipient **SE:** May ↑ cardiac risk, CP, hypo-/hypertension, N/V/D, myalgia, arthralgia, dizziness, edema, fatigue, fever, ↑ risk Infxn **Interactions:** None noted **Labs:** Monitor weekly CBC until stable **NIPE:** Longer 1/2-life than Epogen; monitor BP & for Sz activity, shaking vial inactivates drug; needle cover on the prefilled syringe contains a derivative of latex—⊘ handle if latex allergy

Darifenacin (Enablex) [Antispasmodic/Anticholinergic]
Uses: *OAB* Urinary antispasmodic **Action:** Muscarinic receptor antagonist **Dose:** 7.5 mg/d PO; 15 mg/d max (7.5 mg/d w/ mod hepatic impair or w/ CYP3A4 Inhib); w/ drugs metabolized by CYP2D (Table 10); swallow whole **Caution:** [C, ?/–] Hepatic impair **CI:** Urinary/gastric retention, uncontrolled NAG, paralytic ileus **Disp:** Tabs ER 7.5, 15 mg **SE:** Xerostomia/eyes, constipation, dyspepsia, Abd pain, retention, abnormal vision, dizziness, asthenia **Interactions:** ↑ Effects *W/* clarithromycin, itraconazole, ketoconazole, ritonavir, nelfinavir; ↑ effects *OF* digoxin, flecainide, TCAs, thioridazine **Labs:** Monitor LFTs **NIPE:** Take w/ or w/o food & swallow whole; drug will relieve Sxs but not treat cause; may cause heat prostration d/t < sweating; for dry mouth take sips of water or use ice chips, sugarless hard candy, or sugarless gum

Darunavir (Prezista) [Antiretroviral/Protease Inhibitor]
Uses: *Rx HIV w/ resistance to multiple protease Inhib* **Action:** HIV-1 protease Inhib **Dose:** *Adult. Rx-naïve and w/o darunavir resistance substitutions:* 800 mg w/ ritonavir

100 mg qd. *Rx experienced w/o darunavir resistance:* 600 mg w/ ritonavir 100 mg bid w/ food. **Peds (6–18 y and > 20 kg).** Dose based on body weight (see label); do not exceed the Rx experienced adult dose. Do not use qd dosing in peds; w/ food **Caution:** [C, ?/–] Hx sulfa allergy, CYP3A4 substrate, changes levels of many meds (↑ amiodarone, ↑ dihydropyridine, ↑ HMG-CoA reductase Inhib [statins], ↓ SSRIs, ↓ methadone); do not use w/ salmeterol, colchicine w/ renal impair; do not use w/ severe hepatic impair); adjust dose w/ bosentan, tadalafil for PAH **CI:** w/ Astemizole, rifampin, St. John's wort, terfenadine, ergotamine, lovastatin, simvastatin, methylergonovine, pimozide, midazolam, triazolam, alpha 1-adrenoreceptor antagonist (alfuzosin), PDE5 Inhibs (eg, sildenafil) **Disp:** Tabs 75, 150, 400, 600 mg **SE:** ↑ glucose, cholesterol, triglycerides, central redistribution of fat (metabolic synd), N, ↓ neutrophils, ↑ amylase **Interactions:** ↑ Effects *OF* amiodarone, atorvastatin, bepridil, clarithromycin, cyclosporine, dihydropyridine, felodipine, HMG-CoA reductase Inhibs (statins), itraconazole, ketoconazole, lidocaine, nifedipine, pravastatin, quinidine, sildenafil, tacrolimus, trazodone, vardenafil; ↓ effects *W/* carbamazepine, phenobarbital, phenytoin, rifabutin, rifampin, efavirenz, St. John's wort; ↓ effects *OF* methadone, rifampin, SSRI, trazodone, warfarin **Labs:** ↑ Amylase, glucose; cholesterol, triglycerides, LFTs, uric acid; ↓ WBCs, neutrophils **NIPE:** Administer w/ ritonavir & food; contraindicated with numerous medications as listed

Dasatinib (Sprycel) [Antineoplastic/Protein-Tyrosine Kinase Inhibitor] Uses: CML, Ph, ALL **Action:** Multi TKI **Dose:** 100–140 mg PO d; adjust w/ CYP3A4 Inhib/inducers (Table 10) **Caution:** [D, ?/–] **CI:** None **Disp:** Tabs 20, 50, 70, 80, 100 mg **SE:** ↓ BM, edema, fluid retention, pleural effusions, N/V/D, Abd pain, bleeding, fever, ↑ QT **Interactions:** ↑ Effects *W/* atazanavir, clarithromycin, erythromycin, indinavir, itraconazole, ketoconazole, nefazodone, nelfinavir, ritonavir, saquinavir, telithromycin; ↓ effects *W/* antacids, carbamazepine, dexamethasone, phenobarbital, phenytoin, rifampicin, St. John's wort **Labs:** ↑ LFTs, Cr, uric acid, troponin levels; ↓ plts, RBC, neutrophils; monitor CBC weekly for 2 mo, then monthly **NIPE:** ⊘ Chew or crush tabs; may take w or w/o food; replace K+, Mg before Rx

Daunorubicin (Cerubidine) [Antineoplastic/Anthracycline] WARN-ING: Cardiac Fxn should be monitored d/t potential risk for cardiac tox & CHF, renal/hepatic dysfunction Uses: *Acute leukemias* **Action:** DNA-intercalating agent; ↓ topoisomerase II; generates oxygen free radicals **Dose:** 45–60 mg/m²/d for 3 consecutive d; 25 mg/m²/wk (per protocols); ↓ in renal/ hepatic impair **Caution:** [D, ?] **CI:** Component sens **Disp:** Inj 20, 50 mg **SE:** ↓ BM, mucositis, N/V, orange urine, alopecia, radiation recall phenomenon, hepatotox (↑ bili), tissue necrosis w/ extrav, cardiotox (1–2% CHF w/ 550 mg/m² cumulative dose) **Interactions:** ↑ Risk of cardiotox *W/* cyclophosphamide; ↑ myelosuppression *W/* antineoplastic agents; ↓ response to live virus vaccines **Labs:** ↓ Neutrophils, plts **NIPE:** ⊘ ASA, NSAIDs, EtOH, PRG, breast-feeding, immunizations; ↑ risk Infxn; risk of hair loss; prevent cardiotox w/ dexrazoxane (w/ > 300 mg/m² daunorubicin cum dose); IV use only; allopurinol prior to ↑ hyperuricemia

Decitabine (Dacogen) [Nucleoside Analogue] Uses: *MDS* Action: Inhibits DNA methyltransferase Dose: 15 mg/m² cont Inf over 3 h; repeat q8h × 3 d; repeat cycle q6wk, min 4 cycles; delay Tx and ↓ dose if inadequate hematologic recovery at 6 wk (see PI); delay Tx w/ Cr > 2 mg/dL or bili > 2 × ULN **Caution:** [D, ?/−] avoid PRG; males should not father a child during or 2 mo after; renal/hepatic impair **Disp:** Powder 50 mg/vial **SE:** ↓ WBC, ↓ HgB, V plt, febrile neutropenia, edema, petechiae, N/V/D, constipation, stomatitis, dyspepsia, cough, fever, fatigue, ↑ LFTs/bilirubin, hyperglycemia, Infxn, HA **Labs:** ↑ LFTs, bilirubin, glucose; ↑↑ WBC, ↓ Hgb, ↓ plt; check CBC & plt before each cycle & PRN **NIPE:** May premedicate w/ antiemetic; ⊘ PRG; males should not father a child during or 2 mo after use; use appropriate contraception; ↑ risk of Infxn

Deferasirox (Exjade) [Iron-Chelating Agent] **WARNING:** May cause renal and hepatic tox/failure, GI bleed; follow labs Uses: *Chronic iron overload d/t transfusion in pts > 2 y* Action: Oral iron chelator Dose: 20 mg/kg PO/d; adjust by 5–10 mg/kg q3–6mo based on monthly ferritin; 40 mg/kg/d max; on empty stomach 30 min ac; hold dose if ferritin < 500 mcg/L, dissolve in water/orange/apple juice (< 1 g/3.5 oz; > 1 g in 7 oz) drink immediately; resuspend residue and swallow; do not chew, swallow whole tabs or take w/ Al-containing antacids **Caution:** [B, ?/−] Elderly, renal impair, heme disorders; ↑ MDS in pt 60 y **Disp:** Tabs for oral susp 125, 250, 500 mg **SE:** N/V/D, Abd pain, skin rash, HA, fever, cough, ↑ Cr & LFTs, Infxn, hearing loss, dizziness, cataracts, retinal disorders, ↑ IOP **Interactions:** N Combine *W/* other Fe-chelator therapies **Labs:** ↑ Cr & LFTs; ✓ Cr weekly 1st mo then qmo, ✓ CBC, urine protein, LFTs; monitor monthly Cr, urine protein, LFTs **NIPE:** ARF, cytopenias possible; dose to nearest whole tab; auditory/ophthal testing initially & q12mo; tabs are only for suspension in water, juice—do not swallow whole

Deferiprone (Ferriprox) **WARNING:** May cause neutropenia & agranulocytosis w/Infxn & death. Monitor baseline ANC & weekly. D/C if Infxn develops. Advise pts to report any Sx of Infxn. Uses: *Transfusion iron overload in thalassemia synds* Action: Iron chelator Dose: 25 mg/kg PO 3 × day (75 mg/kg/d); 33 mg/kg PO 3 × d (99 mg/kg/day) max; round dose to nearest ½ tab Caution: [D, −] D/C w/ANC < 1.5 × 10⁹/L CI: Hypersens Disp: Tabs (scored) 500 mg SE: N/V, Abd pain, chromaturia, arthralgia, ↑ ALT, neutropenia, agranulocytosis, ↑ QT, HA NIPE: Take with meals to ↓ nausea; separate by 4 h antacids & mineral supplements w/ polyvalent cations (Al, Fe, Zn); V plasma zinc; urine may have reddish/brown discoloration

Degarelix (Firmagon) [GnRH Receptor Antagonist] Uses: *Advanced PCa* Action: Reversible LHRH antagonist, ↓ LH and testosterone w/o flare seen w/ LHRH agonists (transient ↑ in testosterone) **Dose:** Initial 240 mg SQ in two 120 mg doses (40 mg/mL); maint 80 mg SQ (20 mg/mL) q28d **Caution:** [Not for women] **CI:** Women **Disp:** Inj vial 120 mg (initial); 80 mg (maint) **SE:** Inj site Rxns, hot flashes, ↑ wgt, ↑ serum GGT **Notes:** Requires 2 Inj initial (vol); 44% testosterone castrate (< 50 ng/dL) at day 1, 96% day 3 **Interactions:** Caution W/ Class Ia (eg, quinidine, procainamide) or Class III (amiodarone, sotalol) antiarrhythmics; ↑ risk of QT prolongation **Labs:** Monitor PSA; ↑ serum GGT **NIPE:** Give SQ Inj in abdomen—avoid waist & rib areas; reconstitute with sterile water only

Delavirdine (Rescriptor) [Antiretroviral/NNRTI] Uses: *HIV Infxn* **Action:** Nonnucleoside RT Inhib **Dose:** 400 mg PO tid **Caution:** [C, ?] CDC rec: HIV-infected mothers not breast-feed (transmission risk); w/ renal/hepatic impair **CI:** w/ drugs dependent on CYP3A (Table 10) **Disp:** Tabs 100, 200 mg **SE:** Fat redistribution, immune reconstitution synd, HA, fatigue, rash, ↑ transaminases, N/V/D **Interactions:** Numerous drug interactions; ↑ effects W/ fluoxetine; ↑ effects OF benzodiazepines, cisapride, clarithromycin, dapsone, ergotamine, indinavir, lovastatin, midazolam, nifedipine, quinidine, ritonavir, simvastatin, terfena-dine, triazolam, warfarin; ↓ CYP; ↓ effects W/ antacids, barbiturates, carbamazepine, cimetidine, famotidine, lansoprazole, nizatidine, phenobarbital, phenytoin, ranitidine, rifabutin, rifampin; ↓ effects OF didanosine **Labs:** Monitor LFTs, ↑ AST, ALT, ↓ Hgb, Hct, plts, neutrophil counts, WBC **NIPE:** Take w/o regard to food; space antacids 1 h before/after taking dose; okay to dissolve the 100-mg tab in water; swallow 200-mg tab whole; not a cure for HIV—maintain transmission precautions

Demeclocycline (Declomycin) [Antibiotic] Uses: *SIADH* **Action:** Antibiotic, antagonizes ADH action on renal tubules **Dose:** 600–1200 mg/d PO on empty stomach; ↓ in renal failure; avoid antacids **Caution:** [D, ?/–] Avoid in hepatic/renal impair & children **CI:** Tetracycline allergy **Disp:** Tabs 150, 300 mg **SE:** D, Abd cramps, photosens, DI **Interactions:** ↑ Effects OF digoxin, anticoagulants; ↓ effects W/ antacids, Bi salts, Fe, NaHCO₃, barbiturates, carbamazepine, hydantoins, food; ↓ effects OF OCPs, PCN **Labs:** False(−) urine glucose; monitor CBC, LFTs, BUN, Cr **NIPE:** Risk of photosensitivity—use sunblock & avoid sunlight; not for peds < 8 y; take 1 h before or 2 h after meals and/or milk; take with ↑ fluids to avoid esophageal irritation/ulceration; take Al, Ca or Mg antacids 1–2 h before or after dose

Denosumab (Prolia, Xgeva) [Osteoclast Inhibitor (RANKL Inhibitor)] Uses: *Tx osteoporosis postmenopausal women ↑ BMD in men on ADT (Prolia); prevent skeletal events w/ bone mets from solid tumors (Xgeva)* **Action:** RANK ligand (RANKL) Inhib (human IgG2 MoAb); Inhibits osteoclasts **Dose:** Prolia: 60 mg SQ q6mo Xgeva: 120 mg SQ q4w; in upper arm, thigh, Abd **Caution:** [X (Xgeva), D (Prolia), ?/–] **CI:** Hypocalcemia **Disp:** Inj Prolia 60 mg/mL; Xgeva 70 mg/mL; **SE:** ↓ Ca²⁺, hypophosphatemia, serious Infxns, dermatitis, rashes, eczema, jaw osteonecrosis, pancreatitis, pain (musculoskeletal, back), fatigue, asthenia, dyspnea, N, Abd pain, flatulence, hypercholesterolemia, anemia, cystitis **Interactions:** ↑ risk of Infxn **W/** immunosuppressants; ↑ risk of jaw osteonecrosis **W/** corticosteroids **Labs:** ↓ Ca^{2+} **NIPE:** Give Ca 1000 mg & vit D 400 IU/d; w/ D/C BMD levels return to baseline at 1 y; prefilled *Prolia* syringe cap contains a derivative of latex—avoid handling if latex allergy; avoid invasive dental procedures

Desipramine (Norpramin) [Antidepressant/TCA]
WARNING: Closely monitor for worsening depression or emergence of suicidality **Uses:** *Endogenous depression*, chronic pain, peripheral neuropathy **Action:** TCA; ↑ synaptic serotonin or norepinephrine in CNS **Dose:** *Adults.* 100–200 mg/d single or ÷ dose; usually single hs dose (max 300 mg/d) ↓ dose in elderly; *Peds 6–12 y.* 1–3 mg/kg/d ÷ dose, 5 mg/kg/d max; **Caution:** [C, ?/–] CV Dz, Sz disorder, hypothyroidism, elderly, liver impair **CI:** MAOIs w/in 14 d; during AMI recovery phase w/linezolid or IV methylene blue (↑ risk serotonin synd) **Disp:** Tabs 10, 25, 50, 75, 100, 150 mg **SE:** Anticholinergic (blurred vision, urinary retention, xerostomia); orthostatic ↓ BP; ↑ QT, arrhythmias **Interactions:** ↑ Effects **W/** cimetidine, diltiazem, fluoxetine, indinavir, MAOIs, paroxetine, propoxyphene, quinidine, ritonavir ranitidine, EtOH, grapefruit juice; ↑ effects **OF** Li, sulfonylureas; ↓ effects **W/** barbiturates, carbamazepine rifampin, tobacco **NIPE:** Full effect of drug may take 4 wk; blue-green urine; risk of photosensitivity—use sunblock & avoid sunlight; taper D/C; may be taken as single dose for pt compliance; ø EtOH; allow ≥ 14 days to elapse when changing to/from MAOI

Desirudin (Iprivask) [Direct Thrombin Inhibitor (Recombinant Hirudin)]
WARNING: Recent/planned epidural/spinal anesthesia, ↑ epidural/spinal hematoma risk w/ paralysis; consider risk vs benefit before neuraxial intervention **Uses:** *DVT Px in hip replacement* **Action:** Thrombin Inhib **Dose:** *Adults.* 15 mg SQ q12h, initial 5–15 min prior to surgery *CrCl 31–60 mL/min:* 5 mg SQ q12h; CrCl < 31 mL/min: 1.7 mg SQ q12h; aPTT & SCr daily for dosage mod **Caution:** [C, ?/–] **CI:** Active bleeding, irreversible coags, hypersens to hirudins **Disp:** Inj 15 mg; **SE:** Hemorrhage, N/V, Inj site mass, wound secretion, anemia, thrombophlebitis, ↓ BP, dizziness, anaphylactic Rxn, fever **Interactions:** ↑ risk of bleeding **W/** anticoagulants, NSAIDs, plt Inhibs **NIPE:** Monitor for neurologic impair—may indicate spinal/epidural hematoma

Desloratadine (Clarinex) [Antihistamine/Selective H_1-Receptor Antagonist]
Uses: *Seasonal & perennial allergic rhinitis; chronic idiopathic urticaria* **Action:** Active metabolite of Claritin, H_1-antihistamine, blocks inflammatory mediators **Dose:** *Adults & Peds >12 y.* 5 mg PO daily; 5 mg PO q other day w/ hepatic/renal impair **Caution:** [C, ?/–] RediTabs contain phenylalanine **Disp:** Tabs 5 mg; RediTabs (rapid dissolving) 2.5, 5 mg, syrup 0.5 mg/mL **SE:** Allergy, anaphylaxis, somnolence, HA, dizziness, fatigue, pharyngitis, xerostomia, N, dyspepsia, myalgia **Labs:** ↑ LFTs, bilirubin **NIPE:** Take w/o regard to food; avoid EtOH; may cause drowsiness—avoid driving

Desmopressin (DDAVP, Stimate) [Antidiuretic Hormone] **WARNING:** Not for hemophilia B or w/ factor VIII antibody; not for hemophilia A w/ factor VIII levels < 5% **Uses:** *DI; bleeding d/t uremia, hemophilia A, & type I von Willebrand Dz (parenteral), nocturnal enuresis* **Action:** Synthetic analogue of vasopressin (human ADH); ↑ factor VIII **Dose:** *DI: Intranasal: Adults.* 0.1–0.4 mL (10–40 mcg/d in 1–3 ÷ doses) *Peds 3 mo–12 y.* 0.05–0.3 mL/d (5 mcg/d) in 1 or 2 doses *Parenteral: Adults.* 0.5–1 mL (2–4 mcg/d in 2 ÷ doses); converting from nasal to parenteral, use 1/10 nasal dose *PO: Adults.* 0.05 mg bid; ↑ to max of 1.2 mg *Hemophilia A & von Willebrand Dz (type I): Adults & Peds > 10 kg.* 0.3 mcg/kg in 50 mL NS, Inf over 15–30 min *Peds < 10 kg.* As above w/ dilution to 10 mL w/ NS. *Nocturnal enuresis: Peds > 6 y.* 20 mcg intranasally hs **Caution:** [B, M] Avoid overhydration **CI:** Hemophilia B; CrCl < 50 mL/min; severe classic von Willebrand Dz; pts w/ factor VIII antibodies; hyponatremia **Disp:** Tabs 0.1, 0.2 mg; Inj 4 mcg/mL; nasal spray 0.1 mg/mL (10 mcg)/spray; **SE:** Facial flushing, HA, dizziness, vulval pain, nasal congestion, pain at Inj site, ↓ Na⁺, H₂O intoxication **Interactions:** ↑ Antidiuretic effects *W/* carbamazepine, chlorpropamide, clofibrate; ↑ effects *OF* vasopressors; ↓ antidiuretic effects *W/* demeclocycline, Li, norepinephrine **Labs:** ↓ Na⁺ **NIPE:** Monitor I&O, ⊘ EtOH, overhydration; in very young & old pts, ↓ fluid intake to avoid H₂O intoxication & ↓ Na⁺

Desvenlafaxine (Pristiq) [Serotonin-Norepinephrine Reuptake Inhibitor (SNRI)] **WARNING:** Monitor for worsening or emergence of suicidality, particularly in ped, adolescent, and young adult pts **Uses:** *MDD* **Action:** Selective serotonin and norepinephrine reuptake Inhib **Dose:** 50 mg PO daily, ↓ w/ renal impair **Caution:** [C, ±/M] **CI:** Hypersens, MAOI w/in 14 d of stopping MAOI **Disp:** Tabs 50, 100 mg **SE:** N, dizziness, insomnia, hyperhidrosis, constipation, somnolence, decreased appetite, anxiety, and specific male sexual Fxn disorders **Interactions:** ↑ Effects *W/* CYP3A4 Inhibs; ↑ effects *OF* anticoagulants; ↓ effects *OF* CYP3A4 substrates **NIPE:** Tabs should be taken whole, allow 7 d after stopping before starting an MAOI; ⊘ ETOH; Caution w/ other serotonergics & CNS active drugs; may ↑ BP— ✓ regularly

Dexamethasone, Ophthalmic (AK-Dex Ophthalmic, Decadron Ophthalmic, Maxidex) [Anti-Inflammatory, Immunosuppressant/ Glucocorticoid] **Uses:** *Inflammatory or allergic conjunctivitis* **Action:** Anti-inflammatory corticosteroid **Dose:** Instill 1–2 gtt tid–qid **Caution:** [C, ?/–] **CI:** Active untreated bacterial, viral, & fungal eye Infxns **Disp:** Susp & soln 0.1% **SE:** Long-term use associated w/ cataracts **NIPE:** Eval IOP & lens if prolonged use; wait ≥ 15 min before inserting soft contacts; teach use of eye drops/ointment

Dexamethasone Systemic, Topical (Decadron) [Anti-Inflammatory, Immunosuppressant/Glucocorticoid] See Steroids, Systemic and Steroids, Topical

Dexlansoprazole (Dexilant, Kapidex) [Proton Pump Inhibitor]
Uses: *Heal and maint of erosive esophagitis (EE), GERD* **PUD Action:** PPI, delayed release **Dose:** *EE:* 60 mg qd up to 8 wk; maint healed EE: 30 mg qd up to 6 mo; *GERD:* 30 mg /QD × 4 wk; ↓ w/ hepatic impair **Caution:** [B, +/−] do not use w/ clopidogrel/atazanavir or drugs w/ pH-based absorption (eg, ampicillin, iron salts, ketoconazole); may alter warfarin and tacrolimus levels **CI:** Component hypersensitivity **Disp:** Caps 30, 60 mg **SE:** N/V/D, flatulence, Abd pain, URI **Interactions:** Avoid w/ atazanavir; ↓ effects *OF* atazanavir; ↓ absorption *OF* ketoconazole, digoxin, Fe, ampicillin **Labs:** Monitor INR if on warfarin **NIPE:** w/ or w/o food; swallow whole or open caps, sprinkle on applesauce & swallow stat; ↑ Risk of fxs w/ all PPI; risk of hypomagnesemia w/ long-term use, monitor; take at ≥ 30 min before sucralfate.

Dexmedetomidine (Precedex) [Sedative/Selective Alpha-2-Agonist]
Uses: *Sedation in intubated & nonintubated pts* **Action:** Sedative; selective α_2-agonist **Dose:** *Adults. ICU sedation:* 1 mcg/kg IV over 10 min, then 0.2–0.7 mcg/kg/h *Procedural sedation:* 0.5–1 mcg/kg IV over 10 min, then 0.2–1 mcg/kg/h; ↓ in elderly, liver Dz **Caution:** [C, ?/−] **CI:** None **Disp:** Inj 200 mcg/2 mL **SE:** Hypotension, bradycardia **NIPE:** Tachyphylaxis & tolerance associated w/ exposure > 24 h; monitor BP

Dexmethylphenidate (Focalin, Focalin XR) [C-II] [Stimulant]
WARNING: Caution w/ Hx drug dependence/alcoholism. Chronic abuse may lead to tolerance, psychological dependence & abnormal behavior; monitor closely during withdrawal **Uses:** *ADHD* **Action:** CNS stimulant, blocks reuptake of norepinephrine & DA **Dose:** *Adults. Focalin:* 2.5 mg PO twice daily, ↑ by 2.5–5 mg weekly; max 20 mg/d *Focalin XR:* 10 mg PO daily, ↑ 10 mg weekly; max 40 mg/d *Peds ≥ 6 y. Focalin:* 2.5 mg PO bid, ↑ 2.5–5 mg weekly; max 20 mg/d *Focalin XR:* 5 mg PO daily, ↑ 5 mg weekly; max 30 mg/d; if already on methylphenidate, start w/ half of current total daily dose **Caution:** [C, ?/−] Avoid w/ known cardiac abnormality; may ↓ metabolism of warfarin/anticonvulsants/antidepressants **CI:** Agitation, anxiety, tension, glaucoma, Hx motor tic, family Hx/Ax Tourette w/in 14 d of MAOI; hypersens to methylphenidate **Disp:** Tabs 2.5, 5, 10 mg; caps ER 5, 10, 15, 20, 25, 30, 35, 40 mg **SE:** HA, anxiety, dyspepsia, ↓ appetite, wgt loss, dry mouth, visual disturbances, ↑ HR, HTN, MI, stroke, sudden death, Szs, growth suppression, aggression, mania, psychosis **Interactions:** ↑ Effects *OF* anticonvulsants, oral anticoagulants, TCA, SSRIs, phenylbutazone; ↓ effects *OF* guanethidine, antihypertensives **Labs:** ✓ CBC w/ prolonged use **NIPE:** Swallow ER caps whole or sprinkle contents on applesauce (do not crush/chew); do not give w/in 14 d of MAOI; avoid abrupt D/C

Dexpanthenol (Ilopan-Choline [Oral], Ilopan) [Cholinergic]
Uses: *Minimize paralytic ileus, Rx post-op distention* **Action:** Cholinergic agent **Dose:** *Adults. Relief of gas:* 2–3 tabs PO tid. *Prevent post-op ileus:* 250–500 mg IM stat, repeat in 2 h, then q6h PRN *Ileus:* 500 mg IM stat, repeat in

2 h, then q6h, PRN **Caution:** [C, ?] **CI:** Hemophilia, mechanical bowel obst **Disp:** Inj 250 mg/mL; cream 2% (Panthoderm Cream [OTC]) **SE:** GI cramps **NIPE:** Monitor BP during IV administration

Dexrazoxane (Zinecard, Totect) [Chelating Agent] Uses: *Prevent anthracycline-induced (eg, doxorubicin) cardiomyopathy (*Zinecard*), extrav of anthracycline chemotherapy (*Totect*)* **Action:** Chelates heavy metals; binds intracellular iron & prevents anthracycline-induced free radicals **Dose:** *Systemic for (cardiomyopathy, Zinecard):* 10:1 ratio dexrazoxane: doxorubicin 30 min before each dose, 5:1 ratio w/ CrCl < 40 mL/min *Extrav (Totect):* IV Inf over 1–2 h qd × 3 d, w/in 6 h of extrav *Day 1:* 1000 mg/m² (max 2000 mg) *Day 2:* 1000 mg/m² (max 2000 mg) *Day 3:* 500 mg/m² (max: 1000 mg) w/ CrCl < 40 mL/min, ↓ dose by 50% **Caution:** [D, –] **CI:** Component sensitivity **Disp:** Inj powder 250, 500 mg (10 mg/mL) **SE:** ↓ BM, fever, Infxn, stomatitis, alopecia, N/V/D, ↑ LFTs, Inj site pain **Interactions:** ↑ Length of muscle relaxation *W/* succinylcholine **Labs:** ↑ LFTs **NIPE:** Inj site pain; may ↑ bone marrow suppression from chemo, ↑ risk Infxn

Dextran 40 (Gentran 40, Rheomacrodex) [Plasma Volume Expander, Glucose Polymer] Uses: *Shock, prophylaxis of DVT & thromboembolism, adjunct in peripheral vascular surgery* **Action:** Expands plasma vol; ↓ blood viscosity **Dose:** *Shock:* 10 mL/kg Inf rapidly; 20 mL/kg max 1st 24 h; beyond 24 h 10 mL/kg max; D/C after 5 d *Prophylaxis of DVT & thromboembolism:* 10 mL/kg IV day of surgery, then 500 mL/d IV for 2–3 d, then 500 mL IV q2–3d based on risk for up to 2 wk **Caution:** [C, ?] Inf Rxns; w/ corticosteroids **CI:** Major hemostatic defects; cardiac decompensation; renal Dz w/ severe oliguria/anuria **Disp:** 10% dextran 40 in 0.9% NaCl or 5% dextrose **SE:** Allergy/anaphylactoid Rxn (observe during 1st min of Inf), arthralgia, cutaneous Rxns, ↑ BP, fever **Interactions:** ↑ Bleeding times *W/* antiplt agents or anticoagulants **Labs:** Monitor Cr & lytes; ↑ ALT, AST **NIPE:** Draw blood before administration of drug; pt should be well hydrated prior to Inf

Dextroamphetamine (Dexedrine, Procentra) [C-II] [Amphetamine] WARNING: Amphetamines have a high potential for abuse. Long-term use may lead to dependence; serious CV events, including death; caution re existing cardiac cond. **Uses:** *ADHD, narcolepsy* **Action:** CNS stimulant; ↑ DA & norepinephrine release **Dose:** *ADHD ≥ 6 y:* 5 mg daily–bid, ↑ by 5 mg/d weekly PRN, max 60 mg/d ÷ bid–tid *Peds < 3 y. Not recommended.* *Narcolepsy 6–12 y:* 5 mg daily, ↑ by 5 mg/d weekly PRN max 60 mg/d ÷ bid–tid *≥ 12 y:* 10–60 mg/d ÷ bid–tid; ER caps once daily **Caution:** [C, +/–] Hx drug abuse; separate 14 d from MAOIs **CI:** Advanced arteriosclerosis, CVD, mod–severe HTN, hyperthyroidism, glaucoma **Disp:** Tabs 5, 10 mg; ER capsules 5, 10, 15 mg; soln 5 mg/5 mL **SE:** HTN, ↓ appetite, insomnia **Interactions:** ↑ Risk of hypertensive crisis *W/* MAOIs; ↑ effects *W/* thiazides, TCAs; ↑ effects *OF* meperidine, norepinephrine, phenobarbital, phenytoin; ↓ effects *W/* Li, psychotropics; ↓ effects *OF* adrenergic blockers, sedatives, antihypertensives **Labs:** Interferes *W/* urinary steroid tests **NIPE:** May open ER caps, do not crush beads; take w/ or w/o food; avoid abrupt D/C ; ↑ risk of peripheral vasculopathy—immed report unexplained wounds on fingers/toes

Dextromethorphan (Benylin DM, Delsym, Mediquell, PediaCare 1, Others) [OTC] [Antitussive]   **Uses:** *Control nonproductive cough* **Action:** Suppresses medullary cough center **Dose:** *Adults.* 10–30 mg PO q4h PRN (max 120 mg/24 h) *Peds 4–6 y.* 2.5–7.5 mg q4–8h (max 30 mg/24 h) *7–12 y.* 5–10 mg q4–8h (max 60 mg/24 h) **Caution:** [C, ?/–] Not for persistent or chronic cough **CI:** < 2 y **Disp:** Caps 30 mg; lozenges 2.5, 5, 7.5, 15 mg; syrup 15 mg/15 mL, 10 mg/5 mL; Liq 10 mg/15 mL, 3.5, 7.5, 15 mg/5 mL; sustained-action Liq 30 mg/5 mL **SE:** GI disturbances **Interactions:** ↑ Effects *W/* amiodarone, fluoxetine, quinidine, terbinafine; ↑ risk of serotonin synd *W/* sibutramine, MAOIs; ↑ CNS depression *W/* antihistamines, antidepressants, sedative, opioids, EtOH **NIPE:** Fluids, humidity to environment, D/C MAOIs for 14 d before administering drug; found in combo OTC products w/ guaifenesin; deaths reported in pts < 2 y; abuse potential; efficacy in children debated

Dextrose 50%/25%   **Uses:** Hypoglycemia, insulin OD **Action:** Sugar source in the form of D-glucose **Dose:** *Adults.* One 50-mL amp of 50% soln IV *Peds. ECC 2010:* Hypoglycemia: 0.5–1 g/kg (25% max IV/IO conc); 50% dextrose (0.5 g/mL): 1–2 mL/kg; 25% dextrose (0.25 g/mL): 2–5 mL/kg; 10% dextrose (0.1 g/mL): 5–10 mL/kg; 5 % dextrose (0.95 g/mL): 10–20 mL/kg if volume tolerated **Caution:** [C, M] w/ Suspected intracranial bleeding can ↑ ICP **CI:** None if used w/ documented hypoglycemia **Disp:** Inj forms **SE:** Burning at IV site, local tissue necrosis w/ extravasation; neurologic Sxs (Wernicke encephalopathy) if pt thiamine deficient **NIPE:** If pt is mentating well enough to protect airway, use oral glucose first; lower concs used in IV fluids

Diazepam (Valium, Diastat) [C-IV] [Anxiolytic, Skeletal Muscle Relaxant, Anticonvulsant, Sedative/Hypnotic/Benzodiazepine]   **Uses:** *Anxiety, EtOH withdrawal, muscle spasm, status epilepticus, panic disorders, amnesia, pre-op sedation* **Action:** Benzodiazepine **Dose:** *Adults. Status epilepticus:* 5–10 mg q 5–10 min to 30 mg max in 8-h period *Anxiety, muscle spasm:* 2–10 mg PO bid–qid or IM/IV q3–4h PRN *Pre-op:* 5–10 mg PO or IM 20–30 min or IV just prior to procedure *EtOH withdrawal:* 10 mg q3–4h × 24 h, then 5 mg PO q3–4h PRN or 5–10 mg IV q10–15min for CIWA withdrawal score ≥ 8, 100 mg/h max; titrate to agitation; avoid excessive sedation; may lead to aspiration or resp arrest *Peds. Status epilepticus:* < 5 y. 0.05–0.3 mg/kg/dose IV q15–30 min up to a max of 5 mg. > 5 y: to max of 10 mg. *Sedation, muscle relaxation:* 0.04–0.3 mg/kg/dose q2–4h IM or IV to max of 0.6 mg/kg in 8 h, or 0.12–0.8 mg/kg/24 h PO ÷ tid–qid; ↓ w/ hepatic impair **Caution:** [D, ?/–] **CI:** Coma, CNS depression, resp depression, NAG, severe uncontrolled pain, PRG **Disp:** Tabs 2, 5, 10 mg; soln, 5 mg/mL; Inj 5 mg/mL; rectal gel 2.5, 5, 10, 20 mg/mL **SE:** Sedation, amnesia, ↓ HR, ↓ BP, rash, ↓ resp rate **Notes:** 5 mg/min IV max in adults or 1–2 mg/min in peds (resp arrest possible) **Interactions:** ↑ Effects W/ antihistamines, azole antifungals, BBs, CNS depressants, cimetidine, ciprofloxin, disulfiram, INH, OCP, omeprazole, phenytoin, valproic acid, verapamil, EtOH, kava kava, valerian; ↑ effects OF digoxin, diuretics; ↓ effects W/ barbiturates, carbamazepine, theophylline, ranitidine, tobacco; ↓ effects OF haloperidol, levodopa **Labs:** Monitor LFTs, BUN, Cr, CBC w/ long-term drug use **NIPE:** Risk ↑ Sz activity; IM absorption erratic; avoid abrupt D/C; avoid EtOH; avoid grapefruit/grapefruit juice; wait ≥ 1 h before taking antacid

Diazoxide (Proglycem) [Antihypertensive/Peripheral Vasodilator] Uses: *Hypoglycemia d/t hyperinsulinism* **Action:** ↓ Pancreatic insulin release; antihypertensive **Dose:** Repeat in 5–15 min until BP controlled; repeat q4–24h; monitor BP closely. *Hypoglycemia: Adults & Peds.* 3–8 mg/kg/24 h PO ÷ q8–12h *Neonates.* 8–10 mg/kg/24 h PO in 2–3 equal doses; **Caution:** [C, ?] ↓ Effect w/ phenytoin; ↑ effect w/ diuretics, warfarin **CI:** Allergy to thiazides or other sulfonamide-containing products; HTN associated w/ aortic coarctation, AV shunt, or pheochromocytoma **Disp:** Caps 50 mg; PO susp 50 mg/mL **SE:** Hyperglycemia, ↓ BP, dizziness, Na$^+$ & H$_2$O retention, N/V, weakness **Interactions:** ↑ Effects W/ carboplatin, cisplatin, diuretics, phenothiazines; ↑ effects OF anticoagulants; ↓ effects W/ sulfonylureas; ↓ effects OF phenytoin, sulfonylureas **Labs:** ↑ Serum uric acid, glucose; can give false(–) insulin response to glucagons; ↓ neutrophil count, Hgb, Hct, WBC **NIPE:** Daily wgt, ↑ reversible body hair growth

Dibucaine (Nupercainal) [Topical Anesthetic] Uses: *Hemorrhoids & minor skin conditions* **Action:** Topical anesthetic **Dose:** Insert PR w/ applicator bid & after each bowel movement; apply sparingly to skin **Caution:** [C, ?] Topical use only **CI:** Component sensitivity **Disp:** 1% oint w/ rectal applicator; 0.5% cream **SE:** Local irritation, rash **Interactions:** None noted **NIPE:** Do not cover w/ occlusive dressing

Diclofenac & Misoprostol (Arthrotec) [Antiarthritic, Anti- Inflammatory/NSAIDs + Prostaglandin E$_1$ (PGE$_1$) Analogue] WARNING: May induce abortion, birth defects; do not take if PRG; may ↑ risk of CV events & GI bleeding; CI in post-op CABG Uses: *OA & RA w/ ↑ risk of CV events & GI bleeding* **Action:** NSAID w/ GI protective PGE$_1$ **Dose:** *OA:* 50–75 mg PO bid–tid; RA 50 mg bid–qid or 75 mg bid; w/ food or milk **Caution:** [X, ?] CHF, HTN, renal/hepatic dysfunction, & Hx PUD, asthma; avoid w/ porphyria **CI:** PRG; GI bleed; renal/hepatic failure; severe CHF; NSAID/ aspirin allergy; following CABG **Disp:** Tabs *Arthrotec* 50: 50 mg diclofenac w/ 200 mcg misoprostol *Arthrotec:* 75 mg diclofenac w/ 200 mcg misoprostol **SE:** *Oral:* Abd cramps, heartburn, GI ulcers, rash, interstitial nephritis **Interactions:** ↑ Risk of GI bleed W/ oral corticosteroids, anticoagulants, prolonged NSAID use, EtOH, smoking; ↓ effects OF ACE Inhibs, diuretics, digoxin, methotrexate, cyclosporine, Li, warfarin **Labs:** ✓ CBC, LFTs **NIPE:** Do not crush tabs; watch for GI bleed; PRG test females before use; immed report any skin rash/blister

Diclofenac Ophthalmic (Voltaren Ophthalmic) [NSAID] Uses: *Inflammation postcataract or pain/photophobia post corneal refractive surgery* **Action:** NSAID **Dose:** *Post-op cataract:* 1 gtt qid, start 24 h p post-op × 2 wk *Post-op refractive:* 1–2 gtt w/in 1 h pre-op and w/in 15 min post-op then qid up to 3 d **Caution:** [C, ?] May ↑ bleed risk in ocular tissues **CI:** NSAID/ASA allergy **Disp:** Ophthal soln 0.1% 2.5 mL bottle **SE:** Burning/stinging/itching, keratitis, ↑ IOP, lacrimation, abnormal vision, conjunctivitis, lid swelling, discharge, iritis **Interactions:** ↑ Effects *OF* oral anticoagulants **NIPE:** ⊘ Wear soft contact lenses; ✓ w/ MD about wearing any contacts ≤ 3 d after surgery; may delay wound healing; teach use of eye drops

Diclofenac, Oral (Cataflam, Voltaren, Voltaren-XR) [Antiarthritic, Anti-Inflammatory/NSAID] WARNING: May ↑ risk of CV events & GI bleeding; CI in post-op CABG **Uses:** *Arthritis (RA/OA) & pain, oral and topical, actinic keratosis* **Action:** NSAID **Dose:** RA/OA: 150–200 mg/d ÷ 2–4 doses DR; 100 mg/d XR; W/ food or milk **Caution:** [C (avoid after 30 wk), –] CHF, HTN, renal/hepatic dysfunction, & Hx PUD, asthma **CI:** NSAID/aspirin allergy; porphyria; following CABG **Disp:** Tabs 50 mg; tabs DR 25, 50, 75, 100 mg; XR tabs 100 mg **SE:** *Oral:* Abd cramps, heartburn, GI ulceration, rash, interstitial nephritis **Interactions:** ↑ Risk of bleeding *W/* feverfew, garlic, ginger, ginkgo; ↑ effects *OF* digoxin, MTX, cyclosporine, Li, insulin, sulfonylureas, K⁺-sparing diuretics, warfarin; ↓ effects *W/* ASA; ↓ effects *OF* thiazide diuretics, furosemide, BBs **Labs:** ↑ LFTs, serum glucose & cortisol; ↑ serum uric acid; monitor LFTs, CBC, BUN, Cr **NIPE:** Risk of photosensitivity—use sunblock; most effective if taken w/o food; ⊘ crush tabs; watch for GI bleed; immed report any skin rash

Diclofenac, Topical (Flector Patch, Pennsaid, Solaraze, Voltaren Gel) [Antiarthritic, Anti-Inflammatory/NSAID + Prostaglandin E₁ Analogue] WARNING: May ↑ risk of CV events & GI bleeding; CI in post-op CABG **Uses:** *Arthritis of the knee (Pennsaid); arthritis of knee/hands (Voltaren Gel); pain due to strain, sprain, and contusions (Flector Patch), actinic keratosis (Solaraze)* **Action:** NSAID **Dose:** *Flector Patch:* 1 patch to painful area bid; *Pennsaid:* 10 drops spread around knee; repeat until 40 drops applied **Usual Dose:** 40 drops/knee qid; wash hands; wait until it dries before dressing *Solaraze:* 0.5 g to each 5 × 5 cm lesion 60–90 d, apply bid; *Voltaren Gel:* upper extremity 2 g qid (max 8 g/d); lower extremity 4 g qid (max 16 g/d) **Caution:** [C < 30 wk gest; D > 30 wk; ?] avoid nonintact skin; CV events possible w/ CHF, ↑ BP, renal/hepatic dysfunct, w/ Hx PUD, asthma; avoid w/ PO NSAID **CI:** NSAID/ASA allergy; following CABG; component allergy **Disp:** *Flector Patch:* 180 mg (10 × 14 cm); *Voltaren Gel 1%; Solaraze 3%;* Pennsaid 1.5% soln **SE:** Pruritus, dermatitis, burning, dry skin, N, HA **Interactions:** ↑ Risk of bleeding *W/* feverfew, garlic, ginger, ginkgo; ↑ effects *OF* digoxin, MTX, cyclosporine, Li, insulin, sulfonylureas, K+-sparing diuretics, warfarin; ↓ effects *W/* ASA; ↓ effects *OF* thiazide diuretics, furosemide, BBs **Labs:** ✓ CBC, LFTs periodically **NIPE:** Do not apply patch/gel to damaged skin or while bathing; no box warning on *Solaraze;* ⊘ cover w/ bandage/dressing

Dicloxacillin (Dynapen, Dycill) [Antibiotic/Penicillin]

Uses: *Rx of pneumonia, skin, & soft-tissue Infxns, & osteomyelitis caused by penicillinase-producing staphylococci* **Action:** Bactericidal; ↓ cell wall synth *Spectrum: S aureus & Streptococcus* **Dose:** *Adults.* 150–500 mg qid (2 g/d max) *Peds < 40 kg.* 12.5–100 mg/kg/d ÷ qid; take on empty stomach **Caution:** [B, ?] **CI:** Component or PCN sensitivity **Disp:** Caps 125, 250, 500 mg **SE:** N/D, Abd pain **Interactions:** ↑ Effects *W/* disulfiram, probenecid; ↑ effects *OF* MTX, ↓ effects *W/* macrolides, tetracyclines, food; ↓ effects *OF* OCPs, warfarin **Labs:** False ↑ urine glucose; ↑ eosinophils; ↓ Hgb, Hct, plts, WBC; monitor PTT if pt on warfarin **NIPE:** Take w/ H2O, 1 h ac or 2 pc

Dicyclomine (Bentyl) [Antimuscarinic, GI Antispasmodic/ Anticholinergic]

Uses: *Functional IBS* **Action:** Smooth-muscle relaxant **Dose:** *Adults.* 20 mg PO qid; ↑ to 160 mg/d max or 20 mg IM q6h, 80 mg/d ÷ qid then ↑ to 160 mg/d, max 2 wk **Caution:** [B, –] **CI:** Infants < 6 mo, NAG, MyG, severe UC, BOO, GI obst, reflux esophagitis **Disp:** Caps 10, 20 mg; tabs 20 mg; syrup 10 mg/5 mL; Inj 10 mg/mL **SE:** Anticholinergic SEs may limit dose **Interactions:** ↑ Anticholinergic effects *W/* anticholinergics, antihistamines, amantadine, MAOIs, TCAs, phenothiazides; ↑ effects *OF* atenolol, digoxin; ↓ effects *W/* antacids; ↓ effects *OF* haloperidol, ketoconazole, levodopa, phenothiazines **NIPE:** Do not administer IV; ⊘ EtOH, CNS depressant; adequate hydration; take 30–60 min ac

Didanosine [ddI] (Videx) [Antiretroviral, NRTI]

WARNING: Allergy manifested as fever, rash, fatigue, GI/resp Sxs reported; stop drug immediately & do not rechallenge; lactic acidosis & hepatomegaly/steatosis reported **Uses:** *HIV Infxn in zidovudine-intolerant pts* **Action:** NRTI **Dose:** *Adults. > 60 kg:* 400 mg/d PO or 200 mg PO bid *< 60 kg:* 250 mg/d PO or 125 mg PO bid; adults should take 2 tabs/administration *Peds. 2 wk–8 mo:* 100 mg/m² *> 8 mo:* 120 mg/m² PO bid; on empty stomach; ↓ w/ renal impair **Caution:** [B, –] CDC rec HIV-infected mothers not breast-feed **CI:** Component sensitivity **Disp:** Chew tabs 100, 150, 200 mg; DR caps 125, 200, 250, 400 mg; powder for soln 2, 4 g **SE:** Pancreatitis, peripheral neuropathy, D, HA **Interactions:** ↑ Effects *W/* allopurinol, ganciclovir; ↓ effects *W/* methadone, food; ↑ risk of pancreatitis *W/* thiazide diuretics, IV pentamidine, EtOH; ↓ effects *OF* azole antifungals, dapsone, delavirdine, ganciclovir, indinavir, quinolone, ranitidine, tetracycline **Labs:** ↑ LFTs, uric acid, amylase, lipase, triglycerides **NIPE:** May cause hyperglycemia; do not take w/ meals; thoroughly chew tabs, do not mix w/ fruit juice or acidic beverages; reconstitute powder w/ H2O; not a cure for HIV—maintain trans precautions

Diflunisal (Dolobid) [Analgesic, Antipyretic, Anti-Inflammatory/ NSAID] **WARNING:** May ↑ risk of CV events & GI bleeding; CI in post-op CABG **Uses:** *Mild–mod pain; OA* **Action:** NSAID **Dose:** *Pain:* 500 mg PO bid *OA:* 500–1000 mg/d PO bid (max 1.5 g/d); ↓ in renal impair, take w/ food/milk **Caution:** [C (D 3rd tri or near delivery), ?] CHF, HTN, renal/hepatic dysfunction, & Hx PUD **CI:** Allergy to NSAIDs or ASA, active GI bleed, post-CABG **Disp:** Tabs 500 mg **SE:** May ↑ bleeding time; HA, Abd cramps, heartburn, GI ulceration, rash, interstitial nephritis, fluid retention **Interactions:** ↑ Effects *W/* probenecid; ↑ effects *OF* APAP, anticoagulants, digoxin, HCTZ, indomethacin, Li, MTX, phenytoin, sulfonamides, sulfonylureas; ↓ effects *W/* antacids, ASA; ↓ effects *OF* furosemide **Labs:** ↑ Salicylate levels **NIPE:** Take w/ food or milk; ⊘ chew or crush tabs

Digoxin (Digitek, Lanoxin) [Antiarrhythmic/Cardiac Glycoside] **Uses:** *CHF, AF & A flutter, & PAT* **Action:** Positive inotrope; AV node refractory period **Dose:** *Adults. PO digitalization:* 0.5–0.75 mg PO, then 0.25 mg PO q6–8h to total 1–1.5 mg. *IV or IM digitalization:* 0.25–0.5 mg IM or IV, then 0.25 mg q4–6h to total 0.125–0.5 mg/d PO, IM, or IV (average daily dose 0.125–0.25 mg) *Peds. Preterm Infants. Digitalization:* 30 mcg/kg PO or 25 mcg/kg IV; give 1/2 of dose initial, then 1/4 of dose at 8–12-h intervals for 2 doses *Maint:* 5–7.5 mcg/kg/24 h PO or 4–6 mcg/kg/24 h IV ÷ q12h *Term Infants. Digitalization:* 25–35 mcg/kg PO or 20–30 mcg/kg IV; give 1/2 the initial dose, then 1/3 of dose at 8–12 h *Maint:* 6–10 mcg/kg/24 h PO or 5–8 mcg/kg/24 h ÷ q12h; *2–5 y: Digitalization:* 30–40 mcg/kg PO or 25–35 mcg/kg IV. *Maint:* 7.5–10 mcg/kg/24 h PO or 6–9 mcg/kg IV ÷ q12h. *5–10 y: Digitalization:* 25–35 mcg/kg PO or 15–30 mcg/ kg IV; *Maint:* 5–10 mcg/kg/24 h PO or 4–8 mcg/kg q12h. *>10 y:* 10–15 mcg/kg PO or 8–12 mcg/kg IV. *Maint:* 2.5–5 mcg/kg PO or 2–3 mcg/kg IV q24h; ↓ in renal impair **Caution:** [C, +] w/ K^+, Mg^{2+}, renal failure **CI:** AV block; IHSS; constrictive pericarditis **Disp:** Tabs 0.125, 0.25 mg; elixir 0.05 mg/mL; Inj 0.1, 0.25 mg/mL **SE:** Can cause heart block; ↓ K^+ potentiates tox; N/V, HA, fatigue, visual disturbances (yellow-green halos around lights), cardiac arrhythmias **Notes:** *Levels: Trough:* Just before next dose *Therapeutic:* 0.8–2.0 mg/mL *Toxic* > 2 ng/mL *1/2-life:* 36 h **Interactions:** ↑ Effects *W/* alprazolam, amiodarone, azole antifungals, BBs, carvedilol, cyclosporine, corticosteroids, diltiazem, diuretics, erythromycin, NSAIDs, quinidine, spironolactone, tetracyclines, verapamil, goldenseal, hawthorn, licorice, quinine, Siberian ginseng; ↓ effects *W/* charcoal, cholestyramine, cisapride, neomycin, rifampin, sucralfate, thyroid hormones, psyllium, St. John's wort **Labs:** Monitor serum electrolytes **NIPE:** Different bioavailability in various brands; IM Inj painful, has erratic absorption & should not be used; monitor for dig toxicity; teach pt to monitor BP and HR daily

Digoxin Immune Fab (DigiFab) [Cardiac Glycoside Antidote/ Antibody Fragment] **Uses:** *Life-threatening digoxin intoxication* **Action:** Antigen-binding fragments bind & inactivate digoxin **Dose:** *Adults & Peds.*

Based on serum level & pt's wgt; see charts provided w/ drug **Caution:** [C, ?] **CI:** Sheep product allergy **Disp:** Inj 40 mg/vial **SE:** Worsening of cardiac output or CHF, ↓ K+, facial swelling, & redness **Notes:** Each vial binds ≈ 0.6 mg of digoxin **Interactions:** ↓ Effects *OF* cardiac glycosides **Labs:** ↓ K+ level **NIPE:** Will take up to 1 wk for accurate serum digoxin levels after use of Digibind; renal failure may require redosing on several days

Diltiazem (Cardizem, Cardizem CD, Cardizem LA, Cardizem SR, Cartia XT, Dilacor XR, Diltia XT, Taztia XT, Tiazac) [Antianginal/ CCB]

Uses: *Angina, prevention of reinfarction, HTN, AF or A flutter, & PAT* **Action:** CCB **Dose:** *Stable angina PO:* Initial, 30 mg PO qid; ↑ to 120–320 mg/d in 3–4 ÷ doses PRN; XR 120 mg/d (540 mg/d max) *LA:* 180–360 mg/d *HTN: SR:* 60–120 mg PO bid; ↑ to 360 mg/d max. *CD or XR:* 120–360 mg/d (max 540 mg/d) or LA 180–360 mg/d; *A-Fib, A-Flutter. PSVT:* 0.25 mg/kg IV bolus over 2 min; may repeat in 15 min at 0.35 mg/kg; begin Inf 5–15 mg/h *ECC 2010: Acute rate control:* 0.25 mg/kg (15–20 mg) over 2 min, followed in 15 min by 0.35 mg/kg (20–25 mg) over 2 min; maint Inf 5–15 mg/h **Caution:** [C, +] ↑ Effect w/ amiodarone, cimetidine, fentanyl, Li, cyclosporine, digoxin, ®-blockers, theophylline **CI:** SSS, AV block, ↓ BP, AMI, pulm congestion **CI:** SSS, AV block, ↓ BP, AMI, pulm congestion **Disp:** *Cardizem CD:* Caps 120, 180, 240, 300, 360 mg *Cardizem LA:* Tabs 120, 180, 240, 300, 360, 420 mg *Cardizem SR:* Caps 60, 90, 120 mg *Cardizem:* Tabs 30, 60, 90, 120 mg *Cartia XT:* Caps 120, 180, 240, 300 mg *Dilacor XR:* Caps 120, 180, 240 mg *Diltia XT:* Caps 120, 180, 240 mg *Tiazac:* Caps 120, 180, 240, 300, 360, 420 mg Inj 5 mg/mL *Taztia XT:* 120, 180, 240, 300, 360 mg **SE:** Gingival hyperplasia, ↓ HR, AV block, ECG abnormalities, peripheral edema, dizziness, HA **Interactions:** ↑ Effects *W/* α-blockers, amiodarone, azole antifungals, BBs, cimetidine, cyclosporine, digoxin, erythromycin, fentanyl, H₂-receptor antagonists, Li, nitroprusside, quinidine, theophylline, EtOH, grapefruit juice; ↑ effects *OF* carbamazepine, cyclosporine, digitalis glycosides, quinidine, phenytoin, prazosin, theophylline, TCAs; ↓ effects *W/* NSAIDs, phenobarbital, rifampin **Labs:** ↑ LFTs **NIPE:** Take before meals; ⊘ chew or crush SR or ER preps; risk of photosensitivity—use sunblock; Cardizem CD, Dilacor XR, & Tiazac not interchangeable—avoid alcohol

Dimenhydrinate (Dramamine, Others) [Antiemetic/Antivertigo/ Anticholinergic]

Uses: *Prevention & Rx of N/V, dizziness, or vertigo of motion sickness* **Action:** Antiemetic, action unknown **Dose:** *Adults.* 50–100 mg PO q4–6h, max 400 mg/d; 50 mg IM/IV PRN *Peds 2–6 y.* 12.5–25 mg q6–8h max 75 mg/d *6–12 y.* 25–50 mg q6–8h max 150 mg/d **Caution:** [B, ?] **CI:** Component sensitivity **Disp:** Tabs 25, 50 mg; chew tabs 50 mg; Inj 50 mg/mL **SE:** Anticholinergic **SE Interactions:** ↑ Effects *W/* CNS depressants, antihistamines, opioids, quinidine, TCAs, EtOH; prolonged anticholinergic effects *W/* MAOIs **Labs:** False allergy skin tests **NIPE:** ⊘ Drug 72 h prior to allergy skin testing; take 30 min before travel for motion sickness; may cause drowsiness—caution driving

Dimethyl Fumarate (Tecfidera) Uses: *Relapsing MS* Action: Activates the nuclear factor (erythroid-derived 2)-like 2 (Nrf2) pathway, exact mechanism unknown Dose: 120 mg PO bid × 7 d, then ↑ to 240 mg PO bid; swallow whole Caution: [C, ?/–] may cause lymphopenia, check CBC at baseline, annually, & prn; withhold Tx w/ severe Infxn CI: None Disp: Caps DR 120, 240 mg SE: N/D, abd pain, flushing, pruritus, rash, ↑ LFTs NIPE: Take w/o regard to food; taking w/ food may ↓ risk of flushing; swallow whole—⊘ chew/crush/split

Dimethyl Sulfoxide [DMSO] (Rimso-50) [GU Agent] Uses: *Interstitial cystitis* Action: Unknown Dose: Intravesical, 50 mL, retain for 15 min; repeat q2wk until relief Caution: [C, ?] CI: Component sensitivity Disp: 50% soln SE: Cystitis, eosinophilia, GI, & taste disturbance Interactions: ↓ Effects *OF* sulindac Labs: Monitor CBC, LFTs, BUN, Cr levels NIPE: ↑ Taste & smell of garlic

Dinoprostone (Cervidil Vaginal Insert, Prepidil Vaginal Gel, Prostin E2) [Prostaglandin/Abortifacient] WARNING: Should only be used by trained personnel in an appropriate hospital setting Uses: *Induce labor; terminate PRG (12–20 wk); evacuate uterus in missed abortion or fetal death* Action: Prostaglandin, changes consistency, dilatation, & effacement of the cervix; induces uterine contraction Dose: *Gel:* 0.5 mg; if no cervical/uterine response, repeat 0.5 mg q6h (max 24-h dose 1.5 mg) *Vag insert:* 1 insert (10 mg = 0.3 mg dinoprostone/h over 12 h); remove w/ onset of labor or 12 h after insertion *Vag supp:* 20 mg repeated q3–5h; adjust *PRN supp:* 1 high in vagina, repeat at 3–5-h intervals until abortion (240 mg max) Caution: [X, ?] CI: Ruptured membranes, allergy to prostaglandins, placenta previa or AUB, when oxytocic drugs CI or if prolonged uterine contractions are inappropriate (Hx C-section, cephalopelvic disproportion, etc) Disp: *Endocervical gel:* 0.5 mg in 3-g syringes (w/ 10- & 20-mm shielded catheter) *Vag gel:* 1 mg/3 g, 2 mg/3 g. *Vag supp:* 20 mg *Vag insert, CR:* 10 mg SE: N/V/D, dizziness, flushing, HA, fever, abnormal uterine contractions Interactions: ↑ Effects of oxytocics; ↓ effects *W/* large amts EtOH NIPE: Pt supine after insertion of supp or gel up to 1/2 h; may have ↑ temp 15–45 min after insertion—fluids, sponge baths

Diphenhydramine (Benadryl) [Antihistamine/Antitussive/ Antiemetic] [OTC] Uses: *Rx & prevent allergic Rxns, motion sickness, potentiate narcotics, sedation, cough suppression, & Rx of extrapyramidal Rxns* Action: Antihistamine, antiemetic Dose: *Adults.* 25–50 mg PO, IV, or IM tid–qid; *Peds > 2 y.* 5 mg/ kg/24 h PO or IM ÷ q6h (max 300 mg/d); ↑ dosing interval w/ mod–severe renal Insuff Caution: [B, –] Elderly, NAG, BPH, w/ MAOI CI: acute asthma Disp: Tabs & caps 25, 50 mg; chew tabs 12.5 mg; elixir 12.5 mg/5 mL; syrup 12.5 mg/5 mL; Liq 12.5 mg/5 mL; Inj 50 mg/mL, cream, gel, liq 2% SE: Anticholinergic (xerostomia, urinary retention, sedation) Interactions: ↑ Effects *W/* CNS depressants, antihistamines, opioids, MAOIs, TCAs, EtOH Labs: ↓

Response to allergy skin testing; ↓ Hgb, Hct, plts **NIPE:** ↑ Risk of photosensitivity—use sunblock; may cause drowsiness; avoid EtOH

Diphenoxylate + Atropine (Lomotil, Lonox) [C-V] [Opioid Antidiarrheal]
Uses: *D* **Action:** Constipating meperidine congener, ↓ GI motility **Dose:** *Adults.* Initial, 5 mg PO tid–qid until controlled, then 2.5–5 mg PO bid; 20 mg/d max *Peds > 2 y.* 0.3–0.4 mg/kg/24 h (of diphenoxylate) bid–qid, 10 mg/d max **Caution:** [C, ?/–] Elderly, w/ renal impair **CI:** Obstructive jaundice, D d/t bacterial Infxn; children < 2 y **Disp:** Tabs 2.5 mg diphenoxylate/0.025 mg atropine; Liq 2.5 mg diphenoxylate/0.025 mg atropine/5 mL **SE:** Drowsiness, dizziness, xerostomia, blurred vision, urinary retention, constipation **Interactions:** ↑ Effects W/ CNS depressants, opioids, EtOH, ↑ risk HTN crisis W/ MAOIs **NIPE:** ↓ Effectiveness w/ D caused by antibiotics; only liquid form to children <13 y; ↑ fluids; avoid EtOH

Diphtheria & Tetanus Toxoids (Td) (Decavac, Tenivac—for > 7 y) [Td Vaccine]
Uses: Primary immunization, booster (peds 7–9 y; peds 11–12 y if 5 y since last shot then q10y); tetanus protection after wound **Actions:** Active immunization **Dose:** 0.5 mL IM × 1; **Caution:** [C, ?/–] **CI:** Component sensitivity **Disp:** Single-dose syringes 0.5 mL **SE:** Inj site pain, redness, swelling; fever, fatigue, HA, malaise, neuro disorders rare **Interactions:** ↑ Risk of suboptimal response W/ concomitant vaccines, radiation, chemotherapy, high-dose steroids **NIPE:** If IM, use only preservative-free Inj; use DTaP (Adacel) rather than TT or Td all adults 19–64 y who have not previously received one dose of DTaP (protection adult pertussis) & Tdap for ages 10–18 y (Boostrix); do not confuse Td (for adults) w/ DT (for children < 7 y)

Diphtheria & Tetanus Toxoids (DT) (Generic Only—for < 7 y) [Tetanus Vaccine]
Uses: Primary immunization ages < 7 y (DTaP is recommended vaccine) **Actions:** Active immunization **Dose:** 0.5 mL IM × 1, 5 dose series for primary immunization if DTaP **Caution:** [C, N/A] **CI:** Component sensitivity **Disp:** Single-dose syringes 0.5 mL **SE:** Inj site pain, redness, swelling; fever, fatigue, myalgias/arthralgias, N/V, Szs, other neurologic SE rare; syncope, apnea in preemies **Interactions:** ↑ Risk of suboptimal response W/ chemotherapy, high-dose corticosteroids > 2 wk, radiation **NIPE:** If IM, use only preservative-free Inj; do not confuse DT (for children < 7 y) w/ Td (for adults); DTaP is recommended for primary immunization

Diphtheria, Tetanus Toxoids, & Acellular Pertussis Adsorbed (Tdap) (Ages > 10–11 y) (Boosters: Adacel, Boostrix)
Uses: "Catch-up" vaccination if 1 or more of the 5 childhood doses of DTP or DTaP missed; all adults 19–64 y who have not received 1 dose previously (adult pertussis protection) or if around infants < 12 mo; booster q10y; tetanus protection after fresh wound **Actions:** Active immunization, ages >10–11 y **Dose:** 0.5 mL IM × 1 **Caution:** [C, ?/–] **CI:** Component sensitivity; if previous pertussis vaccine caused

progressive neurologic disorder/encephalopathy w/in 7 d of shot **Disp:** Single-dose vial 0.5 mL **SE:** Inj site pain, redness, swelling; Abd pain, arthralgias/myalgias, fatigue, fever, HA, N/V/D, rash, tiredness **Interactions:** ↑ Risk of suboptimal response **W/** chemotherapy, high-dose corticosteroids > 2 wk, radiation **NIPE:** If IM, use only preservative-free Inj; ACIP rec: Tdap for ages 10–18 y (*Boostrix*) or 11–64 y (*Adacel*); Td should be used in children 7–9 y; CDC recommends pts > age 65 who have close contact with infants get a dose of Tdap (protection against pertussis)

Diphtheria, Tetanus Toxoids, & Acellular Pertussis Adsorbed (DTaP) (Ages < 7 y) (Daptacel, Infanrix, Tripedia)

Uses: Primary vaccination; 5 Inj at 2, 4, 6, 15–18 mo, & 4–6 y **Actions:** Active immunization **Dose:** 0.5 mL IM × 1 as in previous above **Caution:** [C, N/A] **CI:** Component sensitivity; if previous pertussis vaccine caused progressive neurologic disorder/encephalopathy w/in 7 d of shot **Disp:** Single-dose vials 0.5 mL **SE:** Inj site nodule/pain/swelling/ redness; drowsiness, fatigue, fever, fussiness, irritability, lethargy, V, prolonged crying; rare ITP and neurologic disease **Interactions:** ↑ Risk of suboptimal response **W/** chemotherapy, high-dose corticosteroids > 2 wk, radiation **NIPE:** If IM, use only preservative-free Inj; DTaP recommended for primary immunization age < 7 y, if age 7–9 y use Td, ages > 10–11 y use Tdap; if encephalopathy or other neurologic disorder w/in 7 d of previous dose. **Do not use** DTaP use DT or Td depending on age

Diphtheria, Tetanus Toxoids, Acellular Pertussis Adsorbed, Inactivated Poliovirus Vaccine [IPV], & Haemophilus b Conjugate Vaccine Combined (Pentacel) [Vaccine, Activated]

Uses: *Immunization against diphtheria, tetanus, pertussis, poliomyelitis and invasive Dz due to *Haemophilus influenzae* type b* **Action:** Active immunization **Dose:** *Infants:* 0.5 mL IM at 2, 4, 6, and 15–18 mo of age. **Caution:** [C, N/A] w/ Fever > 40.5°C (105°F), hypotonic-hyporesponsive episode (HHE) or persistent, inconsolable crying > 3 h w/in 48 h after a previous pertussis-containing vaccine; Sz w/in 3 d after a previous pertussis-containing vaccine; Guillain-Barré w/in 6 wk of previous tetanus toxoid vaccine; w/ Hx Sz antipyretic may be administered w/ vaccine × 24 h w/ bleeding disorders **CI:** Allergy to any components; encephalopathy w/in 7 d of previous pertussis vaccine; caution progressive neurologic disorders **Disp:** Single-dose vials 0.5 mL **SE:** Fussiness/irritability and inconsolable crying; fever > 38.0°C Inj site Rxn; **interactions:** ↓ effects **W/** immunosuppressants, corticosteroids **NIPE:** Use only preservative-free Inj

Diphtheria, Tetanus Toxoids, & Acellular Pertussis Adsorbed, Hep B (Recombinant), & Inactivated Poliovirus Vaccine [IPV] Combined (Pediarix) [Vaccine, Inactivated]

Uses: *Vaccine against diphtheria, tetanus, pertussis, HBV, polio (types 1, 2, 3) as a 3-dose primary series in infants & children < 7 y, born to HBsAg(−) mothers* **Actions:** Active immunization

Dose: *Infants:* Three 0.5-mL doses IM, at 6–8-wk intervals, start at 2 mo; child given 1 dose of hep B vaccine, same; previously vaccinated w/ 1 or more doses inactivated poliovirus vaccine, use to complete series **Caution:** [C, N/A] w/Bleeding disorders **CI:** HBsAg(+) mother, adults, children > 7 y, immunosuppressed, component sensitivity or allergy to yeast/neomycin/polymyxin B; encephalopathy, or progressive neurologic disorders **Disp:** Single-dose syringes 0.5 mL **SE:** Drowsiness, restlessness, fever, fussiness, ↓ appetite, Inj site pain/swelling/nodule/redness **Interactions:** ↑ Effects W/ immunosuppressants, corticosteroids **NIPE:** Use only preservative-free Inj

Dipivefrin (Propine) [Alpha-Adrenergic Agonist/Glaucoma Agent] **Uses:** *Open-angle glaucoma* **Action:** α-Adrenergic agonist **Dose:** 1 gtt in eye q12h **Caution:** [B, ?] **CI:** NAG **Disp:** 0.1% soln **SE:** HA, local irritation, blurred vision, photophobia, HTN **Interactions:** ↑ Effects W/ BBs, ophthal anhydrase Inhibs, osmotic drugs, sympathomimetics, ↑ risk of cardiac arrhythmias W/ digoxin, TCAs **NIPE:** Discard discolored solns; teach use of eye drops; wait ≥ 15 m before inserting contacts

Dipyridamole (Persantine) [Coronary Vasodilator/Platelet Aggregation Inhibitor] **Uses:** *Prevent postop thromboembolic disorders, often in combo w/ ASA or warfarin (eg, CABG, vascular graft); w/ warfarin after artificial heart valve; chronic angina; w/ ASA to prevent coronary artery thrombosis; dipyridamole IV used in place of exercise stress test for CAD* **Action:** Antiplt activity; coronary vasodilator **Dose:** *Adults.* 75–100 mg PO qid; stress test 0.14 mg/kg/min (max 60 mg over 4 min) *Peds > 12 y.* 3–6 mg/kg/d ÷ tid (safety/efficacy not established) **Caution:** [B, ?/–] w/ Other drugs that affect coagulation **CI:** Component sensitivity **Disp:** Tabs 25, 50, 75 mg; Inj 5 mg/mL **SE:** HA, ↓ BP, N, Abd distress, flushing rash, dizziness, dyspnea **Interactions:** ↑ Effects W/ anticoagulants, heparin, evening primrose oil, feverfew, garlic, ginger, ginkgo, ginseng, grapeseed extract; ↑ effects *OF* adenosine; ↑ bradycardia W/ BBs; ↓ effects W/ aminophylline **NIPE:** IV use can worsen angina; ⊘ EtOH or tobacco because of vasoconstriction effects; + effects may take several mo

Dipyridamole & Aspirin (Aggrenox) [Platelet Aggregation Inhibitor] **Uses:** *Reinfarction after MI; prevent occlusion after CABG; ↓ risk of stroke* **Action:** ↓ Plt aggregation (both agents) **Dose:** 1 cap PO bid **Caution:** [D, ?] **CI:** Ulcers, bleeding diathesis **Disp:** Dipyridamole (XR) 200 mg/ASA 25 mg **SE:** *ASA component:* Allergic Rxns, skin Rxns, ulcers/GI bleed, bronchospasm *dipyridamole component:* dizziness, HA, rash **Interactions:** ↑ Risk of GI bleed W/ EtOH, NSAIDs; ↑ effects *OF* acetazolamide, adenosine, anticoagulants, methotrexate, oral hypoglycemics; ↓ effects *OF* ACEIs, BB, cholinesterase Inhibs, diuretics **NIPE:** Swallow caps whole

Disopyramide (Norpace, Norpace CR, NAPAmide, Rythmodan) [Antiarrhythmic/Pyridine Derivative] **WARNING:** Excessive mortality or nonfatal cardiac arrest rate w/ use in asymptomatic non-life-threatening ventricular arrhythmias w/ MI 6 d–2 y prior. Restrict use to life-threatening arrhythmias only **Uses:** *Suppression & prevention of VT* **Action:** Class Ia antiarrhythmic; stabilizes membranes, ↓ action potential **Dose:** *Adults.* Immediate < 50 kg 200 mg, > 50 kg 300 mg, maint 400–800 mg/d ÷ q6h or q12h for CR, max 1600 mg/d *Peds < 1 y.* 10–30 mg/kg/24 h PO (÷ qid) *1–4 y.* 10–20 mg/kg/24 h PO (÷ qid) *4–12 y.* 10–15 mg/kg/24 h PO (÷ qid) *12–18 y.* 6–15 mg/kg/24 h PO (÷ qid); ↓ in renal/hepatic impair **Caution:** [C, +] Elderly, w/ abnormal ECG, lytes, liver/renal impair, NAG **CI:** AV block, cardiogenic shock, ↓ BP, CHF **Disp:** Caps 100, 150 mg; CR caps 100, 150 mg **SE:** Anticholinergic SEs; negative inotrope, may induce CHF **Notes:** *Levels: Trough:* Just before next dose *Therapeutic:* 2–5 mcg/mL *Toxic* > 5 mcg/mL *1/2-life:* 4–10 h **Interactions:** ↑ Effects *W/* cimetidine, clarithromycin, erythromycin, quinidine; ↑ effects *OF* digoxin, hypoglycemics, insulin, warfarin; ↑ risk of arrhythmias *W/* pimozide; ↓ effects *W/* barbiturates, phenytoin, phenobarbital, rifampin **Labs:** ↑ LFTs, lipids, BUN, Cr; ↓ serum glucose, Hgb, Hct **NIPE:** Risk of photosensitivity—use sunblock; daily wgt; may cause drowsiness; avoid EtOH

Dobutamine (Dobutrex) [Inotropic/Adrenergic, Beta-1 Agonist] **Uses:** *Short-term in cardiac decompensation secondary to ↓ contractility* **Action:** Positive inotrope **Dose:** *Adults. ECC 2010:* 2.5–20 mcg/kg/min; titrate to HR not > 10% of baseline **Peds.** *ECC 2010: Shock w/ high SVR*: 2–20 mcg/kg/min; titrate **Caution:** [B, ?/–] w/ Arrhythmia, MI, severe CAD, ↓ vol **CI:** Sensitivity to sulfites, IHSS **Disp:** Inj 250 mg/20 mL, 500 mg/40 mL; **SE:** CP, HTN, dyspnea **Interactions:** ↑ Effects *W/* furazolidone, methyldopa, MAOIs, TCAs; ↓ effects *W/* BBs, NaHCO₃; ↓ effects *OF* guanethidine **Labs:** ↓ K⁺ **NIPE:** Eval for adequate hydration; monitor I&O; monitor PWP & cardiac output if possible; continuous monitoring of BP and ECG for ↑ HR or ectopic activity

Docetaxel (Taxotere) [Antineoplastic/Antimitotic Agent] **WARNING:** Do not administer if neutrophil count < 1500 cell/mm³; severe Rxns possible in hepatic dysfunction **Uses:** *Breast (anthracycline-resistant), ovarian, lung, & prostate CA* **Action:** Antimitotic agent; promotes microtubular aggregation; semisynthetic taxoid **Dose:** 100 mg/m² over 1 h IV q3wk (per protocols); dexamethasone 8 mg bid prior & continue for 3–4 d; ↓ dose w/ ↑ bili levels **Caution:** [D, –] **CI:** Sensitivity to meds w/ polysorbate 80, component sensitivity **Disp:** Inj 20 mg/0.5 mL, 80 mg/2 mL **SE:** ↓ BM, neuropathy, N/V, alopecia, fluid retention synd; cumulative doses of 300–400 mg/m² w/o steroid prep & post-Tx & 600–800 mg/m² w/ steroid prep; allergy possible (rare w/ steroid prep) **Interactions:** ↑ Effects *W/* cyclosporine, ketoconazole, erythromycin, terfenadine **Labs:** ↑ AST, ALT, alk phos, bilirubin; ↓ plts, WBCs; frequent CBC during therapy; ✓ bilirubin, AST and ALT prior to each cycle **NIPE:** ↑ Fluids to 2–3 L/d, ↑ risk of hair loss, ↑ susceptibility to Infxn; urine may become reddish-brown; pts should be premedicated with oral corticosteroids for 3 d prior to Rx to ↓ risk of fluid retention

Docusate Calcium (Surfak)/Docusate Potassium (Dialose)/Docusate Sodium (DOSS, Colace) [Emollient Laxative/Fecal Softener] Uses: *Constipation; adjunct to painful anorectal conditions (hemorrhoids)* Action: Stool softener Dose: *Adults.* 50–500 mg PO ÷ daily–qid *Peds Infants–3 y.* 10–40 mg/24 h ÷ daily–qid *3–6 y.* 20–60 mg/24 h ÷ daily–qid. *6–12 y.* 40–150 mg/24 h ÷ daily–qid Caution: [C, ?] CI: Use w/ mineral oil; intestinal obst, acute Abd pain, N/V Disp: *Ca:* Caps 50, 240 mg *K:* Caps 100, 240 mg. *Na:* Caps 50, 100 mg; syrup 50, 60 mg/15 mL; Liq 150 mg/15 mL; soln 50 mg/mL; enema 283 mg/mL SE: Rare Abd cramping, D Interactions: ↑ Absorption of mineral oil NIPE: Take w/ full glass of water; no laxative action; do not use > 1 wk; short-term use

Dofetilide (Tikosyn) [Antiarrhythmic] WARNING: To minimize the risk of induced arrhythmia, hospitalize for minimum of 3 d to provide calculations of CrCl, cont ECG monitoring, & cardiac resuscitation Uses: *Maint nl sinus rhythm in AF/A flutter after conversion* Action: Class III antiarrhythmic, prolongs action potential Dose: Based on CrCl & QTc; CrCl > 60 mL/min 500 mcg PO q12h, ✓ QTc 2–3 h after, if QTc > 15% over baseline or > 500 ms, ↓ to 250 mcg q12h, ✓ after each dose; if CrCl < 60 mL/min, see PI; D/C if QTc > 500 ms after dosing adjustments Caution: [C, –] w/ AV block, renal Dz, electrolyte imbalance CI: Baseline QTc > 440 ms, CrCl < 20 mL/min; w/ verapamil, cimetidine, trimethoprim, ketoconazole, quinolones, ACE Inhib/HCTZ combo Disp: Caps 125, 250, 500 mcg SE: Ventricular arrhythmias, QT ↑, torsades de pointes, rash, HA, CP, dizziness Interactions: ↑ Effects *W/* amiloride, amiodarone, azole antifungals, cimetidine, diltiazem, macrolides, metformin, megestrol, nefazodone, norfloxacin, SSRIs, TCAs, triamterene, TMP, verapamil, zafirlukast, quinine, grapefruit juice Labs: Correct K+ & Mg2+ before use; monitor LFTs, BUN, Cr NIPE: Must be hospitalized before initiating; take w/o regard to food; avoid w/ other drugs that ↑ QT interval; hold Class I/III antiarrhythmics for 3 1/2-lives prior to dosing; amiodarone level should be < 0.3 mg/L before use; do not initiate if HR < 60 BPM; may cause drowsiness; restricted to participating prescribers

Dolasetron (Anzemet) [Antiemetic/Selective Serotonin 5-HT3 Receptor Antagonist] Uses: *Prevent chemotherapy & post-op-associated N/V* Action: 5-HT3 receptor antagonist Dose: *Adults.* *PO:* 100 mg PO as a single dose 1 h prior to chemotherapy *Post-op:* 12.5 mg IV, 100 mg PO 2 h pre-op *Peds 2–16 y.* 1.8 mg/kg PO (max 100 mg) as single dose *Post-op:* 0.35 mg/kg IV or 1.2 mg/kg PO Caution: [B, ?] w/ Cardiac conduction problems CI: IV use with chemo; component sensitivity Disp: Tabs 50, 100 mg; Inj 20 mg/mL SE: ↑ QT interval, D, HTN, HA, Abd pain, urinary retention, transient ↑ LFTs Interactions: ↑ Effects *W/* cimetidine; ↑ risk of arrhythmias *W/* diuretics; ↓ effects *W/* rifampin Labs: Transient ↑ LFTs NIPE Monitor ECG for prolonged QT interval; frequently causes HA; IV form no longer approved for chemotherapy-induced

N&V d/t heart rhythm abnormalities; for peds—injectable soln may be given PO mixed in apple-grape or apple juice

Dolutegravir (Tivicay) Uses: *HIV-1 Infxn w/ other antiretrovirals* Action: Integrase strand transfer Inhib (INSTI) Dose: *Adults.* Tx-naive or Tx-experienced INSTI naive: 50 mg PO 1 ×/d; Tx-naive or Tx-experienced INSTI naive w/ a potent UGT1A/CYP3A inducer (efavirenz, fosamprenavir/ritonavir, tipranavir/ritonavir, or rifampin): 50 mg PO 2 ×/d; INSTI-experienced with certain INSTI-associated resistance substitutions or suspected INSTI resist: 50 mg PO 2 ×/d *Peds ≥ 12 y & ≥ 40 kg.* Tx-naive or Tx-experienced INSTI-naive: 50 mg PO 1 ×/d; w/ efavirenz, fosamprenavir/ritonavir, tipranavir/ritonavir, or rifampin: 50 mg PO 2 ×/d Caution: [B, ?/–] CDC rec HIV infect mothers not breast-feed; D/C w/ hypersens rxn (rash, constitutional findings, organ dysfunction); ↑ LFTs w/ underlying hep B or C (monitor LFTs); w/ other antiretroviral therapy, may cause fat redistribution/ accumulation and immune reconstitution synd CI: w/ dofetilide Disp: Tabs 50 mg SE: HA, insomnia, N/V/D, abd pain, ↑ serum lipase, hypersens Rxn, ↑ glucose, ↑ bilirubin, pruritus NIPE: Take w/ or w/o food; take 2 h before or 6 h after antacids or laxatives, sucralfate, iron & calcium suppl, buffered meds; not a cure for HIV—continue transmission prec; ⊘ for children < 8 y or < 88 lb (40 kg)

Donepezil (Aricept) [Reversible Acetylcholinesterase Inhibitor] Uses: *Severe Alzheimer dementia* ADHD; behavioral synds in dementia; dementia w/ Parkinson Dz; Lewy-body dementia Action: ACH Inhib Dose: *Adults.* 5 mg qhs, ↑ to 10 mg PO qhs after 4–6 wk *Peds. ADHD:* 5 mg/d Caution: [C, ?] Risk for ↓ HR w/ preexisting conduction abnormalities, may exaggerate succinylcholine-type muscle relaxation w/ anesthesia, ↑ gastric acid secretion CI: Hypersens Disp: Tabs 5, 10, 23 mg; ODT 5, 10 mg SE: N/V/D, insomnia, Infxn, muscle cramp, fatigue, anorexia Interactions: Drugs that affect CYP2D6 & CYP3A4 may affect rate of elimination; ↑ effects *OF* succinylcholine-type muscle relaxants, other cholinesterase Inhibs, cholinergic agonists (eg, bethanechol); ↓ effects *OF* anticholinergic drugs; concomitant NSAIDs may ↑ risk of GI bleed NIPE: Take at bedtime, w/ or w/o food; follow oral disintegrating tabs with 8 oz water; N/V/D dose-related & resolves in 1–3 wk

Dopamine (Intropin) [Vasopressor/Adrenergic] WARNING: Tissue vesicant, give phentolamine w/ extrav Uses: *Short-term use in cardiac decompensation secondary to ↓ contractility;* ↑ *organ perfusion (at low dose)* Action: Positive inotropic agent w/ dose respon 1–10 mcg/kg/min β effects (↑ CO); 10–20 mcg/kg/min β-effects (peripheral vasoconstriction, pressor); > 20 mcg/ kg/min peripheral & renal vasoconstriction Dose: *Adults.* 5 mcg/kg/min by cont Inf, ↑ by 5 mcg/kg/min to 50 mcg/kg/min max to effect *ECC 2010:* 2–20 mcg/kg/min Peds. *ECC 2010: Shock w/ adequate intravascular volume and stable rhythm:* 2–20 mcg/kg/min; titrate, if > 20 mcg/kg/min needed, consider alternative adrenergic Caution: [C, ?] ↓ Dose w/ MAOI CI: Pheochromocytoma, VF, sulfite sensitivity **Disp:** Inj 40, 80, 160 mg/mL, premixed 0.8, 1.6, 3.2 mg/mL **SE:** Tachycardia, vasoconstriction, ↓ BP, HA, N/V, dyspnea **Notes:** > 10 mcg/kg/min ↓ renal perfusion **Interactions:** ↑ Effects W/ α-blockers, diuretics, ergot alkaloids, MAOIs, BBs, anesthetics, phenytoin; ↓ effects W/ guanethidine **Labs:** ↑ Glucose, urea levels **NIPE:** Maint adequate hydration; monitor urinary output & ECG for ↑ HR, BP, ectopy; monitor PCWP & cardiac output if possible; ↑ risk peripheral ischemia; phentolamine used for extrav 10–15 mL NS w/ 5–10 mg of phentolamine

Doripenem (Doribax) [Carbapenem] Uses: *Complicated intra-Abd Infxn and UTI including pyelo* **Action:** Carbapenem, ↓ cell wall synth, a β-lactam *Spectrum:* Excellent gram(+) (except MRSA & *Enterococcus* sp), excellent gram(−) coverage including β-lactamase producers, good anaerobic **Dose:** 500 mg IV q8h, ↓ w/ renal impair **Caution:** [B, ?] **CI:** Carbapenems β-lactams hypersens **Disp:** 250, 500 mg vial **SE:** HA, N/D, rash, phlebitis **Interactions:** ↑ Effects W/ probenecid; may ↓ valproic acid levels; overuse may ↑ bacterial resistance **NIPE:** Monitor for *C difficile*–associated D

Dornase Alfa (Pulmozyme, DNase) [Respiratory Inhalant/ Enzyme/Recombinant Human DNAse] Uses: *↓ Frequency of resp Infxns in CF* **Action:** Enzyme cleaves extracellular DNA, ↓ mucous viscosity **Dose:** *Adults.* Inh 2.5 mg/daily–bid dosing w/ FVC > 85% w/ recommended nebulizer *Peds* > 5 y. Inh 2.5 mg/daily–bid if forced vital capacity > 85% **Caution:** [B, ?] **CI:** Chinese hamster product allergy **Disp:** Soln for Inh 1 mg/mL **SE:** Pharyngitis, voice alteration, CP, rash **NIPE:** Teach pt to use nebulizer; do not mix w/ other drugs in nebulizer

Dorzolamide (Trusopt) [Carbonic Anhydrase Inhibitor, Sulfonamide/Glaucoma Agent] Uses: *Open-angle glaucoma, ocular hypertension* **Action:** Carbonic anhydrase Inhib **Dose:** 1 gtt in eye(s) tid **Caution:** [C, ?] w/ NAG, CrCl < 30 mL/min **CI:** Component sensitivity **Disp:** 2% soln **SE:** Irritation, bitter taste, punctate keratitis, ocular allergic Rxn **Interactions:** ↑ Effects W/ oral carbonic anhydrase Inhibs, salicylates **NIPE:** ⊘ Wear soft contact lenses; teach use of eye drops

Dorzolamide & Timolol (Cosopt) [Carbonic Anhydrase Inhibitor/Beta-Adrenergic Blocker] Uses: *Open-angle glaucoma, ocular hypertension* **Action:** Carbonic anhydrase Inhib w/ β-adrenergic blocker **Dose:** 1 gtt in eye(s) bid **Caution:** [C, ?] CrCl < 30mL/min **CI:** Component sensitivity, asthma, severe COPD, sinus bradycardia, AV block **Disp:** Soln dorzolamide 2% & timolol 0.5% **SE:** Irritation, bitter taste, superficial keratitis, ocular allergic Rxn **NIPE:** ⊘ Wear soft contact lenses; teach use of eye drops

Doxazosin (Cardura, Cardura XL) [Antihypertensive/Alpha-Blocker] Uses: *HTN & symptomatic BPH* **Action:** α₁-Adrenergic blocker; relaxes bladder neck smooth muscle **Dose:** *HTN:* Initial 1 mg/d PO; may be ↑ to 16 mg/d PO *BPH:* Initial 1 mg/d PO, may ↑ to 8 mg/d; XL 4–8 mg q AM **Caution:**

[C, ?] w/ Liver impair **CI:** Component sensitivity; use w/ PDE5 Inhib (eg, sildenafil), can cause ↓ BP **Disp:** Tabs 1, 2, 4, 8 mg; XL 4, 8 mg **SE:** Dizziness, HA, drowsiness, fatigue, malaise, sexual dysfunction, doses > 4 mg ↑ postural ↓ BP risk; intraoperative floppy iris synd **Interactions:** ↑ Effects *W/* nitrates, antihypertensives, EtOH; ↓ effects *W/* NSAIDs, butcher's broom; ↓ effects *OF* clonidine **NIPE:** May be taken w/ food; 1st dose and ↑ dose at hs; syncope may occur w/in 90 min of initial dose; may cause dizziness/drowsiness—caution driving

Doxepin (Adapin) [Antidepressant/TCA]   WARNING: Closely monitor for worsening depression or emergence of suicidality **Uses:** *Depression, anxiety, chronic pain* **Action:** TCA; ↑ synaptic CNS serotonin or norepinephrine **Dose:** 25–150 mg/d PO, usually hs but can ÷ doses; up to 300 mg/d for depression; ↓ in hepatic impair **Caution:** [C, ?/–] w/ EtOH abuse, elderly, w/ MAOI **CI:** NAG, urinary retention, MAOI use w/in 14 d, in recovery phase of MI **Disp:** Caps 10, 25, 50, 75, 100, 150 mg; PO conc 10 mg/mL **SE:** Anticholinergic SEs, ↓ BP, tachycardia, drowsiness, photosens **Interactions:** ↑ Effects *W/* fluoxetine, MAOIs, albuterol, CNS depressants, anticholinergics, propoxyphene, quinidine, EtOH, grapefruit juice; ↑ effects *OF* carbamazepine, anticoagulants, amphetamines, thyroid drugs, sympathomimetics; effects *W/* ascorbic acid, cholestyramine, tobacco; ↓ effects *OF* bretylium, guanethidine, levodopa **Labs:** ↑ Serum bilirubin, alk phos, glucose **NIPE:** Risk of photosensitivity—use sunblock; urine may turn blue-green; may take 4–6 wk for full effect; mix oral conc w/ 4 oz water or milk, or juice (except grape); may give qhs to ↓ daytime sedation; ↑ fluids, fiber; avoid EtOH

Doxepin (Silenor) [H₁-Receptor Antagonist] Uses: *Insomnia* **Action:** TCA **Dose:** Take w/in 30 min HS 6 mg qd; 3 mg in elderly; 6 mg/d max; not w/in 3 h of a meal. **Caution:** [C, ?/–] w/ EtOH abuse/elderly/sleep apnea/CNS depressants; may cause abnormal thinking and hallucinations; may worsen depression **CI:** NAG, urinary retention, MAOI w/in 14 d **Disp:** Tabs 3, 6 mg **SE:** Somnolence/sedation, N, URI **Interactions:** ↑ Effects *W/* CNS depressants, antihistamines, cimetidine, EtOH; ↑ risk of hypoglycemia *W/* tolazamide **NIPE:** Monitor for new onset behavioral changes

Doxepin, Topical (Prudoxin, Zonalon) [Antipruritic] Uses: *Short-term Rx pruritus (atopic dermatitis or lichen simplex chronicus)* **Action:** Antipruritic; H₁- & H₂-receptor antagonism **Dose:** Apply thin coating tid–qid, 8 d max **Caution:** [B, ?/–] **CI:** Component sensitivity **Disp:** 5% cream **SE:** ↓ BP, tachycardia, drowsiness, photosens **NIPE:** Limit application area to avoid systemic tox; do not bandage or cover; photosensitivity—use sunblock

Doxorubicin (Adriamycin, Rubex) [Antineoplastic/Anthracycline Antibiotic] Uses: *Acute leukemias; Hodgkin Dz & NHLs; soft tissue, osteo- & Ewing sarcoma; Wilms tumor; neuroblastoma; bladder, breast, ovarian, gastric, thyroid, & lung CAs* **Action:** Intercalates DNA; ↓ DNA topoisomerases I & II **Dose:** 60–75 mg/m² q3wk; ↓ w/ hepatic impair; IV use only ↓ cardiotox w/

weekly (20 mg/m^2/wk) or cont Inf (60–90 mg/m^2 over 96 h); (per protocols) **Caution:** [D, ?] **CI:** Severe CHF, cardiomyopathy, preexisting ↓ BM, previous Rx w/ total cumulative doses of doxorubicin, idarubicin, daunorubicin **Disp:** Inj 10, 20, 50, 150, 200 mg **SE:** ↑ BM, venous streaking & phlebitis, N/V/D, mucositis, radiation recall phenomenon, cardiomyopathy rare (dose-related) **Notes:** Limit of 550 mg/m^2 cumulative dose (400 mg/m^2 w/ prior mediastinal irradiation); dexrazoxane may limit cardiac tox **Interactions:** ↑ Effects **W/** streptozocin, verapamil, green tea; ↑ BM depression **W/** antineoplastic drugs & radiation; ↓ effects ↑ **W/** phenobarbital; ↓ effects **OF** digoxin, phenytoin, live virus vaccines **Labs:** ↑ Bilirubin, glucose, urine, & plasma uric acid levels; ↓ Ca, Hgb, Hct, plts, WBCs **NIPE:** ⊘ PRG, use contraception at least 4 mo after drug Rx; red/orange urine; tissue damage w/ extrav; vesicant w/ extrav, Rx w/ dexrazoxane; ↑ risk of Infxn

Doxycycline (Adoxa, Periostat, Oracea, Vibramycin, VibraTabs) [Antibiotic/Tetracycline] Uses: *Broad-spectrum antibiotic* acne vulgaris,
uncomplicated GC, chlamydia, PID, Lyme Dz, skin Infxns, anthrax, malaria prophylaxis **Action:** Tetracycline; bacteriostatic; ↓ protein synth *Spectrum:* Limited gram(+) & (–), *Rickettsia* sp, *Chlamydia, M pneumoniae, B anthracis* **Dose:** *Adults.* 100 mg PO q12h on 1st d, then 100 mg PO daily–bid or 100 mg IV q12h; acne: qd, chlamydia × 7 d, Lyme × 21 d, PID × 14 d *Peds > 8 y.* 5 mg/kg/24 h PO, 200 mg/d max ÷ daily–bid **Caution:** [D, –] hepatic impair **CI:** Children < 8 y, severe hepatic dysfunction **Disp:** Tabs 20, 50, 75, 100, 150 mg; caps 50, 75, 100, 150 mg; Oracea 40 mg caps (30 mg timed release, 10 mg DR); syrup 50 mg/5 mL; susp 25 mg/5 mL; Inj 100/vial **SE:** D, GI disturbance, photosens **Interactions:** ↑ Effects **OF** digoxin, warfarin; ↓ effects **W/** antacids, Fe, barbiturates, carbamazepine, phenytoins, food; ↓ effects **OF** PCN **Labs:** ↑ LFTs, BUN, eosinophils; ↓ Hgb, Hct, plts, neutrophils, WBC **NIPE:** Take with 8 oz water; take 1 h before or 2 h after antacids; ↑ risk of super Infxn, ⊘ PRG, use barrier contraception; tetracycline of choice w/ renal impair; for inhalational anthrax use w/ 1–2 additional antibiotics, not for CNS anthrax

Doxylamine/Pyridoxine (Diclegis) Uses: * Morning sickness * Action:
Antihistamine & vit B$_6$ **Dose:** 2 tabs PO qhs; max 4 tabs/d (1 q AM, 1 mid-afternoon, 2 qhs) **Caution:** [A, –] CNS depression; anticholinergic (caution w/ asthma, ↑ IOP, NAG, peptic ulcer, pyloroduodenal or bladder-neck obst) **CI:** Component hypersens, w/ MAOIs **Disp:** Tabs DR (doxylamine/pyridoxine): 10/10 mg **SE:** Somnolence, dizziness, HA, urinary retention, blurred vision, palpitation, ↑ HR, dyspnea **NIPE:** Take on empty stomach with 8 oz water; ⊘ chew/crush/split; ⊘ EtOH; may cause drowsiness—caution driving

Dronabinol (Marinol) [C-II] [Antiemetic, Appetite Stimulant/Antivertigo] Uses: *N/V associated w/ CA chemotherapy; appetite stimulation*
Action: Antiemetic; ↓ V center in the medulla **Dose:** *Adults & Peds.* Antiemetic: 5–15 mg/m^2/dose q4–6h PRN. *Adults.* Appetite stimulant: 2.5 mg PO before lunch

& dinner; max 20 mg/d **Caution:** [C, ?] Elderly, Hx psychological disorder, Sz disorder, substance abuse **CI:** Hx schizophrenia, sesame oil hypersens **Disp:** Caps 2.5, 5, 10 mg **SE:** Drowsiness, dizziness, anxiety, mood change, hallucinations, depersonalization, orthostatic ↓ BP, tachycardia **Interactions:** ↑ Effects *W/* anticholinergics, CNS depressants, EtOH; ↓ effects *OF* theophylline **NIPE:** Swallow whole—⊘ chew/crust/split; principal psychoactive substance present in marijuana; avoid EtOH; caution driving

Dronedarone (Multaq) [Antiarrhythmic/Benzofurans] WARNING: CI w/ NYHA Class IV HF or NYHA Class II–III HF w/ decompensation **Uses:** *A Fib/A flutter* **Action:** Antiarrhythmic **Dose:** 400 mg PO bid w/ AM and PM meal **Caution:** [X, –] w/ Other drugs (see PI) **CI:** See Warning; 2nd/3rd-degree AV block or SSS (unless w/ pacemaker), HR < 50 BPM, w/ strong CYP3A Inhib, w/ drugs/herbals that ↑ QT interval, QTc interval ≥ 500 ms, severe hepatic impair, PRG **Disp:** Tabs 400 mg **SE:** N/V/D, Abd pain, asthenia, heart failure, ↑ K^+, ↑ Mg^{2+}, ↑ QTc, ↓ HR, ↑SCr, rash **Interactions:** ↑ Risk of prolonged QT Interval *W/* antidepressants, antipsychotics, macrolides, phenothiazine, TCA; ↑ risk of CV Rxns *W/* amiodarone, BB, CCB, disopyramide, dofetilide, flecainide, propafenone, quinidine, sotalol, grapefruit juice; ↑ effects *OF* SSRIs, statins, TCA ↓ effects *W/* carbamazepine, phenobarbital, phenytoin, rifampin, St. John's wort **Labs:** ↑ SCr; ↑ ↑ K^+, ↑ Mg^{2+} **NIPE:** ⊘ Grapefruit/grapefruit juice

Droperidol (Inapsine) [General Anesthetic/Butyrophenone] WARNING: Cases of QT interval prolongation and torsades de pointes (some fatal) reported **Uses:** *N/V; anesthetic premedication* **Action:** Tranquilizer, sedation, antiemetic **Dose: Adults.** *N:* Initial max 2.5 mg IV/IM, may repeat 1.25 mg based on response. **Peds.** *Premed:* 0.1–0.15 mg/kg/dose (max 1.25 mg); N Tx 0.1 mg/kg/dose (max 2.5 mg) **Caution:** [C, ?] w/ Hepatic/renal impair **CI:** Component sensitivity **Disp:** Inj 2.5 mg/mL **SE:** Drowsiness, ↓ BP, occasional tachycardia & extrapyramidal Rxns, ↑ QT interval, arrhythmias **Interactions:** ↑ Effects *W/* CNS depressants, fentanyl, EtOH; ↑ hypotension *W/* antihypertensives, nitrates **NIPE:** Give IV push slowly over 2–5 min

Droxidopa (Northera) WARNING: Monitor supine BP (↓ dose or D/C if raising head of bed does not ↓ supine BP) **Uses:** *Neurogenic orthostatic hypotension* **Action:** Norepinephrine precursor; caution peripheral arterial/venous vasoconstriction **Dose:** 100 mg PO tid; max 600 mg PO tid; last dose 3 h prior to hs & elevate head of bed **Caution:** [C, –] supine HTN may ↑ CV risk; w/ h/o CHF, arrhythmias, ischemic heart Dz; w/ DOPA decarboxylase Inhib **CI:** None **Disp:** Caps 100, 200, 300 mg **SE:** HA, dizziness, N, HTN, fatigue, syncope, hyperpyrexia, confusion, UTI **Notes:** Contains FD&C Yellow No. 5 (tartrazine), may cause allergic-type Rxn **NIPE:** Take consistently w/ or w/o food; swallow whole—⊘ crush/chew/split; may need to keep head ↑ when sleeping; check BP when supine and then when head elevated

Duloxetine (Cymbalta) [Antidepressant/SSNRI] **WARNING:** Antidepressants may ↑ risk of suicidality; consider risks/benefits of use. Closely monitor for clinical worsening, suicidality, or behavior changes **Uses:** *Depression, DM peripheral neuropathic pain, generalized anxiety disorder (GAD) fibromyalgia, chronic OA, & back pain* **Action:** Selective serotonin & norepinephrine reuptake Inhib (SSNRI) **Dose:** *Depression:* 40–60 mg/d PO ÷ bid. *DM neuropathy:* 60 mg/d PO *GAD:* 60 mg/d, max 120 mg/d *Fibromyalgia, OA/back pain:* 30–60 mg/d, 60 mg/d max **Caution:** [C, ?/–]; use in 3rd tri; avoid if CrCl < 30 mL/min, NAG, w/ fluvoxamine, Inhib of CYP2D6 (Table 10), TCAs, phenothiazines, type class Ic antiarrhythmics (Table 9) **CI:** ↑ Risk serotonin synd w/MAOIs [linezolid or IV meth blue] MAOI use w/in 14 d, w/ thioridazine, NAG, hepatic Insuff **Disp:** Caps delayed-response 20, 30, 60 mg **SE:** N, dry mouth, somnolence, fatigue, constipation, ↓ appetite, hyperhidrosis **Interactions:** ↑ Effects *OF* flecainide, propafenone, phenothiazines, TCAs; ↓ effects *W/* cimetidine, fluvoxamine, quinolones; ↑ risk *OF* hypertensive crisis *W/* MAOIs w/in 14 d of taking duloxetine **Labs:** ? ↑ LFTs **NIPE:** ↑ Risk of liver damage *W/* EtOH use; ⊘ D/C drug abruptly; swallow whole; monitor BP

Dutasteride (Avodart) [Androgen Hormone Inhibitor/BPH Agent] **Uses:** *Symptomatic BPH to improve Sxs, ↓ risk of retention and BPH surgery alone or in combo w/ tamsulosin* **Action:** 5α-Reductase Inhib; ↓ intracellular dihydrotestosterone (DHT) **Dose:** *Monotherapy:* 0.5 mg PO/d *Combo:* 0.5 mg PO qd w/ tamsulosin 0.4 mg q day **Caution:** [X, –] Hepatic impair; pregnant women should not handle pills; R/O CA before starting **CI:** Women, peds **Disp:** Caps 0.5 mg **SE:** ↑ Testosterone, ↑ TSH, impotence, ↓ libido, gynecomastia, ejaculatory disturbance, may ↑ risk of high-grade prostate CA **Interactions:** ↑ Effects *W/* cimetidine, ciprofloxacin, diltiazem, ketoconazole, ritonavir, verapamil **Labs:** ↓ PSA levels; ✓ new baseline PSA at 6 mo (corrected PSA × 2); any PSA rise on dutasteride suspicious for CA **NIPE:** ⊘ Handling by PRG women; take w/o regard to food; swallow whole; no blood donation until 6 mo after D/C; under FDA review for PCa chemotherapy prevention; now available in fixed dose combo w/ tamsulosin (see Jalyn)

Dutasteride & Tamsulosin (Jalyn) [BPH Agent/Type I & II 5 Alpha-Reductase Inhibitor + Alpha-1A-Blocker] **Uses:** *Symptomatic BPH to improve Sxs* **Action:** 5 α-Reductase Inhib (↓ intracellular DHT) w/ α-blocker **Dose:** 1 capsule daily after same meal **Caution:** [X, –] w/CYP3A4 and CYP2D6 Inhib may ↑ SEs; pregnant women should not handle pills; R/O CA before starting; IFIS (tamsulosin) discuss w/ ophthalmologist before cataract surgery; rare priapism; w/ warfarin; may ↑ risk of high grade prostatic CA **CI:** Women, peds, component sensitivity **Disp:** Caps 0.5 mg dutasteride w/ 0.4 mg tamsulosin **SE:** Impotence, decreased libido, ejaculation disorders, and breast disorders **Interactions:** ↑ Effects *W/* cimetidine, diltiazem, erythromycin, terbinatine

Labs: ↓ PSA, ✓ new baseline PSA at 6 mo **NIPE:** Swallow whole; no blood donation until 6 mo after D/C therapy; any PSA rise on dutasteride suspicious for CA (see also Dutasteride & Tamsulosin); may cause drowsiness/dizziness—caution changing positions/driving

Ecallantide (Kalbitor) [Plasma Kallikrein Inhibitor] WARNING: Anaphylaxis reported, administer in a setting able to manage anaphylaxis and HAE, monitor closely **Uses:** *Acute attacks of hereditary angioedema (HAE)* **Action:** Plasma kallikrein Inhibitor **Dose:** *Adult & > 16 y.* 30 mg SC in three 10-mg injections; if attack persists may repeat 30-mg dose w/in 24 h **Caution:** [C, ?/–] Hypersens Rxns **CI:** Hypersens to ecallantide **Disp:** Inj 10 mg/mL **SE:** HA, N/V/D, pyrexia, Inj site Rxn, nasopharyngitis, fatigue, Abd pain **NIPE:** Administer in a medical setting

Echothiophate Iodine (Phospholine Ophthalmic) [Cholinesterase Inhibitor/Glaucoma Agent] Uses: *Glaucoma* **Action:** Cholinesterase Inhib **Dose:** 1 gtt eye(s) bid w/ 1 dose h **Caution:** [C, ?] **CI:** Active uveal inflammation, inflammatory Dz of iris/ciliary body, glaucoma iridocyclitis **Disp:** Powder for reconstitution 6.25 mg/5 mL (0.125%); **SE:** Local irritation, myopia, blurred vision, ↓ BP ↓ HR **Interactions:** ↑ Effects W/ cholinesterase Inhibs, pilocarpine, succinylcholine, carbamate, or organophosphate insecticides; ↑ effects OF cocaine; ↓ effects W/ anticholinergics, atropine, cyclopentolate, ophthal adrenocorticoids **NIPE:** ⊘ Drug 2 wk before surgery if succinylcholine is to be administered; keep drug refrigerated; monitor for lens opacities; teach use of eye drops; may cause blurry vision – caution driving

Econazole (Spectazole) [Topical Antifungal] Uses: *Tinea, cutaneous Candida, & tinea versicolor Infxns* **Action:** Topical antifungal **Dose:** Apply to areas bid Candida (daily for tinea versicolor) for 2–4 wk **Caution:** [C, ?] **CI:** Component sensitivity **Disp:** Topical cream 1% **SE:** Local irritation, pruritus, erythema **Interactions:** ↓ Effects W/ corticosteroids **NIPE:** Topical use only; ⊘ cover, wrap, bandage area; ⊘ eye area; early Sx/clinical improvement; complete course to avoid recurrence

Eculizumab (Soliris) [Complement Inhibitor] WARNING: ↑ Risk of meningococcal Infxns (give meningococcal vaccine 2 wk prior to 1st dose and revaccinate per guidelines) **Uses:** *Rx paroxysmal nocturnal hemoglobinuria* **Action:** Complement Inhib **Dose:** 600 mg IV q7d × 4 wk, then 900 mg IV 5th dose 7 d later, then 900 mg IV q14d **Caution:** [C, ?] **CI:** Active N meningitidis Infxn; if not vaccinated against N meningitidis **Disp:** 300-mg vial **SE:** Meningococcal Infxn, HA, nasopharyngitis, N, back pain, Infxns, fatigue, severe hemolysis on D/C **NIPE:** IV over 35 min (2-h max Inf time); monitor for 1 h for S/Sx of Inf Rxn; should have meningococcal vaccine ≥ 2wk prior to Rx

Edrophonium (Enlon) [Cholinergic Muscle Stimulant/Anticholinesterase] Uses: *Diagnosis of MyG; acute MyG crisis; curare antagonist, reverse of nondepolarizing neuromuscular blockers* **Action:** Anticholinesterase **Dose:** *Adults. Test for MyG:* 2 mg IV in 1 min; if tolerated, give 8 mg IV; (+) test is brief ↑ in strength. *Peds.* See label **Caution:** [C, ?] **CI:** GI or GU obst; allergy to sulfite **Disp:** Inj 10 mg/mL **SE:** N/V/D, excessive salivation, stomach cramps, ↑ aminotransferases **Interactions:** ↑ Effects *W/* tacrine; ↑ cardiac effects *W/* digoxin; ↑ effects *OF* neostigmine, pyridostigmine, succinylcholine, jaborandi tree, pill-bearing spurge; ↓ effects *W/* corticosteroids, procainamide, quinidine **Labs:** ↑ AST, ALT; serum amylase **NIPE:** ↑ Risk uterine irritability & premature labor in PRG pts near term; can cause severe cholinergic effects; keep atropine available

Efavirenz (Sustiva) [Antiretroviral/NNRTI] Uses: *HIV Infxns* **Action:** Antiretroviral; nonnucleoside RT Inhib **Dose:** *Adults.* 600 mg/d PO qd hs *Peds ≥ 3 y 10–< 15 kg:* 200 mg PO qd; *15–< 20 kg:* 250 mg PO qd *20–< 25 kg.* 300 mg PO qd *25–< 32.5 kg:* 350 mg PO qd; *32.5–< 40 kg:* 400 mg PO qd *> 40 kg:* 600 mg PO qd; on empty stomach **Caution:** [D, ?] CDC rec HIV-infected mothers not breast-feed **CI:** w/ Astemizole, bepridil, cisapride, midazolam, pimozide, triazolam, ergot derivatives, voriconazole **Disp:** Caps 50, 200; 600 mg tab **SE:** Somnolence, vivid dreams, depression, CNS Sxs, dizziness, rash, N/V/D **Interactions:** ↑ Effects *W/* ritonavir; ↑ effects *OF* CNS depressants, ergot derivatives, midazolam, ritonavir, simvastatin, triazolam, warfarin; ↓ effects *W/* carbamazepine, phenobarbital, rifabutin, rifampin, saquinavir, St. John's wort; ↓ effects *OF* amprenavir, carbamazepine, clarithromycin, indinavir, phenobarbital, saquinavir, warfarin; may alter effectiveness of OCPs **Labs:** ↑ LFTs, cholesterol; monitor LFT, cholesterol; ✓ LFTs (esp w/ underlying liver Dz), cholesterol **NIPE:** ⊘ High-fat foods; take w/o regard to food; use barrier contraception; maintain transmission precautions; not for monotherapy; ⊘ PRG

Efavirenz, Emtricitabine, Tenofovir (Atripla) [Combination Anti-retroviral] **WARNING:** Lactic acidosis and severe hepatomegaly w/ steatosis, including fatal cases, reported w/ nucleoside analogues alone or combo w/ other antiretrovirals Uses: *HIV Infxns* **Action:** Triple fixed-dose combo NNRTI/ nucleoside analogue **Dose:** *Adults.* 1 tab qd on empty stomach; hs dose may ↓ CNS SE **Caution:** [D, ?] CDC rec HIV-infected mothers not breast-feed, w/ obesity **CI:** < 12 y or > 40 kg, w/ astemizole, midazolam, triazolam, or ergot derivatives (CYP3A4 competition by efavirenz could cause serious/life-threatening SE) **Disp:** Tab efavirenz 600 mg/emtricitabine 200 mg/tenofovir 300 mg **SE:** Somnolence, vivid dreams, HA, dizziness, rash, N/V/D, ↓ BMD **Interactions:** ↑ Effects *OF* ritonavir, tenofovir, ethinyl estradiol levels ↓ effects *W/* phenobarbital, rifampin, rifabutin, saquinavir, ↓ effects *OF* indinavir, amprenavir, clarithromycin, methadone, rifabutin, sertraline, statins, saquinavir; monitor warfarin levels **Labs:** Monitor LFT, cholesterol **NIPE:** Swallow tablet whole w/o food; cap contents may be sprinkled/mixed with small amt food; ⊘ EtOH; ⊘ PRG & breast-feeding; do not use in HIV & hep B coinfection; maintain transmission precautions; see individual agents for additional info

Eletriptan (Relpax) [Analgesic/Antimigraine Agent] Uses: *Acute Rx of migraine* **Action:** Selective serotonin receptor (5-HT$_{1B/1D}$) agonist **Dose:**

20–40 mg PO, may repeat in 2 h; 80 mg/24 h max **Caution:** [C, +/–] **CI:** Hx ischemic heart Dz, coronary artery spasm, stroke or TIA, peripheral vascular Dz, IBD, uncontrolled HTN, hemiplegic or basilar migraine, severe hepatic impair, w/in 24 h of another 5-HT$_1$ agonist or ergot, w/in 72 h of CYP3A4 Inhibs **Disp:** Tabs 20, 40 mg **SE:** Dizziness, somnolence, N, asthenia, xerostomia, paresthesias; pain, pressure, or tightness in chest, jaw, or neck; serious cardiac events **Interactions:** ↑ Risk of serotonin synd **W/** SSRIs; ↑ risks of prolonged vasospasms **W/** ergot-containing medications **Labs:** None known **NIPE:** Not for migraine prevention; ⊘ EtOH; ⊘ use for more than 3 migraine attacks/mo; if overused, may cause rebound headache

Eltrombopag (Promacta) [Thrombopoietin Receptor Agonist]
WARNING: May cause hepatotox ✓ baseline ALT/AST/bilirubin, q2wk w/ dosage adjustment, then monthly. D/C if ALT is > 3 × ULN w/ ↑ bilirubin, or Sx of liver injury **Uses:** *Tx plt in idiopathic ↓ plt refractory to steroids, immune globulins, splenectomy* **Action:** Thrombopoietin receptor agonist **Dose:** 50 mg PO daily, adjust to keep plt ≥ 50,000 cells/mm³; 75 mg/d max; start 25 mg/d if East-Asian or w/ hepatic impair; on an empty stomach; not w/in 4 h of product w/ polyvalent cations **Caution:** [C, ?/–] ↑ Risk for BM reticulin fiber deposition, heme malignancies, rebound ↓ plt ↑ on D/C, thromboembolism **CI:** None **Disp:** Tabs 12.5, 25, 50, 75 mg **SE:** Rash, bruising, menorrhagia, N/V, dyspepsia, ↓ plt, ↑ ALT/AST, limb pain, myalgia, paresthesia, cataract, conjunctival hemorrhage **Interactions:** ↑ Effects **W/** ciprofloxacin, fluvoxamine, gemfibrozil, TMP; ↑ effects **OF** benzylpenicillin, most statins, methotrexate, nateglinide, repaglinide, rifampine **Labs:** ↑ plt, ↑ ALT/AST **NIPE:** D/C If no ↑ plt count after 4 wk; restricted distribution PROMACTA® *Cares (1-877-9-PROMACTA)*; take w/o food 1 h before or 2 h after meal; allow 4-h interval if taking food/med high in Ca or supplements with Ca, Fe, Zn, Mg

Emedastine (Emadine) [Antihistamine]
Uses: *Allergic conjunctivitis* **Action:** Antihistamine; selective H$_1$-antagonist **Dose:** 1 gtt in eye(s) up to qid **Caution:** [B, ?] **CI:** Allergy to ingredients (preservatives benzalkonium, tromethamine) **Disp:** 0.05% soln **SE:** HA, blurred vision, burning/stinging, corneal infiltrates/ staining, dry eyes, foreign body sensation, hyperemia, keratitis, tearing, pruritus, rhinitis, sinusitis, asthenia, bad taste, dermatitis, discomfort **NIPE:** Do not use contact lenses if eyes are red; may reinsert contact lenses 10 min after administration if eyes not red; teach use of eye drops

Emtricitabine (Emtriva) [Antiretroviral/NRTI]
WARNING: Lactic acidosis, & severe hepatomegaly w/ steatosis reported; not for HBV Infxn **Uses:** HIV-1 Infxn **Action:** NRTI **Dose:** 200 mg caps or 240 mg soln PO daily; ↓ w/ renal impair **Caution:** [B, –] risk of liver Dz **CI:** Component sensitivity **Disp:** Soln 10 mg/ mL, caps 200 mg **SE:** HA, N/D, rash, rare hyperpigmentation of feet & hands, post-Tx exacerbation of hep **Interactions:** None noted **W/** additional NRTIs **Labs:** ↑ LFTs, bilirubin, triglycerides, glucose **NIPE:** Take w/o regard to food;

causes redistribution & accumulation of body fat; take w/ other antiretrovirals; not a cure for HIV or prevention of opportunistic Infxns; 1st one-daily NRTI; caps/soln not equivalent; not recommended as monotherapy; screen for hep B, do not use w/ HIV & HBV coinfection

Enalapril (Vasotec) [Antihypertensive/ACEI] **WARNING:** ACE Inhib used during PRG can cause fetal injury & death **Uses:** *HTN, CHF, LVD*, DN **Action:** ACE Inhib **Dose:** *Adults.* 2.5–40 mg/d PO; 1.25 mg IV q6h **Peds.** 0.05–0.08 mg/kg/d PO q12–24h; ↓ w/ renal impair **Caution:** [C (1st tri), D (2nd & 3rd tri), +] D/C immediately w/ PRG, w/ NSAIDs, K⁺ supls **CI:** Bilateral RAS, angioedema **Disp:** Tabs 2.5, 5, 10, 20 mg; IV 1.25 mg/mL (1, 2 mL) **SE:** ↓ BP w/ initial dose (esp w/ diuretics), ↑ K+, ↑ Cr, nonproductive cough, angioedema **Interactions:** ↑ Effects *W/* loop diuretics; ↑ risk of cough *W/* capsaicin; ↑ effects *OF* α-blockers, insulin, Li; ↑ risk of hyperkalemia *W/* K⁺ supls, K⁺-sparing diuretics, salt substitutes, TMP; ↓ effects *W/* ASA, NSAIDs, rifampin **Labs:** May cause ↑ K⁺, ↑ Cr—monitor levels **NIPE:** Several wk needed for full hypotensive effect; D/C diuretic for 2–3 d prior to start; may cause dizziness—caution driving

Enfuvirtide (Fuzeon) [Antiretroviral/Fusion Inhibitor] **WARNING:** Rarely causes allergy; never rechallenge **Uses:** *w/ Antiretroviral agents for HIV-1 in Tx-experienced pts w/ viral replication despite ongoing Rx* **Action:** Viral fusion Inhib **Dose:** *Adults.* 90 mg (1 mL) SQ bid in upper arm, anterior thigh, or Abd; rotate site **Peds.** See package insert **Caution:** [B, –] **CI:** Previous allergy to drug **Disp:** 90 mg/mL recons; pt kit w/ supplies × 1 mo **SE:** Inj site Rxns; pneumonia, D, N, fatigue, insomnia, peripheral neuropathy **Interactions:** None noted *W/* other antiretrovirals **Labs:** ↑ LFTs, triglycerides; ↓ Hgb, Hct, eosinophils **NIPE:** Does not cure HIV; does not ↓ risk of transmission or prevent opportunistic Infxns; available via restricted distribution system; use stat on recons or refrigerate (24 h max); each vial is for single use only; teach SQ Inj technique

Enoxaparin (Lovenox) [Anticoagulant/Low-Molecular-Weight Heparin Derivative] **WARNING:** Recent or anticipated epidural/spinal anesthesia, ↑ risk of spinal/epidural hematoma w/ subsequent paralysis **Uses:** *Prevention & Rx of DVT; Rx PE; unstable angina & non-Q-wave MI* **Action:** LMW heparin; Inhib thrombin by complexing w/ antithrombin III **Dose:** *Adults. Prevention:* 30 mg SQ bid or 40 mg SQ q24h *DVT/PE Rx:* 1 mg/kg SQ q12h or 1.5 mg/kg SQ q24h *Angina:* 1 mg/kg SQ q12h *Ancillary to AMI fibrinolysis:* 30 mg IV bolus, then 1 mg/kg SQ bid; CrCl < 30 mL/min ↓ to 1 mg/kg SQ qd **Peds.** *Prevention:* 0.5 mg/kg SQ q12h *DVT/PE Rx:* 1 mg/kg SQ q12h; ↓ dose w/ CrCl < 30 mL/min **Caution:** [B, ?] Not for prophylaxis in prosthetic heart valves **CI:** Active bleeding, HIT Ab, heparin, pork sens **Disp:** Inj 10 mg/0.1 mL (30-, 40-, 60-, 80-, 100-, 120-, 150-mg syringes); 300-mg/mL multidose vial **SE:** Bleeding, hemorrhage, bruising, thrombocytopenia, fever, pain/hematoma at site, AST/ALT **Interactions:** ↑ Bleeding effects *W/* ASA, anticoagulants, cephalosporins,

NSAIDs, PCN, chamomile, garlic, ginger, ginkgo, feverfew, horse chestnut **Labs:** ↑ AST, ALT; no effect on bleeding time, plt Fxn, PT, or aPTT; monitor plt for HIT, clinical bleeding; may monitor antifactor Xa **NIPE:** Administer deep SQ; ⊘ IM; bleeding precautions

Entacapone (Comtan) [Antiparkinsonian Agent/COMT Inhibitor]
Uses: *Parkinson Dz* **Action:** Selective & reversible catechol-O-methyltransferase Inhib **Dose:** 200 mg w/ each levodopa/carbidopa dose; max 1600 mg/d; ↓ levodopa/carbidopa dose 25% w/ levodopa dose > 800 mg **Caution:** [C, ?] Hepatic impair **CI:** Use w/ MAOI **Disp:** Tabs 200 mg **SE:** Dyskinesia, hyperkinesia, N, D, dizziness, hallucinations, orthostatic ↓ BP **Interactions:** ↑ Effects *W/* ampicillin, chloramphenicol cholestyramine, erythromycin, MAOIs, probenecid, rifampin; ↑ risk of arrhythmias & HTN *W/* bitolterol, DA, dobutamine, epinephrine, isoetharine, methyldopa, norepinephrine **Labs:** Monitor LFTs **NIPE:** Take w/ or w/o food; ⊘ D/C abruptly, breast-feed; brownish-orange urine

Enzalutamide (Xtandi)
Uses: *Metastatic castration-resistant prostate cancer w/ previous docetaxel* **Action:** Androgen receptor inhibitor **Dose (men only):** 160 mg daily, do not chew/open caps **Caution:** [X, –] Sz risk **CI:** PRG **Disp:** Caps 40 mg **SE:** HA, dizziness, insomnia, fatigue, anxiety, MS pain, muscle weakness, paresthesia, back pain, spinal cord compression, cauda equina synd, arthralgias, edema, URI, lower resp Infxn, hematuria, ↑ BP **Notes:** Avoid w/ strong CYP2C8 Inhib, strong/mod CYP3A4 or CYP2C8 induc, avoid CPY3A4, CYP2C9, CYP2C19 substrates w/ narrow therapeutic index; if on warfarin check INR **NIPE:** Take w/ or w/o food; ⊘ crush, chew, split, swallow whole; use condom + 1 other form of birth control; ↑ risk Szs

Ephedrine [Vasopressor/Decongestant/Bronchodilator]
Uses: *Acute bronchospasm, bronchial asthma, nasal congestion*, ↓ BP, narcolepsy, enuresis, & MyG **Action:** Sympathomimetic; stimulates alpha- and beta-receptors; bronchodilator **Dose: Adults.** *Congestion:* 1 2.5–25 mg PO q4h PRN w/ expectorant; ↓ *BP:* 25–50 mg IV q5–10min, 150 mg/d max **Peds.** 0.2–0.3 mg/kg/dose IV q4–6h PRN **Caution:** [C, ?/–] **CI:** Arrhythmias, NAG **Disp:** Caps 25 mg; Inj 50 mg/mL; nasal spray 0.25% **SE:** CNS stimulation (nervousness, anxiety, trembling), tachycardia, arrhythmia, HTN, xerostomia, dysuria **Interactions:** ↑ Effects *W/* acetazolamide, antacids, MAOIs, TCAs, urinary alkalinizers; ↑ effects *OF* sympathomimetics; ↓ response *W/* diuretics, methyldopa, reserpine, urinary acidifiers; ↓ effects *OF* antihypertensives, BBs, dexamethasone, guanethidine **Labs:** False ↑ urine amino acids; can cause false(+) amphetamine EMIT **NIPE:** ⊘ EtOH; store away from light/heat; protect from light; monitor BP, HR, urinary output; take last dose 4–6 h before hs; abuse potential, OTC sales mostly banned/restricted; may cause dizziness—caution driving

Epinastine (Elestat) [Antihistamine/Mast Cell Stabilizer]
Uses: Itching w/ allergic conjunctivitis **Action:** Antihistamine **Dose:** 1 gtt bid **Caution:**

[C, ?/–] **Disp:** Soln 0.05% **SE:** Burning, folliculosis, hyperemia, pruritus, URI, HA, rhinitis, sinusitis, cough, pharyngitis **NIPE:** Remove contacts before, reinsert in 10 min

Epinephrine (Adrenalin, EpiPen, EpiPen Jr, Others) [Vasopressor/ Bronchodilator/Cardiac Stimulant, Local Anesthetic] Uses: *Cardiac arrest, anaphylactic Rxn, bronchospasm, open-angle glaucoma* **Action:** Beta-adrenergic agonist, some α effects **Dose: Adults. ECC 2010:** 1-mg (10 mL of 1:10,000 soln) IV/IO push, repeat q3–5min (0.2 mg/kg max) if 1 mg dose fails *Inf:* 0.1–0.5 mcg/kg/min, titrate. ET 2–2.5 mg in 5–10 mL NS *Profound bradycardia/ hypotension:* 2–10 mcg/min (1 mg in 250 mL D₅W) *Allergic Rxn:* 0.3–0.5 mg (0.3–0.5 mL of 1:1000 soln) SQ *Anaphylaxis:* 0.3–0.5 (3–5 mL of 1:1000 soln) IV *Asthma:* 0.1–0.5 mL SQ of 1:1000 dilution, repeat q20min to 4 h, or 1 Inh (metered-dose) repeat in 1–2 min, or susp 0.1–0.3 mL SQ for extended effect **Peds. ECC 2010:** *Pulseless arrest:* (0.1 mL/kg 1:1000) IV/IO q3–5 min; max dose 1 mg; OK via ET tube (0.1 mL/kg 1:1000) until IV/IO access *Symptomatic bradycardia:* 0.01 mg/ kg (0.1 mL/kg 1:1000) cont Inf: typical 0.1–1 mcg/kg/min, titrate. *Anaphylaxis/Status Asthmaticus:* 0.01 mg/kg (0.01 mL/kg 1:1000) IM, repeat PRN; max single dose 0.3 mg **Caution:** [C, ?] ↓ Bronchodilation w/ β-blockers **CI:** Cardiac arrhythmias, NAG **Disp:** Inj 1:1000; 1:2000; 1:10,000; nasal inhal 0.1%; oral inhal 2.25% soln; Epipen Autoinjector 1 dose = 0.30 mg; EpiPen Jr 1 dose = 0.15 mg **SE:** CV (tachycardia, HTN, vasoconstriction), CNS stimulation (nervousness, anxiety, trembling), ↓ renal blood flow **Interactions:** ↑ HTN effects *W/* α-blockers, BBs, ergot alkaloids, furazolidone, MAOIs; ↑ cardiac effects *W/* antihistamines, cardiac glycosides, levodopa, HTN, thyroid hormones, TCAs; ↑ effects *OF* sympathomimetics; ↓ effects *OF* diuretics, guanethidine, hypoglycemics, methyldopa **Labs:** ↑ BUN, glucose, & lactic acid w/ prolonged use **NIPE:** ⊘ OTC Inh drugs; can give via ET tube if no central line (use 2–2.5 × IV dose); EpiPen for pt self-use (www.EpiPen .com)

Epirubicin (Ellence) [Antineoplastic/Anthracycline] WARNING: Do not give IM or SQ. Extrav causes tissue necrosis; potential cardiotox; severe myelosuppression; ↓ dose w/ hepatic impair Uses: *Adjuvant therapy for + axillary nodes after resection of primary breast CA* *secondary AML* **Actions:** Anthracycline cytotoxic agent **Dose:** Per protocols; ↓ dose w/ hepatic impair **Caution:** [D, –] **CI:** Baseline neutrophil count < 1500 cells/mm³, severe cardiac Insuff, recent MI, severe arrhythmias, severe hepatic dysfunction, previous anthracyclines Rx to max cumulative dose **Disp:** Inj 50 mg/25 mL, 200 mg/100 mL **SE:** Mucositis, N/V/D, alopecia, ↓ BM, cardiotox, secondary AML, tissue necrosis w/ extrav (see Adriamycin for Rx), lethargy **Interactions:** ↑ Effects *W/* cimetidine; ↑ effects *OF* cytotoxic drugs, radiation therapy; ↑ risk of HF w/ CCBs, trastuzumab; incompatible chemically *W/* 5-FU, heparin **Labs:** ✓ CBC, bilirubin, AST, Cr, cardiac Fxn before/during each cycle; ↓ Hgb, Hct, neutrophils, plts, WBC **NIPE:** ⊘ Handle if PRG breast-feeding; urine reddish up to 2 d after Tx, use

contraception during Tx, burning at Inj site indicates infiltration; menstruation may cease permanently; ↑ risk Infxn

Eplerenone (Inspra) [Antihypertensive/Selective Aldosterone Receptor Antagonist] **Uses:** HTN, survival after MI w/ LVEF < 40% and CHF **Action:** Selective aldosterone antagonist **Dose:** *Adults.* 50 mg PO daily–bid, doses > 100 mg/d no benefit w/ ↑ K+; ↓ to 25 mg PO daily if giving w/ CYP3A4 Inhibs **Caution:** [B, +/–] w/ CYP3A4 Inhibs (Table 10); monitor K+ w/ ACE Inhib, ARBs, NSAIDs, K+-sparing diuretics; grapefruit juice, St. John's Wort. **CI:** K+ > 5.5 mEq/L; non-insulin-dependent diabetes mellitus (NIDDM) w/ microalbuminuria; SCr > 2 mg/dL (males), > 1.8 mg/dL (females); CrCl < 30 mL/min; w/ K+ supls/K+-sparing diuretics, ketoconazole **Disp:** Tabs 25, 50 mg **SE:** cholesterol/triglycerides, K+, HA, dizziness, gynecomastia, D, orthostatic ↓ BP **Interactions:** ↑ Risk hyperkalemia **W/** ACEIs; ↑ risk of toxic effects **W/** azole antifungals, erythromycin, saquinavir, verapamil, ↑ effects **OF** Li; ↓ effects **W/** NSAIDs **Labs:** ↑ K+, cholesterol, triglycerides; monitor K+ w/ ACE Inhib, ARBs, NSAIDs, K+-sparing diuretics; grapefruit juice, St. John's wort **NIPE:** ⊘ High-K+ foods; ⊘ K+ or salt substitutes; may cause reversible breast pain or enlargement w/ use; may take 4 wk for full effect; may cause dizziness—caution driving; ✓ BP reg

Epoetin Alfa [Erythropoietin, EPO] (Epogen, Procrit) [Recombinant Human Erythropoietin] **WARNING:** ↑ Mortality, serious CV/thromboembolic events, and tumor progression. Renal failure pts experienced greater risks (death/CV events) on erythropoiesis-stimulating agents (ESAs) to target higher Hgb levels 11 g/dL; maint Hgb 10–12 g/dL. In CA pt, ESAs ↓ survival/time to progression in some CAs when dosed Hgb ≥ 12 g/dL. Use lowest dose needed. Use only for myelosuppressive chemotherapy. D/C following chemotherapy. Pre-op ESA ↑ DVT. Consider DVT prophylaxis **Uses:** *CRF-associated anemia, zidovudine Rx in HIV-infected pts, CA chemotherapy; ↓ transfusions associated w/ surgery* **Action:** Induces erythropoiesis **Dose:** *Adults & Peds.* 50–150 units/kg IV/SQ 3 ×/wk; adjust dose q4–6wk PRN *Surgery:* 300 units/kg/d × 10 d before to 4 d after; ↓ dose if Hct ~ 36% or Hgb, ↑ > ≅12 g/dL or Hgb ↑ > 1 g/dL in 2-wk period; hold dose if Hgb > 12 g/dL **Caution:** [C, ?/–] **CI:** Uncontrolled HTN **Disp:** Inj 2000, 3000, 4000, 10,000, 20,000, 40,000 units/mL **SE:** HTN, HA, fatigue, fever, tachycardia, N/V **Interactions:** None noted **Labs:** ↑ WBCs, plts; monitor baseline & post-Tx Hct/ Hgb, ferritin **NIPE:** Monitor for access line clotting; ⊘ shake vial; refrigerate; monitor post-Tx BP, lytes, Hgb

Epoprostenol (Flolan, Veletri) [Antihypertensive] **Uses:** *Pulm HTN** **Action:** Dilates pulm/systemic arterial vascular beds; ↓ plt aggregation **Dose:** Initial 2 ng/kg/min; ↑ by 2 ng/kg/min q15min until dose-limiting SE (CP, dizziness, N/V, HA, ↓ BP, flushing); IV cont Inf 4 ng/kg/min < max tolerated rate; adjust based on response; see PI **Caution:** [B, ?] ↑ tox w/ diuretics, vasodilators, acetate in dialysis fluids, anticoagulants **CI:** Chronic use in CHF 2nd degree, if pt develops pulm edema w/ dose initiation, severe LVSD **Disp:** Inj 0.5, 1.5 mg **SE:** Flushing, tachycardia, CHF, fever, chills, nervousness, HA, N/V/D, jaw pain, flu-like Sxs **Interactions:** ↑ Risk of bleeding w/ anticoagulants, antiplts; ↑ effects *OF* digoxin; ↓ BP *W/* antihypertensives, diuretics, vasodilators **NIPE:** First dose administered in medical setting; ⊘ Mix or administer w/ other drugs; abrupt D/C can cause rebound pulm HTN; monitor bleeding w/ other antiplt/anticoagulants; watch ↓ BP *W/* other vasodilators/diuretics

Eprosartan (Teveten) [Antihypertensive/ARB] Uses: *HTN*, DN, CHF **Action:** ARB **Dose:** 400–800 mg/d single dose or bid **Caution:** [C (1st tri), D (2nd & 3rd tri), D/C immediately when PRG detected] w/ Li, ↑ K⁺ w/ K⁺-sparing diuretics/supls/high-dose trimethoprim **CI:** Bilateral RAS, 1st-degree aldosteronism **Disp:** Tabs 400, 600 mg **SE:** Fatigue, depression, URI, UTI, Abd pain, rhinitis/pharyngitis/cough, hypertriglyceridemia **Interactions:** ↑ Risk of hyperkalemia *W/* K⁺-sparing diuretics, K⁺ supls, TMP; ↑ effects *OF* Li **Labs:** ↑ BUN, triglycerides; ↓ Hgb, Hct, neutrophils **NIPE:** Monitor CBC & differential, renal Fxn; ⊘ PRG, breast-feeding; may cause dizziness; caution driving

Eptifibatide (Integrilin) [Antiplatelet Agent] Uses: *ACS, PCI* **Action:** Glycoprotein IIb/IIIa Inhib **Dose:** 180 mcg/kg IV bolus, then 2 mcg/kg/min cont Inf; ↓ in renal impair (CrCl < 50 mL/min: 180 mcg/kg, then 1 mcg/kg/min) *ECC 2010:* ACS: 180 mcg/kg/min IV bolus over 1–2 min, then 2 mcg/kg/min, then repeat bolus in 10 min; continue Inf 18–24 h post PCI **Caution:** [B, ?] Monitor bleeding w/ other anticoagulants **CI:** Other glycoprotein IIb/IIIa Inhibs, Hx abnormal bleeding, hemorrhagic stroke (w/in 30 d), severe HTN, major surgery (w/in 6 wk), plt count < 100,000 cells/mm³, renal dialysis **Disp:** Inj 0.75, 2 mg/mL **SE:** Bleeding, ↓ BP, Inj site Rxn, thrombocytopenia **Interactions:** ↑ Bleeding *W/* ASA, cephalosporins, clopidogrel, heparin, NSAIDs, thrombolytics, ticlopidine, warfarin, evening primrose oil, feverfew, garlic, ginger, ginkgo, ginseng **Labs:** ↓ Plts; monitor bleeding, coagulants, plts, SCr, ACT w/ prothrombin consumption index (keep ACT 200–300 s) **NIPE:** Bleeding precautions

Eribulin (Halaven) [Non-Taxane Microtubule Dynamics Inhibitor] Uses: *Met breast CA after 2 chemo regimens (including anthracycline & taxane)* **Action:** Microtubule Inhib **Dose:** *Adults.* 1.4 mg/m² IV (over 2–5 min) days 1 & 8 of 21-d cycle; ↓ dose w/ hepatic & mod renal impair; delay/↓ for tox (see label) **Caution:** [D, –] **CI:** None **Disp:** Inj 0.5 mg/mL **SE:** ↓ WBC/ Hct/plt, fatigue/asthenia, neuropathy, N/V/D, constipation, pyrexia, alopecia, ↑ QT, arthralgia/myalgia, back pain, cough, dyspnea, UTI **Labs:** ↓ WBC/Hct/plt; ✓ CBC & monitor **NIPE:** Monitor for neuropathy & neutopenia prior to dosing; ↑ risk Infxn

Erlotinib (Tarceva) [Antineoplastic] Uses: *NSCLC after failing 1 chemotherapy; maint NSCLC who have not progressed after 4 cycles cisplatin-based therapy; CA pancreas* **Action:** HER2/EGFR TKI **Dose:** *CA pancreas:* 100 mg, *others:* 150 mg/d PO 1 h ac or 2 h pc; ↓ (in 50-mg decrements) w/ severe Rxn or w/ CYP3A4 Inhibs (Table 10); per protocols **Caution:** [D, ?/–]; Avoid PRG;

w/ CYP3A4 (Table 10) Inhibs **Disp:** Tabs 25, 100, 150 mg **SE:** Rash, N/V/D, anorexia, Abd pain, fatigue, cough, dyspnea, edema, stomatitis, conjunctivitis, pruritus, skin/nail changes, Infxn, LFTs, interstitial lung Dz **Interactions:** ↓ Drug plasma levels *W/* CYP3A4 Inhibs (clarithromycin, ritonavir, ketoconazole); ↓ drug plasma levels *W/* CYP3A4 inducers (carbamazepine, phenytoin, phenobarbital, St. John's wort); ↑ risk of bleeding *W/* anticoagulants, NSAIDs **Labs:** ↑ LFTs; monitor LFTs, PT, INR; may ↑ INR w/ warfarin **NIPE:** Take on empty stomach; ⊘ PRG or lactation; use adequate contraception; ↑ drug metabolism in smokers; separate antacids by several hours; diarrhea common SE—↑ fluids

Ertapenem (Invanz) [Anti-Infective/Carbapenem] Uses: *Complicated intra-Abd, acute pelvic, & skin Infxns, pyelonephritis, CAP* **Action:** α–carbapenem; β-lactam antibiotic, ↓ cell wall synth *Spectrum:* Good gram(+/–) & anaerobic coverage, not *Pseudomonas*, PCN-resistant pneumococci, MRSA, Enterococcus, β-lactamase (+) *H influenzae, Mycoplasma, Chlamydia* **Dose: Adults.** 1 g IM/IV daily; 500 mg/d in CrCl < 30 mL/min *Peds 3 mo–12 y.* 15 mg/kg bid IM/IV, max 1 g/d **Caution:** [B, ?/–] Sz Hx, CNS disorders, β-lactam & multiple allergies, probenecid ↓ renal clearance **CI:** Component hypersens or amide anesthetics **Disp:** Inj 1 g/vial **SE:** HA, N/V/D, Inj site Rxns, thrombocytosis, LFTs **Notes:** Can give IM × 7 d, IV × 14 d; 137 mg Na$^+$ (6 mEq)/g ertapenem **Interactions:** ↑ Effects *W/* probenecid **Labs:** ↑ LFTs, glucose, K$^+$, Cr, PT, PTT, RBCs, urine WBCs **NIPE:** Monitor for super Infxn

Erythromycin (E-Mycin, E.E.S., Ery-Tab, EryPed, Ilotycin) [Antibiotic/Macrolide] Uses: *Bacterial Infxns; bowel prep*; ↑ GI motility (prokinetic); *acne vulgaris* **Action:** Bacteriostatic; interferes w/ protein synth *Spectrum:* Group A streptococci (*S pyogenes*), *S pneumoniae, N gonorrhoeae* (if PCN-allergic), *Legionella, M pneumoniae* **Dose: Adults.** Base 250–500 mg PO q6–12h or ethylsuccinate 400–800 mg q6–12h; 500 mg–1 g IV q6h *Prokinetic:* 250 mg PO tid 30 min ac **Peds.** 30–50 mg/kg/d PO ÷ q6–8h or 20–40 mg/kg/d IV ÷ q6h, max 2 g/d **Caution:** [B, +] Pseudomembranous colitis risk, ↑ tox of carbamazepine, cyclosporine, digoxin, methylprednisolone, felodipine, theophylline, warfarin, simvastatin/lovastatin; ↓ sildenafil dose w/ use **CI:** Hepatic impair, preexisting liver Dz (estolate), use w/ pimozide ergotamine dihydroergotamine **Disp:** *Lactobionate (Ilotycin):* Powder for Inj 500 mg, 1 g *Base:* Tabs 250, 333, 500 mg; caps 250 mg *Stearate (Erythrocin):* Tabs 250, 500 mg *Ethylsuccinate (EES, EryPed):* Chew tabs 200 mg; tabs 400 mg; susp 200, 400 mg/5 mL **SE:** HA, Abd pain, N/V/D; QT, torsades de pointes, ventricular arrhythmias/tachycardias (rarely)]; cholestatic jaundice (estolate) **Notes:** 400 mg ethylsuccinate = 250 mg base/estolate **Interactions:** ↑ Effects *W/* amprenavir, indinavir, ritonavir, saquinavir, grapefruit juice; ↑ effects *OF* alprazolam, benzodiazepines, buspirone, carbamazepine, clozapine, colchicines, cyclosporine, digoxin, felodipine, lovastatin, midazolam, quinidine, sildenafil, simvastatin, tacrolimus, theophylline, triazolam, valproic acid; ↑

QT *W/* astemizole, cisapride; ↓ effects *OF* PCN, zafirlukast **Labs:** ↑ LFTs, eosinophils, neutrophils, plts; ↓ bicarbonate levels **NIPE:** Take w/ food to ↓ GI upset, monitor for super Infxn & ototox; lactobionate contains benzyl alcohol (caution in neonates)

Erythromycin, Ophthalmic (Ilotycin Ophthalmic) [Anti-Infective, Macrolide, Opthalmic Agent] Uses: *Conjunctival/corneal Infxns* **Action:** Macrolide antibiotic **Dose:** 1/2 in 2–6 × /d **Caution:** [B, +] **CI:** Erythromycin hypersensitivity **Disp:** 0.5% oint **SE:** Local irritation **NIPE:** May cause burning, stinging, blurred vision; teach use of eye ointment; ⊘ contact lenses for ≥ 15 min after application

Erythromycin, Topical (A/T/S, Eryderm, Erycette, T-Stat) [Topical Anti-Infective, Macrolide] Uses: *Acne vulgaris* **Action:** Macrolide antibiotic **Dose:** Wash & dry area, apply 2% product over area bid **Caution:** [B, +] Pseudomembranous colitis possible **CI:** Component sensitivity **Disp:** Soln 1.5%, 2%; gel 2%; pads & swabs 2% **SE:** Local irritation **NIPE:** Apply w/o rubbing; may take up to 12 wk to see ↓ Sx

Erythromycin & Benzoyl Peroxide (Benzamycin) [Anti-Infective, Macrolide/Keratolytic] Uses: *Topical for acne vulgaris* **Action:** Macrolide antibiotic w/ keratolytic **Dose:** Apply bid (AM & PM) **Caution:** [C, ?] **CI:** Component sensitivity **Disp:** Gel erythromycin 30 mg/benzoyl peroxide 50 mg/g **SE:** Local irritation, dryness **Interactions:** ↑ Irritation *W/* other topical agents; ↑ transient skin discoloration *W/* PABA sunscreen **NIPE:** May cause super Infxn; D/C if irritation or dryness occurs; may bleach hair or fabrics

Erythromycin & Sulfisoxazole (E.S.P.) [Anti-Infective, Macrolide/Sulfonamide] Uses: *Upper & lower resp tract; bacterial Infxns; H influenzae otitis media in children* Infxns in PCN-allergic pts **Action:** Macrolide antibiotic w/ sulfonamide **Dose:** *Adults.* Based on erythromycin content; 400 mg erythromycin/1200 mg sulfisoxazole PO q6h *Peds > 2 mo.* 40–50 mg/ kg/d erythromycin & 150 mg/kg/d sulfisoxazole PO ÷ q6h; max 2 g/d erythromycin or 6 g/d sulfisoxazole × 10 d; ↓ in renal impair **Caution:** [C (D if near term), +] w/ PO anticoagulants, hypoglycemics, phenytoin, cyclosporine **CI:** Infants < 2 mo **Disp:** Susp erythromycin ethylsuccinate 200 mg/sulfisoxazole 600 mg/5 mL (100, 150, 200 mL) **SE:** GI upset **Interactions:** ↑ Effects of sulfonamides *W/* ASA, diuretics, NSAIDs, probenecid **Labs:** False(+) urine protein **NIPE:** ↑ Risk of photosensitivity—use sunblock, ↑ fluid intake

Escitalopram (Lexapro) [Antidepressant/SSRI] **WARNING:** Closely monitor for worsening depression or emergence of suicidality, particularly in ped pts Uses: *Depression, anxiety* **Action:** SSRI **Dose:** *Adults.* 10–20 mg PO daily; 10 mg/d in elderly & hepatic impair **Caution:** [C, +/−] Serotonin synd (Table 11); use w/ escitalopram, NSAID, ASA, or other drugs affecting coagulation associated w/ ↑ bleeding risk **CI:** w/in 14 d of MAOI **Disp:** Tabs 5, 10, 20 mg; soln 1 mg/mL

SE: N/V/D, sweating, insomnia, dizziness, xerostomia, sexual dysfunction **Interactions:** ↑ Risk of serotonin synd *W/* linezolid; ↑ risk of bleeding *W/* anticoagulants, ASA, NSAIDs; may ↑ CNS effects *W/* CNS depressants **NIPE:** ⊘ D/C abruptly; full effects may take 3 wk; take w/o regard to food; may cause ↑ appetite & wgt gain; do not take tryptophan

Eslicarbazepine (Aptiom)   **Uses:** *Partial-onset Sz* **Action:** Inhib voltage-gated Na⁺ channels **Dose:** 400 mg PO daily × 1/wk, then 800 mg PO daily; max 1200 mg/d; CrCl < 50 mL/min: 200 mg PO daily × 2 wk, then 400 mg PO daily, max 600 mg/d **Caution:** [C, –] suicidal behavior/ideation; TEN; SJS; DRESS; ↓ Na⁺; anaphylactic Rxn/angioedema; hepatotox **CI:** Hypersens to eslicarbazepine, oxcarbazepine **Disp:** Tabs 200, 400, 600, 800 mg **SE:** See W/P, N/V, dizziness, somnolence, HA, diplopia, fatigue, vertigo, ataxia, blurred vision, tremor, abnormal TFTs **NIPE:** Take w/ or w/o food; swallow whole; report changes in mood; use birth control; w/ PRG enroll in the North American Antiepileptic Drug Pregnancy Registry (1-888-233-2334 or http://www.aedpregnancyregistry.org/); w/ D/C withdrawal gradually

Esmolol (Brevibloc) [Antiarrhythmic/Beta-Blocker]   **Uses:** *SVT & noncompensatory sinus tachycardia, AF/A flutter* **Action:** β₁-Adrenergic blocker; Class II antiarrhythmic **Dose:** *Adults & Peds. ECC 2010:* 0.5 mg/kg (500 mcg/kg) over 1 min, then 0.05 mg/kg/min (50 mcg/kg/min) Inf; if inadequate response after 5 min, repeat 0.5 mg/kg bolus then titrate Inf up to 0.2 mg/kg/min (200 mcg/kg/min); max 0.3 mg/kg/min (300 mcg/kg/min) **Caution:** [C (1st tri), D (2nd or 3rd tri), ?] **CI:** Sinus bradycardia, heart block, uncompensated CHF, cardiogenic shock, ↓ BP **Disp:** Inj 10, 20, 250 mg/mL; premix Inf 10 mg/mL **SE:** ↓ BP; ↓ HR, diaphoresis, dizziness, pain on Inj **Interaction:** ↑ Effects *W/* verapamil; ↑ effects *OF* digoxin, antihypertensives, nitrates; ↑ HTN *W/* amphetamines, cocaine, ephedrine, epinephrine, MAOIs, norepinephrine, phenylephrine, pseudoephedrine; ↓ effects *OF* glucagons, insulin, hypoglycemics, theophylline; ↓ effects *W/* NSAIDs, thyroid hormones **Labs:** ↑ Glucose, cholesterol **NIPE:** Monitor BS of pts w/ DM; pain on Inj; hemodynamic effects back to baseline w/in 30 min after D/C Inf

Esomeprazole (Nexium) [Gastric Acid Inhibitor/Proton Pump Inhibitor]   **Uses:** *Short-term (4–8 wk) for erosive esophagitis/GERD; H pylori Infxn in combo w/ antibiotics* **Action:** PPI, ↓ gastric acid **Dose:** *Adults. GERD/ erosive gastritis:* 20–40 mg/d PO × 4–8 wk; 20–40 mg IV 10–30 min Inf or > 3 min IV push, 10 d max *Maint:* 20 mg/d PO. *H pylori Infxn:* 40 mg PO, plus clarithromycin 500 mg PO bid & amoxicillin 1000 mg/bid for 10 d **Caution:** [B, ?/–] **CI:** Component sensitivity; do not use w/ clopidogrel (↓ effect) **Disp:** Caps 20, 40 mg; IV 20, 40 mg **SE:** HA, D, Abd pain **Interactions:** ↑ Effects *W/* amoxicillin, clarithromycin; ↑ effects *OF* benzodiazepines, saquinavir, warfarin; ↓ effects *OF* digoxin, ketoconazole, Fe salts; may affect drugs metabolized by CYP2C19 **Labs:** ↑ SCr, uric acid, LFTs, Hgb, WBCs, plts, K⁺, thyroxine levels;

risk of hypomagnesemia w/ long-term use, monitor **NIPE:** Take drug 1 h before food; ⊘ EtOH; do not chew; may open caps & sprinkle on applesauce—do not chew; see pkg insert for NGT admin; ↑ risk of fxs w/ all PPIs; may give antacids concomitantly

Estazolam (ProSom) [Hypnotic/Benzodiazepine] [C-IV] Uses: *Short-term management of insomnia* **Action:** Benzodiazepine **Dose:** 1–2 mg PO qhs PRN; ↓ in hepatic impair/elderly/debilitated **Caution:** [X, –] ↑ Effects w/ CNS depressants; cross-sensitivity w/ other benzodiazepines **CI:** PRG, component hypersensitivity, w/ itraconazole or ketoconazole **Disp:** Tabs 1, 2 mg **SE:** Somnolence, weakness, palpitations, anaphylaxis, angioedema, amnesia **Interactions:** ↑ Effects *W/* amoxicillin, clarithromycin; ↑ effects *OF* diazepam, phenytoin, warfarin; ↓ effects *W/* food; ↓ effects *OF* azole antifungals, digoxin **Labs:** ↑ LFTs **NIPE:** Take at least 1 h ac; take only when ready for several h sleep; may cause psychological/physical dependence; avoid abrupt D/C after prolonged use

Esterified Estrogens (Menest) [Estrogen Supplement] **WARNING:** ↑ Risk endometrial CA. Do not use to prevent CV Dz or dementia; ↑ risk of MI, stroke, breast CA, PE, & DVT. in postmenopausal Uses: *Vasomotor Sxs or vulvar/Vag atrophy w/ menopause*; female hypogonadism, PCa* **Action:** Estrogen supls **Dose:** *Menopausal vasomotor Sx:* 0.3–1.25 mg/d, cyclically 3 wk on, 1 wk off; add progestin 10–14 d w/ 28-d cycle w/ uterus intact *Vulvovaginal atrophy:* Same regimen except use 0.3–1.25 mg *Hypogonadism:* 2.5–7.5 mg/d PO × 20 d, off × 10 d; add progestin 10–14 d w/ 28-d cycle w/ uterus intact **Caution:** [X, –] **CI:** Undiagnosed genital bleeding, breast CA, estrogen-dependent tumors, thromboembolic disorders, thrombophlebitis, recent MI, PRG, severe hepatic Dz **Disp:** Tabs 0.3, 0.625, 1.25, 2.5 mg **SE:** N, HA, bloating, breast enlargement/tenderness, edema, venous thromboembolism, hypertriglyceridemia, gallbladder Dz **Interactions:** ↑ Effects *OF* corticosteroids, cyclosporine, TCAs, theophylline, caffeine, tobacco; ↓ effects *W/* barbiturates, phenytoin, rifampin; ↓ effects *OF* anticoagulants, hypoglycemics, insulin, tamoxifen **Labs:** ↑ Prothrombin & factors VII, VIII, IX, X, plt aggregation, thyroid-binding globulin, T₄, triglycerides; ↓ antithrombin III, folate **NIPE:** ⊘ PRG, breast-feeding; use lowest dose for shortest time (see WHI data [www.whi.org])

Estradiol, Gel (Divigel) [Estrogen Supplement] **WARNING:** ↑ Risk endometrial CA. Do not use to prevent CV Dz or dementia; ↑ risk MI, stroke, breast CA, PE, & DVT in postmenopausal (50–79 y). ↑ Dementia risk in postmenopausal (≥ 65 y) Uses: *Vasomotor Sx in menopause* **Action:** Estrogen **Dose:** 0.25 g qd on right or left upper thigh (alternate) **Caution:** [X, +/–] May ↑ thyroid binding globulin (TBD) w/ thyroid Dz **CI:** Undiagnosed genital bleeding, breast CA, estrogen-dependent tumors, thromboembolic disorders, thrombophlebitis, recent MI, PRG, severe hepatic Dz **Disp:** 0.1% gel 0.25/0.5/1 g single-dose foil packets w/ 0.25-, 0.5-, 1-mg estradiol, respectively **SE:** N, HA, bloating, breast enlargement/tenderness, edema, venous thromboembolism, ↑ BP, hypertriglyceridemia, gallbladder Dz

NIPE: If person other than pt applies, glove should be used, keep dry stat after, rotate site; contains alcohol, caution around flames until dry, not for Vag use

Estradiol, Gel (Elestrin) [Estrogen Supplement] WARNING: ↑ Risk endometrial CA. Do not use to prevent CV Dz or dementia; ↑ risk MI, stroke, breast CA, PE, & DVT in postmenopausal (50–79 y) women. ↑ Dementia risk in postmenopausal (≥ 65 y) **Uses:** *Postmenopausal vasomotor Sxs* **Action:** Estrogen **Dose:** Apply 0.87–1.7 g to skin qd; add progestin × 10–14 d/28-d cycle w/ intact uterus; use lowest effective estrogen dose **Caution:** [X, ?] **CI:** AUB, breast CA, estrogen-dependent tumors, hereditary angioedema, thromboembolic disorders, recent MI, PRG, severe hepatic Dz **Disp:** Gel 0.06%; metered dose/activation **SE:** Thromboembolic events, MI, stroke, ↑ BP, breast/ovarian/endometrial CA, site Rxns, Vag spotting, breast changes, Abd bloating, cramps, HA, fluid retention **NIPE:** Apply to upper arm, wait > 25 min before sunscreen; avoid concomitant use for > 7 d; ✓ BP, breast exams

Estradiol, Oral (Estrace, Delestrogen, Femtrace) [Estrogen Supplement] WARNING: ↑ Risk of endometrial CA; do not use to prevent CV Dz or dementia; ↑ risk MI, stroke, breast CA, PE, and DVT in postmenopausal (50–79 y). ↑ Demential risk in postmenopausal (× 65 y) **Uses:** *Atrophic vaginitis, menopausal vasomotor Sxs, prevent osteoporosis, ↑ low estrogen levels, palliation breast & PCa** **Action:** Estrogen **Dose:** *PO:* 1–2 mg/d, adjust PRN to control Sxs *Vag cream:* 2–4 g/d × 2 wk, then 1 g 1–3×/wk *Vasomotor Sx/Vag atrophy:* 10–20 mg IM q4wk, D/C or taper at 3- to 6-mo intervals *Hypoestrogenism:* 10–20 mg IM q4wk *PCa:* 30 mg IM q12wk **Caution:** [X, –] **CI:** Genital bleeding of unknown cause, breast CA, porphyria, estrogen-dependent tumors, thromboembolic disorders, thrombophlebitis; recent MI; hepatic impair **Disp:** Tabs 0.5, 1, 2 mg; Vag cream 0.1 mg/g, depot Inj (Delestrogen) 10, 20, 40 mg/mL **SE:** N, HA, bloating, breast enlargement/tenderness, edema, ↑ triglycerides, venous thromboembolism, gallbladder Dz **Interactions:** ↑ Effects *W/* grapefruit juice; ↑ effects *OF* corticosteroids, cyclosporine, TCAs, theophylline, caffeine, tobacco; ↓ effects *W/* barbiturates, carbamazepine, phenytoin, primidone, rifampin; ↓ effects *OF* clofibrate, hypoglycemics, insulin, tamoxifen, warfarin **Labs:** ↑ Prothrombin & factors VII, VIII, IX, X, plt aggregation, thyroid-binding globulin, T_4, triglycerides; ↓ antithrombin III, folate **NIPE:** ⊘ PRG, breast-feeding

Estradiol, Spray (Evamist) [Estrogen Supplement] WARNING: ↑ Risk of endometrial CA. Do not use to prevent CV Dz or dementia; ↑ risk MI, stroke, breast CA, PE, & DVT in postmenopausal (50–79 y). ↑ Dementia risk in postmenopausal (× 65 y) **Uses:** *Vasomotor Sx in menopause** **Action:** Estrogen supl **Dose:** 1 spray on inner surface of forearm **Caution:** [X, +/–] May ↑ PT/PTT/plt aggregation w/ thyroid Dz **CI:** Undiagnosed genital bleeding, breast CA, estrogen-dependent tumors, thromboembolic disorders, thrombophlebitis, recent MI, PRG, severe hepatic Dz **Disp:** 1.53 mg/spray (56-spray container) **SE:** N, HA, bloating, breast enlargement/tenderness, edema, venous thromboembolism, ↑ BP, hypertriglyceridemia, gallbladder Dz **NIPE:** Contains alcohol, caution around flames until dry; not for Vag use; let dry before washing

Estradiol, Transdermal (Alora, Climara, Estraderm, Vivelle Dot) [Estrogen Supplement] **WARNING:** ↑ Risk of endometrial CA. Do not use to prevent CV Dz or dementia; ↑ risk MI, stroke, breast CA, PE, & DVT in postmenopausal (50–79 y). ↑ Dementia risk in postmenopausal (≥ 65 y) **Uses:** *Severe menopausal vasomotor Sxs; female hypogonadism* **Action:** Estrogen supls **Dose:** Start 0.0375–0.05 mg/d patch 2 × /wk based on product (Climara 1×/wk; Alora 2×/wk; adjust PRN to control Sxs; w/ intact uterus cycle 3 wk on 1 wk off or use cyclic progestin 10–14 d **Caution:** [X, –] See Estradiol **CI:** PRG, AUB, porphyria, breast CA, estrogen-dependent tumors, Hx thrombophlebitis, thrombosis **Disp:** Transdermal patches (mg/24 h) 0.025, 0.0375, 0.05, 0.06, 0.075, 0.1 **SE:** N, bloating, breast enlargement/tenderness, edema, HA, hypertriglyceridemia, gallbladder Dz; **NIPE:** Do not apply to breasts, place on trunk, rotate sites

Estradiol, Vaginal (Estring, Femring, Vagifem) [Estrogen Supplement] **WARNING:** ↑ Risk of endometrial CA. Do not use to prevent CV Dz or dementia; ↑ risk MI, stroke, breast CA, PE, and DVT in postmenopausal (50–79 y). Dementia risk in postmenopausal (× 65 y) **Uses:** *Postmenopausal Vag atrophy (Estring)* *vasomotor Sxs and vulvar/Vag atrophy associated w/ menopause (Femring)* *Atrophic vaginitis (Vagifem)* **Action:** Estrogen supl **Dose:** Estring: Insert ring into upper third of Vag vault; remove and replace after 90 d; reassess 3–6 mo; Femring: Use lowest effective dose, insert vaginally, replace q3mo; Vagifem: 1 tab vaginally qd × 2 wk, then maint 1 tab 2 × /wk, D/C or taper at 3–6 mo **Caution:** [X, –] May ↑ PT/PTT/plt aggregation w/ thyroid Dz, toxic shock reported **CI:** Undiagnosed genital bleeding, breast CA, estrogen-dependent tumors, thromboembolic disorders, thrombophlebitis, recent MI, PRG, severe hepatic Dz **Disp:** Estring ring: 0.0075 mg/24 h; Femring ring: 0.05 and 0.1 mg/d Vagifem tab (Vag): 10 mcg **SE:** HA, leukorrhea, back pain, candidiasis, vaginitis, Vag discomfort/hemorrhage, arthralgia, insomnia, Abd pain; see estradiol, oral notes **Labs:** May ↑ PT/PTT/plt aggregation w/ thyroid Dz **NIPE:** Remove during Vag Infxn Tx & during Tx w/ other vaginally administered preps; if ring falls out, rinse with warm water and re-insert

Estradiol/Levonorgestrel Transdermal (Climara Pro) [Estrogen & Progesterone Supplement] **WARNING:** ↑ Risk of endometrial CA. Do not use to prevent CV Dz or dementia; ↑ risk MI, stroke, breast CA, PE, & DVT in postmenopausal (50–79 y). ↑ Dementia risk in postmenopausal (≥ 65 y) **Uses:** *Menopausal vasomotor Sx; postmenopausal osteoporosis* **Action:** Estrogen & progesterone **Dose:** 1 patch 1 × /wk **Caution:** [X, –] w/ ↓ thyroid **CI:** AUB, estrogen-sensitive tumors, Hx thromboembolism, liver impair, PRG, hysterectomy **Disp:** Estradiol 0.045 mg/levonorgestrel 0.015/mg d patch **SE:** Site Rxn, Vag bleed/spotting, breast changes, Abd bloating/cramps, HA, retention fluid, edema, ↑

BP **NIPE:** Apply lower Abd; for osteoporosis give Ca²⁺/vit D supls; follow breast exams; intolerance to contact lenses; D/C use at least 2 wk before surgery

Estradiol/Norethindrone Acetate (Activella, Generic) [Estrogen & Progesterone Supplement] WARNING: ↑ Risk of endometrial CA.

Do not use to prevent CV Dz or dementia; ↑ risk MI, stroke, breast CA, PE, & DVT in postmenopausal (50–79 y). ↑ Dementia risk in postmenopausal (≥ 65 y) **Uses:** *Menopause vasomotor Sxs; prevent osteoporosis* **Action:** Estrogen/progestin; plant derived **Dose:** 1 tab/d start w/ lowest dose combo **Caution:** [X, –] w/ ↓ Ca²⁺/thyroid **CI:** PRG; Hx breast CA; estrogen-dependent tumor; abnormal genital bleeding; Hx DVT, PE, or related disorders; recent (w/in past year) arterial thromboembolic Dz (CVA, MI) **Disp:** *Femhrt* tabs (mcg/mg) 2.5/0.5, 5 mg/1 mg; *Activella* tabs (mg/mg) 1/0.5, 0.5 mg/0.1 mg. **SE:** Thrombosis, dizziness, HA, libido changes, insomnia, emotional instability, breast pain **Interactions:** ↑ Effects W/ vit C, APAP, atorvastatin; ↓ effects W/ rifampin, troglitazone, anticonvulsants; ↓ effects OF temazepam, morphine, clofibrate; monitor use of theophylline, cyclosporine **Labs:** Monitor serum lipids **NIPE:** Use in women w/ intact uterus; caution in heavy smokers; intolerance to contact lenses; D/C 2 wk before surgery

Estramustine Phosphate (Emcyt) [Antimicrotubule Agent] Uses:

Advanced PCa **Action:** Estradiol w/ nitrogen mustard; exact mechanism unknown **Disp:** Caps 140 mg **Caution:** [NA, not used in females] **CI:** Active thrombophlebitis or thromboembolic disorders **Disp:** Caps 140 mg **SE:** N/V, exacerbation of preexisting CHF, edema, hepatic disturbances, thrombophlebitis, MI, PE, gynecomastia in 20–100% **Interactions:** ↓ Absorption & effects W/ antacids, Ca supls, Ca-containing foods; ↓ effects OF anticoagulants **Labs:** Monitor bilirubin & LFTs during & 2 mo after Tx is D/C **NIPE:** Take on empty stomach, ⊘ take with milk or dairy; several wk may be needed for full effects, store in refrigerator; low-dose breast irradiation before may ↓ gynecomastia; use barrier/effective contraception

Estrogen, Conjugated (Premarin) [Estrogen/Hormone] WARNING:

↑ Risk of endometrial CA. Do not use to prevent CV Dz or dementia; ↑ risk MI, stroke, breast CA, PE, and DVT in postmenopausal (50–79 y). ↑ Dementia risk in postmenopausal (≥ 65 y) **Uses:** *Mod–severe menopausal vasomotor Sxs; atrophic vaginitis; dyspareunia; palliative advanced CAP; prevention & Tx of estrogen-deficiency osteoporosis* **Action:** Estrogen replacement **Dose:** 0.3–1.25 mg PO; intravaginal cream 0.5–2 g × 21 d, then off × 7 d or 0.5 mg twice weekly **Caution:** [X, –] **CI:** Severe hepatic impair, genital bleeding of unknown cause, breast CA, estrogen-dependent tumors, thromboembolic disorders, thrombosis, thrombophlebitis, recent MI **Disp:** Tabs 0.3, 0.45, 0.625, 0.9, 1.25, 2.5 mg; Vag cream 0.625 mg/g **SE:** ↑ Risk of endometrial CA, gallbladder Dz, thromboembolism, HA, & possibly breast CA **Interactions:** ↑ Effects OF corticosteroids, cyclosporine, TCAs, theophylline, tobacco; ↓ effects OF anticoag-ulants, clofibrate; ↓ effects W/ barbiturates, carbamazepine, phenytoin, rifampin **Labs:** ↑ Prothrombin &

factors VII, VIII, IX, X, plt aggregation, thyroid-binding globulin, T$_4$, triglycerides; ↓ antithrombin III, folate **NIPE:** ⊘ PRG, breast-feeding; generic products not equivalent

Estrogen, Conjugated + Medroxyprogesterone (Prempro, Premphase) [Estrogen/Progestin Hormones]

WARNING: Risk of endometrial CA. Do not use for the prevention of CV Dz or dementia; ↑ risk MI, stroke, breast CA, PE, and DVT; ↑ dementia risk in postmenopausal (> 65) **Uses:** *Mod–severe menopausal vasomotor Sxs; atrophic vaginitis; prevent postmenopausal osteoporosis* **Action:** Hormonal replacement **Dose:** *Prempro:* 1 tab PO daily *Premphase:* 1 tab PO daily **CI:** [X, –] **CI:** Severe hepatic impair, genital bleeding of unknown cause, breast CA, estrogen-dependent tumors, thromboembolic disorders, thrombosis, thrombophlebitis **Disp:** (As estrogen/medroxyprogesterone) *Prempro:* Tabs 0.3/1.5, 0.45/1.5, 0.625/2.5, 0.625/5 mg *Premphase:* Tabs 0.625/0 mg (d 1–14) & 0.625/5 mg (d 15–28) **SE:** Gallbladder Dz, thromboembolism, HA, breast tenderness **NIPE:** Intolerance to contact lenses; see WHI (www.whi.org); use lowest dose/shortest time possible

Estrogen, Conjugated Synthetic (Cenestin, Enjuvia) [Estrogen/Hormone]

WARNING: ↑ Risk endometrial CA. Do not use to prevent CV Dz or dementia; ↑ risk MI, stroke, breast CA, PE, and DVT in postmenopausal (50–79 y). ↑ Dementia risk in postmenopausal (≥ 65 y) **Uses:** *Vasomotor menopausal Sxs, vulvovaginal atrophy* **Action:** Multiple estrogen replacement **Dose:** For all w/ intact uterus progestin × 10–14 d/28-d cycle *Vasomotor:* 0.3–1.25 mg (Enjuvia) 0.625–1.25 mg (Cenestin) PO daily *Vag atrophy:* 0.3 mg/d *Osteoporosis:* (Cenestin) 0.625 mg/d **Caution:** [X, –] **CI:** See Estrogen, Conjugated **Disp:** Tabs *Cenestin* 0.3, 0.45, 0.625, 0.9 mg; 1.25; *Enjuvia* ER 0.3, 0.45, 0.625, 1.25 mg **SE:** ↑ Risk endometrial/breast CA, gallbladder Dz, thromboembolism **NIPE:** D/C if jaundice occurs & 2 wk before surgery

Eszopiclone (Lunesta) [Hypnotic/Nonbenzodiazepine] [C-IV]

Uses: *Insomnia* **Action:** Nonbenzodiazepine hypnotic **Dose:** 2–3 mg/d hs *Elderly:* 1–2 mg/d hs; w/ hepatic impair use w/ CYP3A4 Inhib (Table 10); 1 mg/d hs **Caution:** [C, ?/–] **Disp:** Tabs 1, 2, 3 mg **SE:** HA, xerostomia, dizziness, somnolence, hallucinations, rash, Infxn, unpleasant taste, anaphylaxis, angioedema **Interactions:** ↑ Effects W/ itraconazole, ketoconazole, ritonavir; ↑ CNS effects W/ CNS depressants; ↓ effects W/ rifampin **NIPE:** High-fat meals ↓ absorption; take right before bed—must be able to sleep 7–8 h; ⊘ EtOH

Etanercept (Enbrel) [Antirheumatic/TNF Blocker]

WARNING: Serious Infxns (bacterial sepsis, TB, reported); D/C w/ severe Infxn. Eval for TB risk; test for TB before use; lymphoma/other CA possible in children/adolescents from use **Uses:** *↓ Sxs of RA in pts who fail other DMARD*, Crohn Dz **Action:** TNF receptor blocker **Dose:** *Adults.* RA 50 mg SQ weekly or 25 mg SQ 2 ×/wk (separated by at least 72–96 h) *Peds 4–17 y.* 0.8 mg/kg/wk (max 50 mg/wk) or 0.4 mg/kg (max 25 mg/dose) 2 ×/wk 72–96 h apart **Caution:** [B, ?] w/ Predisposition to Infxn (ie, DM); may ↑ risk of malignancy in peds & young adults **CI:** Active Infxn **Disp:** Inj 25 mg/vial, 50 mg/mL syringe **SE:** HA, rhinitis, Inj site Rxn, URI, new-onset psoriasis **Interactions:** ↓ Response to live virus vaccine **NIPE:** Rotate Inj sites; ⊘ live vaccines; ↑ risk Infxn; teach SC Inj tech

Ethambutol (Myambutol) [Antitubercular Agent] Uses: *Pulm TB* & other mycobacterial Infxns, MAC **Action:** ↓ RNA synth **Dose:** *Adults & Peds > 12 y.* 15–25 mg/kg/d PO single dose; ↓ in renal impair, take w/ food, avoid antacids **Caution:** [C, +] **CI:** Unconscious pts, optic neuritis **Disp:** Tabs 100, 400 mg **SE:** HA, hyperuricemia, acute gout, Abd pain, optic neuritis **Interactions:** ↑ Neurotox *W/* neurotoxic drugs; ↓ effects *W/* Al salts **Labs:** ↑ LFTs **NIPE:** Monitor visual acuity; take 1 h before or 2 h after antacids

Ethinyl Estradiol & Norelgestromin (Ortho Evra) [Estrogen & Progestin Hormones] **WARNING:** Cigarette smoking ↑ risk of serious CV events. ↑ Risk w/ age & no. of cigarettes smoked. Hormonal contraceptives should not be used by women who are > 35 y and smoke. Different from OCP pharmacokinetics Uses: *Contraceptive patch* **Action:** Estrogen & progestin **Dose:** Apply patch to abdomen, buttocks, upper torso (not breasts), or upper outer arm at the beginning of the menstrual cycle; new patch is applied weekly for 3 wk; wk 4 is patch-free **Caution:** [X, +/−] **CI:** PRG, h/o or current DVT/PE, stroke, MI, CV Dz, CAD; SBP ≥ 160 systolic mm Hg or DBP ≥ 100 diastolic mm Hg severe HTN; severe HA w/ focal neurologic Sx; breast/endometrial CA; estrogen-dependent neoplasms; hepatic dysfunction; jaundice; major surgery w/ prolonged immobilization; heavy smoking if > 35 y **Disp:** 20 cm² patch (6 mg norelgestromin [active metabolite norgestimate] & 0.75 mg of ethinyl estradiol) **SE:** Breast discomfort, HA, site Rxns, N, menstrual cramps; thrombosis risks similar to OCP **Labs:** ↑ Serum amylase, Na, Ca, protein **NIPE:** Less effective in women > 90 kg; instruct pt does not protect against STD/HIV; discourage smoking

Ethosuximide (Zarontin) [Anticonvulsant] Uses: *Absence (petit mal) Szs* **Action:** Anticonvulsant; ↑ Sz threshold **Dose:** *Adults & Peds > 6 y. Initial:* 500 mg PO ÷ bid; ↑ by 250 mg/d q4–7d PRN (max 1500 mg/d) usual maint 20–30 mg/kg *Peds 3–6 y.* 250 mg/d; ↑ by 250 mg/d q4–7d PRN; maint 20–30 mg/kg/d ÷ bid; max 1500 mg/d **Caution:** [D, +] In renal/hepatic impair; antiepileptics may ↑ risk of suicidal behavior or ideation **CI:** Component sensitivity **Disp:** Caps 250 mg; syrup 250 mg/5 mL **SE:** Blood dyscrasias, GI upset, drowsiness, dizziness, irritability **Notes:** *Levels: Trough:* Just before next dose *Therapeutic: Peak:* 40–100 mcg/mL *Toxic trough:*> 100 mcg/mL *1/2-life:* 25–60 h **Interactions:** ↑ Effects *W/* INH, phenobarbital, EtOH; ↑ effects *OF* CNS depressants, phenytoin; ↓ effects *W/* carbamazepine, valproic acid, ginkgo; ↓ effects *OF* phenobarbital **Labs:** Monitor BUN, Cr, LFTs **NIPE:** Take w/ food; ⊘ EtOH; ⊘ D/C abruptly; may cause dizziness—caution driving

Etidronate Disodium (Didronel) [Hormone/Bisphosphonates]
Uses: *↑ Ca²⁺ of malignancy, Paget Dz, & heterotopic ossification* **Action:** ↓ Nl & abnormal bone resorption **Dose:** *Paget Dz:* 5–10 mg/kg/d PO ÷ doses (for 3–6 mo). ↑ *Ca²⁺:* 20 mg/kg/d IV × 30–90 d; **Caution:** [B PO (C parenteral), ?] Bisphosphonates may cause severe musculoskeletal pain **CI:** Overt osteomalacia, SCr > 5 mg/dL **Disp:** Tabs 200, 400 mg; **SE:** GI intolerance (↓ by ÷ daily doses); hyperphosphatemia, hypomagnesemia, bone pain, abnormal taste, fever, convulsions, nephrotox **Interactions:** ↓ Effects W/ antacids, foods that contain Ca; monitor warfarin **NIPE:** Take PO on empty stomach 2 h before or 2 h pc; esp. avoid milk/dairy within 2 of taking; swallow whole—⊘ chew/crush

Etodolac [Antiarthritic/NSAID]   WARNING: May ↑ risk of CV events & GI bleeding; may worsen ↑ BP **Uses:** *OA & pain*, RA **Action:** NSAID **Dose:** 200–400 mg PO bid–qid (max 1200 mg/d) **Caution:** [C (D 3rd tri), ?] ↑ Bleeding risk w/ ASA, warfarin; ↑ nephrotox w/ cyclosporine; Hx CHF, HTN, renal/hepatic impair, PUD **CI:** Active GI ulcer **Disp:** Tabs 400, 500 mg; ER tabs 400, 500, 600 mg; caps 200, 300 mg **SE:** N/V/D, gastritis, Abd cramps, dizziness, HA, depression, edema, renal impair **Interactions:** ↑ Risk of bleeding W/ anticoagulants, antiplts; ↑ effects *OF* Li, MTX, digoxin, cyclosporine; ↓ effects W/ ASA; ↓ effects *OF* antihypertensives **Labs:** ↑ LFTs, BUN, Cr; ↓ Hgb, Hct, plts, WBC, uric acid **NIPE:** Take w/ food; do not crush tabs; avoid EtOH; ↑ risk photosensivity—use sunscreen

Etomidate (Amidate) [Hypnotic]   Uses: *Induce general or short-procedure anesthesia* **Action:** Short-acting hypnotic **Dose:** *Adults & Peds > 10 y.* Induce anesthesia 0.2–0.6 mg/kg IV over 30–60 s; *Peds < 10 y* Not recommended *Peds. ECC 2010:* Rapid sedation: 0.2–0.4 mg/kg IV/IO over 30–60 s; max dose 20 mg **Caution:** [C; ?] **CI:** Hypersensitivity **Disp:** Inj 2 mg/mL **SE:** Inj site pain, myoclonus **NIPE:** May induce cardiac depression in elderly

Etonogestrel Implant (Implanon) [Hormone]   Uses: *Contraception* **Action:** Transforms endometrium from proliferative to secretory **Dose:** 1 implant subdermally q3y **Caution:** [X, +] Exclude PRG before implant **CI:** PRG, hormonally responsive tumors, breast CA, AUB, hepatic tumor, active liver Dz, Hx thromboembolic Dz **Disp:** 68-mg implant 4 cm long **SE:** Spotting, irregular periods, amenorrhea, dysmenorrhea, HA, tender breasts, N, Wt gain, acne, ectopic PRG, PE, ovarian cysts, stroke, ↑ BP **Interactions:** ↓ Effects W/ ketoconazole, itraconazole, other hepatic enzyme Inhibs **Labs:** Monitor LFTs **NIPE:** 99% Effective; remove implant & replace; restricted distribution; healthcare provider must register & train; does not protect against STDs

Etonogestrel/Ethinyl Estradiol Vaginal Insert (NuvaRing) [Estrogen & Progestin Hormones]   WARNING: Cigarette smoking ↑ risk of serious CV events. ↑ Risk w/ age & number cigarettes smoked. Hormonal contraceptives should not be used by women who are > 35 y and smoke. Different from

OCP pharmacokinetics **Uses:** *Contraceptive* **Action:** Estrogen & progestin combo **Dose:** Rule out PRG 1st; insert ring vaginally for 3 wk, remove for 1 wk; insert new ring 7 d after last removed (even if bleeding) at same time of day ring removed. 1st day of menses is day 1, insert before day 5 even if bleeding. Use other contraception for 1st 7 d of starting Rx. See PI if converting from other contraceptive; after delivery or 2nd tri abortion, insert 4 wk postpartum (if not breast-feeding) **Caution:** [X, ?/–] HTN, gallbladder Dz, ↑ lipids, migraines, sudden HA **CI:** PRG, heavy smokers > 35 y, DVT, PE, cerebro-/CV Dz, estrogen-dependent neoplasm, undiagnosed abnormal genital bleeding, hepatic tumors, cholestatic jaundice **Disp:** *Intravag ring:* Ethinyl estradiol 0.015 mg/d & etonogestrel 0.12 mg/d **NIPE:** If ring removed, rinse w/ cool/lukewarm H_2O (not hot) & reinsert ASAP; if not reinserted w/in 3 h, effectiveness ↓; do not use w/ diaphragm

Etoposide [VP-16] (Etopophos, Toposar, Vepesid, Generic) [Antineoplastic] **Uses:** *Testicular, NSCLC, Hodgkin Dz, & NHLs, peds ALL, & allogeneic/autologous BMT in high doses* **Action:** Topoisomerase II Inhib **Dose:** 50 mg/m²/d IV for 3–5 d; 50 mg/m²/d PO for 21 d (PO availability = 50% of IV); 2–6 g/m² or 25–70 mg/kg in BMT (per protocols); ↓ in renal/hepatic impair **Caution:** [D, –] **CI:** IT administration **Disp:** Caps 50 mg; Inj 20 mg/mL **SE:** N/V (emesis in 10–30%), ↓ BM, alopecia, ↓ BP w/ rapid IV, anorexia, anemia, leukopenia, ↑ risk secondary leukemias **Interactions:** ↑ Bleeding W/ ASA, NSAIDs, warfarin; ↑ BM suppression W/ antineoplastics & radiation; ↑ effects OF cisplatin; ↓ effects OF live vaccines **Labs:** ↑ Uric acid; ↓ Hgb, Hct, plts, RBC, WBC **NIPE:** ⊘ EtOH, immunizations, PRG, breast-feeding; use contraception; 2–3 L/d fluids; avoid grapefruit/grapefruit juice; limit EtOH

Etravirine (Intelence) [Nonnucleoside Reverse Transcriptase Inhibitor] **Uses:** *HIV* **Action:** NNRTI **Dose:** *Adult:* 200 mg PO bid after a meal *Peds: 16–20 kg:* 100 mg, *20–25 kg:* 125 mg, *25–30 kg:* 150 mg, *> 30 kg:* 200 mg all PO bid after a meal **Caution:** [B, ±] **CI:** None **Disp:** Tabs 100, 200 mg **SE:** N/V/D, rash, severe/potentially life-threatening skin Rxns, fat redistribution **Interactions:** substrate/inducer (CYP3A4), substrate/Inhib (CYP2C9, CYP2C19); do not use w/ tipranavir/ritonavir, fosamprenavir/ritonavir, atazanavir/ritonavir, protease Inhibs w/o ritonavir, & non-NRTIs; ↑ effects OF warfarin, diazepam; ↑ effects W/ lopinavir, ritonavir **Labs:** Monitor BS & LFTs **NIPE:** Take after meals; ⊘ crush/chew/split—okay to place tab in glass of water and let dissolve

Everolimus (Afinitor, Afinitor Disperz) [mTOR Kinase Inhibitor] **Uses:** *Advanced RCC w/ sunitinib or sorafenib failure, subependymal giant cell astrocytoma and PNET in nonsurgical candidates w/ tuberous sclerosis, renal angiomyolipoma w/tuberous sclerosis* **Action:** mTOR Inhib **Dose:** 10 mg PO daily, ↓ to 5 mg w/ SE or hepatic impair; avoid with high-fat meal; **Caution:** [D, ?] Avoid w/ or if received live vaccines; w/ CYP3A4 Inhib **CI:** Compound/rapamycin derivative hypersens **Disp:** Tabs 2.5, 5, 7.5, 10 mg; Disperz for suspen 2, 3, 5 mg; **SE:**

Noninfectious pneumonitis, ↑ Infxn risk, oral ulcers, asthenia, cough, fatigue, diarrhea, ↑ glucose/SCr/lipids; ↓ hemoglobin/WBC/plt **Interactions:** ↑ Effects W/ mod–strong CYP3A4 Inhibs: amprenavir, aprepitant, atazanavir, clarithromycin, delavirdine, diltiazem, erythromycin, fluconazole, fosamprenavir, indinavir, itraconazole, ketoconazole, nefazodone, nelfinavir, ritonavir, saquinavir, telithromycin, verapamil, voriconazole, grapefruit juice; ↓ effects W/ strong CYP3A4 inducers: carbamazepine, dexamethasone, phenobarbital, phenytoin, rifabutin, rifampin **Labs:** ↑ Glucose/SCr/lipids; ↓ Hgb/WBC/plt; monitor CBC, LFT, glucose, lipids **NIPE:** ⊘ Live vaccines; swallow whole w/ H$_2$O; monitor for pneumonitis—reduce dose and/or manage w/ corticosteroids; monitor for Infxn & D/C if fungal Infxn occurs; monitor for stomatitis—treat w/ nonalcoholic, non-peroxide mouthwash; see also Everolimus (Zortress)

Everolimus (Zortress) [Immunosuppressant (Macrolide)] Uses: *Prevent renal transplant rejection; combo w/ basiliximab w/ ↓ dose of steroids & cyclosporine* **Action:** mTOR Inhib (mammalian rapamycin target) **Dose:** 0.75 mg PO bid, adjust to trough levels 3–8 ng/mL **Caution:** [D, ?] **CI:** Compound/-rapamycin-derivative hypersensitivity **Disp:** Tabs 0.25, 0.5, 0.75 mg **SE:** Peripheral edema, constipation, ↑ BP, N, ↓ Hct, UTI, ↑ lipids **Interactions:** Avoid live vaccines, simvastatin, lovastatin; ↑ risk of angioedema W/ ACEI; ↑ effects W/ ketoconazole, itraconazole, voriconazole, clarithromycin, telithromycin, ritonavir, grapefruit juice, digoxin; ↓ effects W/ carbamazepine, phenobarbital, phenytoin, rifampin, rifabulin, efavirenz, nevirapine, St. Johns wort **Labs:** ↑ Lipids; ↓ Hct; follow CBC, LFT, glucose, lipids **NIPE:** Swallow whole w/ or w/o food; trough level 3–8 ng/mL w/ cyclosporine; see also Everolimus (Afinitor); avoid sunlight & UV light; ↑ risk of Infxn

Exemestane (Aromasin) [Antineoplastic] Uses: *Advanced breast CA in postmenopausal w/ progression after tamoxifen* **Action:** Irreversible, steroidal aromatase Inhib; ↓ estrogens **Dose:** 25 mg PO daily after a meal **Caution:** [D, ?/–] **CI:** PRG, component sensitivity **Disp:** Tabs 25 mg **SE:** Hot flashes, N, fatigue, ↑ alkaline phosphate **Interactions:** ↓ Effects W/ erythromycin, ketoconazole, phenobarbital, rifampin, other drugs that inhibit P4503A4, St. John's wort, black cohosh, dong quai **Labs:** ↑ Alk phos, bilirubin, alk phos **NIPE:** ⊘ PRG, breast-feeding; take pc & same time each d; monitor BP; limit EtOH; may cause ↓ mental alertness—caution driving

Exenatide (Byetta) [Hypoglycemic/Incretin] Uses: *Type 2 DM combined w/ metformin &/or sulfonylurea* **Action:** Incretin mimetic: ↑ insulin release, ↓ glucagon secretion, ↓ gastric emptying, promotes satiety **Dose:** 5 mcg SQ bid w/in 60 min before AM & PM meals; ↑ to 10 mcg SQ bid after 1 mo PRN; do not give pc **Caution:** [C, ?/–] May ↓ absorption of other drugs (take antibiotics or contraceptives 1 h before) **CI:** CrCl < 30 mL/min **Disp:** Soln 5, 10 mcg/dose in prefilled pen **SE:** Hypoglycemia, N/V/D, dizziness, HA, dyspepsia, ↓ appetite, jittery; acute pancreatitis **Interactions:** May ↓ absorption of oral drugs (take antibiotics/contraceptives 1 h before) **Labs:** Monitor Cr, warfarin **NIPE:** Consider ↓ sulfonylurea & insulin to ↓ risk of hypoglycemia; discard pen 30 d after 1st use; ⊘ use with short-/fast-acting insulins; teach SQ inj technique

Exenatide ER (Bydureon)   **WARNING:** Causes thyroid C-cell tumors in rats, ? human relevance; CI in pts w/ Hx or family Hx medullary thyroid carcinoma (MTC) or multiple endocrine neoplasia synd type 2 (MEN2); counsel pts on thyroid tumor risk & Sx **Uses:** *Type 2 DM* **Acts:** Glucagon-like peptide-1 (GLP-1) receptor agonist **Dose:** *Adult.* 2 mg SQ 1 × week; w/ or w/o meals **W/P:** [C, ?/–] w/ mod renal impair; w/ severe GI dz; may cause acute pancreatitis and absorption of PO meds, may ↑ INR w/ warfarin **CI:** MTC, MEN2, hypersens; CrCl < 30 mL/min **Disp:** Inj 2 mg/vial **SE:** N/V/D/C, dyspepsia, ↓ appetite, hypoglycemia, HA, Inj site Rxn, pancreatitis, renal impair, hypersens **NIPE:** not for type 1 DM or DKA; ⊘ use with insulin; teach SQ Inj technique; monitor BS

Ezetimibe (Zetia) [Antilipemic/Selective Cholesterol Absorption Inhibitor]   **Uses:** *Hypercholesterolemia alone or w/ a HMG-CoA reductase Inhib* **Action:** ↓ Cholesterol & phytosterols absorption **Dose:** *Adults & Peds > 10 y.* 10 mg/d PO **Caution:** [C, +/–] Bile acid sequestrants ↓ bioavailability **CI:** Hepatic impair **Disp:** Tabs 10 mg **SE:** HA, D, Abd pain, ↑ transaminases w/ HMG-CoA reductase Inhib, erythema multiforme **Notes:** See Ezetimibe/Simvastatin **Interactions:** ↑ Effects *W/* cyclosporine; ↓ effects *W/* cholestyramine, fenofibrate, gemfibrozil **Labs:** ↑ LFTs **NIPE:** If used w/ fibrates ↑ risk of cholelithiasis; teach ↓ chol diet

Ezetimibe/Atorvastatin (Liptruzet)   **Uses:** *Tx primary & mixed hyperlipidemia* **Acts:** Cholesterol absorption Inhib & HMG-CoA reductase Inhib **Dose:** *Adults.* 10/10–10/80 mg/d PO; w/ clarithromycin, itraconazole, saquinavir/ritonavir, darunavir/ritonavir, fosamprenavir, fosamprenavir/ritonavir: 10/20 mg/d max; w/ nelfinavir, boceprevir: 10/40 mg/d max; use caution/lowest effective dose w/ lopinavir/ritonavir; start 10/40 mg/d for > 55% ↓ in LDL-C **W/P:** [X, –] w/ CYP3A4 Inhib, fenofibrates, niacin > 1 g/d **CI:** Liver Dz, ↑ LFTs; PRG/lactation; w/ cyclosporine, tipranavir/ritonavir, telaprevir, gemfibrozil; component hypersens **Disp:** Tabs (ezetimibe/atorvastatin): 10/10, 10/20, 10/40, 10/80 mg **SE:** ↑ LFTs, musculoskeletal pain, myopathy, Abd pain, dizziness, N/D, HA, insomnia, hot flash, ↑ K⁺ **NIPE:** Take w/ or w/o food; swallow whole—⊘ crush/chew/split; avoid grapefruit/grapefruit juice; ⊘ PRG, breast-feeding; instruct pt to report unusual muscle pain/weakness;

Ezetimibe/Simvastatin (Vytorin) [Antilipemic/HMG-CoA Reductase Inhibitor]   **Uses:** *Hypercholesterolemia* **Action:** ↓ Absorption of cholesterol & phytosterols w/ HMG-CoA-reductase Inhib **Dose:** 10/10–10/80 mg/d PO; w/ cyclosporine/danazol: 10/10 mg/d max; w/ diltiazem/amiodarone or verapamil: 10/10 mg/d max; w/ amlodipine/ranolazine 10/20 max; ↓ w/ severe renal Insuff; give 2 h before or 4 h after bile acid sequestrants **Caution:** [X, −]; w/ CYP3A4

Inhibs (Table 10), gemfibrozil, niacin > 1 g/d, danazol, amiodarone, verapamil; avoid high dose w/ diltiazem; w/ Chinese pt on lipid-modifying meds **CI**: PRG/lactation; w/ cyclosporine & danazol; liver Dz, ↑ LFTs **Disp**: Tabs (mg ezetimibe/mg simvastatin) 10/10, 10/20, 10/40, 10/80 **SE**: HA, GI upset, myalgia, myopathy (muscle pain, weakness, or tenderness w/ creatine kinase 10 × ULN, rhabdomyolysis), hep, Infxn **Interactions**: ↑ Risk of myopathy W/ clarithromycin, erythromycin, itraconazole, ketoconazole **Labs**: Monitor LFTs, lipids **NIPE**: ⊘ PRG or lactation; use adequate contraception; ⊘ EtOH; ezetimibe/simvastatin; ⊘ grapefruit/grapefruit juice

Ezogabine (Potiga) Uses: *Partial-onset Szs* **Action**: ↑ Transmembrane K⁺ currents & augment GABA-mediated currents **Dose**: Adult. 100 mg PO 3 × d; ↑ dose by 50 mg 3 × d qwk, Max dose 400 mg 3 × d (1200 mg/d); ↓ dosage in elderly, renal/hepatic impair (see labeling); swallow whole **W/P**: [C, ?/–] May need to ↓ dose when used w/ phenytoin & carbamazepine; monitor digoxin levels **Disp**: Tabs 50, 200, 300, 400 mg **SE**: Dizziness, somnolence, fatigue, abnormal coordination, gait disturbance, confusion, psychotic Sxs, hallucinations, attention disturbance, memory impair, vertigo, tremor, blurred vision, aphasia, dysarthria, urinary retention, ↑ QT interval, suicidal ideation/behavior, withdrawal Szs **NIPE**: baseline vision exam, then q 6 mo; take w/ or w/o food; swallow whole—⊘ crush, chew, split; D/C over ≥ 3 wk; may cause blurred vision—caution driving

Famciclovir (Famvir) [Antiviral/Synthetic Nucleoside] Uses: *Acute herpes zoster (shingles) & genital herpes* **Action**: ↓ Viral DNA synth **Dose**: Zoster: 500 mg PO q8h × 7 d Simplex: 125–250 mg PO bid; ↓ w/ renal impair **Caution**: [B, –] **CI**: Component sensitivity **Disp**: Tabs 125, 250, 500 mg **SE**: Fatigue, dizziness, HA, pruritus, N/D **Interactions**: ↑ Effects W/ cimetidine, probenecid, theophylline; ↑ effects OF digoxin **NIPE**: Take w/o regard to food, therapy most effective if taken w/in 72 h of initial lesion; use barrier methods of contraception

Famotidine (Fluxid, Pepcid, Pepcid AC) [OTC] [Antisecretory/ H₂-Receptor Antagonist] Uses: *Short-term Tx of duodenal ulcer & benign gastric ulcer; maint for duodenal ulcer, hypersecretory conditions, GERD, & heartburn* **Action**: H₂-antagonist; ↓ gastric acid **Dose**: Adults. Ulcer: 20 mg IV q12h or 20–40 mg PO qhs × 4–8 wk. Hypersecretion: 20–160 mg PO q6h GERD: 20 mg PO bid × 6 wk; maint: 20 mg PO hs. Heartburn: 10 mg PO PRN q12h Peds. 0.5–1 mg/kg/d; ↓ in severe renal Insuff **Caution**: [B, M] **CI**: Component sensitivity **Disp**: Tabs 10, 20, 40 mg; chew tabs 10 mg; susp 40 mg/5 mL; gelatin caps 10 mg, Fluxid ODT 20 mg; Inj 10 mg/2 mL **SE**: Dizziness, HA, constipation, N/V/D, ↓ plt, hepatitis **Interactions**: ↑ GI irritation W/ caffeinated foods, EtOH, nicotine **Labs**: ↑ BUN, Cr, LFTs **NIPE**: ⊘ ASA, EtOH, tobacco, caffeine—d/t ↑ SEs; take hs; to prevent heartburn, take 15–60 min ac; chew tabs contain phenylalanine

Febuxostat (Uloric) [Antigout/Xanthine Oxidase Inhibitor]
Uses: *Hyperuricemia and gout* **Action:** Xanthine oxidase Inhib (enzyme that converts hypoxanthine to xanthine to uric acid) **Dose:** 40 mg PO 1 × daily, ↑ 80 mg if uric acid not < 6 mg/dL after 2 wk **Caution:** [C, ?/–] **CI:** Use w/ azathioprine, mercaptopurine, theophylline **Disp:** Tabs 40, 80 mg **SE:** ↑ LFTs, rash, myalgia **Interactions:** ↑ Effects *OF* xanthine oxidase substrate drugs: Azathioprine, mercaptopurine, theophylline **Labs:** Monitor uric acid < & 2 wk > start of therapy; monitor LFTs 2 & 4 mo > initiation & periodically; ↑ LFTs, ↑ or ↓ WBC **NIPE:** OK to continue drug w/ gouty flare or use w/ NSAIDs/colchicine on initiation of therapy for up to 6 mo; chronic management of hyperuricemia w/ gout. Not for use in asymptomatic pts

Felodipine (Plendil) [Antihypertensive/CCB] **Uses:** *HTN & CHF* **Action:** CCB **Dose:** 2.5–10 mg PO daily; swallow whole; ↓ in hepatic impair **Caution:** [C, ?] ↑ Effect w/ azole antifungals, erythromycin, grapefruit juice **CI:** Component sensitivity **Disp:** ER tabs 2.5, 5, 10 mg **SE:** Peripheral edema, flushing, tachycardia, HA, gingival hyperplasia **Interactions:** ↑ Effects *W/* azole antifungals, cimetidine, cyclosporine, ranitidine, propranolol, EtOH, grapefruit juice; ↑ effects *OF* digoxin, erythromycin; ↓ effects *W/* barbiturates, carbamazepine, nafcillin, NSAIDS, oxcarbazepine, phenytoin; rifampin; ↓ effects *OF* theophylline **NIPE:** Best taken w/o food–if gastric upset, may take w/ light snack; ⊘ chew/crush/split; ⊘ D/C abruptly; follow BP in elderly & w/ hepatic impair

Fenofibrate (Antara, Lipofen, Lofibra, TriCor, Triglide) [Antilipemic/Fibric Acid Derivative] **Uses:** *Hypertriglyceridemia, hypercholesteremia* **Action:** ↓ Triglyceride synth **Dose:** 43–160 mg/d; ↓ w/ renal impair; take w/ meals **Caution:** [C, ?] **CI:** Hepatic/severe renal Insuff, primary biliary cirrhosis, unexplained ↑ LFTs, gallbladder Dz **Disp:** Caps 35, 40, 43, 48, 50, 54, 67, 105, 107, 130, 134, 145, 160, 200 mg **SE:** GI disturbances, cholecystitis, arthralgia, myalgia, dizziness, ↑ LFTs **Interactions:** ↑ Effects *OF* anticoagulants; ↑ risk of rhabdomyolysis & ARF *W/* statins; ↑ risk of renal dysfunction *W/* immunosuppressants, nephrotoxic agents; ↓ effects *W/* bile acid sequestrants **Labs:** ↑ LFTs, BUN, Cr; ↓ Hgb, Hct, WBCs, uric acid; monitor LFTs **NIPE:** Food ↑ drug absorption; EtOH ↑ triglycerides; may take up to 2 mo to modify lipids; ⊘ switch brands; take 1 h before or 4–6 h after bile acid sequestrants

Fenofibric Acid (Fibricor, Trilipix) [Antilipemic/Fibrate] **Uses:** *Adjunct to diet for ↑ triglycerides, to ↓ LDL-C, cholesterol, triglycerides, & apo B, to ↑ HDL-C in hypercholesterolemia/ mixed dyslipidemia; adjunct to diet w/ a statin to ↓ triglycerides and ↑ HDL-C w/ CHD or w/ CHD risk* **Action:** Agonist of peroxisome proliferator-activated receptor-α (PPAR-α), causes ↑ VLDL catabolism, fatty acid oxidation, and clearing of triglyceride-rich particles w/ ↓ VLDL, triglycerides; ↑ HDL in some **Dose:** *Mixed dyslipidemia w/ a statin:* 135 mg PO × 1 d; *Hypertriglyceridemia:* 45–135 mg 1 × d; maint based on response; *Primary hypercholesterolemia/mixed dyslipidemia:* 135 mg PO 1 × d; 135 mg/d max; **Caution:**

[C,/−], Multiple interactions, ↑ embolic phenomenon **CI:** Severe renal impair, pt on dialysis, active liver/gallbladder Dz, nursing **Disp:** DR caps 35, 45, 105, 135 mg **SE:** HA, back pain, nasopharyngitis, URI, N/D, myalgia, gallstones, ↓ CBC (usually stabilizes) rare myositis/rhabdomyolysis **Interactions:** ↑ Effects of HMG-CoA reductase Inhibits, warfarin; ↑ risk of nephrotox w/ cyclosporine; ↓ effects **W/** bile acid sequestrants **Labs:** ↓ CBC (usually stabilizes), ✓ CBC, lipid panel, LFTs; D/C if LFTs > 3 × ULN **NIPE:** Take w/o regard to food; avoid w/ max dose of a statin—↑ risk of myopathy; take 1 h before or 4–6 h after bile acid sequestrants; use w/ low-fat/low-cholesterol diet & w/ a statin

Fenoldopam (Corlopam) [Antihypertensive/Vasodilator] Uses: *Hypertensive emergency* **Action:** Rapid vasodilator **Dose:** Initial 0.03–0.1 mcg/kg/min IV Inf, titrate q15min by 0.05–0.1 mcg/kg/min to max 1.6 mcg/kg/min; **Caution:** [B, ?] ↓ BP w/ β-blockers **CI:** Allergy to sulfites **Disp:** Inj 10 mg/mL **SE:** ↓ BP, edema, facial flushing, N/V/D, atrial flutter/fibrillation, ↑ IOP **Interactions:** ↑ Effects **W/** APAP ↑ hypotension **W/** BBs; ↓ effects **W/** DA antagonists, metoclopramide **Labs:** ↓ Serum urea nitrogen, Cr, LFTs, LDH, K⁺ **NIPE:** Continuously monitor BP HR; avoid concurrent BBs; asthmatics have ↑ risk of sulfite sensitivity

Fenoprofen (Nalfon) [Analgesic/NSAID] WARNING: May ↑ risk of CV events and GI bleeding **Uses:** *Arthritis & pain* **Action:** NSAID **Dose:** 200–600 mg q4–8h, to 3200 mg/d max; w/ food **Caution:** [B (D 3rd tri), +/−] CHF, HTN, renal/hepatic impair, Hx PUD **CI:** NSAID sensitivity **Disp:** Caps 200, 400, 600 mg **SE:** GI disturbance, dizziness, HA, rash, edema, renal impair, hep **Interactions:** ↑ Effects **W/** ASA, anticoagulants; ↑ hyperkalemia **W/** K⁺-sparing diuretics; ↑ effects **OF** anticoagulants, MTX; ↓ effects **W/** phenobarbital; ↓ effects **OF** antihypertensives **Labs:** False ↑ free & total T₃ levels **NIPE:** Swallow whole; take with food or 8–12 oz water to ↓ GI SEs; ⊘ supine position ≤ 10 min after taking; ⊘ ASA, EtOH, OTC drugs

Fentanyl (Sublimaze) [C-II] [Opioid Analgesic] Uses: *Short-acting analgesic* in anesthesia & PCA **Action:** Narcotic analgesic **Dose:** *Adults.* 1–2 mcg/kg or 25–100 mcg/dose IV/IM titrated; *Anesthesia:* 5–15 mcg/kg *Pain:* 200 mcg over 15 min, titrate to effect *Peds.* 1–2 mcg/kg IV/IM q1–4h titrate; ↓ in renal impair **Caution:** [B, +] **CI:** Paralytic ileus ↑ ICP, resp depression, severe renal/hepatic impair **Disp:** Inj 0.05 mg/mL **SE:** Sedation, ↓ BP, ↓ HR, constipation, N, resp depression, miosis **Interactions:** ↑ Effects **W/** CNS depressants, cimetidine, erythromycin, ketoconazole, phenothiazine, ritonavir, TCAs, EtOH, grapefruit juice; ↑ risks of HTN crisis **W/** MAOIs; ↑ risk of CNS & resp depression **W/** protease Inhibs; ↓ effects **W/** buprenorphine, dezocine, nalbuphine, pentazocine **Labs:** ↑ Serum amylase, lipase; ↓ Hgb, Hct, plts, WBCs **NIPE:** 0.1 mg fentanyl = 10 mg morphine IM

Fentanyl, Transdermal (Duragesic) [C-II] [Opioid Analgesic] WARNING: Potential for abuse and fatal OD **Uses:** *Persistent mod–severe chronic pain in pts already tolerant to opioids* **Action:** Narcotic **Dose:** Apply patch to upper torso q72h; dose based on narcotic requirements in previous 24 h; start 25 mcg/h patch q72h; ↓ in renal impair **Caution:** [B, +] w/ CYP3A4 Inhib (Table 10) may ↑ fentanyl effect, w/ Hx substance abuse **CI:** Not opioid tolerant, short-term pain management, post-op pain in outpatient surgery, mild pain, PRN use ↑ ICP, resp depression, severe renal/hepatic impair, pts < 2 y **Disp:** Patches 12.5, 25, 50, 75, 100 mcg/h **SE:** Resp depression (fatal), sedation, ↓ BP, ↓ HR, constipation, N, miosis **Interactions:** ↑ Effects W/ CNS depressants, cimetidine, erythromycin, ketoconazole, phenothiazine, ritonavir, TCAs, EtOH, grapefruit juice; ↑ risks of HTN crisis W/ MAOIs; ↑ risk of CNS & resp depression W/ protease Inhibs; ↓ effects W/ buprenorphine, dezocine, nalbuphine, pentazocine **Labs:** ↑ Serum amylase, lipase; ↓ Hgb, Hct, plts, WBCs **NIPE:** 0.1 mg fentanyl = 10 mg morphine IM; do not cut patch; peak level 24–72 h; ↑ risk of ↑ absorption w/ elevated temperature ⊘ heating pad/lamp, hot water; cleanse skin only w/ H₂O; ⊘ soap, lotions, or EtOH because they may ↑ absorption; ⊘ use in children < 110 lb; not for PRN use

Fentanyl, Transmucosal (Abstral, Actiq, Fentora, Lazanda, Onsolis) [C-II] [Opioid Analgesic] **WARNING:** Potential for abuse and fatal OD; use only in pts w/ chronic pain who are opioid tolerant; CI in acute/post-op pain; do not substitute for other fentanyl products; fentanyl can be fatal to children, keep away; use w/ strong CYP3A4 Inhib may ↑ fentanyl levels. *Abstral, Onsolis* restricted distribution **Uses:** *Breakthrough CA pain w/ tolerance to opioids* **Action:** Narcotic analgesic, transmucosal absorption **Dose:** Titrate to effect *Abstral:* Start 100 mcg SL, 2 doses max per pain breakthrough episode; wait 2 h for next breakthrough dose; limit to < 4 breakthrough doses w/ successful baseline dosing. *Actiq:* Start 200 mcg PO × 1, may repeat × 1 after 30 min *Fentora:* Start 100-mcg buccal tab × 1, may repeat in 30 min, 4 tabs/dose max *Lazanda:* Through TIRF REMS Access Program; initial 1 × 100 mcg spray; if no relief, titrate for breakthrough pain as follows: 2 × 100 mcg spray (1 in each nostril); 1 × 400 mcg; 2 × 400 mcg (1 in each nostril); wait 2 h before another dose; max 4 doses/24 h *Onsolis:* Start 200 mcg film, ↑ 200 mcg increments to max of four 200-mcg films or single 1200-mcg film **Caution:** [B, +] resp/CNS depression possible; CNS depressants/CYP3A4 Inhib may ↑ effect; may impair tasks (driving, machinery); w/ severe renal/hepatic impair **CI:** Opioid intolerant pt, acute/post-op pain **Disp:** *Abstral:* SL tab 100, 200, 300, 400, 600, 800 mcg *Actiq:* Lozenges on stick 200, 400, 600, 800, 1200, 1600 mcg *Fentora:* Buccal tabs 100, 200, 400, 600, 800 mcg *Lazanda:* Nasal spray metered dose audible and visual counter, 8 doses/ bottle, 100/400 mcg/spray *Onsolis:* Buccal soluble film 200, 400, 600, 800, 1200 mcg **SE:** Sedation, ↓ BP, ↓ HR, constipation, N/V, ↓ resp, dyspnea, HA, miosis, anxiety, confusion, depression, rash, dizziness **Interactions:** ↑ Effects W/ CNS depressants, cimetidine, erythromycin, ketoconazole, phenothiazine, ritonavir, TCAs, EtOH, grapefruit juice; ↑ risks of HTN crisis W/ MAOIs; ↑ risk of CNS & resp depression W/ protease Inhibs; ↓ effects W/

buprenorphine, dezocine, nalbuphine, pentazocine **Labs:** ↑ Serum amylase, lipase; ↓ Hgb, Hct, plts, WBCs **NIPE:** 0.1 mg fentanyl = 10 mg IM morphine; for use in pts already tolerant to opioid therapy; ⊘ switch brands; ⊘ consume grapefruit/grapefruit juice; ⊘ use w/in 14 d of MAOI

Ferric Carboxymaltose (Injectafer) Uses: *Iron-deficiency anemia* **Action:** Fe Supl **Dose: Adults.** ≥ 50 kg: 2 doses 750 mg IV separated by 7 days; < 50 kg: 2 doses of 15 mg/kg IV separated by 7 days **Caution:** [C, M] Hypersens Rxn (monitor during & 30 min after Inf) **CI:** Component hypersens **Disp:** Inj 750 mg iron/ 15 mL single-use vial **SE:** N, HTN, flushing, hypophosphatemia, dizziness, HTN; **NIPE:** Give by IV push—monitor during and 30 min after for allergic Rxn; may cause dizziness—caution driving

Ferrous Gluconate (Fergon [OTC], Others) [Oral Iron Supplement] **WARNING:** Accidental OD of iron-containing products is a leading cause of fatal poisoning in children < 6. Keep out of reach of children **Uses:** *Iron-deficiency anemia* & Fe supls **Action:** Dietary supl **Dose: Adults.** 100–200 mg of elemental Fe/d ÷ doses **Peds.** 4–6 mg/kg/d ÷ doses; on empty stomach (OK w/ meals if GI upset occurs); avoid antacids **Caution:** [A, ?] **CI:** Hemochromatosis, hemolytic anemia **Disp:** Tabs Fergon 240 mg (27 mg Fe), 246 (28 mg Fe), 300 (34 mg Fe), 324 mg (38 mg Fe) **SE:** GI upset, constipation, dark stools, discoloration of urine, may stain teeth **Interactions:** ↑ Effects W/ chloramphenicol, citrus fruits or juices, vit C; ↓ effects W/ antacids, levodopa, black cohosh, chamomile, feverfew, gossypol, hawthorn, nettle, plantain, St. John's wort, whole-grain breads, cheese, eggs, milk, coffee, tea, yogurt; ↓ effects OF fluoroquinolones, tetracycline **Labs:** False(+) stool guaiac test **NIPE:** ⊘ Antacids, dairy, coffee/tea w/in 2 h before/after taking; ⊘ tetracyclines, take Liq form in Liq & through a straw to prevent teeth staining; 12% elemental Fe; keep away from children; severe tox in OD; measures to ↓ constipation

Ferrous Gluconate Complex (Ferrlecit) [Iron Supplement] **Uses:** *Iron-deficiency anemia or supl to erythropoietin Rx therapy* **Action:** Fe supl **Dose:** Test dose: 2 mL (25 mg Fe) IV over 1 h, if OK, 125 mg (10 mL) IV over 1 h Usual cumulative Dose: 1 g Fe over 8 sessions (until favorable Hct) **Caution:** [B, ?] **CI:** Non–Fe-deficiency anemia; CHF; Fe overload **Disp:** Inj 12.5 mg/mL **SE:** ↓ BP, serious allergic Rxns, GI disturbance, Inj site Rxn **Interactions:** ↑ Effects W/ chloramphenicol, citrus fruits or juices, vit C; ↓ effects W/ antacids, levodopa, black cohosh, chamomile, feverfew, gossypol, hawthorn, nettle, plantain, St. John's wort, whole-grain breads, cheese, eggs, milk, coffee, tea, yogurt; ↓ effects OF fluoroquinolones, tetracycline **Labs:** False(+) stool guaiac test **NIPE:** Dose expressed as mg Fe; may infuse during dialysis

Ferrous Sulfate (OTC) [Iron Supplement] Uses: *Fe-deficiency anemia & Fe supl* **Action:** Dietary supl **Dose: Adults.** 100–200 mg elemental Fe/d in ÷ doses **Peds.** 1–6 mg/kg/d ÷ daily–tid; on empty stomach (OK w/ meals if GI upset occurs); avoid antacids **Caution:** [A, ?] ↑ Absorption w/ vit C; ↓ absorption w/

tetracycline, fluoroquinolones, antacids, H$_2$-blockers, proton pump Inhib **CI:** Hemochromatosis, hemolytic anemia **Disp:** Tabs 187 mg (60 mg Fe), 200 (65 mg Fe), 324 (65 mg Fe), 325 mg (65 mg Fe); SR caplets & tabs 160 (50 mg Fe), 200 mg (65 mg Fe); gtt 75 mg/0.6 mL (15 mg Fe/0.6 mL); elixir 220 mg/5 mL (44 mg Fe/5 mL); syrup 90 mg/5 mL (18 mg Fe/5 mL) **SE:** GI upset, constipation, dark stools, discolored urine **Interactions:** ↑ Effects **W/** chloramphenicol, citrus fruits or juices, vit C; ↓ effects **W/** antacids, levodopa, black cohosh, chamomile, feverfew, gossypol, hawthorn, nettle, plantain, St. John's wort, whole-grain breads, cheese, eggs, milk, coffee, tea, yogurt; ↓ effects **OF** fluoroquinolones, tetracycline **Labs:** False(+) stool guaiac test **NIPE:** Take w/ meals if GI upset; can cause severe tox; see Ferrous gluconate OTC

Ferumoxytol (Feraheme) [Hematinic]   Uses: *Iron-deficiency anemia in chronic kidney Dz* **Action:** Fe replacement **Dose:** *Adults.* 510 mg IV × 1, then 510 mg IV × 1 3–8 d later; give 1 mL/s **Caution:** [C, ?/–] Monitor for hypersens & ↓ BP for 30 min after dose, may alter MRI studies **CI:** Iron overload; hypersens to ferumoxytol **Disp:** IV soln 30 mg/mL (510 mg elemental Fe/17 mL) **SE:** N/D, constipation, dizziness, hypotension, peripheral edema, hypersens Rxn **Interactions:** May ↓ absorption **OF** oral Fe Prep **Labs:** May transiently (up to 3 mo) affect diagnostic ability of MRI **NIPE:** ✓ Hematologic response 1 mo after 2nd dose

Fesoterodine (Toviaz) [Muscarinic Receptor Antagonist] Uses: *OAB w/ urge urinary incontinence, urgency, frequency* **Action:** Competitive muscarinic receptor antagonist, ↓ bladder muscle contractions **Dose:** 4 mg PO qd, ↑ to 8 mg PO daily PRN **Caution:** [C, /?] Avoid > 4 mg w/ severe renal Insuff or w/ CYP3A4 Inhib (eg, ketoconazole, clarithromycin); w/ BOO, ↓ GI motility/constipation, NAG, MyG **CI:** Urinary/gastric retention, or uncontrolled NAG, hypersens to class **Disp:** Tabs 4, 8 mg **SE:** Dry mouth, constipation, ↓ sweating can cause heat prostration **Interactions:** ↑ Effects **W/** CYP3A4 Inhibs: Amiodarone, amprenavir, atazanavir, ciprofloxacin, cisapride, clarithromycin, diltiazem, erythromycin, fluconazole, fluvoxamine, indinavir, itraconazole, ketoconazole, nefazodone, nelfinavir, norfloxacin, ritonavir, telithromycin, troleandomycin, verapamil voriconazole, grapefruit juice; ↑ CNS depression **W/** EtOH, other CNS depressants **NIPE:** Take w/o regard to food; swallow whole, in elderly (> 75 y)—↑ risk of anticholinergic SEs; measures to ↓ dry mouth, constipation

Fexofenadine (Allegra, Allegra-D) [Antihistamine/H$_1$-Receptor Antagonist] Uses: *Allergic rhinitis; chronic idiopathic urticaria* **Action:** Selective antihistamine, antagonizes H$_1$-receptors; Allegra-D contains pseudo-ephedrine **Dose:** *Adults & Peds > 12 y.* 60 mg PO bid or 180 mg/d; 12-h ER form bid, 24-h ER form qd *Peds 2–11 y.* 30 mg PO bid; ↓ in renal impair **Caution:** [C, +] w/ Nevirapine **CI:** Component sensitivity **Disp:** Tabs 30, 60, 180 mg; susp 6 mg/mL; *Allegra-D* 12-h ER tab (60 mg fexofenadine/120 mg pseudoephedrine), *Allegra-D* 24-h ER (180 mg fexofenadine/240 mg pseudoephedrine) **SE:**

Drowsiness (rare), HA, ischemic colitis **Interactions:** ↑ Effects W/ erythromycin, ketoconazole; ↓ absorption & effects W/ antacids, apples, OJ, grapefruit juice **NIPE:** ⊗ take with fruit juice; ⊘ antacids w/in 2 h before/after taking; ⊗ EtOH or CNS depressants

Fidaxomicin (Dificid) [Macrolide/Antibiotic] Uses: *Clostridium diffi-cile*–associated diarrhea* **Action:** Macrolide antibiotic **Dose:** 200 mg PO bid × 10 d **Caution:** [B, +/–] Not for systemic Infxn or < 18 y; ⊗ resistance, use only when diagnosis suspected/proven **Disp:** Tabs 200 mg **SE:** N/V, Abd pain, GI bleed, anemia, neutropenia **NIPE:** Take w/o regard to food; minimal systemic absorption

Filgrastim [G-CSF] (Neupogen) [Hematopoietic/Colony-Stimulating Factor] Uses: *↑↓ Incidence of Infxn in febrile neutropenic pts; Rx chronic neutropenia* **Action:** Recombinant G-CSF **Dose:** *Adults & Peds.* 5 mcg/kg/d SQ or IV single daily dose; D/C when ANC > 10,000 cells/mm³ **Caution:** [C, ?] w/ Drugs that potentiate release of neutrophils (eg, Li) **CI:** Allergy to *E coli*–derived proteins or G-CSF **Disp:** Inj 300 mcg/mL, 480 mg/1.6 mL **SE:** Fever, alopecia, N/V/D, splenomegaly, bone pain, HA, rash **Interactions:** ↑ Interference W/ cyto-toxic drugs; ↑ release of neutrophils W/ Li **Labs:** Monitor CBC & plts **NIPE:** Monitor for cardiac events; no benefit w/ ANC > 10,000 cells/mm³

Finasteride (Proscar [Generic], Propecia) [Androgen Hormone Inhibitor/Steroid] Uses: *BPH & androgenetic alopecia* **Action:** ↓ 5-α-reductase **Dose:** *BPH:* 5 mg/d PO *Alopecia:* 1 mg/d PO; food ↓ absorption **Caution:** [X, –] Hepatic impair **CI:** Pregnant women should avoid handling pills, teratogen to male fetus **Disp:** Tabs 1 mg (*Propecia*), 5 mg (*Proscar*) **SE:** ↓ Libido, vol ejaculate, ED, gynecomastia **Interactions:** ↑ Effects W/ saw palmetto; ↓ effects W/ anticholinergics, adrenergic bronchodilators, theophylline **Labs:** ↓ PSA by 50%; reestablish PSA baseline 6 mo (double PSA for "true" reading) **NIPE:** May take 6–12 mo for effect; continue to maint new hair, not for use in women; potential chemoprevention for PCa; no role in diagnosed PCa

Fingolimod (Gilenya) [Sphingosine 1-Phosphate Receptor Modulator] Uses: *Relapsing MS* **Action:** Sphingosine 1-phosphate receptor modulator; ↓ lymphocyte migration into CNS **Dose:** *Adults.* 0.5 mg PO 1 × d; monitor for 6 h after 1st dose for bradycardia; monitor **Caution:** [C, –] Monitor w/ severe hepatic impair; avoid live vaccines during & 2 mo after D/C; ketoconazole ↑ level **Disp:** Caps 0.5 mg **SE:** HA, D, back pain, dizziness, bradycardia, AV block, HTN, Infxns, macular edema, ↑ LFTs, cough, dyspnea **Interactions:** ↑ Risk of rhythm disturbances W/ Class Ia or III; ↑ levels W/ ketoconazole **Labs:** ↑ LFTs; obtain baseline CBC, LFTs **NIPE:** Monitor HR & BP for at least 6 h after 1st dose; obtain ECG before/after 1st dose; continue monitoring HR& BP if HR < 45 bpm; obtain baseline eye exam; women of childbearing potential should use contraception during & 2 mo after D/C; ⊘ abrupt D/C

Flavoxate (Generic) [Antispasmodic] Uses: *Relief of Sx of dysuria, urgency, nocturia, suprapubic pain, urinary frequency, incontinence* **Action:** Antispasmodic **Dose:** 100–200 mg PO tid–qid **Caution:** [B, ?] **CI:** GI obst, GI hemorrhage, ileus, achalasia, BPH **Disp:** Tabs 100 mg **SE:** Drowsiness, blurred vision, xerostomia **Interactions:** ↑ Effects *OF* CNS depressants **NIPE:** Take w/ food if GI upset; ↑ risk of heat stroke w/ exercise & in hot weather; measures to relieve dry mouth/constipation

Flecainide (Tambocor) [Antiarrhythmic/Benzamide Anesthetic] **WARNING:** ↑ Mortality in pts w/ ventricular arrhythmias and recent MI; pulm effects reported; ventricular proarrhythmic effects in AF/A flutter, not OK for chronic AF Uses: Prevent AF/A flutter & PSVT, *prevent/suppress life-threatenng ventricular arrhythmias* **Action:** Class IC antiarrhythmic **Dose:** *Adults.* Start 50 mg PO q 12h; ↑ by 50 mg q12h q4d to max 400 mg/d **Peds.** 3–6 mg/kg/d in 3 ÷ doses; ↓ w/ renal impair **Caution:** [C, +] Monitor w/ hepatic impair, ↑ conc w/ amiodarone, digoxin, quinidine, ritonavir/ amprenavir, β-blockers, verapamil; may worsen arrhythmias **CI:** 2nd-/3rd-degree AV block, right BBB w/ bifascicular or trifascicular block, cardiogenic shock, CAD, ritonavir/amprenavir, alkalinizing agents **Disp:** Tabs 50, 100, 150 mg **SE:** Dizziness, visual disturbances, dyspnea, palpitations, edema, CP, tachycardia, CHF, HA, fatigue, rash, N **Notes:** *Levels: Trough:* Just before next dose; *Therapeutic:* 0.2–1 mcg/mL; *Toxic:* > 1 mcg/mL; *1/2-life:* 11–14 h **Interactions:** ↑ Effects *W/* alkalinizing drugs, amiodarone, cimetidine, propranolol, quinidine; ↑ effects *OF* digoxin; ↑ risk of arrhythmias *W/* CCBs, antiarrhythmics, disopyramide; ↓ effects *W/* acidifying drugs, tobacco **Labs:** ↑ Alk phos **NIPE:** Take w/ or w/o food; limit alcohol; initiate Rx in hospital; dose q8h if pt is intolerant/uncontrolled at q12h; full effects may take 3–5 d

Floxuridine (Generic) [Pyrimidine Antimetabolite] **WARNING:** Administration by experienced physician only; pts should be hospitalized for 1st course d/t risk for severe Rxn Uses: *GI adenoma, liver, renal CAs*; colon & pancreatic CAs **Action:** Converted to 5-FU; Inhibits thymidylate synthase; ↓ DNA synthase (S-phase specific) **Dose:** 0.1–0.6 mg/kg/d for 1–6 wk (per protocols) usually intra-arterial for liver mets **Caution:** [D, −] Interaction w/ vaccines **CI:** BM suppression, poor nutritional status, serious Infxn, PRG, component sensitivity **Disp:** Inj 500 mg **SE:** ↓ BM, anorexia, Abd cramps, N/V/D, mucositis, alopecia, skin rash, & hyperpigmentation; rare neurotox (blurred vision, depression, nystagmus, vertigo, & lethargy); intra-arterial catheter-related problems (ischemia, thrombosis, bleeding, & Infxn) **Interactions:** ↑ Effects *W/* metronidazole **Labs:** ↑ LFTs, 5-HIAA urine excretion; ↓ plasma albumin **NIPE:** Need effective birth control; palliative Rx for inoperable/incurable pts; ↑ risk of photosensitivity—use sunscreen; ↑ risk Infxn

Fluconazole (Diflucan) [Antifungal/Synthetic Azole] Uses: *Candidiasis (esophageal, oropharyngeal, urinary tract, Vag prophylaxis); cryptococcal meningitis, prophylaxis w/ BMT* **Action:** Antifungal; ↓ cytochrome P-450 sterol demethylation *Spectrum:* All *Candida* sp except *C krusei* **Dose:** *Adults.* 100–400 mg/d PO or IV *Vaginitis:* 150 mg PO daily *Crypto:* Doses up to 800 mg/d reported: 400 mg × 1, then 200 mg × 10–12 wk after CSF(−) **Peds.** 3–6 mg/kg/d PO or IV; 12 mg/kg/d/ systemic Infxn; ↓ in renal impair **Caution:** [C, Vag candidiasis (D high or prolonged dose), −] Do not use w/ clopidogrel (↓ effect) **CI:** None **Disp:** Tabs 50, 100, 150, 200 mg; susp 10, 40 mg/mL; Inj 2 mg/mL **SE:** HA, rash, GI upset, ↓ K^+, ↑ LFTs **Interactions:** ↑ Effects W/ HCTZ, anticoagulants; ↑ effects *OF* amitriptyline, benzodiazepines, carbamazepine, cyclosporine, hypoglycemics, losartan, methadone, phenytoin, quinidine, tacrolimus, TCAs, theophylline, caffeine, zidovudine; ↓ effects W/ cimetidine, rifampin **Labs:** ↑ LFTs; ↓ K^+ **NIPE:** PO (preferred) = IV levels; monitor ECG for hypokalemia (flattened T waves)

Fludarabine (Generic) [Antineoplastic] **WARNING:** Administer only under supervision of qualified physician experienced in chemotherapy. Can ↓ BM & cause severe CNS effects (blindness, coma, & death). Severe/fatal autoimmune hemolytic anemia reported; monitor for hemolysis. Use w/ pentostatin not OK (fatal pulm tox) **Uses:** *Autoimmune hemolytic anemia, CLL, cold agglutinin hemolysis*, low-grade lymphoma, mycosis fungoides **Action:** ↓ Ribonucleotide reductase; blocks DNA polymerase-induced DNA repair **Dose:** 18–30 mg/m² for 5 d, as a 30-min Inf (per protocols); ↓ w/ renal impair **Caution:** [D, −] Give cytarabine before fludarabine (↓ its metabolism) **CI:** w/ Pentostatin, severe Infxns, CrCl < 30 mL/min, hemolytic anemia **Disp:** Inj 50 mg **SE:** ↓ BM, N/V/D, ↑ LFTs, edema, CHF, fever, chills, fatigue, dyspnea, nonproductive cough, pneumonitis, severe CNS tox rare in leukemia, autoimmune hemolytic anemia **Interactions:** ↑ Effects W/ other myelosuppressive drugs; ↑ risk of pulm effects W/ pentostatin **Labs:** ↑ LFTs **NIPE:** May take several wk for full effect, use barrier contraception

Fludrocortisone Acetate (Florinef) [Steroid/Mineralocorticoid] **Uses:** *Adrenocortical Insuff, Addison Dz, salt-wasting synd* **Action:** Mineralocorticoid **Dose:** *Adults.* 0.1–0.2 mg/d PO **Peds.** 0.05–0.1 mg/d PO **Caution:** [C, ?] **CI:** Systemic fungal Infxns; known allergy **Disp:** Tabs 0.1 mg **SE:** HTN, edema, CHF, HA, dizziness, convulsions, acne, rash, bruising, hyperglycemia, hypothalamic-pituitary-adrenal suppression, cataracts **Interactions:** ↑ Risk of hypokalemia W/ amphotericin B, thiazide diuretics, loop diuretics; ↓ effects W/ rifampin, barbiturates, hydantoins; ↓ effects *OF* ASA, INH **Labs:** ↓ Serum K^+ **NIPE:** Eval for fluid retention; for adrenal Insuff, use w/ glucocorticoid; dose changes based on plasma renin activity; monitor ECG for hypokalemia (flattened T waves); monitor salt intake—may need restriction to ↓ risk of edema, wgt gain,↑ BP

Flumazenil (Romazicon) [Antidote/Benzodiazepine] **Uses:** *Reverse sedative effects of benzodiazepines & general anesthesia* **Action:** Benzodiazepine receptor antagonist **Dose:** *Adults.* 0.2 mg IV over 15 s; repeat PRN, to 1 mg max

(5 mg max in benzodiazepine OD) *Peds.* 0.01 mg/kg (0.2 mg/dose max) IV over 15 s; repeat 0.005 mg/kg at 1-min intervals to max 1 mg total; ↓ in hepatic impair **Caution:** [C, ?] **CI:** TCA OD; if pts given benzodiazepines to control life-threatening conditions (ICP/status epilepticus) **Disp:** Inj 0.1 mg/mL **SE:** N/V, palpitations, HA, anxiety, nervousness, hot flashes, tremor, blurred vision, dyspnea, hyperventilation, withdrawal synd **Interactions:** ↑ Risk of Szs & arrhythmias when benzodiazepine action is reduced **NIPE:** Food given during IV administration will reduce drug serum level; does not reverse narcotic Sx or amnesia; use associated w/ Szs; ○ driving, EtOH, OTC preps ≥ 24 h after Rx

Fluorouracil, Injection [5-FU] (Adrucil) [Antineoplastic/Antimetabolite] **WARNING:** Administration by experienced chemotherapy physician only; pts should be hospitalized for 1st course d/t risk for severe Rxn **Uses:** *Colorectal, gastric, pancreatic, breast, basal cell*, head, neck, bladder, CAs **Action:** Inhibits thymidylate synthetase (↓ DNA synth, S-phase specific) **Dose:** 370–1000 mg/m²/d × 1–5 d IV push to 24-h cont Inf; protracted venous Inf of 200–300 mg/m²/d (per protocol); 800 mg/d max **Caution:** [D, ?] ↑ Tox w/ allopurinol; do not give live vaccine before 5-FU Rx **CI:** Poor nutritional status, depressed BM Fxn, thrombocytopenia, major surgery w/in past mo, G6PD enzyme deficiency, PRG, serious Infxn, bili > 5 mg/dL **Disp:** Inj 50 mg/mL **SE:** Stomatitis, esophagopharyngitis, N/V/D, anorexia, ↓ BM, rash/dry skin/photosens, tingling in hands/feet w/ pain (palmar–plantar erythrodysesthesia), phlebitis/discoloration at Inj sites **Interactions:** ↑ Effects *W/* leucovorin Ca **Labs:** ↑ LFTs **NIPE:** ↑ Thiamine intake; N EtOH, ↑ risk of photosensitivity—use sunscreen, ↑ fluids 2–3 L/d, use barrier contraception

Fluorouracil, Topical [5-FU] (Carac, Efudex, Fluoroplex) [Antineoplastic/Antimetabolite] **Uses:** *Basal cell carcinoma (when standard therapy impractical); actinic/solar keratosis** **Action:** Inhibits thymidylate synthetase (↓ DNA synth, S-phase specific) **Dose:** 5% cream bid × 2–6 wk **Caution:** [D, ?] Irritant chemotherapy **CI:** Component sensitivity **Disp:** Cream 0.5%, 1%, 5%; soln 1, 2, 5% **SE:** Rash, dry skin, photosens **NIPE:** Healing may not be evident for 1–2 mo; wash hands thoroughly; avoid occlusive dressings; do not overuse; ○ PRG—use effective method of birth control

Fluoxetine (Gaboxetine, Prozac, Prozac Weekly, Sarafem) [Antidepressant/SSRI] **WARNING:** Closely monitor for worsening depression or emergence of suicidality, particularly in ped pt **Uses:** *Depression, OCD, panic disorder, bulimia (Prozac)** **PMDD (Sarafem)** **Action:** SSRI **Dose:** 20 mg/d PO (max 80 mg/d ÷ dose); weekly 90 mg/wk after 1–2 wk of standard dose *Bulimia:* 60 mg q AM *Panic disorder:* 20 mg/d *OCD:* 20–80 mg/d *PMDD:* 20 mg/d or 20 mg intermittently, start 14 d prior to menses, repeat w/ each cycle; ↓ in hepatic failure **Caution:** [C, ?/−] Serotonin synd w/ MAOI, SSRI, serotonin agonists, linezolid; QT prolongation w/phenothiazines; do not use w/ clopidogrel (↓ effect) **CI:**

w/ MAOI/thioridazine (wait 5 wk after D/C before MAOI) **Disp:** *Prozac:* Caps 10, 20, 40 mg; scored tabs 10, 20 mg; SR weekly caps 90 mg; soln 20 mg/5 mL *Sarafem:* Caps 10, 15, 20 mg **SE:** N, nervousness, wt loss, HA, insomnia **Interactions:** ↑ Effects W/ CNS depressants, MAOIs, EtOH, St. John's wort; ↑ effects *OF* alprazolam, BBs, carbamazepine, clozapine, cardiac glycosides, diazepam, dextromethorphan, loop diuretics, haloperidol, phenytoin, Li, ritonavir, thioridazine, tryptophan, warfarin, sympathomimetic drugs; ↓ effects W/ cyproheptadine; ↓ effects *OF* buspirone, statins **Labs:** ↑ LFTs, BUN, Cr, urine albumin **NIPE:** ↑ Risk of serotonin synd W/ St. John's wort; may take > 4 wk for full effects; ⊘ abrupt D/C; ⊘ EtOH

Fluoxymesterone (Androxy) [CIII] [Hormone] Uses: Androgen-responsive metastatic *breast CA, hypogonadism* **Action:** ↓ Secretion of LH & FSH (feedback inhibition) **Dose:** *Breast CA:* 10–40 mg/d ÷ × 1–3 mo *Hypogonadism:* 5–20 mg/d **Caution:** [X, ?/–] ↑ Effect w/ anticoagulants, cyclosporine, insulin, Li, narcotics **CI:** Serious cardiac, liver, or kidney Dz; PRG **Disp:** Tabs 10 mg **SE:** Priapism, edema, virilization, amenorrhea & menstrual irregularities, hirsutism, alopecia, acne, N, cholestasis; suppression of factors II, V, VII, & X, & polycythemia; ↑ libido, HA, anxiety **Interactions:** ↑ Effects W/ narcotics, EtOH, echinacea; ↑ effects *OF* anticoagulants, cyclosporine, insulin, hypoglycemics, tacrolimus; ↓ effects W/ anticholinergics, barbiturates **Labs:** ↑ Cr, CrCl; ↓ thyroxine-binding globulin, ↓ serum total T4 **NIPE:** Radiographic exam of hand/wrist q6mo in prepubertal children; ⊘ abrupt D/C

Flurazepam (Dalmane) [C-IV] [Sedative/Hypnotic/Benzodiazepine] Uses: *Insomnia* **Action:** Benzodiazepine **Dose:** *Adults & Peds > 15 y.* 15–30 mg PO qhs PRN; ↓ in elderly **Caution:** [X, ?/–] Elderly, low albumin, hepatic impair **CI:** NAG; PRG **Disp:** Caps 15, 30 mg **SE:** "Hangover" d/t accumulation of metabolites, apnea, anaphylaxis, angioedema, amnesia **Interactions:** ↑ CNS depression W/ antidepressants, antihistamines, opioids, EtOH; ↑ effects *OF* digoxin, phenytoin; ↑ effects W/ cimetidine, disulfiram, fluoxetine, INH, ketoconazole, metoprolol, OCPs, propranolol, SSRIs, valproic acid, chamomile, kava kava, passion flower, valerian; ↓ effects *OF* levodopa; ↓ effects W/ barbiturates, rifampin, theophylline, nicotine **Labs:** ↑ LFTs **NIPE:** ⊘ In PRG or lactation; use adequate contraception; ⊘ EtOH; N D/C abruptly w/ long-term use; may cause dependency

Flurbiprofen (Ansaid, Ocufen) [Analgesic/NSAID] **WARNING:** May ↑ risk of CV events and GI bleeding Uses: *Arthritis, ocular surgery* **Action:** NSAID **Dose:** 50–300 mg/d ÷ bid-qid, max 300 mg/d w/ food, *Ocufen:* Ocular 1 gtt q30 min × 4, beginning 2 h pre-op **Caution:** [C (D in 3rd tri), ?/–] **CI:** PRG (3rd tri); ASA allergy **Disp:** Tabs 50, 100 mg; Ocufen 0.03% opthal soln **SE:** Dizziness, GI upset, peptic ulcer Dz, ocular irritation **Interactions:** ↑ Effects W/ amprenavir, anticonvulsants, azole antifungals, BBs, CNS depressants, cimetidine, ciprofloxin, clozapine, digoxin, disulfiram, diltiazem, INH, levodopa, macrolides,

OCPs, rifampin, ritonavir, SSRIs, valproic acid, verapamil, EtOH, grapefruit juice, kava kava, valerian; ↓ effects W/ aminophylline, carbamazepine, rifampin, rifabutin, theophylline; ↓ effects OF levodopa **Labs:** ↑ LFTs **NIPE:** ⊘ PRG, breast-feeding; take w/ food to ↓ GI upset

Flutamide (Generic) [Antineoplastic/Antiandrogen] WARNING: Liver failure & death reported. Measure LFTs before, monthly, & periodically during therapy; D/C immediately if ALT 2 × ULN or jaundice develops **Uses:** Advanced *PCa* (w/ LHRH agonists, eg, leuprolide or goserelin); w/ radiation & GnRH for localized CAP **Action:** Nonsteroidal antiandrogen **Dose:** 250 mg PO tid (750 mg total) **Caution:** [D, ?] **CI:** Severe hepatic impair **Disp:** Caps 125 mg **SE:** Hot flashes, loss of libido, impotence, N/V/D, gynecomastia, hepatic failure **Interactions:** ↑ Effects W/ anticoagulants **Labs:** ↑ LFTs (monitor) **NIPE:** ⊘ EtOH; urine amber/yellow-green in color; diarrhea common SE – ↑ fluids to ↓ risk dehydration

Fluticasone Furoate, Nasal (Veramyst) [Steroid] Uses: *Seasonal allergic rhinitis* **Action:** Topical steroid **Dose:** *Adults & Peds > 12 y.* 2 sprays/nostril/d, then 1 spray/d maint *Peds 2–11 y.* 1–2 spray/nostril/d **Caution:** [C, M] Avoid w/ ritonavir, other steroids, recent nasal surgery/trauma **CI:** None **Disp:** Nasal spray 27.5 mcg/actuation **SE:** HA, epistaxis, nasopharyngitis, pyrexia, pharyngolaryngeal pain, cough, nasal ulcers, back pain, anaphylaxis **Interactions:** N Ritonavir & caution w/ potent CYP3A4 Inhib (Table 10) **NIPE:** Monitor for growth suppression in children; ↑ risk of *Candida* Infxns; prime nasal pump; may take 3–4 d to see full benefit

Fluticasone Propionate, Inhalation (Flovent HFA, Flovent Diskus) [Anti-Inflammatory/Corticosteroid] Uses: *Chronic asthma* **Action:** Topical steroid **Dose:** *Adults & Peds > 12 y.* 2–4 puffs bid *Peds 4–11 y.* 44 or 50 mcg bid **Caution:** [C, M] **CI:** Status asthmaticus **Disp:** *Diskus* dry powder: 50, 100, 250 mcg/action; *HFA*: MDI 44/110/220 mcg/Inh **SE:** HA, dysphonia, oral candidiasis **Interactions:** ↑ Effects W/ ketoconazole **Labs:** ↑ Cholesterol **NIPE:** Risk of thrush, rinse mouth after; counsel on use of devices; ⊘ for acute asthma attack

Fluticasone Propionate, Nasal (Flonase) [Anti-Inflammatory/ Corticosteroid] Uses: *Seasonal allergic rhinitis* **Action:** Topical steroid **Dose:** *Adults & Peds > 12 y.* 2 sprays/nostril/d *Peds 4–11 y.* 1–2 sprays/nostril/d **Caution:** [C, M] **CI:** Primary Rx of status asthmaticus **Disp:** Nasal spray 50 mcg/ actuation **SE:** HA, dysphonia, oral candidiasis **Interactions:** ↑ Effects W/ ketoconazole **Labs:** ↑ Glucose **NIPE:** Clear nares of exudate before use; prime nasal pump; may take 3–4 d to see full benefit

Fluticasone Propionate & Salmeterol Xinafoate (Advair Diskus, Advair HFA) [Anti-Inflammatory/Corticosteroid] WARNING: ↑ Risk of worsening wheezing or asthma-related death w/ long-acting β₂-adrenergic agonists; use only if asthma not controlled on agent such as inhaled steroid **Uses:**

Maint Rx for asthma & COPD **Action:** Corticosteroid w/ LA bronchodilator β_2 agonist **Dose:** *Adults & Peds > 12 y.* 1 Inh bid q12h; titrate to lowest effective dose (4 Inh or 920/84 mcg/d max) **Caution:** [C, M] **CI:** Acute asthma attack; conversion from PO steroids; w/ phenothiazines **Disp:** Diskus = metered-dose Inh powder (fluticasone/salmeterol in mcg) 100/50, 250/50, 500/50; HFA = aerosol 45/21, 115/21, 230/21 mg **SE:** URI, pharyngitis, HA **Interactions:** ↑ Bronchospasm *W/* BBs; ↑ hypokalemia *W/* loop & thiazide diuretics; ↑ effects *W/* ketoconazole, MAOIs, TCAs **Labs:** ↑ Cholesterol **NIPE:** Combo of Flovent & Serevent; do not wash mouthpiece; do not exhale into device; Advair HFA for pts not controlled on other meds (eg, low-medium dose Inh steroids) or whose Dz severity warrants 2 maint therapies; rinse mouth after use; ⊘ for acute asthma attack → ↑ risk asthma-related death

Fluticasone/Vilanterol (Breo Ellipta) WARNING: LABAs may ↑ risk of asthma-related death; not indicated for Tx of asthma Uses: *COPD* Action: Inhaled steroid & LABA **Dose:** *Adults.* 1 Inh 1 × day **Caution:** [C, ?/–] not for acute Sx; ↑ risk pneumonia & other Infxns; adrenal suppression/hypercorticism w/ high doses; w/ CV Dz, Sz disorders, thyrotoxicosis, DM, ketoacidosis; w/ strong CYP3A4 Inhib, MAOIs, TCAs, beta-blockers, diuretics, other LABAs **CI:** Hypersens to milk protein/components **Disp:** Inh powder (fluticasone/vilanterol) 100 mcg/25 mcg/blister **SE:** Nasopharyngitis, URI, HA, oral candidiasis, ↑ glucose, ↓ K⁺, glaucoma, cataracts, ↓ BMD, paradoxical bronchospasm **NIPE:** After Inh rinse mouth w/o swallowing to ↓ risk of candidiasis; ⊘ for acute asthma attack

Fluvastatin (Lescol) [Antilipemic/HMG-CoA Reductase Inhibitor]
Uses: *Atherosclerosis, primary hypercholesterolemia, heterozygous familial hypercholesterolemia hypertriglyceridemia* **Action:** HMG-CoA reductase Inhib **Dose:** 20–40 mg bid PO or XL 80 mg/d ↓ w/ hepatic impair **Caution:** [X, –] **CI:** Active liver Dz, ↑ LFTs, PRG, breast-feeding **Disp:** Caps 20, 40 mg; XL 80 mg **SE:** HA, dyspepsia, N/D, Abd pain **Interactions:** ↑ Effects *W/* azole antifungals, cimetidine, danazol, glyburide, macrolides, phenytoin, ritonavir, EtOH; ↑ effects *OF* diclofenac, glyburide, phenytoin, warfarin; ↓ effects *W/* cholestyramine, colestipol, isradipine, rifampin **Labs:** ↑ LFTs, (monitor) **NIPE:** Dose no longer limited to hs; ↑ photosensitivity—use sunblock; OK w/ grapefruit; follow ↓ fat, ↓ chol diet; limit EtOH

Fluvoxamine (Luvox CR) [Antidepressant/SSRI] WARNING: Closely monitor for worsening depression or emergence of suicidality, particularly in ped pts
Uses: *OCD, SAD* **Action:** SSRI **Dose:** Initial 50-mg single qhs dose, ↑ to 300 mg/d in ÷ doses; CR: 100–300 mg PO qhs, may ↑ by 50 mg/d qwk, max 300 mg/d ↓ in elderly/hepatic impair, titrate slowly; ÷ doses > 100 mg **Caution:** [C, ?/–] Multiple interactions (see PI: MAOIs, phenothiazines, SSRIs, serotonin agonists, others); do not use w/ clopidogrel **CI:** MAOI w/in 14 d; w/ alosetron, tizanidine, thioridazine, pimozide **Disp:** Tabs 25, 50, 100 mg; caps ER 100, 150 mg **SE:** HA, N/D, somnolence, insomnia **Interactions:** ↑ Effects *W/* melatonin,

MAOIs; ↑ effects *OF* BBs, benzodiazepines, methadone, carbamazepine, haloperidol, Li, phenytoin, TCAs, theophylline, warfarin, St. John's wort; ↑ risks of serotonin synd *W/* buspirone, dexfenfluramine, fenfluramine, tramadol, nefazodone, sibutramine, tryptophan; ↓ effects *W/* buspirone, cyproheptadine, tobacco; ↓ effects *OF* buspirone, HMG-CoA reductase Inhibs **Labs:** ↓ Na⁺ **NIPE:** ⊘ MAOIs for 14 d before start of drug; take hs; ⊘ EtOH; gradual taper to D/C

Folic Acid, Injectable, Oral (Generic) [Vitamin Supplement]
Uses: *Megaloblastic anemia; folate deficiency* **Action:** Dietary supls **Dose:** *Adults. Supls:* 0.4 mg/d PO *PRG:* 0.8 mg/d PO *Folate deficiency:* 1 mg PO daily–tid *Peds. Supls:* 0.04–0.4 mg/24 h PO, IM, IV, or SQ *Folate deficiency:* 0.5–1 mg/24 h PO, IM, IV, or SQ **Caution:** [A, +] **CI:** Pernicious, aplastic, normocytic anemias **Disp:** Tabs 0.4, 0.8, 1 mg; Inj 5 mg/mL **SE:** Well tolerated **Interactions:** ↓ Effects *W/* anticonvulsants, sulfasalazine, aminosalicyclic acid, chloramphenicol, MTX, OCPs, pyrimethamine, triamterene, TMP; ↓ effects *OF* phenobarbital, phenytoin **NIPE:** OK for all women of child-bearing age; ↓ fetal neural tube defects by 50%; no effect on normocytic anemias; take with full glass water

Fondaparinux (Arixtra) [Anticoagulant/Factor X Inhibitor]
WARNING: When epidural/spinal anesthesia or spinal puncture is used, pts anticoagulated or scheduled to be anticoagulated w/ LMW heparins, heparinoids, or fondaparinux are at risk for epidural or spinal hematoma, which can result in long-term or permanent paralysis **Uses:** *DVT prophylaxis* w/ hip fracture, hip or knee replacement, Abd surgery; w/ DVT or PE in combo w/ warfarin **Action:** Synth Inhib of activated factor X; a pentasaccharide **Dose:** Prophylaxis 2.5 mg SQ daily, up to 5–9 d; start > 6 h post-op; Tx: 7.5 mg SQ daily (< 50 kg; 5 mg SQ daily; > 100 kg: 10 mg SQ daily); ↓ w/ renal impair **Caution:** [B, ?] ↑ Bleeding risk w/ anticoagulants, anti-plts, drotrecogin alfa, NSAIDs **CI:** Wgt < 50 kg, CrCl < 30 mL/min, active bleeding, SBE ↓ plt w/ anti-plt Ab **Disp:** Prefilled syringes w/ 27-gauge needle: 2.5/0.5, 5/0.4, 7.5/0.6, 10/0.8 mg/mL **SE:** Thrombocytopenia, anemia, fever, N **Interactions:** ↑ Effects *W/* anticoagulants, cephalosporins, NSAIDs, PCNs, salicylates **Labs:** ↑ LFTs; ↓ HMG, Hct, plts **NIPE:** D/C if plts < 100,000 cells/mm³; only give SQ; may monitor antifactor Xa levels; ⊘ give if < 110 lbs; bleeding precautions

Formoterol Fumarate (Foradil, Performist) [Bronchodilator/ Beta-2-Adrenergic Agonist] **WARNING:** May ↑ risk of asthma-related death **Uses:** *Long-term Rx of bronchoconstriction in COPD, EIB (only Foradil)* **Action:** LA β₂ agonist **Dose:** *Adults. Performist:* 20-mcg Inh q12h *Foradil:* 12-mcg Inh q12h, 24 mcg/d max *EIB:* 12 mcg 15 min before exercise *Peds > 5 y. Foradil:* See Adults **Caution:** [C, M] Not for acute Sx, w/ CV Dz, w/ adrenergic meds, xanthine derivatives meds that ↑ QT; BBs may ↓ effect, D/C w/ ECG change **CI:** None **Disp:** *Foradil* caps 12 mcg for Aerolizer inhaler (12 & 60 doses); *Performist:* 20 mcg/2 mL for inhaler **SE:** N/D, nasopharyngitis, dry mouth, angina, HTN, ↓ BP, tachycardia, arrhythmias, nervousness, HA, tremor, muscle cramps, palpitations, dizziness **Interactions:** ↑ Effects *W/* adrenergics; ↑ effects *OF* BBs; ↑ risk of hypokalemia *W/* corticosteroids, diuretics, xanthins; ↑ risk of arrhythmias *W/* MAOIs, TCAs **Labs:** ↑ Glucose; ↓ K+ **NIPE:** Do not swallow caps; only use w/ inhaler; do not start w/ worsening or acutely deteriorating asthma; excess use may ↑ CV risks; not for oral use

Fosamprenavir (Lexiva) [Antiretroviral/Protease Inhibitor]
WARNING: Do not use w/ severe liver dysfunction, reduce dose w/ mild–mod liver impair (fosamprenavir 700 mg bid w/o ritonavir) **Uses:** HIV Infxn **Action:** Protease Inhib **Dose:** 1400 mg bid w/o ritonavir; w/ ritonavir, fosamprenavir 1400 mg + ritonavir 200 mg daily or fosamprenavir 700 mg + ritonavir 100 mg bid; w/ efavirenz & ritonavir: fosamprenavir 1400 mg + ritonavir 300 mg daily **Caution:** [C, ?/–] Do not use w/ salmeterol, colchicine (w/ renal/hepatic failure); adjust dose w/ bosentan, tadalafil for PAH **CI:** w/ CYP3A4 drugs (Table 10) such as w/ rifampin, lovastatin, simvastatin, delavirdine, ergot alkaloids, midazolam, triazolam, or pimozide; sulfa allergy; w/ alpha 1-adrenoceptor antagonist (alfuzosin); w/ PDE5 Inhibitor sildenafil **Disp:** Tabs 700 mg; susp 50 mg/mL **SE:** N/V/D, HA, fatigue, rash **Interactions:** ↑ Effects *W/* indinavir, nelfinavir; ↑ effects *OF* antiarrhythmics, amitriptyline, atorvastatin, benzodiazepine, bepridil, CCBs, cyclosporine, ergotamine, ethinyl estradiol, imipramine, itraconazole, ketoconazole, midazolam, norethindrone, rapamycin, rifabutin, sildenafil, tacrolimus, TCA, vardenafil, warfarin; ↓ effects *W/* antacids, carbamazepine, dexamethasone, didanosine, efavirenz, H₂-receptor antagonists, nevirapine, phenobarbital, phenytoin, PPIs, rifampin St. John's wort; ↓ effects *OF* methadone **Labs:** ↑ LFTs; triglycerides, lipase; ↓ neutrophils **NIPE:** Take tabs w/o regard to food; adult liquid – take w/o food; pediatric liquid—okay to take w/ food; use barrier contraception; monitor for opportunistic Infxn; inform about fat redistribution/accumulation; replaced amprenavir

Fosaprepitant (Emend, Injection) [Substance P/Neurokinin-1 Receptor Antagonist] **Uses:** *Prevent chemotherapy-associated N/V* **Action:** Substance P/neurokinin 1 receptor antagonist **Dose:** *Chemotherapy:* 150 mg IV 30 min before chemotherapy on d 1 (followed by aprepitant [*Emend, Oral*] 80 mg PO days 2 and 3) in combo w/ other antiemetics **Caution:** [B, ?/–] Potential for drug interactions, substrate and mod CYP3A4 Inhib (dose dependent); ↓ effect of OCP and warfarin **CI:** w/ Pimozide, terfenadine, astemizole, or cisapride **Disp:** Inj 115 mg **SE:** N/D, weakness, hiccups, dizziness, HA, dehydration, hot flushing, dyspepsia, Abd pain, neutropenia, ↑ LFTs; Inf site discomfort **Interactions:** ↑ Effects *OF* dexamethasone, methylprednisolone, midazolam, alprazolam, triazolam; ↓ effect *OF* OCP & warfarin, phenytoin, tolbutamide **Labs:** ↑ LFTs; monitor INR **NIPE:** Inj site discomfort; see also Aprepitant (*Emend, Oral*)

Foscarnet (Foscavir) [Antiviral] **Uses:** *CMV retinitis; acyclovir-resistant *herpes Infxns* **Action:** ↓ Viral DNA polymerase & RT **Dose:** *CMV retinitis: Induction:* 90 mg/kg q12h or 60 mg/kg IV q8h × 14–21 d *Maint:* 90–120 mg/kg/d IV (Mon–Fri). *Acyclovir-resistant HSV: Induction:* 40 mg/kg IV q8–12h ×

14–21 d; use central line; ↓ w/ renal impair **Caution:** [C, –] ↑ Sz potential w/ fluoroquinolones; avoid nephrotoxic Rx (cyclosporine, aminoglycosides, amphotericin B, protease Inhib) **CI:** CrCl < 0.4 mL/min/kg **Disp:** Inj 24 mg/mL **SE:** Nephrotox, electrolyte abnormalities **Interactions:** ↑ Risks of Sz w/ quinolones; ↑ risks of nephrotox W/ aminoglycosides, amphotericin B, didanosine, pentamidine, vancomycin **Labs:** ↑ LFTs, BUN, SCr; ↓ Hgb, Hct, Ca^{2+}, Mg^{2+}, K^+, P; monitor ionized Ca^{2+} **NIPE:** ↑ Fluids; perioral tingling, extremity numbness & paresthesia indicates lytes imbalance; Na loading (500 mL 0.9% NaCl) before & after helps minimize nephrotox; infuse over 1–2 h

Fosfomycin (Monurol) [Antibiotic]
Uses: *Uncomplicated UTI* **Action:** ↓ Cell wall synth *Spectrum:* Gram(+) *Enterococcus*, staphylococci, pneumococci; gram(–) (*E coli, Salmonella, Shigella, H influenzae, Neisseria*), indole(–) *Proteus, Providencia*); *B fragilis* & anaerobic gram(–) cocci are resistant **Dose:** 3 g PO in 90–120 mL of H_2O single dose; ↓ in renal impair **Caution:** [B, ?] ↓ Absorption w/ antacids/Ca salts **CI:** Component sensitivity **Disp:** Granule packets 3 g **SE:** HA, GI upset **Interactions:** ↓ Effects W/ antacids, metoclopramide **Labs:** ↑ LFTs; ↓ Hgb, Hct **NIPE:** May take w/o food; mix powder with 3–4 oz cold water–⊘ hot water; may take 2–3 d for Sxs to improve

Fosinopril (Monopril) [Antihypertensive/ACEI]
Uses: *HTN, CHF*, DN **Action:** ACE Inhib **Dose:** 10 mg/d PO initial; max 40 mg/d PO; ↓ in elderly; ↓ in renal impair **Caution:** [D, +] ↑ K^+ w/ K^+ supls, ARBs, K^+-sparing diuretics; ↑ renal after effects w/ NSAIDs, diuretics, hypovolemia **CI:** Hereditary/idiopathic angioedema or angioedema w/ ACE Inhib, bilateral RAS **Disp:** Tabs 10, 20, 40 mg **SE:** Cough, dizziness, angioedema, ↑ K^+ **Interactions:** ↑ Effects W/ antihypertensives, diuretics; ↑ effects OF Li; ↑ risk of hyperkalemia W/ K^+-sparing diuretics, salt substitutes; ↑ cough W/ capsaicin; ↓ effects W/ antacids, ASA, NSAIDs **Labs:** ↑ LFTs, K^+; ↓ Hgb, Hct **NIPE:** ⊘ PRG, breast-feeding; avoid EtOH to ↓ risk of hypotension

Fosphenytoin (Cerebyx) [Anticonvulsant/Hydantoin]
Uses: *Status epilepticus* **Action:** ↓ Sz spread in motor cortex **Dose:** As phenytoin equivalents (PE) *Load:* 15–20 mg PE/kg *Maint:* 4–6 mg PE/kg/d; ↓ dosage, monitor levels in hepatic impair **Caution:** [D, +] May ↑ phenobarbital **CI:** Sinus bradycardia, SA block, 2nd-/3rd-degree AV block, Adams–Stokes synd, rash during Rx **Disp:** Inj 75 mg/mL **SE:** ↓ BP, dizziness, ataxia, pruritus, nystagmus **Interactions:** ↑ Effects W/ amiodarone, chloramphenicol, cimetidine, diazepam, disulfiram, estrogens, INH, omeprazole, phenothiazine, salicylates, sulfonamides, tolbutamide; ↓ effects W/ TCAs, anti-TB drugs, carbamazepine, EtOH, nutritional supls, ginkgo; ↓ effects OF anticoagulants, corticosteroids, digitoxin, doxycycline, OCPs, folic acid, Ca, vit D, rifampin, quinidine, theophylline **Labs:** ↑ Serum glucose, alk phos; ↓ serum thyroxine, Ca **NIPE:** Breast-feeding, for short-term use; 15 min to convert fosphenytoin to phenytoin; administer < 150 mg PE/min to prevent ↓ BP; administer w/ cardiac monitoring

Frovatriptan (Frova) [Migraine Suppressant/5-HT Agonist]
Uses: *Rx acute migraine* Action: Vascular serotonin receptor agonist Dose: 2.5 mg PO repeat in 2 h PRN; max 7.5 mg/d Caution: [C, ?/–] Angina, ischemic heart Dz, coronary artery vasospasm, hemiplegic or basilar migraine, uncontrolled HTN, ergot use, MAOI use w/in 14 d Disp: Tabs 2.5 mg SE: N, V, dizziness, hot flashes, paresthesias, dyspepsia, dry mouth, hot/cold sensation, CP, skeletal pain, flushing, weakness, numbness, coronary vasospasm Interactions: ↑ Vasoactive Rxn W/ ergot drugs; serotonin 5-HT₁ agonists; ↑ effects W/ hormonal contraceptives, propranolol; ↑ risk of serotonin synd W/ SSRIs NIPE: Risk of photosensitivity; reports of severe cardiac events w/ this drug; overuse ↑ risk rebound headache

Fulvestrant (Faslodex) [Antineoplastic/Antiestrogen] Uses: *HR(+) metastatic breast CA in postmenopausal women w/ progression following antiestrogen Rx therapy* Action: Estrogen receptor antagonist Dose: 500 mg days 1, 15, & 29; maint 500 mg IM mo Inj in buttocks Caution: [X, ?/–] ↑ Effects w/ CYP3A4 Inhib (Table 10); w/ hepatic impair CI: PRG Disp: Prefilled syringes 50 mg/mL (single 5 mL, dual 2.5 mL) SE: N/V/D, constipation, Abd pain, HA, back pain, hot flushes, pharyngitis, Inj site Rxns Interactions: ↑ Risk of bleeding W/ anticoagulants NIPE: ⊘ PRG, breast-feeding; use barrier contraception; only use IM

Furosemide (Lasix) [Antihypertensive/Loop Diuretic] Uses: *CHF, HTN, edema*, ascites Action: Loop diuretic; ↓ Na & Cl reabsorption in ascending loop of Henle & distal tubule Dose: Adults. 20–80 mg PO or IV bid Peds. 1 mg/kg/ dose IV q6–12h; 2 mg/kg/dose PO q12–24h (max 6 mg/kg/dose); ↑ doses w/ renal impair Caution: [C, +] ↓ K⁺, ↑ risk digoxin tox & ototox w/ aminoglycosides, cisplatin (especially in renal dysfunction) CI: Sulfonylurea allergy; anuria; hepatic coma; electrolyte depletion Disp: Tabs 20, 40, 80 mg; soln 10 mg/mL, 40 mg/5 mL; Inj 10 mg/mL SE: ↓ BP, hyperglycemia, ↓ K⁺ Interactions: ↑ Nephrotoxic effects W/ cephalosporins; risk of digoxin tox & ototox W/ aminoglycosides, cisplatin (esp in renal dysfunction); ↑ risk of hypokalemia W/ antihypertensives, carbenoxolone, corticosteroids, digitalis glycosides, terbutaline; ↓ effects W/ barbiturates, cholestyramine, colestipol, NSAIDs, phenytoin, dandelion, ginseng; ↓ effects OF hypoglycemics Labs: ↑ BUN, Cr; cholesterol, glucose, uric acid, ↓ serum K⁺, Na⁺, Ca²⁺, Mg²⁺, monitor lytes, renal Fxn NIPE: Risk of photosensitivity—use sunblock; high doses IV may cause ototox; monitor BP with IV; monitor ECG for hypokalemia (flattened T waves); monitor lytes; may cause dizziness—caution driving, changing positions

Gabapentin (Neurontin) [Anticonvulsant] Uses: Adjunct in *partial Szs; postherpetic neuralgia (PHN)*; chronic pain synds Action: Anticonvulsant; GABA analogue Dose: Adults & Peds > 12 y. Anticonvulsant: 300 mg PO tid, ↑ max 3600 mg/d. PHN: 300 mg d 1, 300 mg bid d 2, 300 mg tid d 3, titrate (1800–3600 mg/d) Peds 3–12 y. 10–15 mg/kg/d ÷ tid, ↑ over 3 d; 3–4 y. 40 mg/kg/d given tid; ≥ 5 y. 25–35 mg/kg/d ÷ tid, 50 mg/kg/d max; ↓ w/ renal impair Caution: [C, ?] Use in peds 3–12 y w/ epilepsy may ↑ CNS-related adverse events CI:

Component sensitivity **Disp:** Caps 100, 300, 400 mg; soln 250 mg/5 mL; scored tab 600, 800 mg **SE:** Somnolence, dizziness, ataxia, fatigue **Interactions:** ↑ Effects *W/* CNS depressants; ↓ effects *W/* antacids, ginkgo **Labs:** ↓ WBCs; **NIPE:** Take w/o regard to food; not necessary to monitor levels; do not stop suddenly, taper ↑ or ↓ over 1 wk; report mood changes, thoughts of suicide

Gabapentin Enacarbil (Horizant)   **Uses:** *RLS* **Action:** GABA analog; ? mechanism **Dose:** Adult. CrCl > 60 mL/min: 600 mg PO 1 ×/d; 30–59 mL/min: 300 mg 1 ×/d (max 600 mg/d); 15–29 mL/min: 300 mg 1 ×/d; < 15 mL/min: 300 mg qod **Caution:** [C, ?/–] **Disp:** Tabs ER 300, 600 mg **SE:** Somnolence, sedation, fatigue, dizziness, HA, blurred vision, feeling drunk, disorientation; ↓ libido, depression, suicidal thoughts/ behaviors, multiorgan hypersensitivity; ↑ effects *W/* CNS depressants; ↓ effects *W/* antacids, ginkgo **Labs:** ↓ WBCs **NIPE:** Not recommended w/ hemodialysis; regular night time sleepers take w/ food at 5 PM, daytime sleepers take in AM; swallow whole; do not cut/crush/chew

Galantamine (Razadyne, Razadyne ER) [Cholinesterase Inhibitor]   **Uses:** *Mild–mod Alzheimer Dz* **Action:** ? Acetylcholinesterase Inhib **Dose:** *Razadyne:* 4 mg PO bid, ↑ to 8 mg bid after 4 wk; may ↑ to 16 mg bid in 4 wk; target 16–24 mg/d ÷ bid. *Razadyne ER:* Start 8 mg/d, ↑ to 16 mg/d after 4 wk, then to 24 mg/d after 4 more wk; give qAM w/ food **Caution:** [B, ?] w/ Heart block, ↑ effect w/ succinylcholine, bethanechol, amiodarone, diltiazem, verapamil, NSAIDs, digoxin; ↓ effect w/ anticholinergics; ↑ risk of death w/ mild impair **CI:** Severe renal/hepatic impair **Disp:** *Razadyne* Tabs 4, 8, 12 mg; soln 4 mg/mL; *Razadyne ER* caps 8, 16, 24 mg **SE:** GI disturbances, ↓ wgt, sleep disturbances, dizziness, HA **Interactions:** ↑ Effects *W/* amiodarone, amitriptyline, bethanechol, cimetidine, digoxin, diltiazem, erythromycin, fluoxetine, fluvoxamine, ketoconazole, NSAIDs, paroxetine, quinidine, succinylcholine, verapamil; ↓ effect *W/* anticholinergics **Labs:** ↓ HMG, Hct **NIPE:** ↑ Dosage q4wk, if D/C several d then restart at lowest dose; take in AM w/food & maint adequate fluid intake; do no cut/crush/chew; limit alcohol; caution w/ urinary outflow obst, Parkinson Dz, severe asthma/COPD, severe heart Dz or ↓ BP; monitor ECG for conduction abnormalities

Gallium Nitrate (Ganite) [Hormone]   **WARNING:** ↑ Risk of severe renal Insuff w/ concurrent use of nephrotoxic drugs (eg, aminoglycosides, amphotericin B). D/C if use of potentially nephrotoxic drug is indicated; hydrate several d after administration. D/C w/ SCr > 2.5 mg/dL **Uses:** *↑ Ca²⁺ of malignancy*; bladder CA **Action:** ↓ Bone resorption of Ca²⁺ **Dose:** ↑ Ca²⁺: 100–200 mg/m²/d × 5 d. *CA:* 350 mg/m² cont Inf × 5 d to 700 mg/m² rapid IV Inf q2wk in antineoplastic settings (per protocols), Inf over 24 h **Caution:** [C, ?] Do not give w/ live or rotavirus vaccine **CI:** SCr > 2.5 mg/dL **Disp:** Inj 25 mg/mL **SE:** Renal Insuff, ↓ Ca²⁺, hypophosphatemia, ↓ bicarb, < 1% acute optic neuritis **Interactions:** ↑ Risks of nephrotox *W/* amphotericin B, aminoglycosides, vancomycin **NIPE:** Monitor BUN, SCr, adequate fluids; avoid foods ↑ in calcium; bladder

CA, use in combo w/ vinblastine & ifosfamide; monitor ECG for cardiac conduction abnormalities

Ganciclovir (Cytovene, Vitrasert) [Antiviral/Synthetic Nucleoside] Uses: *Rx & prevent CMV retinitis, prevent CMV Dz* in transplant recipients **Action:** ↓ viral DNA synth **Dose:** *Adults & Peds. IV:* 5 mg/kg IV q12h for 14–21 d, then maint 5 mg/kg/d IV × 7 d/wk or 6 mg/kg/d IV × 5 d/wk. *Ocular implant:* 1 implant q5–8mo *Adults.* PO: Following induction, 1000 mg PO tid. *Prevention:* 1000 mg PO tid; w/ food; ↓ in renal impair **Caution:** [C, −] ↑ Effect w/ immunosuppressives, imipenem/cilastatin, zidovudine, didanosine, other nephrotoxic Rx **CI:** ANC < 500 cells/mm³, plt < 25,000 cells/mm³, intravitreal implant **Disp:** Caps 250, 500 mg; Inj 500 mg, ocular implant 4.5 mg **SE:** Granulocytopenia & thrombocytopenia, fever, rash, GI upset **Interactions:** ↑ Effects *W/* cytotoxic drugs, immunosuppressive drugs, probenecid; ↑ risks of nephrotox *W/* amphotericin B, cyclosporine; ↑ effects *W/* didanosine **Labs:** ↑ LFTs; ↓ blood glucose **NIPE:** Take w/ food; ⊘ PRG, breast-feeding, EtOH, NSAIDs; photosensitivity— use sunblock; not a cure for CMV; handle Inj w/ cytotoxic cautions; no systemic benefit w/ implant

Ganciclovir, Ophthalmic Gel (Zirgan) [Nucleoside Analogue] Uses: *Acute herpetic keratitis (dendritic ulcers)* **Action:** ↓ Viral DNA synth **Dose:** *Adult & Peds ≥ 2 y.* 1 gtt affected eye/s 5 × daily (q3h while awake) until ulcer heals, then 1 gtt tid × 7 d **Caution:** [C, ?/−] Remove contacts during Tx **CI:** None **Disp:** Gel, 5-g tube **SE:** Blurred vision, eye irritation, punctate keratitis, conjunctival hyperemia **Labs:** Correct ↓ Ca²⁺ before use; ✓ Ca²⁺ **NIPE:** Remove contact lenses during Tx; may cause blurred vision—caution driving

Gemcitabine (Gemzar) [Antineoplastic/Nucleoside Analogue] Uses: *Pancreatic CA (single agent), breast CA w/ paclitaxel, NSCLC w/ cisplatin, ovarian CA w/ carboplatin*, gastric CA **Action:** Antimetabolite; nucleoside metabolic inhibitor; ↓ ribonucleotide reductase; produces false nucleotide base-inhibiting DNA synth **Dose:** 1000–1250 mg/m² over 30 min–1 h IV Inf/wk × 3–4 wk or 6–8 wk; modify dose based on hematologic Fxn (per protocol) **Caution:** [D, ?/−] **CI:** PRG **Disp:** Inj 200 mg, 1 g **SE:** ↓ BM, N/V/D, drug fever, skin rash **Interactions:** ↑ BM depression *W/* radiation Tx, antineoplastic drugs; ↓ live virus vaccines **Labs:** ↑ LFTs, BUN, SCr (monitor) **NIPE:** ⊘ EtOH, NSAIDs, immunizations, PRG; reconstituted soln stable 38 mg/mL

Gemfibrozil (Lopid) [Antilipemic/Fibric Acid Derivative] Uses: *Hypertriglyceridemia, coronary heart Dz* **Action:** Fibric acid **Dose:** 1200 mg/d PO ÷ bid 30 min ac AM & PM **Caution:** [C, ?] ↑ Warfarin effect, sulfonylureas; ↑ risk of myopathy w/ HMG-CoA reductase inhib; ↓ effects w/ cyclosporine **CI:** Renal/hepatic impair (SCr > 2.0 mg/dL), gallbladder Dz, primary biliary cirrhosis, use w/ repaglinide (↓ glucose) **Disp:** Tabs 600 mg **SE:** Cholelithiasis, GI upset **Interactions:** ↑ Effects *OF* anticoagulants, sulfonylureas; ↑ risk of rhabdomyolysis *W/* HMG-CoA reductase Inhibs; ↓ effects *W/* rifampin; ↓ effects

OF cyclosporine **Labs:** ↑ LFTs & serum lipids (monitor) **NIPE:** Avoid w/ HMG-CoA reductase Inhib; take 30 min before AM or PM meal

Gemifloxacin (Factive) [Antibiotic/Fluoroquinolone]

Uses: *CAP, acute exacerbation of chronic bronchitis* **Action:** ↓ DNA gyrase & topoisomerase IV *Spectrum:* S pneumoniae (including multidrug-resistant strains), H influenzae, H parainfluenzae, M catarrhalis, M pneumoniae, C pneumoniae, K pneumoniae **Dose:** 320 mg PO daily × 5–7 d; CrCl < 40 mL/min: 160 mg PO/d **Caution:** [C, ?/–]; Peds < 18 y; Hx of ↑ QTc interval, electrolyte disorders, w/ class IA/III antiarrhythmics, erythromycin, TCAs, antipsychotics, ↑ INR and bleeding risk w/ warfarin **CI:** Fluoroquinolone allergy **Disp:** Tabs 320 mg **SE:** Rash, N/V/D, C difficile enterocolitis, ↑ risk of Achilles tendon rupture, tendonitis, Abd pain, dizziness, xerostomia, arthralgia, allergy/anaphylactic Rxns, peripheral neuropathy, tendon rupture **Interactions:** ↑ Risk of prolonged QT interval *W/* amiodarone, antipsychotics, erythromycin, procainamide, quinidine, sotalol, TCAs; ↑ effect *OF* warfarin; ↑ effects *W/* probenecid; ↓ effects *W/* antacids, didanosine, Fe, sucralfate **Labs:** ↑ LFTs **NIPE:** ↑ Fluid intake; D/C if c/o tenderness/pain in muscles/tendons; ⊘ excessive sunlight exposure—use sunblock; take 3 h before or 2 h after Al/Mg antacids, Fe^{2+}, Zn^{2+} or other metal cations; ↑ rash risk w/ ↑ duration of therapy; monitor ECG for ↑ QT interval; ↑ risk ↑ or ↓ BG—closely monitor BG in DM

Gentamicin, Injectable (Generic) [Antibiotic/Aminoglycoside]

Uses: *Septicemia, serious bacterial Infxn of CNS, urinary tract, resp tract, GI tract, including peritonitis, skin, bone, soft tissue, including burns; severe Infxn P aeruginosa w/ carbenicillin; group D streptococci endocarditis w/ PCN-type drug; serious staphylococcal Infxns, but not the antibiotic of 1st choice; mixed Infxn w/ staphylococci & gram(–)* **Action:** Aminoglycoside, bactericidal; ↓ protein synth *Spectrum:* gram(–) (not Neisseria, Legionella, Acinetobacter); weaker gram(+) but synergy w/ PCNs **Dose: Adults.** *Standard:* 1–2 mg/kg IV q8–12h or daily dosing 4–7 mg/kg q24h IV. *Gram(+) Synergy:* 1 mg/kg q8h **Peds. Infants < 7 d < 1200 g.** 2.5 mg/kg/dose q18–24h **Infants > 1200 g.** 2.5 mg/kg/dose q12–18h **Infants > 7 d.** 2.5 mg/kg/dose IV q8–12h **Children.** 2.5 mg/kg/d IV q8h; ↓ w/ renal Insuff; if obese, dose based on IBW **Caution:** [C, +/–] Avoid other nephrotoxics **CI:** Aminoglycoside sensitivity **Disp:** Premixed Inf 40, 60, 70, 80, 90, 100, 120 mg; ADD-Vantage Inj vials 10 mg/mL; Inj 40 mg/mL; IT preservative-free 2 mg/mL **SE:** Nephro-/oto-/neurotox **Notes:** *Levels: Peak:* 30 min after Inf; *Trough:* < 0.5 h before next dose; *Therapeutic: Peak:* 5–8 mcg/mL; *Trough:* < 2 mcg/mL, if > 2 mcg/mL associated w/ renal tox **Interactions:** ↑ Ototox, neurotox, nephrotox *W/* aminoglycosides, amphotericin B, cephalosporins, loop diuretics, PCNs; ↑ effects *W/* NSAIDs; ↓ effects *W/* carbenicillin **Labs:** Monitor CrCl, SCr, & serum conc for dose adjustments; ↑ LFTs, BUN, Cr; ↓ HMG, Hct, plts, WBC **NIPE:** Photosensitivity—use sunblock; use IBW to dose (use adjusted if obese > 30% IBW); OK to use intraperitoneal for peritoneal dialysis-related Infxns; report hearing problems

Gentamicin, Ophthalmic (Garamycin, Genoptic, Gentak, Generic) [Antibiotic] Uses: *Conjunctival Infxns* Action: Bactericidal; ↓ protein synth **Dose:** *Oint:* Apply 1/2 in bid–tid. *Soln:* 1–2 gtt q2–4h, up to 2 gtt/h for severe Infxn **Caution:** [C, ?] CI: Aminoglycoside sensitivity **Disp:** Soln & oint 0.1% & 0.3% **SE:** Local irritation **NIPE:** Do not use other eye drops w/in 5–10 min; ⊘ touch dropper to eye

Gentamicin, Topical (Generic) [Antibiotic] Uses: *Skin Infxns* caused by susceptible organisms **Action:** Bactericidal; ↓ protein synth **Dose:** *Adults & Peds > 1 y.* Apply tid–qid **Caution:** [C, ?] CI: Aminoglycoside sensitivity **Disp:** Cream & oint 0.1% **SE:** Irritation **NIPE:** ⊘ apply to large denuded areas

Gentamicin & Prednisolone, Ophthalmic (Pred-G Ophthalmic) [Antibiotic/Anti-Inflammatory] Uses: *Steroid-responsive ocular & conjunctival Infxns* sensitive to gentamicin **Action:** Bactericidal; ↓ protein synth w/ anti-inflammatory. *Spectrum: Staphylococcus, E coli, H influenzae, Klebsiella, Neisseria, Pseudomonas, Proteus, & Serratia* sp **Dose:** *Oint:* 1/2 in in conjunctival sac daily–tid. *Susp:* 1 gtt bid–qid, up to 1 gtt/h for severe Infxns **CI:** Aminoglycoside sensitivity **Caution:** [C, ?] **Disp:** *Oint, ophthal:* Prednisolone acetate 0.6% & gentamicin sulfate 0.3% (3.5 g). *Susp, ophthal:* Prednisolone acetate 1% & gentamicin sulfate 0.3% (2, 5, 10 mL) **SE:** Local irritation **NIPE:** Systemic effects w/ long-term use; ⊘ use > 10 d

Glimepiride (Amaryl, Generic) [Hypoglycemic/Sulfonylurea] Uses: *Type 2 DM* Action: Sulfonylurea; ↑ pancreatic insulin release; ↑ peripheral insulin sensitivity; ↓ hepatic glucose output/production **Dose:** 1–4 mg/d, max 8 mg **Caution:** [C, –] CI: DKA **Disp:** Tabs 1, 2, 4 mg **SE:** HA, N, hypoglycemia **Interactions:** ↑ Effects W/ ACEIs, adrenergic antagonists, BBs, chloramphenicol, MAOIs, NSAIDs, probenecid, salicylates, sulfonamides, warfarin, ginseng, garlic; ↓ effects W/ corticosteroids, estrogens, INH, OCPs, nicotinic acid, phenytoin, sympathomimetics, thiazide diuretics, thyroid hormones **Labs:** ↑ LFTs, BUN, Cr; ↓ HMG, Hct, plts, WBC, RBC, glucose **NIPE:** Antabuse-like effect w/ EtOH (rare); give w/ 1st meal of d; BB may mask hypoglycemia; photosensitivity—use sunscreen

Glimepiride/Pioglitazone (Duetact) [Hypoglycemic/Sulfonylurea/Thiazolidinedione] WARNING: Thiazolidinediones, including pioglitazone, cause or exacerbate CHF. Not recommended in pts w/ symptomatic heart failure. CI w/ NYHA Class III or IV heart failure. **Uses:** *Adjunct to exercise type 2 DM not controlled by single agent* **Action:** Sulfonylurea (↓ glucose) w/ agent that ↑ insulin sensitivity & ↓ gluconeogenesis **Dose:** Initial 30 mg/2 mg PO qAM; 45 mg pioglitazone/8 mg glimepiride/d max; w/ food **Caution:** [C, ?/–] w/ Liver impair, elderly, w/ Hx bladder CA **CI:** Component hypersens, DKA **Disp:** Tabs 30/2, 30 mg/4 mg **SE:** Hct, ↑ ALT, ↓ glucose, URI, ↑ wgt, edema, HA, N/D, may ↑ CV mortality **Interactions:** ↑ Effects W/ ACEIs, adrenergic antagonists, BBs, chloramphenicol, MAOIs, NSAIDs, probenecid, salicylates, sulfonamides, warfarin, ginseng, garlic; ↓ effects W/ corticosteroids, estrogens, INH, OCPs, nicotinic acid, phenytoin, sympathomimetics, thiazide diuretics, thyroid hormones **Labs:** ↑ LFTs, BUN, Cr; ↓ HMG, Hct, plts, WBC, RBC, glucose; monitor CBC, ALT, Cr **NIPE:** Monitor wgt; monitor BG; BB may mask hypoglycemia; photosensitivity—use sunscreen

Glipizide (Glucotrol, Glucotrol XL, Generic) [Hypoglycemic/Sulfonylurea]

Uses: *Type 2 DM* **Action:** Sulfonylurea; ↑ pancreatic insulin release; ↑ peripheral insulin sensitivity; ↓ hepatic glucose output/production; ↓ intestinal glucose absorption **Dose:** 5 mg initial, ↑ by 2.5–5 mg/d, max 40 mg/d; XL max 20 mg; 30 min ac; hold if NPO **Caution:** [C, ?/–] Severe liver Dz **CI:** DKA, type 1 DM, sulfonamide sensitivity **Disp:** Tabs 5, 10 mg; XL tabs 2.5, 5, 10 mg **SE:** HA, anorexia, N/V/D, constipation, fullness, rash, urticaria, photosensitivity **Interactions:** ↑ Effects W/ azole antifungals, anabolic steroids, BB, chloramphenicol, cimetidine, clofibrate, MAOIs, NSAIDs, probenecid, salicylates, sulfonamides, TCAs, warfarin, celery, coriander, dandelion root, fenugreek, ginseng, garlic, juniper berries; ↓ effects W/ amphetamines, corticosteroids, epinephrine, estrogens, glucocorticoids, OCPs, rifampin, sympathomimetics, thiazide diuretics, thyroid hormones, tobacco **Labs:** ↑ BUN, Cr, AST, lipids; ↓ glucose, HMG, WBC, plts **NIPE:** Antabuse-like effect w/ EtOH (rare); give 30 min ac; hold dose if pt NPO; counsel about DM management; wait several d before adjusting dose; monitor glucose; BB can mask hypoglycemia; photosensitivity—use sunscreen

Glucagon, Recombinant (GlucaGen) [Antihypoglycemic/Hormone]

Uses: Severe *hypoglycemic Rxns in DM*; radiologic GI tract diagnostic aid β-blocker/CCB OD **Action:** Accelerates liver gluconeogenesis **Dose:** **Adults.** 0.5–1 mg SQ, IM, or IV; repeat in 20 min PRN **ECC 2010:** β-Blocker or CCB overdose: 3–10 mg slow IV over 3–5 min; follow w/ Inf of 3–5 mg/h Hypoglycemia: 1 mg IV, IM, or SQ. **Peds. Neonates.** 30 mcg/kg/dose SQ, IM, or IV q4h PRN **Children.** 0.025–0.1 mg/kg/dose SQ, IM, or IV; repeat in 20 min PRN **Caution:** [B, M] **CI:** Pheochromocytoma **Disp:** Inj 1 mg **SE:** N/V, ↓ BP **Interactions:** ↑ Effect W/ epinephrine, phenytoin; ↑ effects OF anticoagulants **Labs:** ↓ Serum K+ **NIPE:** Response w/in 20 min after Inj; administration of dextrose IV if necessary; ineffective in starvation, adrenal Insuff, or chronic hypoglycemia

Glucarpidase (Voraxaze)

Uses: *Tx toxic plasma MTX conc (> 1 micromole/L) in pts w/ ↓ clearance* **Action:** Carboxypeptidase enzyme converts MTX to inactive metabolites **Dose:** 50 units/kg IV over 5 min × 1 **Caution:** [C, ?/–] Serious allergic/anaphylactic Rxns; do not administer leucovorin w/n 2 h before/after dose **Disp:** Inj (powder) 1000 units/vial **SE:** N/V/D, HA, ↓/↑ BP, flushing, paresthesias, hypersensitivity, blurred vision, rash, tremor, throat irritation **Note:** Measure MTX conc by chromatographic method w/n 48 h of admin; continue leucovorin until methotrexate conc below leucovorin Tx threshold × 3 d; hydrate &

alkalinize urine **NIPE:** ⊘ administer leucovorin w/in 2 h before/after glucarpidase; give as a single IV bolus injection over 5 min

Glyburide (DiaBeta Glynase, Generic) [Hypoglycemic/Sulfonylurea] Uses: *Type 2 DM* Action: Sulfonylurea; ↑ pancreatic insulin release; ↑ peripheral insulin sensitivity; ↓ hepatic glucose output/production; ↓ intestinal glucose absorption **Dose:** 1.25–10 mg qd–bid, max 20 mg/d. *Micronized:* 0.75–6 mg qd or bid, max 12 mg/d **Caution:** [C, ?] Renal impair, sulfonamide allergy, ? CV risk **CI:** DKA, type 1 DM **Disp:** Tabs 1.25, 2.5, 5 mg; micronized tabs (Glynase) 1.5, 3, 6 mg **SE:** HA, hypoglycemia, cholestatic jaundice, & hepatitis; may cause liver failure **Interactions:** Many medications can enhance hypoglycemic effects such as: ↑ Effects **W/** anticoagulants, anabolic steroids, BBs, chloramphenicol, cimetidine, clofibrate, MAOIs, NSAIDs, probenecid, salicylates, sulfonamides, TCAs, EtOH, celery, coriander, dandelion root, fenugreek, ginseng, garlic, juniper berries; ↓ effects **W/** amphetamines, corticosteroids, baclofen, epinephrine, glucocorticoids, OCPs, phenytoin, rifampin, sympathomimetics, thiazide diuretics, thyroid hormones, tobacco **Labs:** ↑ LFTs, BUN; ↓ glucose, HMG, Hct, plts, WBC **NIPE:** Antabuse-like effect w/ EtOH (rare); not OK for CrCl < 50 mL/min; hold dose if NPO, hypoglycemia may be difficult to recognize; many medications can enhance hypoglycemic effects; monitor BG; photosensitivity—use sunscreen

Glyburide/Metformin (Glucovance, Generic) [Hypoglycemic/ Sulfonylurea & Biguanide] Uses: *Type 2 DM* Action: *Sulfonylurea:* ↑ Pancreatic insulin release. *Metformin:* ↑ Peripheral insulin sensitivity; ↓ hepatic glucose output/production; ↓ intestinal glucose absorption **Dose:** 1st-line (naïve pts), 1.25/250 mg PO daily–bid; 2nd-line, 2.5/500 mg or 5/500 mg bid (max 20/2000 mg); take w/ meals, slowly ↑ dose; hold before & 48 h after ionic contrast media **Caution:** [C, –] **CI:** SCr > 1.4 mg/dL in females or > 1.5 mg/dL in males; hypoxemic conditions (sepsis, recent MI); alcoholism; metabolic acidosis; liver Dz **Disp:** Tabs (glyburide/metformin) 1.25/250, 2.5/500, 5/500 mg **SE:** HA, hypoglycemia, lactic acidosis, anorexia, N/V, rash **Interactions:** ↑ Effects **W/** amiloride, ciprofloxacin cimetidine, digoxin, miconazole, morphine, nifedipine, procainamide, quinidine, quinine, ranitidine, triamterene, TMP, vancomycin; ↓ effects **W/** CCBs, INH, phenothiazines **Labs:** Monitor folate levels (megaloblastic anemia) **NIPE:** Avoid EtOH; hold dose if NPO, see Glyburide

Glycerin Suppository [Laxative] Uses: *Constipation* Action: Hyper osmolar laxative **Dose:** *Adults.* 1 adult supp PR PRN *Peds.* 1 infant supp PR daily—bid PRN **Caution:** [C, ?] **Disp:** Supp (adult, infant); Liq 4 mL/applicator full **SE:** D **Interactions:** ↑ Effects **W/** diuretics **Labs:** ↑ Serum triglycerides, phosphatidyl-glycerol in amniotic fluid; ↓ serum Ca **NIPE:** Insert & retain for 15 min

Golimumab (Simponi) [Antirheumatics/DMARDs/TNF Blocker] **WARNING:** Serious Infxns (bacterial, fungal, TB, opportunistic) possible. D/C w/ severe Infxn/sepsis, test and monitor for TB w/ Tx; lymphoma/other CA possible in children/adolescents Uses: *Mod–severe RA w/ methotrexate, psoriatic arthritis* w/ or w/o methotrexate, ankylosing spondylitis* **Action:** TNF blocker **Dose:** 50 mg SQ 1 ×/mo **Caution:** [B, ?/–] Do use w/ active Infxn; w/ malignancies, CHF, demyelinating Dz; do use w/ abatacept, anakinra, live vaccines **CI:** None **Disp:** Prefilled syringe & SmartJect auto-injector 50 mg/0.5 mL **SE:** URI, nasopharyngitis, Inj site Rxn, ↑ LFTs, Infxn, hep B reactivation, new-onset psoriasis **Interactions:** ↑ Risk of serious Infxns *W/* abatacept, anakinra, corticosteroids, methotrexate; immunosuppressants; ↓ effects *W/* live virus vaccines; monitor CYP450 substrates w/ narrow therapeutic index: cyclosporine, theophylline, warfarin **Labs:** ↑ LFTs; monitor CBC; **NIPE:** ⊘ w/ live virus vaccines; monitor for signs serious Infxn (fever, malaise, wgt loss, sweats, cough, dyspnea); monitor for new or > CHF; monitor for exacerbation or new-onset psoriasis

Goserelin (Zoladex) [Antineoplastic/Gonadotropin-Releasing Hormone] Uses: *Advanced CA prostate* & w/ radiation and flutamide for localized high-risk Dz, *endometriosis, breast CA* **Action:** LHRH agonist, transient ↑ then ↓ in LH, w/ ↓ testosterone **Dose:** 3.6 mg SQ (implant) q28d or 10.8 mg SQ q3mo; usually upper Abd wall **Caution:** [X, –] **CI:** PRG, breast-feeding, 10.8-mg implant not for women **Disp:** SQ implant 3.6 (1 mo), 10.8 mg (3 mo) **SE:** Hot flashes, ↓ libido, gynecomastia, & transient exacerbation of CA-related bone pain ("flare Rxn" 7–10 d after 1st dose) **Interactions:** None noted **Labs:** ↑ LFTs, glucose, cholesterol, triglycerides; initial ↑ then ↓ after 1–2 wk FSH, LH, testosterone **NIPE:** Inject SQ into fat in Abd wall; do not aspirate; females must use contraception; monitor S/Sx ↑ BG

Granisetron (Generic) [Antiemetic/5-HT₃ Antagonist] Uses: *Rx & prevention of N/V (chemo/radiation/post-operation)* **Action:** Serotonin (5-HT₃) receptor antagonist **Dose:** *Adults & Peds. Chemotherapy:* 10 mcg/kg/dose IV 30 min prior to chemotherapy *Adults. Chemotherapy:* 2 mg PO qd 1 h before chemotherapy, then 12 h later. *Post-op N/V:* 1 mg IV over 30 s before end of case **Caution:** [B, +/–] St. John's wort ↓ levels **CI:** Liver Dz, children < 2 y **Disp:** Tabs 1 mg; Inj 1 mg/mL; soln 2 mg/10 mL **SE:** HA, asthenia, somnolence, D, constipation, Abd pain, dizziness, insomnia **Interactions:** ↑ Serotonergic effects *W/* horehound; ↑ extrapyramidal Rxns *W/* drugs causing these effects **Labs:** ↑ ALT, AST; ↓ HMG, Hct, plts, WBC **NIPE:** May cause anaphylactic Rxn; may cause QT prolongation w/ Hx cardiac disease; may cause drowsiness—caution driving

Guaifenesin (Robitussin, Others, Generic) [Expectorant/Propanediol Derivative] Uses: *Relief of dry, nonproductive cough* **Action:** Expectorant **Dose:** *Adults.* 200–400 mg (10–20 mL) PO q4h SR 600–1200 mg PO bid (max 2.4 g/d) *Peds 2–5 y.* 50–100 mg (2.5–5 mL) PO q4h (max 600 mg/d) *6–11 y.* 100–200 mg (5–10 mL) PO q4h (max 1.2 g/d) **Caution:** [C, ?] **Disp:** Tabs 100, 200 mg; SR tabs 600, 1200 mg; caps 100 mg; SR caps 300 mg; Liq 100 mg/5 mL **SE:** GI upset **Interactions:** ↑ Bleeding *W/* heparin **Labs:** ↓ Serum uric acid level, HMG, plts, WBCs **NIPE:** Give w/ large amount of H₂O; some dosage forms contain EtOH; ⊘ use > 7 d

Guaifenesin/Codeine (Robafen AC, Others, Generic) [Expectorant/Analgesic/Antitussive] [C-V] Uses: *Relief of dry cough* Action: Antitussive w/ expectorant Dose: *Adults.* 5–10 mL or 1 tab PO q6–8h (max 60 mL/24 h) *Peds > 6 y.* 1–1.5 mg/kg codeine/d ÷ dose q4–6h (max 30 mg/24 h) *6–12 y.* 5 mL q4h (max 30 mL/24 h) Caution: [C, +] Disp: Brontex tab 10 mg codeine/300 mg guaifenesin; Liq 2.5 mg codeine/75 mg guaifenesin/5 mL; others 10 mg codeine/100 mg guaifenesin/5 mL SE: Somnolence, constipation Interactions: ↑ CNS depression W/ barbiturates, antihistamines, glutethimide, methocarbamol, cimetidine, EtOH; ↓ effects W/ quinidine Labs: ↑ Urine morphine; ↓ serum uric acid level, HMG, plts, WBCs NIPE: Take w/ food; ↑ fluid intake; may cause drowsiness

Guaifenesin/Dextromethorphan (Many OTC Brands) [Expectorant/Antitussive] Uses: *Cough* d/t upper resp tract irritation Action: Antitussive w/ expectorant Dose: *Adults & Peds > 12 y.* 10 mL PO q6–8h (max 40 mL/24 h) *Peds 2–6 y.* Dextromethorphan 1–2 mg/kg/24 h ÷ 3–4 × d (max 10 mL/d) *6–12 y.* 5 mL q6–8h (max 20 mL/d) Caution: [C, +] CI: Administration w/ MAOI Disp: Many OTC formulations SE: Somnolence Interactions: ↑ Effects W/ quinidine, terbinafine; ↑ effects OF isocarboxazid, MAOIs, phenelzine; ↑ risk of serotonin synd W/ sibutramine Labs: ↓ Serum uric acid level, HMG, plts, WBCs NIPE: Give w/ plenty of fluids; some forms contain EtOH

Guanfacine (Intuniv, Tenex, Generic) [Central Alpha-2A Agonist/Hypertension] Uses: *ADHD (peds > 6 y)*; *HTN (adults)* Action: Central α_{2a}-adrenergic agonist Dose: *Adults.* 1–3 mg/d IR PO h (*Tenex*), ↑ by 1 mg q3–4wk PRN 3 mg/d max; *Peds.* 1–4 mg/d XR PO (*Intuniv*), ↑ by 1 mg q1wk PRN 4 mg/d max Caution: [B; +/–] Disp: Tabs IR 1, 2 mg; tabs XR 1, 2, 3, 4 mg SE: Somnolence, dizziness, HA, fatigue, constipation, Abd pain, xerostomia, hypotension, bradycardia, syncope Interactions: ↑ Effects W/ CYP3A4/5 Inhibs (eg, ketoconazole), antihypertensives, CNS depressants; ↑ effects OF valproic acid; ↓ effects W/ CYP3A4 inducers (eg, rifampin) NIPE: Rebound ↑ BP, anxiety, nervousness w/ abrupt D/C; ↑ fluid intake/measures to relieve dry mouth

Haemophilus B Conjugate Vaccine (ActHIB, HibTITER, Hiberix, Pedvax HIB, Others) [Vaccine/Inactivated] Uses: *Immunize children against H influenzae type B Dzs* Action: Active immunization Dose: *Peds.* 0.5 mL (25 mg) IM (deltoid or vastus lateralis muscle) 2 doses 2 & 4 mo; booster at 12–15 mo or 2, 4, & 6 mo booster at 12–15 mo depending on formulation Caution: [C, +] CI: Component sensitivity, febrile illness, immunosuppression, thimerosal allergy Disp: Inj 7.5, 10, 15, 25 mg/0.5 mL SE: Fever, restlessness, fussiness, anorexia, pain/redness Inj site; observe for anaphylaxis; edema, ↑ risk of *Haemophilus* B Infxn the wk after vaccination Interactions: ↓ Effects W/ immunosuppressives, steroids NIPE: Prohibit & TriHIBit cannot be used in children < 12 mo; *Hiberix*-approved ages 15 mo–4 y, single dose; booster beyond 5 y not required; report SAE to Vaccine Adverse Events Reporting System (VAERS: 1-800-822-7967); dosing varies, check w/ each product; pain/redness at Inj site

Haloperidol (Haldol) [Antipsychotic/Butyrophenone] WARNING: ↑ Mortality in elderly w/ dementia-related psychosis. Risk for torsade de pointes and QT prolongation, death w/ IV administration at higher doses **Uses:** *Psychotic disorders, agitation, Tourette disorders, hyperactivity in children* **Action:** Butyrophenone; antipsychotic, neuroleptic **Dose:** *Adults. Mod Sxs:* 0.5–2 mg PO bid–tid *Severe Sxs/agitation:* 3–5 mg PO bid–tid or 1–5 mg IM q4h PRN (max 100 mg/d) *ICU psychosis:* 2–10 mg IV q 30 min to effect, the 25% max dose q6h *Peds 3–6 y.* 0.01–0.03 mg/kg/24 h PO daily *6–12 y. Initial:* 0.5–1.5 mg/24 h PO; ↑ by 0.5 mg/24 h to maint of 2–4 mg/24 h (0.05–0.1 mg/kg/24 h) or 1–3 mg/dose IM q4–8h to 0.1 mg/kg/24 h max; Tourette Dz may require up to 15 mg/24 h PO; ↓ in elderly **Caution:** [C, ?] ↑ Effects w/ SSRIs, CNS depressants, TCA, indomethacin, metoclopramide; avoid levodopa (↓ antiparkinsonian effects) **CI:** NAG, severe CNS depression, coma, Parkinson Dz, ↓ BM suppression, severe cardiac/hepatic Dz **Disp:** Tabs 0.5, 1, 2, 5, 10, 20 mg; conc Liq 2 mg/mL; Inj 5 mg/mL; decanoate Inj 50, 100 mg/mL **SE:** Extrapyramidal Sxs (EPS), tardive dyskinesia, neuroleptic malignant synd, ↓ BP, anxiety, dystonias, risk for torsades de pointes, & QT prolongation **Interactions:** ↑ Effects *W/* Azole antifungals, buspirone, CNS depressants, macrolides, quinidine, EtOH; ↑ hypotension *W/* antihypertensives, nitrates; ↑ anticholinergic effects *W/* antihistamines, antidepressants, atropine, phenothiazine, quinidine, disopyramide; risk of ↑ CNS depression *W/* chamomile, kava-kava, valerian; ↓ effects *W/* antacids, carbamazepine, rifampin, nutmeg, tobacco; ↓ effects *OF* anticoagulants, levodopa, guanethidine; Li ↑ risk of acute encephalopathy; methyldopa ↑ risk of dementia **Labs:** ↑ LFTs, monitor for leukopenia, neutropenia, & agranulocytosis; follow CBC if WBC counts ↓ **NIPE:** ↑ Risk of photosensitivity—use sunblock; do not give decanoate IV; dilute PO conc Liq w/ H₂O/juice; monitor for EPS; ECG monitoring w/ off-label IV use; causes dry mouth

Hep A Vaccine (Havrix, Vaqta) [Vaccine/Inactivated] **Uses:** *Prevent hep A* in high-risk individuals (eg, travelers, certain professions, day-care workers if 1 or more children or workers are infected, high-risk behaviors, children at ↑ risk), in chronic liver Dz **Action:** Active immunity **Dose:** *Adults. Havrix* 1.0 mL IM w/ 1.0 mL booster 6–12 mo later *Vaqta:* 1.0 mL IM w/ 1.0-mL IM booster 6–18 mo later *Peds > 12 mo. Havrix:* 0.5 mL IM, w/ 0.5-mL booster 6–18 mo later; *Vaqta:* 0.5 mL IM w/ 0.5-mL booster 6–18 mo later **Caution:** [C, +] **CI:** Component sensitivity **Disp:** *Havrix:* Inj 720 E.L.U./0.5 mL, 1440 EL.U./1 mL *Vaqta:* 50 units/mL **SE:** Fever, fatigue, HA, Inj site pain **NIPE:** Give primary at least 2 wk before anticipated exposure; do not give Havrix in gluteal region; report SAE to VAERS (1-800-822-7967)

Hep A (Inactivated) & Hep B (Recombinant) Vaccine (Twinrix) [Vaccine/Inactivated] **Uses:** *Active immunization against hep A/B in pts > 18 y* **Action:** Active immunity **Dose:** 1 mL IM at 0, 1, & 6 mo; accelerated regimen

1 mL IM d 0, 7, & 21– 30 then booster at 12 mo; 720 ELISA EL.U. units hep A antigen, 20 mcg/mL hep B surface antigen **Caution:** [C, +/–] **CI:** Component sensitivity **Disp:** Single-dose vials, syringes **SE:** Fever, fatigue, pain/redness at site, HA **Interactions:** ↓ Immune response W/ corticosteroids, immunosuppressants **NIPE:** ↑ Response if Inj in deltoid vs gluteus; booster OK 6–12 mo after vaccination; report SAE to Vaccine Adverse Events Reporting System (VAERS: 1-800-822-7967)

Hep B Immune Globulin (HyperHep, HepaGam B, Nabi-HB, H-BIG) [Hepatitis B Prophylaxis/Immunoglobulin] **Uses:** *Exposure to HBsAg(+) material (eg, blood, accidental needlestick, mucous membrane contact, PO, or sexual contact), prevent hep B in HBsAg(+) liver Tx pt* **Action:** Passive immunization **Dose:** *Adults & Peds.* 0.06 mL/kg IM 5 mL max; w/in 24 h of exposure; w/in 14 d of sexual contact; repeat 1 mo if nonresponder or refused initial Tx; liver Tx per protocols **Caution:** [C, ?] **CI:** Allergies to γ-globulin anti-immunoglobulin Ab or thimerosol; IgA deficiency **Disp:** Inj **SE:** Inj site pain, dizziness, HA, myalgias, arthralgias, anaphylaxis **Interactions:** ↓ Immune response if given W/ live virus vaccines **NIPE:** IM in gluteal or deltoid; W/ continued exposure, give hep B vaccine; not for active hep B; ineffective for chronic hep B

Hep B Vaccine (Engerix-B, Recombivax HB) [Vaccine/Inactivated] **Uses:** *Prevent hep B*: men who have sex w/ men, people who inject street drugs; chronic renal/liver Dz, healthcare workers exposed to blood, body fluids; sexually active not in monogamous relationship, people seeking eval for or w/ STDs, household contacts & partners of hep B infected persons, travelers to countries w/ ↑ hep B prevalence, clients/staff working w/ people w/ developmental disabilities **Action:** Active immunization; recombinant DNA **Dose:** *Adults.* 3 IM doses 1 mL each; 1st 2 doses 1 mo apart; the 3rd 6 mo after the 1st *Peds.* 0.5 mL IM adult schedule **Caution:** [C, +] **CI:** Yeast allergy, component sensitivity **Disp:** *Engerix-B:* Inj 20 mcg/mL; peds Inj 10 mcg/0.5 mL *Recombivax HB:* Inj 10 & 40 mcg/mL; peds Inj 5 mcg/0.5 mL **SE:** Fever, HA, Inj site pain **Interactions:** ↓ Immune response W/ corticosteroids, immunosuppressants **NIPE:** ↑ Response Inj in deltoid vs gluteus; deltoid IM Inj adults/older peds; younger peds, use anterolateral thigh

Heparin (Generic) [Anticoagulant/Antithrombotic] **Uses:** *Rx & prevention of DVT & PE*, unstable angina, AF w/ emboli, & acute arterial occlusion **Action:** Acts w/ antithrombin III to inactivate thrombin & ↓ thromboplastin formation **Dose:** *Adults. Prophylaxis:* 3000–5000 units SQ q8–12h *DVT/PE Rx:* Load 50–80 units/kg IV (max 10,000 units), then 10–20 units/kg/h IV qh (adjust based on PTT) *ECC 2010: STEMI:* Bolus 60 units/kg (max 4000 units); then 12 units/kg/h (max 1000 units/h) round to nearest 50 units; keep aPTT 1.5–2 × control 48 h or until angiography *Peds. Infants.* Load 50 units/kg IV bolus, then 20 units/kg/h IV by cont Inf *Children.* Load 50 units/kg IV, then 15–25 units/kg cont Inf or 100 units/kg/dose q4h IV intermittent bolus (adjust based on PTT) **Caution:** [C, +]

↑ Risk of hemorrhage w/ anticoagulants, ASA, antiplts, cephalosporins w/ MTT side chain **CI:** Uncontrolled bleeding, severe thrombocytopenia, suspected ICH **Disp:** Unfractionated Inj 10, 100, 1000, 2000, 2500, 5000, 7500, 10,000, 20,000, 40,000 units/mL **SE:** Bruising, bleeding, thrombocytopenia **Interactions:** ↑ Effects *W/* anticoagulants, antihistamines, ASA, clopidogrel, cardiac glycosides, cephalosporins, pyridamole, NSAIDs, quinine, tetracycline, ticlopidine, arnica, capsicum, chamomile, feverfew, garlic, ginkgo, ginseng, ginger, licorice, onion; ↓ effects *W/* digoxin, nitroglycerine, penicillins, nicotine, ↓ effects *OF* insulin **Labs:** ↑ LFTs; follow PTT, thrombin time, or ACT; little PT effect; therapeutic PTT 1.5–2 × control for most conditions; monitor for HIT w/ plt counts **NIPE:** Monitor for signs bleeding: Bleeding gums, nosebleed, unusual bruising, black tarry stools, hematuria, < Hct, guaiac + stool; new "USP" formulation heparin is approximately 10% less effective than older formulations

Hetastarch (Hespan) [Plasma Volume Expander] **Uses:** *Plasma vol expansion* adjunct for leukapheresis **Action:** Synthetic colloid; acts similar to albumin **Dose:** *Vol expansion:* 500–1000 mL (1500 mL/d max) IV (20 mL/kg/h max rate) *Leukapheresis:* 250–700 mL; ↓ in renal failure **Caution:** [C, +] **CI:** Severe bleeding disorders, CHF, oliguric/anuric renal failure **Disp:** Inj 6 g/100 mL **SE:** Bleeding (↑ PT, PTT, bleeding time) **Labs:** ↑ PT, PTT, bleed time; monitor CBC, PT, PTT **NIPE:** Observe for anaphylactic Rxns; not blood or plasma substitute

Human Papillomavirus Recombinant Vaccine (Cervarix [Types 16, 18], Gardasil [Types 6, 11, 16, 18]) **Uses:** *Prevent cervical CA, precancerous genital lesions (Cervarix & Gardasil), genital warts, anal CA & oral CA (Gardasil) d/t HPV types 16, 18 (Cervarix) & types 6, 11, 16, 18 (Gardasil) in females 9–26 y*; prevent genital warts, anal CA, & anal intraepithelial neoplasia in males 9–26 y (Gardasil) **Action:** Recombinant vaccine, passive immunity **Dose:** 0.5 mL IM, then 1 & 6 mo (Cervarix), or 2 & 6 mo (Gardasil) (upper thigh or deltoid) **Caution:** [B, ?/–] **Disp:** SDV & prefilled syringe: 0.5 mL **SE:** Erythema, pain at Inj site, fever, syncope, venous thromboembolism **Interactions:** May be ↓ response *W/* immunosuppressants and antineoplastics, may get ↓ antibody response **NIPE:** 1st CA prevention vaccine; 90% effective in preventing CIN 2 or more severe dx in HPV-naïve populations; report adverse events to Vaccine Adverse Events Reporting System (VAERS: 1-800-822-7967); IM in upper thigh or deltoid; continue cervical CA screening; h/o genital warts, abnormal Pap smear, or (+) HPV DNA test is not CI to vaccination

Hydralazine (Apresoline, Others) [Antihypertensive/Vasodilator] **Uses:** *Mod–severe HTN; CHF* (w/ Isordil) **Action:** Peripheral vasodilator **Dose:** *Adults.* Initial 10 mg PO 3–4 ×/d, ↑ to 25 mg 3–4 ×/d, 300 mg/d max *Peds.* 0.75–3 mg/kg/24 h PO ÷ q6–12h; ↓ in renal impair; ✓ CBC & ANA before **Caution:** [C, +] ↓ Hepatic Fxn & CAD; ↑ tox w/ MAOI, indomethacin, BBs **CI:** Dissecting aortic aneurysm, mitral valve/rheumatic heart Dz **Disp:** Tabs 10, 25, 50, 100 mg; Inj 20 mg/mL **SE:** SLE-like synd w/ chronic high doses; SVT following

IM route, peripheral neuropathy **Interactions:** ↑ Effects W/ antihypertensives, diazoxide, diuretics, MAOIs, nitrates, EtOH; ↓ pressor response W/ epinephrine; ↓ effects W/ NSAIDs **LABs:** ↓ WBC, RBC, Hgb, plts, neutrophils—monitor CBC; may cause + ANA titer **NIPE:** Take w/ food to ↑ drug absorption; compensatory sinus tachycardia eliminated w/ BBs, elderly may experience ↑ hypotensive effects.

Hydrochlorothiazide (HydroDIURIL, Esidrix, Others) [Antihypertensive/Thiazide Diuretic]

Uses: *Edema, HTN* prevent stones in hypercalciuria **Action:** Thiazide diuretic; ↓ distal tubule Na^+ reabsorption **Dose: Adults.** 25–100 mg/d PO single or ÷ doses; 200 mg/d max **Peds < 6 mo.** 2–3 mg/kg/d in 2 ÷ doses *> 6 mo.* 2 mg/kg/d in 2 ÷ doses **Caution:** [D, +] **CI:** Anuria, sulfonamide allergy, renal Insuff **Disp:** Tabs 25, 50, mg; caps 12.5 mg; PO soln 50 mg/5 mL **SE:** ↓ K^+, hyperglycemia, hyperuricemia ↓ Na^+ **Interactions:** ↑ Hypotension W/ ACEIs, antihypertensives, nitrates, EtOH; ↑ hypokalemia W/ amphotericin B, corticosteroids; ↑ hyperglycemia W/ BBs, diazoxide, hypoglycemic drugs; ↑ risk of digoxin & Li tox; ↑ effects OF Li; ↓ effects W/ amphetamines, cholestyramine, colestipol, NSAIDs, quinidine, dandelion **Labs:** ↑ Glucose, cholesterol, Ca, uric acid levels; ↓ K^+, Na^+, HMG, Hct, plts, WBCs; follow K^+, may need supplementation **NIPE:** Take w/ food; ↑ risk of photosensitivity—use sunblock; monitor ECG for hypokalemia (flattened T waves)

Hydrochlorothiazide & Amiloride (Moduretic/Generic) [Antihypertensive/Thiazide & K^+-Sparing Diuretic]

Uses: *HTN* **Action:** Combined thiazide & K^+-sparing diuretic **Dose:** 1–2 tabs/d PO **Caution:** [D, ?] **CI:** Renal failure, sulfonamide allergy **Disp:** Tabs (amiloride/ HCTZ) 5 mg/50 mg **SE:** ↓ BP, hyperglycemia, ↓ hyperlipidemia, hyperuricemia **Interactions:** ↑ Hypotension W/ ACEIs, antihypertensives, carbenoxolone, ↑ hypokalemia W/ amphotericin B, carbenoxolone, corticosteroids, licorice; ↑ risk of hyperkalemia W/ ACE-I, K^+-sparing diuretics, NSAIDs, & K^+ salt substitutes; ↑ hyperglycemia W/ BBs, diazoxide, hypoglycemic drugs; ↑ effects OF amantadine, antihypertensives, digoxin, Li, MTX; ↑ effects W/ CNS depressants; ↑ effects W/ amphetamines, cholestyramine, colestipol, NSAIDs, quinidine, dandelion **Labs:** ↑ Glucose, cholesterol, Ca, uric acid levels; ↓ Na^+, HMG, Hct, plts, WBCs; ↑ K^+/↓ K^+; interferes w/ GTT; monitor lytes, LFTs, uric acid **NIPE:** Take w/ food, I&O, daily wgt, ∅ salt substitutes, bananas, & oranges ↑ risk of photosensitivity—use sunblock; monitor ECG for hypo-/hyperkalemia (flattened or peaked T waves)

Hydrochlorothiazide & Spironolactone (Aldactazide, Generic) [Antihypertensive/Thiazide & K^+-Sparing Diuretic]

Uses: *Edema, HTN* **Action:** Thiazide & K^+-sparing diuretic **Dose:** 25–200 mg each compound/d, ÷ doses **Caution:** [D, +] **CI:** Sulfonamide allergy **Disp:** Tabs (HCTZ mg/spironolactone) 25/25, 50/50 **SE:** ↓ BP, hyperglycemia, hyperlipidemia, hyperuricemia **Interactions** ↑ Risk of hyperkalemia W/ ACEIs, K^+-sparing diuretics, K^+ supls, salt substitutes; ↓ effects OF digoxin **Labs:** ↑ or ↓ K^+, ↓ Na^+ **NIPE:** DC drug 3 d before GTT;

monitor ECG for hypo-/hyperkalemia (flattened or peaked T waves), ↑ risk of photosensitivity—use sunblock

Hydrochlorothiazide & Triamterene (Dyazide, Maxzide, Generic) [Antihypertensive/Thiazide & K⁺-Sparing Diuretic]

Uses: *Edema & HTN* Action: Combo thiazide & K⁺-sparing diuretic Dose: *Dyazide:* 1–2 caps PO daily-bid. *Maxzide:* 1 tab/d PO Caution: [D, +/−] CI: Sulfonamide allergy Disp: (Triamterene mg/HCTZ mg) 37.5/25, 75/50 SE: Photosensitivity, ↓ BP, ↑ or ↓ K⁺, ↑ Na⁺ hyperglycemia, hyperlipidemia, hyperuricemia Interactions: ↑ Risk of hyperkalemia *W/* ACEIs, K⁺-sparing diuretics, K⁺ supls, salt substitutes; ↑ effects *W/* cimetidine, licorice root, ↓ effects *OF* digoxin Labs: ↑ or ↓ Na⁺, ↑ serum glucose, BUN, Cr, Mg²⁺, uric acid, urinary Ca²⁺; interference w/ assay of quinidine & lactic dehydrogenase NIPE: Urine may turn blue; HCTZ component in Maxzide more bioavailable than in Dyazide; monitor ECG for hypo-/hyperkalemia (flattened or peaked T waves), ↑ risk of photosensitivy—use sunblock

Hydrocodone (Zohydro) [C-II]

WARNING: Addiction risk, risk of resp depression. Accidental consumption, esp. peds, can be fatal. Use during PRG can cause neonatal opioid withdrawal. Contains acetaminophen, associated with liver failure, transplant, and death Uses: *Severe pain requiring around the clock long-term opiod treatment where alternatives are inadequate* Action: Opioid agonist Dose: Opioid naïve/opioid intolerant 10 mg PO q12h; ↑ 10 mg q12 h PRN every 3–7 d Caution: w/other CNS depressants, MAOI, TCA, elderly, debilitated, w/ hepatitic impair; may ↑ ICP (✓ pupils); impairs mental/physical abilities; drugs that ↓ CYP3A4 may ↓ clearance; may prolong GI obstruction CI: Component hypersens; resp dep, severe asthma/ hypercarbia, ileus Disp: ER caps 10, 15, 20, 30, 40, 50 mg SE: constipation, N/V, somnolence, fatigue, HA, dizziness, dry mouth, pruritus, Abd pain, edema, URI, spasms, UTI, back pain, tremor NIPE: Monitor for respiratory depression during 1st 72 h; taper D/C; swallow whole with H₂O; ⊘ crush/chew; do not use EtOH; not for PRN use; may cause drowsiness—caution driving; ↑ fluids/fiber to prevent constipation

Hydrocodone & Acetaminophen (Hycet, Lorcet, Vicodin, Generic) [C-III] [Narcotic Analgesic/Antitussive]

Uses: *Mod–severe pain* Action: Narcotic analgesic w/ nonnarcotic analgesic Dose: *Adults.* 1–2 caps or tabs PO q4–6h PRN; soln 15 mL q4–6h *Peds.* Soln (Hycet) 0.27 mL/kg q4–6h Caution: [C, M] CI: CNS depression, severe resp depression Disp: Many formulations; specify hydrocodone/APAP dose; caps 5/500; tabs 2.5/500, 5/300, 5/325, 5/500, 7.5/300, 7.5/325, 7.5/500, 7.5/650, 7.5/750, 10/300, 10/325, 10/500, 10/650, 10/660, 10/750 mg; soln *Hycet* (fruit punch) 7.5 mg hydrocodone/325 mg acetaminophen/15 mL SE: GI upset, sedation, fatigue Interactions: ↑ Effects *W/* antihistamines, cimetidine, CNS depressants, dextroamphetamines, glutethimide, MAOIs, protease Inhibs, TCAs, EtOH, St. John's wort; ↑ effects *OF* warfarin; ↓ effects *W/* phenothiazine Labs: False ↑ amylase, lipase NIPE: Take w/ food, ↑ fluid intake; do not exceed > 4 g APAP/d

Hydrocodone & Homatropine (Hycodan, Hydromet, Generic) [C-III] [Narcotic Analgesic/Antitussive] Uses: *Relief of cough* Action: Combo antitussive Dose: (Based on hydrocodone) *Adults.* 5–10 mg q4–6h *Peds.* 0.6 mg/kg/d ÷ tid–qid Caution: [C, M] CI: NAG, ↑ ICP, depressed ventilation Disp: Syrup 5 mg hydrocodone/5 mL; tabs 5 mg hydrocodone SE: Sedation, fatigue, GI upset Labs: ↑ ALT, AST NIPE: Do not give < q4h; see individual drugs

Hydrocodone & Ibuprofen (Vicoprofen, Generic) [C-III] [Narcotic Analgesic/NSAID] Uses: *Mod–severe pain (< 10 d)* Action: Narcotic w/ NSAID Dose: 1–2 tabs q4–6h PRN Caution: [C, M] Renal Insuff ↓ effect w/ ACE inhib & diuretics; ↑ effect w/ CNS depressants, EtOH, MAOI, ASA, TCA, anticoagulants CI: Component sensitivity Disp: Tabs 7.5 mg hydrocodone/200 mg ibuprofen SE: Sedation, fatigue, GI upset Interactions: ↑ Effect *W/* CNS depressants, EtOH, MAOI, ASA, TCA, anticoagulants; ↓ effects *OF* ACEIs, diuretics; ↓ effect *W/* ACE Inhibs & diuretics; ↑ risk of bleeding *W/* heparin

Hydrocodone & Pseudoephedrine (Detussin, Histussin-D, Generics) [C-III] [Antitussive/Decongestant] Uses: *Cough & nasal congestion* Action: Narcotic cough suppressant w/ decongestant Dose: 5 mL qid, PRN Caution: [C, M] CI: MAOIs Disp: Hydrocodone/pseudoephedrine 5/60, 3/15 mg 5 mL; tabs 5/60 mg SE: ↑ BP, GI upset, sedation, fatigue Interactions: ↑ Effects *W/* sympathomimetics NIPE: ↑ Bleeding w/ heparin

Hydrocortisone, Rectal (Anusol-HC Suppository, Cortifoam Rectal, Proctocort, Others, Generic) [Corticosteroid] Uses: *Painful anorectal conditions*, radiation proctitis, UC Action: Anti-inflammatory steroid Dose: *Adults. UC:* 10–100 mg PR daily–bid for 2–3 wk Caution: [B, ?/–] CI: Component sensitivity Disp: *Hydrocortisone acetate:* Rectal aerosol 90 mg/applicator; supp 25 mg *Hydrocortisone base:* Rectal 0.5%, 1%, 2.5%; rectal susp 100 mg/60 mL SE: Minimal systemic effect NIPE: Administer after BM, insert supp blunt end 1st, administer enema w/ pt lying on side & retain for 1 h

Hydrocortisone, Topical & Systemic (Cortef, Solu-Cortef, Generic) [Corticosteroid] See Steroids Systemic and Topical, *Peds. ECC 2010:* Adrenal insufficiency: 2 mg/kg IV/IO bolus; max dose 100 mg Caution: [B, –] CI: Viral, fungal, or tubercular skin lesions; serious Infxns (except septic shock or TB meningitis) SE: *Systemic:* ↑ Appetite, insomnia, hyperglycemia, bruising Notes: May cause hypothalamic-pituitary-adrenal axis suppression Interactions: ↑ Effects *W/* cyclosporine, estrogens; ↑ effects *OF* cardiac glycosides, cyclosporine; ↑ risk of GI bleed *W/* NSAIDs; ↓ effects *W/* aminoglutethimide, antacids, barbiturates, cholestyramine, colestipol, ephedrine, phenobarbital, phenytoin, rifampin; ↓ effects *OF* anticoagulants, hypoglycemics, insulin, INH, salicylates Labs: ↑ Glucose, cholesterol; ↓ K+, Ca+ NIPE: ⊘ EtOH, live virus vaccines, abrupt D/C of drug; take w/ food; may mask S/Sxs Infxn

Hydromorphone (Dilaudid, Dilaudid HP) [C–II] [Narcotic Analgesic] **WARNING:** A potent Schedule II opioid agonist; highest potential for abuse & risk of resp depression. HP formula is highly concentrated; do not confuse w/ standard formulations, OD & death could result. Alcohol, other opioids, CNS depressants ↑ resp depressant effects **Uses:** *Mod/severe pain* **Action:** Narcotic analgesic **Dose:** 1–4 mg PO, IM, IV, or PR q4–6h PRN; 3 mg PR q6–8h PRN; ↓ w/ hepatic failure **Caution:** [B (D if prolonged use or high doses near term), ?] ↑ Resp depression & CNS effects CNS depressants, phenothiazines, TCA **CI:** ICP lesion w/ ↑ ICP, COPD, cor pulmonale, emphysema, kyphoscoliosis, status asthmaticus; HP-Inj form in OB analgesia **Disp:** Tabs 2, 4 mg, 8 mg scored; Liq 5 mg/5 mL or 1 mg/mL; Inj 1, 2, 4, Dilaudid HP is 10 mg/mL; supp 3 mg **SE:** Sedation, dizziness, GI upset **Interactions:** ↑ Effects **W/** CNS depressants, phenothiazines, TCAs, EtOH, chamomile, St. John's wort, valerian; ↑ risk of urinary retention/constipation with anticholinergics; ↓ effects **W/** nalbuphine, pentazocine **Labs:** ↑ Serum amylase, lipase **NIPE:** Take w/ food; ↑ fluids & fiber to prevent constipation; morphine 10 mg IM = hydromorphone 1.5 mg IM

Hydromorphone, Extended Release (Exalgo) [C–II] [Opioid Analgesic] **WARNING:** Use in opioid tolerant only; high potential for abuse, criminal diversion & resp depression. Not for post-op pain or PRN use. OD & death esp in children. Do not break/crush/chew tabs, may result in OD **Uses:** *Mod/severe chronic pain requiring around the clock opioid analgesic* **Action:** Narcotic analgesic **Dose:** 8–64 mg PO/d titrate to effect; ↓ w/ hepatic/renal impair & elderly **Caution:** [C, –] Abuse potential; ↑ resp depression & CNS effects, w/ CNS depressants, pts susceptible to intracranial effects of CO_2 retention **CI:** Opioid intolerant patients, ↓ pulmonary function, ileus, GI tract narrowing/obst, component hypersensitivity; w/in 14 d of MAOI; anticholinergics may ↑ SE **Disp:** Tabs 8, 12, 16 mg **SE:** Constipation, N/V, somnolence, HA, dizziness; **Interactions:** Anticholinergics may ↑ risk of urinary retention Abd SE; ↑ effects **W/** CNS depressants, TCA, phenothiazines, EtOH **NIPE:** See label for opioid conversion; do not use w/in 14 d of MAOI. Not for opioid naïve; swallow whole; withdraw gradually

Hydroxocobalamin (Cyanokit) [Antidote] **Uses:** *Cyanide poisoning* **Action:** Binds cyanide to form nontoxic cyanocobalamin excreted in urine **Dose:** 5 g IV over 15 min, repeat PRN 5 g IV min–2 h, total dose 10 g **Caution:** [C, ?] **CI:** None known **Disp:** Kit 2-, 2.5-g vials w/ Inf set **SE:** ↑ BP (can be severe) anaphylaxis, chest tightness, edema, urticaria, rash, chromaturia, N, HA **NIPE:** Inj site Rxns

Hydroxychloroquine (Plaquenil) **WARNING:** Healthcare providers should familiarize themselves with the complete contents of the FDA package insert before prescribing **Uses:** *Malaria: Plasmodium vivax, P malariae, P ovale, and P falciparum* (NOT all strains of *falciparum*); malaria prophylaxis; discoid lupus, SLE, RA* **Acts:** Unknown/antimalarial **Dose:** *Acute Malaria: Adults.* 800 mg, 600 mg 6–8 h later, then 400 mg/d × 2 d *Peds.* 25 mg base/kg over 3 d

(200 mg = 155 mg base) 10 mg/kg d 1 (max 620 mg), then 5 mg/kg 6 h after 1st dose (max 310 mg), then 5 mg/kg 18 h after 2nd dose and then 5 mg/kg 24 h after 3rd dose **Suppression Malaria: Adults.** 400 mg/d same day of wk, 2 wk before arrival through 8 wk leaving endemic area **Peds.** 5 mg base/kg, same dosing schedule **Lupus:** 400 mg/d or bid, reevaluate at 4–12 wk, then 200–400 mg/d **RA: Adults.** 400–600 mg/d, reevaluate at 4–12 wk, reduce by 50%; take w/ milk or food; Caution: [D, ?/–] CI: Hx eye changes from any 4-aminoquinoline, hypersens **Disp:** Tabs 200 mg **SE:** HA, dizziness, N/V/D, Abd pain, anorexia, irritability, mood changes, psychosis, seizures, myopathy, blurred vision, corneal changes, visual field defects, retinopathy, aplastic anemia, leukopenia, derm Rxns including Stevens-Johnson synd **Interactions:** ↑ Risk of digoxin toxicity; ↑ risk of toxicity **W/** cimetidine **Labs:** ↓ WBC, Hgb, plts—monitor CBC **NIPE:** Do not use long-term in children; cardiomyopathy rare; need for baseline & periodic ophthalmic exams

Hydroxyurea (Droxia, Hydrea, Generic) [Antineoplastic/Antimetabolite]
Uses: *CML, head & neck, ovarian & colon CA, melanoma, ALL, sickle cell anemia, polycythemia vera, HIV* **Action:** ↓ Ribonucleotide reductase **Dose:** (Per protocol) 50–75 mg/kg for WBC > 100,000 cells/mL; 20–30 mg/kg in refractory CML **HIV:** 1000–1500 mg/d in single or ÷ doses; ↓ in renal Insuff **Caution:** [D, –] **CI:** Severe anemia, BM suppression, WBC < 2500 cells/mL or plt < 100,000 cells/mm³, PRG **Disp:** Caps 200, 300, 400, 500 mg **SE:** ↓ BM (mostly leukopenia), N/V, rashes, facial erythema, radiation recall Rxns, renal impair **Interactions:** ↑ Effects **W/** zidovudine, zalcitabine, didanosine, stavudine, 5-FU, ↑ risk of pancreatitis **W/** didanosine, indinavir, stavudine; ↑ BM suppression **W/** antineoplastic drugs or radiation therapy **Labs:** ↑ Serum uric acid, BUN, Cr; ↓ WBC, HMG, plts **NIPE:** ↑ Fluids 10–12 glasses/d, empty caps into H₂O, use barrier contraception, ↑ risk of infertility

Hydroxyzine (Atarax, Vistaril, Generic) [Antipsychotic, Sedative/Hypnotic/Antihistamine]
Uses: *Anxiety, sedation, itching* **Action:** Antihistamine, antianxiety **Dose:** **Adults.** *Anxiety/sedation:* 50–100 mg PO or IM qid or PRN (max 600 mg/d) *Itching:* 25–50 mg PO or IM tid–qid **Peds.** 0.5–1.0 mg/kg/24 h PO or IM q6h; ↓ w/ hepatic impair **Caution:** [C, +/–] **CI:** Component sensitivity **Disp:** Tabs 10, 25, 50 mg; caps 25, 50 mg; syrup 10 mg/5 mL; susp 25 mg/5 mL; Inj 25, 50 mg/mL **SE:** Drowsiness, anticholinergic effects **Interactions:** ↑ Effects **W/** antihistamines, anticholinergics, CNS depressants, opioids, EtOH, valerian, chamomile; ↓ vasopressor effect of epinephrine **Labs:** False(−) skin allergy tests; false ↑ in urinary 17-hydroxycorticosteroid levels **NIPE:** Used to potentiate narcotic effects; not for IV/SQ (thrombosis & digital gangrene possible); concurrent use with EtOH will ↑ CNS suppression

Hyoscyamine (Anaspaz, Cystospaz, Levsin, Others, Generic) [Antispasmodic/Anticholinergic]
Uses: *Spasm w/ GI & bladder disorders* **Action:** Anticholinergic **Dose:** **Adults.** 0.125–0.25 mg (1–2 tabs) SL/PO tid–qid, ac & hs; 1 SR caps q12h **Caution:** [C, +] ↑ Effects w/ amantadine,

antihistamines, antimuscarinics, haloperidol, phenothiazines, TCA, MAOI **CI:** BOO, GI obst, NAG, MyG, paralytic ileus, UC, MI **Disp:** (Cystospaz-M, Levsinex) time-release caps 0.375 mg; elixir (EtOH); soln 0.125 mg/5 mL; Inj 0.5 mg/mL; tab 0.125 mg; tab (Cystospaz) 0.15 mg; XR tab (Levbid) 0.375 mg; SL (Levsin SL) 0.125 mg **SE:** Dry skin, xerostomia, constipation, anticholinergic SE, heat prostration w/ hot weather **Interactions:** ↑ Effects *W/* amantadine, antimuscarinics, haloperidol, phenothiazine, quinidine, TCAs, MAOIs; ↓ effects *W/* antacids, antidiarrheals; ↓ effects *OF* levodopa, ketoconazole **NIPE:** ↑ Risk of heat intolerance/ exhaustion/stroke; photophobia; administer tabs ac/food

Hyoscyamine, Atropine, Scopolamine, & Phenobarbital (Donnatal, Others, Generic) [Antispasmodic Anticholinergic]
Uses: *Irritable bowel, spastic colitis, peptic ulcer, spastic bladder* **Action:** Anticholinergic, antispasmodic **Dose:** 0.125–0.25 mg (1–2 tabs) tid–qid, 1 caps q12h (SR), 5–10 mL elixir tid–qid or q8h **Caution:** [D, M] **CI:** NAG **Disp:** Many combos/manufacturers Caps *(Donnatal, others):* Hyoscyamine 0.1037 mg/atropine 0.0194 mg/scopolamine 0.0065 mg/phenobarbital 16.2 mg Tabs *(Donnatal, others):* Hyoscyamine 0.1037 mg/atropine 0.0194 mg/scopolamine 0.0065 mg/phenobarbital 16.2 mg. *LA (Donnatal):* Hyoscyamine 0.311 mg/atropine 0.0582 mg/scopolamine 0.0195 mg/phenobarbital 48.6 mg. Elixirs *(Donnatal, others):* Hyoscyamine 0.1037 mg/atropine 0.0194 mg/scopolamine 0.0065 mg/phenobarbital 16.2 mg/5 mL **SE:** Sedation, xerostomia, constipation **Interactions:** ↑ Anticholinergic effects *W/* amantadine, antihistamines, disopyramide; merperidine, procainamide, quinidine, TCA; ↑ effects *OF* atenolol; ↓ effects *W/* antacids **NIPE:** Take drug w/o food; ↑ Risk of heat intolerance/exhaustion/stroke; photophobia

Ibandronate (Boniva, Generic) [Bone Resorption Inhibitor/Bisphosphonate]
Uses: *Rx & prevent osteoporosis in postmenopausal women* **Action:** Bisphosphonate, ↓ osteoclast-mediated bone resorption **Dose:** 2.5 mg PO qd or 150 mg 1 × mo on same d (do not lie down for 60 min after); 3 mg IV over 15–30 s q3mo **Caution:** [C, ?/–] Avoid w/ CrCl < 30 mL/min **CI:** Uncorrected ↓ Ca²⁺; inability to stand/sit upright for 60 min (PO) **Disp:** Tabs 2.5, 150 mg, Inj IV 3 mg/3 mL **SE:** Jaw osteonecrosis (avoid extensive dental procedures) N/D, HA, dizziness, asthenia, HTN, Infxn, dysphagia, esophagitis, esophageal/gastric ulcer, musculoskeletal pain **Interactions:** ↑ GI upset *W/* ASA, NSAIDs; ↓ absorption *W/* antacids, vits, supl or other drugs containing Ca⁺, Mg⁺, Fe; EtOH, food, milk **Labs:** ↑ Cholesterol; ↓ alk phos **NIPE:** ↑ Risk of photophobia, constipation, urinary hesitancy; take 1st thing in ᴀᴍ w/ water (6–8 oz) > 60 min before 1st food/beverage & any meds w/ multivalent cations; give adequate Ca²⁺ & vit D supls; possible association between bisphosphonates & severe muscle/bone/Jt pain; may ↑ atypical subtrochanteric femur fxs; may cause profound hypocalcemia; evaluate ECG for heart conduction abnormalities

Ibrutinib (Imbruvica)
Uses: *Mantle cell lymphoma (MCL) & CLL after 1 prior therapy* **Action:** TKI **Dose:** *Adults.* MCL: 560 mg PO 1 ×/d; CLL: 420 mg

PO 1 ×/d; swallow whole; see label dose mod w/ tox **Caution:** [D, –] embryo-fetal tox; may cause new primary malignancies, ↑ bleeding risk, Infxns, ↓ BM, renal tox; avoid w/ hepatic impair or w/ mod/strong CYP3A Inhib & strong CYP3A inducers, ↓ dose w/CYP3A Inhib **CI:** None **Disp:** Caps 140 mg **SE:** N/V/D, constipation, Abd pain, ↓ plts/WBC, bruising, anemia, fatigue, MS pain, arthralgia, edema, URI, sinusitis, dyspnea, rash, ↓ appetite, pyrexia, stomatitis, dizziness **NIPE:** Swallow whole; ⊘ crush/chew; ⊘ fluids; do not consume grapefruit/grapefruit juice/Seville oranges; limit alcohol; monitor S/Sx Infxn; caution driving

Ibuprofen, Oral (Advil, Motrin, Motrin IB, Rufen, Others, Generic) [OTC] [Anti-Inflammatory, Antipyretic, Analgesic/ NSAID] **WARNING:** May ↑ risk of CV events & GI bleeding **Uses:** *Arthritis, pain, fever* **Action:** NSAID **Dose:** *Adults.* 200–800 mg PO bid–qid (max 2.4 g/d) *Peds.* 30–40 mg/kg/d in 3–4 ÷ doses (max 40 mg/kg/d); w/ food **Caution:** [C (D > 30 wk gestation), +] May interfere w/ ASA's antiplt effect if given < 8 h before ASA **CI:** 3rd tri PRG, severe hepatic impair, allergy, use w/ other NSAIDs, upper GI bleeding, ulcers **Disp:** Tabs 100, 200, 400, 600, 800 mg; chew tabs 50, 100 mg; caps 200 mg; susp 50 mg/1.25 mL, 100 mg/2.5 mL, 100 mg/5 mL, 40 mg/ mL (Motrin IB & Advil OTC 200 mg are the OTC forms) **SE:** Dizziness, peptic ulcer, plt inhibition, worsening of renal Insuff **Interactions:** ↑ Effects *W/* corticosteroids, probenecid, EtOH; ↑ effects *OF* aminoglycosides, anticoagulants, digoxin, hypoglycemics, Li, MTX; ↑ risks of bleeding *W/* abciximab, cefotetan, corticosteroids, valproic acid, thrombolytic drugs, warfarin, ticlopidine, garlic, ginger, ginkgo; ↓ effects *W/* ASA, feverfew; ↓ effects *OF* antihypertensives, diuretics **Labs:** ↑ BUN, Cr, LFTs; ↑ HMG, Hct, BS, plts, WBCs **NIPE:** Take w/ food, may cause hypoglycemia, liver failure, and nystagmus; ↑ risk of photosensitivity

Ibuprofen, Parenteral (Caldolor) [NSAID/Propionic Acid Derivative] **WARNING:** May ↑ risk of CV events & GI bleeding **Uses:** *Mild/mod pain, as adjunct to opioids, ↓ fever* **Action:** NSAID **Dose:** *Pain:* 400–800 mg IV over 30 min q6h PRN *Fever:* 400 mg IV over 30 min, then 400 mg q4–6h or 100– 200 mg q4h PRN **Caution:** [C < 30 wk, D after 30 wk, ?/–] May avoid w/ ASA, & < 17 y **CI:** Hypersensitivity NSAIDs; asthma, urticaria, or allergic Rxns w/ NSAIDs, perioperative CABG **Disp:** Vials 400 mg/4 mL, 800 mg/8 mL **SE:** N/V, HA, flatulence, hemorrhage, dizziness **Interactions:** ↑ risk of GI bleed *W/* anticoagulants; oral corticosteroids, EtOH, tobacco; ↑ Li, methotrexate; ↓ effects *OF* ACEI, diuretics **Labs:** Monitor LFTs, BUN/SCr **NIPE:** Make sure pt well hydrated; use lowest dose & shortest duration possible; prepare and administer w/ in 30 min of reconstitution; infuse over 30 min or greater

Ibutilide (Corvert, Generic) [Antiarrhythmic/Ibutilide Derivative] **Uses:** *Rapid conversion of AF/A flutter* **Action:** Class III antiarrhythmic **Dose:** *Adults.* > 60 kg 1 mg IV over 10 min; may repeat × 1; < 60 kg use 0.01 mg/kg *ECC 2010:* SVT (AFib & Aflutter): *Adults ≥ 60 kg.* 1 mg (10 mL) over 10 min; a 2nd dose may be used; < 60 kg, 0.01 mg/kg over 10 min. Consider DC cardioversion **Caution:** [C, −] **CI:** w/ Class I/III antiarrhythmics (Table 9); QTc > 440 ms **Disp:** Inj 0.1 mg/mL **SE:** Arrhythmias, HA **Interactions:** ↑ Refractory effects **W/** amiodarone, disopyramide, procainamide, quinidine, sotalol; ↑ QT interval **W/** antihistamines, antidepressants, erythromycin, phenothiazine, TCAs **Labs:** Monitor K⁺, Mg²⁺ **NIPE:** Give w/ ECG monitoring; may cause ↑ repolarization leading to arrhythmias, bradycardia; may ↓ BP and lead to cardiac arrest; monitor for rebound hypertension after 1–2 h; wait 10 min between doses

Icatibant (Firazyr) [Bradykinin Inhibitor] Uses: *Hereditary angioedema* **Action:** Bradykinin B2 receptor antag **Dose:** *Adult.* 30 mg SQ in abdomen; repeat q6h × 3 doses/max/24 h **Caution:** [C, ?/–] Seek medical attention after Tx of laryngeal attack **Disp:** Inj 10 mg/mL (30 mg/syringe) **SE:** Inj site Rxns, pyrexia, dizziness, rash **Interactions:** May ↓ the effects *OF/* ACEI **Labs:** ↑ LFTs **NIPE:** May cause drowsiness; administer over 30 sec

Icosapent Ethyl (Vascepa) [Lipid-Regulating Agent] Uses: *Hypertriglyceridemia w/ triglycerides > 500 mg/dL* **Acts:** ↓ Hepatic VLDL-triglyceride synth/secretion & ↑ triglyceride clearance **Dose:** *Adults.* 2 caps bid w/ food **Caution:** [C, M] Caution w/ fish/shellfish allergy **CI:** Component hypersensitivity **Disp:** Caps 1 g **SE:** Arthralgias **Interactions:** Monitor periodically with concomitant drugs that affect coagulation (eg, antiplatelet agents), may ↑ bleeding time **Labs:** If hepatic Dx ✓ ALT/AST baseline and periodically; **NIPE:** (Ethyl ester of eicosapentaenoic); ↓ risk of pancreatitis or CV morbidity/mortality not proven

Idarubicin (Idamycin, Generic) [Antineoplastic; Antibiotic/Anthracycline] WARNING: Administer only under supervision of an MD experienced in leukemia & in an institution w/ resources to maint a pt compromised by drug tox Uses: *Acute leukemias* (AML, ALL), *CML in blast crisis, breast CA* **Action:** DNA intercalating agent; ↓ DNA topoisomerases I & II **Dose:** (Per protocol) 10–12 mg/m²/d for 3–4 d; ↓ in renal/hepatic impair **Caution:** [D, –] **CI:** Bilirubin > 5 mg/dL, PRG **Disp:** Inj 1 mg/mL (5-, 10-, 20-mg vials) **SE:** ↓ BM, cardiotox, N/V, mucositis, alopecia, & IV site Rxns, rarely ↓ renal/hepatic Fxn **Interactions:** ↑ Myelosuppression **W/** antineoplastic drugs & radiation therapy; ↓ effects *OF* live virus vaccines **Labs:** ↑ Uric acid; ↓ WBC, HMG, plts; monitor Cr, LFTs CBC, platelets **NIPE:** ↑ Fluids to 2–3 L/d; avoid extrav, potent vesicant; IV only; may cause a reddish color to urine; avoid OTC products—✓ with provider

Ifosfamide (Ifex, Generic) [Antineoplastic/Alkylating Agent] WARNING: Administer only under supervision by an MD experienced in chemotherapy; hemorrhagic cystitis, myelosuppression; confusion, coma possible Uses: *Testis*, lung, breast, pancreatic & gastric CA, Hodgkin lymphoma/NHL, soft-tissue sarcoma **Action:** Alkylating agent **Dose:** (Per protocol) 1.2 g/m²/d for 5 d bolus or cont Inf; 2.4 g/m²/d for 3 d; w/ mesna uroprotection; ↓ in renal/hepatic impair **Caution:** [D, M] **CI:** ↓ BM Fxn, PRG **Disp:** Inj 1, 3 g **SE:** Hemorrhagic cystitis, nephrotox, N/V, mild–mod leukopenia, lethargy & confusion, alopecia,; **Interactions:** ↑ Risk of bleeding **W/** anticoagulants, ASA,

NSAIDs, thrombolytics; ↑ effects W/ allopurinol, barbiturates, carbamazepine, chloral hydrate, phenobarbital, phenytoin, CYP3A4 inducers; ↑ myelosuppression W/ antineoplastic drugs & radiation therapy; ↓ effects **OF** live virus vaccines; ↓ effects W/ corticosteroids, CYP3A4 Inhibs, St. John's wort **Labs:** ↑ LFTs, uric acid; ↓ plts, WBCs **NIPE:** ↑ Fluids to 2–3 L/d; administer w/ mesna to prevent hemorrhagic cystitis; WBC nadir 10–14 d; recovery 21–28 d; antiemetic before therapy may ↓ N; eval for infection

Iloperidone (Fanapt) [Antipsychotics/Benzisoxazole Derivative] WARNING: Risk for torsades de pointes & ↑ QT. Elderly pts at risk of death, CVA **Uses:** *Acute schizophrenia* **Action:** Atypical antipsychotic **Dose:** *Initial:* 1 mg PO, ↑ daily to goal 6–12 mg bid, max titration 4 mg/d **Caution:** [?, –] **CI:** Component hypersensitivity **Disp:** Tabs: 1, 2, 4, 6, 8, 10, 12 mg **SE:** Orthostatic ↓ BP, dizziness, dry mouth, ↑ wgt **Interactions:** ↑ risk of prolonged QTc W/ amiodarone, antiarrhythmics, antipsychotics, chlorpromazine, gatifloxacin, levomethadyl, methadone, moxifloxacin, pentamidine, procainamide, quinidine, thioridazine; ↑ effect W/ CYP2D6, CYP3A4 inducers (carbamazepine, barbiturates, phenytoins, rifampin); ↑ effects **OF** CYP2D6 & CYP3A4 Inhibs (delavirdine, indinavir, isoniazid, itraconazole, dalfopristin, ritonavir, tipranavir); clarithromycin, fluoxetine, ketoconazole, paroxetine; ↑ risks of orthostatic hypotension W/ antihypertensives; ↑ risks of impaired thermoregulation W/ anticholinergics; ↑ risk of serotonin synd W/ SSRI, SNRIs **Labs:** ↑ Prolactin level; monitor CBC, K+, Mg **NIPE:** Titrate to ↓ BP risk; monitor ECG for prolonged QT interval; avoid OTC meds; may cause drowsiness, tachycardia, syncope; in geriatric pts may cause pneumonia, heart failure, sudden death

Iloprost (Ventavis) [Prostaglandin Analog] WARNING: Associated w/ syncope; may require dosage adjustment **Uses:** *NYHA Class III/IV pulm arterial HTN* **Action:** Prostaglandin analogue **Dose:** Initial 2.5 mcg; if tolerated, ↑ to 5 mcg Inh 6–9 × /d at least 2 h apart while awake **Caution:** [C, ?/–] Antiplt effects, ↑ bleeding risk w/ anticoagulants; additive hypotensive effects **CI:** SBP < 85 mm Hg **Disp:** Inh soln 10, 20 mcg/mL **SE:** Syncope, ↓ BP, vasodilation, cough, HA, trismus, D, dysgeusia, rash, oral irritation **Interactions:** ↑ Effects **OF** anticoagulants, antihypertensives, antiplts **Labs:** ↑ Alk phos **NIPE:** Instruct pt of syncope risk; monitor BP; requires *Pro-Dose AAD* or *I-neb ADD* system nebulizer; counsel on syncope risk; do not mix w/ other drugs; monitor vital signs during initial Rx

Imatinib (Gleevec) [Antineoplastic/Tyrosine Kinase Inhibitor] **Uses:** *Rx CML Ph(+), CML blast crisis, ALL Ph(+), myelodysplastic/myeloproliferative Dz, aggressive systemic mastocytosis, chronic eosinophilic leukemia, GIST, dermatofibrosarcoma protuberans* **Action:** ↓ BCL-ABL; TKI **Dose:** **Adults.** *Typical.* 400–600 mg PO qd; w/ meal **Peds.** *CML Ph(+) newly diagnosed:* 340 mg/m^2/d, 600 mg/d max *Recurrent:* 260 mg/m^2/d PO ÷ qd–bid, to 340 mg/m^2/d max **Caution:** [D, ?/–] Warfarin **CI:** Component sensitivity **Disp:** Tab 100,

400 mg **SE:** GI upset, fluid retention, muscle cramps, musculoskeletal pain, arthralgia, rash, HA, neutropenia, thrombocytopenia **Interactions:** ↑ Effects W/ CYP3A4 inhibitors (ketoconazole, itraconazole, erythromycin, clarithromycin), grapefruit; ↑ effects *OF* CCB, simvastatin, ergots; ↑ risk of liver tox W/ APAP; ↓ effects W/ CYP3A4 inducers (carbamazepine, dexamethasone, phenobarbital, phenytoin, rifampin, carbamazepin, St. John's wort) **Labs:** ↑ LFTs; ↓ HMG, Hct, neutrophils, plts; follow CBCs & LFTs baseline & monthly **NIPE:** Take w/ large glass of H$_2$O & food to ↓ GI irritation; use barrier contraception; ↓ growth noted in children/preadolescents

Imipenem–Cilastatin (Primaxin, Generic) [Antibiotic/Carbapenems]

Uses: *Serious Infxns* d/t susceptible bacteria **Action:** Bactericidal; ↓ cell wall synth. *Spectrum:* Gram(+) (*S aureus,* group A & B streptococci), gram(−) (not *Legionella*), anaerobes **Dose:** *Adults.* 250–1000 mg (imipenem) IV q6–8h, 500–750 mg IM *Peds.* 60–100 mg/kg/24 h IV ÷ q6h; ↓ if CrCl is < 70 mL/min Caution: [C, +/−] **CI:** Ped pts w/ CNS Infxn (↑ Sz risk) & < 30 kg w/ renal impair **Disp:** Inj (imipenem/cilastatin mg) 250/250, 500/500 **SE:** Szs if drug accumulates, GI upset, thrombocytopenia **Interactions:** ↑ Risks of Szs W/ aminophylline, cyclosporine, ganciclovir, theophylline; ↑ effects W/ probenecid; ↓ effect *OF* valproic acid **Labs:** ↑ LFTs, BUN, Cr; ↓ plts, WBCs **NIPE:** Eval for super Infxn; ↑ risk of Sz

Imipramine (Tofranil) [Antidepressant/TCA]

WARNING: Close observation for suicidal thinking or unusual changes in behavior **Uses:** *Depression, enuresis*, panic attack, chronic pain **Action:** TCA; ↑ CNS synaptic serotonin or norepinephrine **Dose:** *Adults.* Hospitalized: Initial 100 mg/24 h PO in ÷ doses; ↑ over several wk 300 mg/d max *Outpatient:* Maint 50–150 mg PO hs, 300 mg/24 h max *Peds. Antidepressant:* 1.5–5 mg/kg/24 h ÷ daily–qid. *Enuresis:* **> 6 y:** 10–25 mg PO qhs; ↑ by 10–25 mg at 1–2-wk intervals (max 50 mg for 6–12 y, 75 mg for > 12 y); Rx for 2–3 mo, then taper Caution: [D, ?/−] **CI:** Use w/ MAOIs, NAG, recovery from AMI, PRG, CHF, angina, CV Dz, arrhythmias **Disp:** Tabs 10, 25, 50 mg; caps 75, 100, 125, 150 mg **SE:** CV Sxs, dizziness, xerostomia, discolored urine **Interactions:** ↑ Effects W/ amiodarone, anticholinergics, BBs, cimetidine, diltiazem, Li, OCPs, quinidine, phenothiazine, ritonavir, verapamil, EtOH, evening primrose oil; ↑ effects *OF* barbiturates, benzodiazepines, CNS depressants, hypoglycemics, warfarin, EtOH; ↑ risk of serotonin synd W/ MAOIs, St. John's Wort; ↓ effects W/ tobacco; ↓ effects *OF* clonidine, ephedrine, guanethidine **Labs:** ↑ Serum glucose, alk phos, bilirubin **NIPE:** D/C 48 h before surgery; D/C MAOIs 2 wk before administration of this drug; 4–6 wk for full effects; take w/ food; less sedation than amitriptyline; therapeutic effects may take 2–3 wk, risk of photosensitivity

Imiquimod Cream (Aldara, Zyclara) [Topical Immunomodulator]

Uses: *Anogenital warts, HPV, condylomata acuminata* **Action:** Unknown; ? cytokine induction **Dose:** *Adults/Peds > 12 y. Warts:* 1 ×/d up to 8 wk

(Zyclara); apply 3 ×/wk, leave on 6–10 h & wash off w/ soap & water, continue 16 wk max (Aldara) *Actinic keratosis:* Apply daily two 2 ×/wk cycle separate by 2 wk *Basal cell:* Apply 5 d/wk × 6 wk, dose based on lesion size (see label) **Caution:** [B, ?] Topical only **CI:** Component sensitivity **Disp:** 2.5% packet, 3.75% packet or pump (Zyclara); single-dose packets 5% (250 mg cream Aldara) **SE:** Local skin Rxns, flu-like synd **NIPE:** Not a cure; may weaken condoms/Vag diaphragms, wash hands before & after use

Immune Globulin, IV (Gamimune N, Gammaplex, Gammar IV, Sandoglobulin, Others) [Immune Serum/Immunologic Agent] **Uses:** *IgG deficiency Dz states, B-cell CLL, CIDP, HIV, hep A prophylaxis, ITP*, Kawasaki Dz, travel to ↑ prevalence area & hep A vaccination w/in 2 wk of travel **Action:** IgG supl **Dose:** *Adults & Peds. Immunodeficiency:* 200–(300 *Gammaplex*)–800 mg/kg/mo IV at 0.01–0.04 (0.08 *Gammaplex*) mL/kg/min; initial dose 0.01 mL/kg/min *B-cell CLL:* 400 mg/kg/dose IV q3wk, *CIDP:* 2000 ÷ doses over 2–4 d *ITP:* 400 mg/kg/dose IV daily × 5 d *BMT:* 500 mg/kg/wk; ↓ in renal Insuff **Caution:** [C, ?] Separate live vaccines by 3 mo **CI:** IgA deficiency w/ Abs to IgA, severe ↓ plt, coagulation disorders **Disp:** Inj SE: Associated mostly w/ Inf rate; GI upset, thrombotic events, hemolysis, renal failure/dysfunction, TRALI **Interactions:** ↓ Effects *OF* live virus vaccines **Labs:** ↑ BUN, Cr **NIPE:** Monitor vitals during Inf; do not give if volume depleted; Infus only if soln clear & at room temp; hep A prophylaxis w/ immunoglobulin is no better than w/ vaccination; advantages to using vaccination, cost similar; wait at least 3 mo before administering live virus vaccine

Immune Globulin, Subcutaneous (Hizentra) [Immune Serum] **Uses:** *Primary immunodeficiency* **Action:** IgG supl **Dose:** See label for dosage calculation/adjustment; for SQ Inf only **Caution:** [C, ?] **CI:** Hx anaphylaxis to immune globulin; some IgA deficiency **Disp:** Soln for SQ Inj 0.2 g/mL (20%) **SE:** Inj site Rxns, HA, GI complaint, fatigue, fever, N, D, rash, sore throat **Interactions:** ↓ Effects *OF* live virus vaccines **Labs:** Falsely elevated serum glucose level, + Coombs' test **NIPE:** May instruct in home administration; keep refrigerated; discard unused drug; use up to 4 Inj sites, max flow rate not > 50 mL/h for all sites combined

Inamrinone [Amrinone] (Inocor) [Inotropic/Vasodilator] **Uses:** *Acute CHF, ischemic cardiomyopathy* **Action:** Inotrope w/ vasodilator **Dose:** *Adults.* IV bolus 0.75 mg/kg over 2–3 min; maint 5–10 mcg/kg/min, 10 mg/kg/d max; ↓ if CrCl < 30 mL/min *Peds. ECC 2010:* CHF in post-op CV surgery pts, shock w/ ↑ SVR: 0.75–1 mg/kg IV/IO load over 5 min; repeat × 2 PRN; max 3 mg/kg; cont Inf 5–10 mcg/kg/min **Caution:** [C, ?] Bisulfite allergy **Disp:** Inj 5 mg/mL **SE:** Monitor fluid, lytes, & renal changes **Interactions:** Diuretics cause sig hypovolemia; ↑ effects *OF* cardiac glycosides; excessive hypotension *W/* disopyramide **Labs:** Monitor LFTs, lytes, plts **NIPE:** Monitor I&O, daily wgt, BP, pulse; incompatible w/ dextrose solns; observe for arrhythmias, bleeding, bruising

Indacaterol Inhalation Powder (Arcapta Neohaler) WARNING: LABAs increase risk of asthma-related deaths. Considered a class effect of all LABAs Uses: *Daily maint of COPD (chronic bronchitis/emphysema)* Acts: Long-acting β₂-adrenergic agonist (LABA) Dose: 75-mcg capsule inhaled 1 ×/d w/ Neohaler inhaler only Caution: [C, ?/–] Not for acute deterioration of COPD or asthma; paradoxical bronchospasm possible; excessive use or use w/ other LABA can cause cardiac effects and can be fatal; caution w/ Sz disorders, thyrotoxicosis or sympathomimetic sensitivity CI: All LABA CI in asthma w/o use of long-term asthma control med; not indicated for asthma Disp: Inhal hard cap 75 mcg (30 blister pack w/ 1 Neohaler) SE: Cough, oropharyngeal pain, nasopharyngitis, HA, N Interactions: ↑ Effects W/ adrenergic drugs; ↓ effect W/ β-blockers; ↑ risk of prolonged QT interval W/ MAOI, TCA; ↑ risk of hypokalemia W/ caffeine, theophylline, non-potassium-sparing diuretics; Labs: ↑ Glucose; ↓ K⁺ NIPE: Inform patient not to swallow caps

Indapamide (Lozol, Generic) [Antihypertensive/Thiazide Diuretic] Uses: *HTN, edema, CHF* Action: Thiazide diuretic; ↑ Na, Cl, & H₂O excretion in distal tubule Dose: 1.25–5 mg/d PO Caution: [D, ?] ↑ Effect w/ loop diuretics, ACE Inhibs, cyclosporine, digoxin, Li CI: Anuria, thiazide/sulfonamide allergy, renal Insuff, PRG Disp: Tabs 1.25, 2.5 mg SE: ↓ BP, dizziness, photosensitivity Interactions: ↑ Effects W/ antihypertensives, diazoxide, nitrates, EtOH; ↑ effects OF ACEIs, Li; ↑ risk of hypokalemia W/ amphotericin B, corticosteroids, mezlocillin, piperacillin, ticarcillin; ↓ effects W/ cholestyramine, colestipol, NSAIDs Labs: ↑ Serum glucose, cholesterol, uric acid, ↓ K⁺, Na, Cl NIPE: ↑ Risk photosensitivity—use sunblock; take w/ food or milk; no additional effects w/ doses > 5 mg; take early to avoid nocturia

Indinavir (Crixivan) [Antiretroviral/Protease Inhibitor] Uses: *HIV Infxn* Action: Protease Inhib; ↑ maturation of noninfectious virions to mature infectious virus Dose: Typical 800 mg PO q8h in combo w/ other antiretrovirals (dose varies); on empty stomach; ↓ w/ hepatic impair Caution: [C, ?] Numerous interactions, esp CYP3A4 Inhib (Table 10) CI: w/ triazolam, midazolam, pimozide, ergot alkaloids, simvastatin, lovastatin, sildenafil, St. John's wort, amiodarone, salmeterol, PDE5 Inhib, alpha 1-adrenoreceptor antagonist (alfuzosin); colchicine Disp: Caps 200, 400 mg SE: Nephrolithiasis, dyslipidemia, lipodystrophy, N/V Interactions: ↑ Effects W/ azole antifungals, clarithromycin, delavirdine, ILs, quinidine, zidovudine; ↑ effects OF amiodarone, cisapride, clarithromycin, ergot alkaloids, fentanyl, HMG-CoA reductase Inhibs, INH, OCPs, phenytoin, rifabutin, ritonavir, sildenafil, stavudine, zidovudine; ↓ effects W/ efavirenz, fluconazole, phenytoin, rifampin, St. John's wort, high-fat/-protein foods, grapefruit juice; ↓ effects OF midazolam, triazolam Labs: ↑ Bilirubin, serum glucose, LFTs, ↓ plts, neutrophils NIPE: ↑ Fluids—drink six 8-oz glasses of H₂O/d; caps moisture sensitive—keep desiccant in container

Indomethacin (Indocin, Generic) [Analgesic, Anti-Inflammatory, Antipyretic/NSAID] **WARNING:** May ↑ risk of CV events & GI bleeding **Uses:** *Arthritis; close ductus arteriosus; ankylosing spondylitis* **Action:** ↓ Prostaglandins **Dose:** *Adults.* 25–50 mg PO bid–tid, max 200 mg/d *Infants.* 0.2–0.25 mg/kg/dose IV; may repeat in 12–24 h max 3 doses; w/ food **Caution:** [C, +] **CI:** ASA/NSAID sensitivity, peptic ulcer/active GI bleed, precipitation of asthma/urticaria/rhinitis by NSAIDs/ASA, premature neonates w/ NEC ↓ renal Fxn, active bleeding, thrombocytopenia, 3rd tri PRG **Disp:** Inj 1 mg/vial; caps 25, 50 mg; SR caps 75 mg; susp 25 mg/5 mL **SE:** GI bleeding or upset, dizziness, edema **Interactions:** ↑ Effects *W/* APAP, anti-inflammatories, gold compounds, diflunisal, probenecid; ↑ effects *OF* aminoglycosides, anticoagulants, digoxin, hypoglycemics, Li, MTX, nifedipine, phenytoin, penicillamine, verapamil; ↑ risk of bleeding *W/* anticoagulants, abciximab, cefamandole, cefoperazone, cefotetan, clopidogrel, eptifibatide, plicamycin, ticlopidine, tirofiban, valproic acid, thrombolytics, ASA, SSRIs, SNRIs; ↓ effects *W/* ASA; ↓ effects *OF* antihypertensives **Labs:** ↑ LFTs, serum K⁺, ↓ HMG, Hct; monitor renal Fxn **NIPE:** Take w/ food, monitor ECG for hyperkalemia (peaked T waves); risk of photosensitivity

Infliximab (Remicade) [Anti-Inflammatory/Monoclonal Antibody] **WARNING:** TB, invasive fungal Infxns, & other opportunistic Infxns reported, some fatal; perform TB skin testing prior to use; possible association w/ rare lymphoma **Uses:** *Mod–severe Crohn Dz; fistulizing Crohn Dz; UC; RA (w/ MTX) psoriasis, ankylosing spondylitis* **Action:** IgG1K neutralizes TNF-α **Dose:** *Adults. Crohn Dz: Induction:* 5 mg/kg IV Inf, w/ doses 2 & 6 wk after *Maint:* 5 mg/kg IV Inf q8wk *RA:* 3 mg/kg IV Inf at 0, 2, 6 wk, then q8wk *Peds > 6 y.* 5 mg/kg IV q8wk **Caution:** [B, ?/–] Active Infxn, hepatic impair, Hx or risk of TB, hep B **CI:** Murine allergy, mod–severe CHF, w/ live vaccines (eg, smallpox) **Disp:** 100 mg Inj **SE:** Allergic Rxns, HA, fatigue, GI upset, Inf Rxns; hepatotox; reactivation hep B, pneumonia, BM suppression, systemic vasculitis, pericardial effusion, new psoriasis **Interactions:** ↑ risk of serious infection *W/* TNF blockers; may ↓ effects *OF* live virus vaccines **Labs:** ↑ LFTs, ↓ WBC, HMG, plts; monitor LFTs; PPD at baseline; monitor hep B carrier **NIPE:** ↑ Susceptibility to Infxn; skin exam for malignancy w/ psoriasis; can premedicate w/ antihistamines, APAP, and/or steroids to ↓ Inf Rxns

Influenza Vaccine, Inactivated, Quadrivalent (IIV4) (Fluarix Quadrivalent, Fluzone Quadrivalent) [Influenza Vaccine] See Table 13 **Uses:** *Prevent influenza* all > 6 mo **Action:** Active immunization **Dose:** *Adults and Peds > 9 y.* 0.5 mL/dose IM annually *Peds 6–35 mo. (Fluzone)* 0.25 mL IM annually; 0.25 mL IM 2 doses 4 wk apart for 1st vaccination; give 2 doses in 2nd vaccination y if only 1 dose given in 1st y *3–8 y.* 0.5 mL IM annually; 0.5 mL IM × 2 doses 4 wk apart for 1st vaccination **Caution:** [C, +] Hx Guillain-Barré synd w/in 6 wk of previous flu vaccine; syncope may occur w/ admin **CI:** Hx allergy to egg protein, latex (*Fluarix*); egg protein (*Fluzone*) **Disp:** Based on manufacturer, 0.25-, 0.5-mL prefilled syringe, single-dose vial **SE:** Inj site soreness, fever, chills, HA, insomnia, myalgia, malaise, rash, urticaria, anaphylactoid Rxns, Guillain-Barré synd **Interactions:** Immunocompromised w/ ↓immune response; ↓ response W/ radiation, chemotherapy, high-dose steroids **NIPE:** US Oct–Nov best, protection 1–2 wk after, lasts up to 6 mo; given yearly, vaccines based on predictions of flu season (Nov–April in US, w/ sporadic cases all year); refer to ACIP annual recs (www.cdc.gov/vaccines/acip)

Influenza Vaccine, Inactivated, Quadrivalent (IIV₃) (Afluria, Fluarix, Flucelvax, FluLaval, Fluvirin, Fluzone, Fluzone High Dose, Fluzone Intradermal) [Antiviral/Vaccine] See Table 13
Uses: *Prevent influenza* all persons ≥ 6 mo **Action:** Active immunization **Dose:** *Adults & Peds > 9 y.* 0.5 mL/dose IM annually; or 0.1 mL intradermal Inj annually (Fluzone Intradermal for adults 18–64 y) *Peds 6–35 mo.* 0.25 mL IM annually; 0.25 mL IM × 2 doses 4 wk apart 1st vaccination; give 2 doses in 2nd vaccination y if only 1 dose given in 1st y *3–8 y.* 0.5 mL IM annually; 0.5 mL IM × 2 doses 4 wk apart for 1st vaccination **Caution:** [B, +] Hx Guillain-Barré synd w/in 6 wk of previous influenza vaccine; syncope may occur w/ admin; immunocompromised w/ ↓ immune response **CI:** Hx allergy to egg protein, neomycin, polymyxin (Afluria); egg protein, latex, gentamicin (Fluarix); latex (Flucelvax); egg protein (FluLaval), egg protein, latex, polymyxin, neomycin (Fluvirin); egg protein, latex (Fluzone); thimerosal allergy (FluLaval, Fluvirin, & multidose Fluzone); single-/multi dose vials latex free; acute resp or febrile illness **Disp:** Based on manufacturer, 0.25- & 0.5-mL prefilled syringes **SE:** Inj site soreness, fever, chills, HA, insomnia, myalgia, malaise, rash, urticaria, anaphylactoid Rxns, Guillain-Barré synd **Interactions:** ↑ Effects *OF* theophylline, warfarin; ↓ effects *W/* corticosteroids, immunosuppressants; ↓ effects *OF* aminophylline, phenytoin **NIPE:** Not for swine flu H1N1; can be administered at the same time. Fluarix & Fluzone Intradermal not for peds; US Oct–Nov best, protection 1–2 wk after, lasts up to 6 mo; given yearly, vaccines based on predictions of flu season (Nov–April in US, w/ sporadic cases all year); refer to ACIP annual recs (www.cdc.gov/vaccines/acip)

Influenza Virus Vaccine Live Attenuated, Quadrivalent [LAIV₄] (FluMist) [Antiviral/Vaccine] See Table 13 **Uses:** *Prevent influenza* **Action:** Live attenuated vaccine **Dose:** *Adults and Peds 9–49 y.* 0.1 mL each nostril × 1 annually *Peds 2–8 y.* 0.1 mL each nostril × 1 annually; initial 0.1 mL each nostril × 2 doses 4 wk apart in 1st vaccination y **Caution:** [B, ?/–] Hx Guillain-Barré synd w/in 6 wk of previous influenza vaccine; **CI:** HX allergy to egg protein, gentamicin, gelatin, or arginine; peds 2–17 y on ASA, PRG, known/ suspected immune deficiency, asthma or reactive airway Dz, acute febrile illness **Disp:** Single dose, nasal sprayer 0.2 mL; shipped frozen, store 35–46°F **SE:** Runny nose, nasal congestion, HA, cough, fever, sore throat **Interaction:** ↑ Risk of wheezing w/ asthma; use w/ influenza A/B antiviral drugs may ↓ efficacy

NIPE: Do not give w/ other vaccines; avoid contact w/ immunocompromised individuals for 21 d; live influenza vaccine more effective in children than inactivated influenza vaccine; refer to ACIP annual recs (*www.cdc.gov/vaccines/acip*)

Influenza Vaccine, Recombinant, Trivalent (RIV₃) (FluBlok) [Antiviral/Vaccine] See Table 13 **Uses:** *Prevent influenza* **Action:** Active immunization **Dose:** *Adults 18–49 y.* 0.5 mL/dose IM annually **Caution:** [B, ?/–] Hx Guillain-Barré synd w/in 6 wk of previous flu vaccine **CI:** Hx component allergy (contains no egg protein, antibiotics, preservatives, latex) **Disp:** 0.5-mL single-dose vial **SE:** Inj site soreness, HA, fatigue, myalgia **Interactions:** Immunocompromised w/ ↓ immune response **NIPE:** US Oct–Nov best, protection 1–2 wk after, lasts up to 6 mo; given yearly, vaccines based on predictions of flu season (Nov–April in US, w/ sporadic cases all year); refer to ACIP annual recs (*www.cdc.gov/vaccines/acip*)

Ingenol Mebutate (Picato) **Uses:** *Actinic keratosis* **Action:** Necrosis by neutrophil activation **Dose:** *Adults.* 25 cm² area (1 tube), evenly spread; 0.015% to face qd × 3 d; 0.05% to trunk/neck qd × 2 days **Caution:** [C, ?/–] None **Disp:** Gel; 0.015%, 0.25 g/tube × 3 tubes; 0.05% 0.25 g/tube × 2 tubes **SE:** Local skin reactions **NIPE:** From plant sap *Euphorbia peplus*; allow to dry × 15 min; do not wash/touch × 6 h; avoid contact w/ eye

Insulin, Injectable [Hypoglycemic/Hormone] See Table 4 **Uses:** *Type 1 or 2 DM refractory to diet or PO hypoglycemic agents; acute life-threatening ↑ K⁺* **Action:** Insulin supl **Dose:** Based on serum glucose; usually SQ (upper arms, Abd wall [most rapid absorption site], upper legs, buttocks); can give IV (only regular)/IM; type 1 typical start dose 0.5–1 units/kg/d; type 2 0.3–0.4 units/kg/d; renal failure ↓ insulin needs **Caution:** [B, +] **CI:** Hypoglycemia **Disp:** Table 4; some can be dispensed w/ preloaded insulin cartridge pens w/ 29-, 30-, or 31-gauge needles & dosing adjustments **SE:** Hypoglycemia. Highly purified insulins ↑ free insulin; monitor for several wk when changing doses/agents **Interactions:** ↑ Hypoglycemic effects *W/* α-blockers, anabolic steroids, BBs, clofibrate, fenfluramine, guanethidine, MAOIs, NSAIDs, pentamidine, phenylbutazone, salicylates, sulfinpyrazone, tetracyclines, EtOH, celery, coriander, dandelion root, fenugreek, ginseng, garlic, juniper berries; ↓ hypoglycemic effects *W/* corticosteroids, dextrothyroxine, diltiazem, dobutamine, epinephrine, niacin, OCPs, protease Inhib antiretrovirals, rifampin, thiazide diuretics, thyroid preps, marijuana, tobacco **NIPE:** If mixing insulins, draw up short-acting preps 1st in syringe; specific agent/regimen based on pt/healthcare provider choices for glycemic control. Typical type 1 DM regimens use basal daily insulin w/ premeal Injs of rapidly acting insulins. Insulin pumps may achieve basal insulin levels. ↑ Malignancy risk w/ glargine controversial

Interferon Alfa-2b (Intron-A) [Antineoplastic/Immunomodulator] **WARNING:** Can cause or aggravate fatal or life-threatening neuropsychological, autoimmune, ischemic, & infectious disorders. Monitor closely **Uses:** *HCL,

Kaposi sarcoma, melanoma, CML, chronic hep B & C, follicular NHL, condylomata acuminata* **Action:** Antiproliferative; modulates host immune response; ↓ viral replication in infected cells **Dose:** Per protocols. *Adults.* Per protocols *HCL:* 2 MU/m² IM/SQ 3 ×/wk for 2–6 mo. *Chronic hep B:* 5 MU/d or 10 MU 3 ×/wk IM/SQ × 16 wk *Follicular NHL:* 5 MU SQ 3 ×/wk for 18 mo *Melanoma:* 20 MU/m² IV × 5 d/wk × 4 wk, then 10 MU/m² SQ 3 ×/wk × 48 wk. *Kaposi sarcoma:* 30 MU/m² IM/SQ 3 ×/wk until disease progression or maximal response achieved *Chronic hep C (Intron-A):* 3 MU IM/SQ 3 ×/wk × 16 wk (continue 18–24 mo if response) *Condyloma:* 1 MU/lesion (max 5 lesions) 3 ×/wk (on alternate days) for 3 wk *Peds. Chronic hep B:* 3 MU/m² SQ 3 ×/wk × 1 wk, then 6 MU/m² max 10 MU/dose 3 ×/wk × 16–24 wk **CI:** Benzyl alcohol sensitivity, decompensated liver Dz, autoimmune hep immunosuppressed, PRG, CrCl < 50 mL/min in combo w/ribavirin **Disp:** Inj units: powder 10/18/50 mill IU; soln 6/10 mill IU/mL (see also Polyethylene Glycol [PEG]-Interferon) **SE:** Flu-like Sxs, fatigue, anorexia, neurotox at high doses; up to 40% neutralizing Ab w/ Rx **Interactions:** ↑ Effects *OF* antineoplastics, CNS depressants, doxorubicin, theophylline; ↓ effects *OF* live virus vaccine **Labs:** ↑ LFTs, BUN, SCr, glucose, P; ↓ HMG, Hct, Ca **NIPE:** ASA & EtOH use may cause GI bleed, ↑ fluids to 2–3 L/d

Interferon Alfacon-1 (Infergen) [Immunomodulator] WARNING: Can cause or aggravate fatal or life-threatening neuropsychological, autoimmune, ischemic, & infectious disorders, combo therapy with ribavirin. Monitor closely **Uses:** *Chronic hep C* **Action:** Biologic response modifier **Dose:** *Monotherapy:* 9 mcg SQ 3 ×/wk × 24 wk (initial Rx) or 15 mcg 3 ×/wk up to 48 wk (retreatment). *Combo:* 15 mcg/d w/ribavirin 1000 or 1200 mg (wgt < 75 kg and ≥ 75 kg) qd up to 48 wk (retreatment); ↓ dose w/ SAE **Caution:** [C, M] **CI:** E coli product allergy, decompensated liver Dz, autoimmune hep **Disp:** Inj 30 mcg/mL **SE:** Flu-like synd, depression, blood dyscrasias, colitis, pancreatitis, hepatic decompensation, ↑ SCr, eye disorders ↓ thyroid **Interactions:** ↑ Effects *OF* theophylline **Labs:** ↑ Triglycerides, TSH; ↑ SCr; ↓ HMG, Hct; ↓ thyroid enzymes; monitor CBC, plt, SCr, TFT **NIPE:** Refrigerate; ⊘ shake; use barrier contraception; allow > 48 h between Inj

Interferon Beta-1a (Avonex, Rebif) [Immunomodulator] **Uses:** *MS, relapsing* **Action:** Biologic response modifier **Dose:** *Rebif:* Give SQ for target dose 44 mcg 3 ×/wk; start 8.8 mcg 3 ×/wk × 2 wk then 22 mcg 3 ×/wk × 2 wk then 44 mcg 3 ×/wk × 2 wk; target dose 22 mcg: 4.4 mcg 3 ×/wk × 2 wk, then 11 mcg 3 ×/wk × 2 wk then 22 mcg SQ 3 ×/wk *Avonex:* 30 mcg SQ 1 ×/wk **Caution:** [C, ?] w/ Hepatic impair, depression, Sz disorder, thyroid Dz **CI:** Human albumin allergy **Disp:** 0.5-mL prefilled syringes w/ 29-gauge needle Titrate Pak 8.8 & 22 mcg; 22 or 44 mcg **SE:** Inj site Rxn, HA, flu-like Sxs, malaise, fatigue, rigors, myalgia, depression w/ suicidal ideation, hepatotox, ↓ BM **Interactions:** Caution w/ other hepatotoxic drugs **Labs:** Monitor CBC 1, 3, 6 mo; ✓ TFTs q6mo w/ h/o thyroid Dz **NIPE:** Dose > 48 h apart; D/C if jaundice occurs; may have abortifacient effects

Interferon Beta-1b (Betaseron, Extavia) [Immunomodulator]
Uses: *MS, relapsing/remitting/secondary progressive* Action: Biologic response modifier Dose: 0.0625 mg (2 MU) (0.25 mL) SQ, ↑ by 0.0625 mg q2wk to target dose 0.25 mg (1 mL) qod Caution: [C, –] CI: Human albumin sensitivity Disp: Powder for Inj 0.3 mg (9.6 MU interferon [IFN]) SE: Flu-like synd, depression, blood dyscrasias, Inj site necrosis, anaphylaxis Interactions: ↑ Effects *OF* theophylline, zidovudine Labs: ↑ AST/ALT/GGT, BUN, urine protein; ✓ LFTs, CBC 1, 3, 6 mo, TFT q6mo NIPE: ↑ Risk *OF* photosensitivity—use sunscreen, ↑ risk of abortion; ↑ fluid intake, use barrier contraception; pt self Inj, rotate sites; consider stopping w/ depression

Interferon Gamma-1b (Actimmune) [Immunomodulator]
Uses: *↓ Incidence of serious Infxns in chronic granulomatous Dz (CGD), osteoporosis* Action: Biologic response modifier Dose: 50 mcg/m² SQ (1.5 MU/m²) BSA > 0.5 m²; if BSA < 0.5 m², give 1.5 mcg/kg/dose; given 3 ×/wk Caution: [C, –] CI: Allergy to *E coli*–derived products Disp: Inj 100 mcg (2 MU) SE: Flu-like synd, depression, blood dyscrasias, dizziness, altered mental status, gait disturbance, hepatic tox Interactions: ↑ Myelosuppression *W/* myelosuppressive drugs Labs: ↑ LFTs; ↓ neutrophils, plts NIPE: Small frequent meals may ↓ GI upset; rotate Inj sites; may ↑ deaths in interstitial pulm fibrosis

Ipecac Syrup [OTC] [Antidote] Uses: *Drug OD, certain cases of poisoning* (Note: Usage is falling out of favor & is no longer recommended by some groups) Action: Irritation of the GI mucosa; stimulation of the chemoreceptor trigger zone Dose: Adults. 15–30 mL PO, followed by 200–300 mL of H₂O; if no emesis in 20 min, repeat once Peds 6–12 y. 5–10 mL PO, followed by 10–20 mL/kg of H₂O; if no emesis in 20 min, repeat once 1–12 y. 15 mL PO followed by 10–20 mL/kg of H₂O; if no emesis in 20 min, repeat once Caution: [C, ?] CI: Ingestion of petroleum distillates, strong acid, base, or other caustic agents; comatose/unconscious Disp: Syrup 15, 30 mL (OTC) SE: Lethargy, D, cardiotox, protracted V Interactions: ↑ Effects *OF* myelosuppressives, theophylline, zidovudine NIPE: ↑ Fluids to 2–3 L/d; ⊘ EtOH; caution in CNS depressant OD; activated charcoal considered more effective

Ipilimumab (Yervoy) [Cytotoxic T-Lymphocyte Antigen 4 (CTLA-4)–Blocking Antibody] WARNING: Severe fatal immune Rxns possible; D/C & Tx w/ high-dose steroids w/ severe Rxn; assess for enterocolitis, dermatitis, neuropathy, endocrinopathy before each dose Uses: *Unresectable/ metastactic melanoma* Action: Human cytotoxic T-lymphocyte antigen 4 (CTLA-4)–blocking Ab; ↑ T-cell proliferation/activation Dose: 3 mg/kg IV q3wk × 4 doses. Inf over 90 min Caution: [C, –] Can cause immune-mediated adverse Rxns; endocrinopathies may require Rx; hep dermatologic tox; neuromuscular tox, ophthalmic tox CI: None Disp: IV 50 mg/10 mL, 200 mg/40 mL SE: Fatigue, D, pruritus, rash, colitis Labs: ✓ LFTs, TFT, chemistries baseline/pre-Inf NIPE: ↑ Risk of neuropathy, dermatitis and enterocolitis; infuse over 90 min q3wk for a total of 4 doses.

Ipratropium (Atrovent HFA, Atrovent Nasal) [Bronchodilator/Anticholinergic] Uses: *Bronchospasm w/ COPD, rhinitis, rhinorrhea* **Action:** Synthetic anticholinergic similar to atropine; antagonizes acetylcholine receptors, inhibits mucous gland secretions **Dose:** *Adults & Peds > 12 y.* 2–4 puffs qid, max 12 Inh/d *Nasal:* 2 sprays/nostril bid–tid *Nebulization:* 500 mcg 3–4 × /d *ECC 2010:* **Asthma:** 250–500 mcg by nebulizer/MDI q20min × 3 **Caution:** [B, ?/M] w/ Inhaled insulin **CI:** Allergy to soya lecithin–related foods **Disp:** HFA: Metered-dose inhaler 17 mcg/dose; Inh soln 0.02%; nasal spray 0.03%, 0.06% **SE:** Nervousness, dizziness, HA, cough, bitter taste, nasal dryness, URI, epistaxis **Interactions:** ↑ Effects *W/* albuterol; ↑ effects *OF* anticholinergics, antimuscarinics; ↓ effects *W/* jaborandi tree, pill-bearing spurge **NIPE:** Adequate fluids; separate Inh of other drugs by 5 min; not for acute bronchospasm unless used w/ inhaled β-agonist

Irbesartan (Avapro) [Antihypertensive/ARB] WARNING: D/C stat if PRG detected Uses: *HTN, DN*, CHF **Action:** Angiotensin II receptor antagonist **Dose:** 150 mg/d PO, may ↑ to 300 mg/d **Caution:** [C (1st tri; D 2nd/3rd tri), ?/–] CI: PRG, component sensitivity **Disp:** Tabs 75, 150, 300 mg **SE:** Fatigue, ↓ BP **Interactions:** ↑ Risk of hyperkalemia *W/* K⁺-sparing diuretics, TMP, K⁺ supls; ↑ effects *W/* CYP2C9 inhibitors (amiodarone, fluconazole, fluoxetine, fluvastatin, imatinib, sulfonamides, voriconazole, zafirlukast); ↑ effects *OF* Li; ↓ antihypertensive effect *W/* NSAIDs, guarana, licorice, yohimbe **Labs:** ↑ K⁺ (monitor) **NIPE:** ⊘ PRG, breast-feeding; monitor ECG for hyperkalemia (peaked T waves)

Irinotecan (Camptosar, Generic) [Antineoplastic] WARNING: D & myelosuppression, administered by experienced provider Uses: *Colorectal* & lung CA **Action:** Topoisomerase I Inhib; ↓ DNA synth **Dose:** Per protocol; 125–350 mg/m² qwk–q3wk (↓ hepatic dysfunction, as tolerated per tox) **Caution:** [D, –] CI: Allergy to component **Disp:** Inj 20 mg/mL **SE:** ↑ BM, N/V/D, Abd cramping, alopecia **Interactions:** ↑ Effects *OF* antineoplastics; ↑ risk of akathisia *W/* prochlorperazine; ↑ risk of bleeding *W/* NSAIDs, anticoagulants; ↓ effects *W/* carbamazepine, phenytoin, phenobarbital, St. John's wort; **Labs:** ↑ AST, Alk Phos **NIPE:** Use barrier contraception; ⊘ exposure to Infxn; D is dose limiting; Rx acute D w/ atropine; Rx subacute D w/ loperamide; D correlated to levels of metabolite SN-38

Iron Dextran (Dexferrum, INFeD) [Iron Supplement] WARNING: Anaphylactic Rxn w/ death reported; proper personnel & equipment should be available. Use test dose only if PO Fe not possible Uses: *Iron-deficiency anemia where PO administration not possible* **Dose:** See also label for tables/formula to calculate dose. Estimate Fe deficiency; total dose (mL) = [0.0442 × (desired Hgb–observed Hgb) × lean body wgt] + (0.26 × lean body wgt); Fe replacement, blood loss: Total dose (mg) = blood loss (mL) × Hct (as decimal fraction) max 100 mg/d **IV use:** *Test Dose:* 0.5 mL IV over 30 s, if OK, 2 mL or less daily IV over 1 mL/min to calculated total dose **IM use:** *Test Dose:* 0.5 mL deep IM in buttock.

Administer calculated total dose not to exceed daily doses as follows: Infants < 5 kg: 1 mL Children < 10 kg. All others 2 mL (100 mg of iron) **Caution:** [C, M] w/ Hx allergy/asthma. Keep epi available (1:1000) for acute Rxn **CI:** Component hypersensitivity, non–Fe-deficiency anemia **Disp:** Inj 50 mg Fe/mL in 2 mL vials (*InFeD*) & 1 & 2-mL vials (*Dexferrrum*) **Interactions:** ↓ Effects *W/* chloramphenicol, ↓ absorption *OF* oral Fe **Labs:** False ↓ serum Ca; false(+) guaiac test; ↑ Hgb/ Hct. Also Fe, TIBC, & % saturation transferrin may be used to monitor **NIPE:** Not recorded in infants < 4 mo. Reticulocyte count best early indicator of response (several d). IM use "Z-track" technique; give test dose > 1 h before; ⊘ take oral Fe

Iron Sucrose (Venofer) [Iron Supplement] Uses: *Iron-deficiency anemia in CKD, w/ or w/o dialysis, w/ or w/o erythropoietin* **Action:** Fe supl **Dose:** 100 mg on dialysis; 200 mg slow IV over 25 min × 5 doses over 14-d period. Total cum dose 1000 mg **W/P:** [B, M] Hypersensitivity, ↓ BP, Fe overload, may interfere w/ MRI **CI:** Non–Fe-deficiency anemia; Fe overload; component sensitivity **Disp:** Inj 20 mg Fe/mL, 2.5, 5, 10 mL vials **SE:** Muscle cramps, N/V, strange taste in the mouth, diarrhea, constipation, HA, cough, back/Jt pain, dizziness, swelling of the arms/legs **Interactions:** ↓ Absorption *OF* oral Fe supls **Labs:** ↑ Monitor ferritin, HMG, Hct, transferrin saturation; obtain Fe levels 48 h > IV dose; ↓ LFTs **NIPE:** Safety in peds not established; ⊘ use oral & IV supls together; most pts require cumulative doses of 1000 mg; give slowly

Isoniazid (INH) [Antitubercular] **WARNING:** Severe & sometimes fatal hep may occur—usually w/in 1st 3 mo of Tx Uses: *Rx & prophylaxis of TB* **Action:** Bactericidal; interferes w/ mycolic acid synth, disrupts cell wall **Dose:** *Adults. Active TB:* 5 mg/kg/24 h PO or IM (usually 300 mg/d) or DOT: 15 mg/kg (max 900 mg) 3 ×/wk *Prophylaxis:* 300 mg/d PO for 6–12 mo or 900 mg 2 ×/wk *Peds. Active TB:* 10–15 mg/kg/d daily–bid PO or IM 300 mg/d max *Prophylaxis:* 10 mg/kg/24 h PO; ↓ in hepatic/renal dysfunction **Caution:** [C, +] Liver Dz, dialysis; avoid EtOH **CI:** Acute liver Dz, h/o INH hep **Disp:** Tabs 100, 300 mg; syrup 50 mg/5 mL; Inj 100 mg/mL **SE:** Hep, peripheral neuropathy, GI upset, anorexia, dizziness, skin Rxn **Interactions:** ↑ Effects *OF* APAP, anticoagulants, carbamazepine, cycloserine, diazepam, meperidine, hydantoins, theophylline, valproic acid, EtOH; ↑ effects *W/* rifampin; ↓ effects *W/* Al salts; ↓ effects *OF* anticoagulants, ketoconazole **Labs:** ↑ LFTs, glucose; ↓ HMG, plts, WBCs **NIPE:** ⊘ EtOH; only take w/ food if GI upset; use w/ 2–3 other drugs for active TB, based on INH resistance patterns when TB acquired & sensitivity results; prophylaxis usually w/ INH alone. IM rarely used. ↓ Peripheral neuropathy w/ pyridoxine 50–100 mg/d. See CDC guidelines (*http://www.cdc.gov/tb/*) for current recommendations

Isoproterenol (Isuprel) [Bronchodilator/Sympathomimetic] Uses: *Shock, cardiac arrest, AV nodal block* **Action:** β_1- & β_2-receptor stimulant **Dose:** *Adults.* 2–10 mcg/min IV Inf; titrate; 2–10 mcg/min titrate (*ECC 2010*) *Peds.* 0.2–2 mcg/kg/min IV Inf; titrate **Caution:** [C, ?] **CI:** Angina, tachyarrhythmias (digitalis-induced or others) **Disp:** 0.02 mg/mL, 0.2 mg/mL **SE:** Insomnia, arrhythmias, HA, trembling, dizziness **Interactions:** ↑ Effects *W/* albuterol, guanethidine, oxytocic drugs, sympathomimetics, TCAs; ↑ risk of arrhythmias *W/* amitriptyline, bretylium, cyclopropane, epinephrine; cardiac glycosides, K⁺-depleting drugs, theophylline; ↓ effects *W/* BBs **Labs:** ↑ Serum glucose **NIPE:** Saliva may turn pink in color, ↑ fluids to 2–3 L/d; more specific β₂-agonists preferred d/t excessive β₁ cardiac stimulation of drug; drug induces ischemia & dysrhythmias; pulse > 130 BPM may induce arrhythmias; monitor ECG during administration.

Isosorbide Dinitrate (Isordil, Sorbitrate, Dilatrate-SR, Generic) [Antianginal/Nitrate]

Uses: *Rx & prevent angina*, CHF (w/ hydralazine) **Action:** Relaxes vascular smooth muscle **Dose:** *Acute angina:* 5–10 mg PO (chew tabs) q2–3h or 2.5–10 mg SL PRN q5–10 min; do not give > 3 doses in a 15–30-min period *Angina prophylaxis:* 5–40 mg PO q6h; do not give nitrates on a chronic q6h or qid basis > 7–10 d; tolerance may develop; provide 10–12-h drug-free intervals *CHF:* Initial 20 mg 3–4 ×/d, target 120–160 mg/d **Caution:** [C, ?] **CI:** Severe anemia, NAG, postural ↓ BP, cerebral hemorrhage, **Disp:** Tabs 5, 10, 20, 30 mg; SR tabs 40 mg; SL tabs 2.5, 5 mg; SR caps 40 mg **SE:** HA, ↓ BP, flushing, tachycardia, dizziness **Interactions:** ↓ Hypotension *W/* antihypertensives, ASA, CCBs, phenothiazides, sildenafil, EtOH; life-threatening hypotension *W/* sildenafil, tadalafil, vardenafil **Labs:** False ↓ serum cholesterol **NIPE:** ⊘ Nitrates for an 8–12-h period/d to avoid tolerance; higher PO dose needed for same results as SL forms; head trauma (can ↑ ICP)

Isosorbide Mononitrate (Ismo, Imdur, Monoket) [Antianginal/ Nitrate]

Uses: *Prevention/Rx of angina pectoris* **Action:** Relaxes vascular smooth muscle **Dose:** 5–10 mg PO bid, w/ doses 7 h apart or XR (Imdur) 30–60 mg/d PO, max 240 mg **Caution:** [B, ?] Severe hypotension w/ paradoxical bradycardia, hypertrophic cardiomyopathy **CI:** Sildenafil, tadalafil, vardenafil **Disp:** Tabs 10, 20 mg; XR 30, 60, 120 mg **SE:** HA, dizziness, ↓ BP **Interactions:** ↑ Hypotension *W/* ASA, CCB, nitrates, sildenafil, EtOH; life-threatening hypotension *W/* sildenafil, tadalafil, vardenafil **Labs:** False ↓ serum cholesterol **NIPE:** Metabolite of isosorbide dinitrate; head trauma/cerebral hemorrhage (can ↑ ICP)

Isotretinoin [13-cis Retinoic Acid] (Amnesteem, Claravis, Myorisan, Sotret, Zentane, Generic) [Antiacne Agent]

WARNING: Do not use in pts who are/may become PRG; ↑ risk of severe birth defects; available only through iPLEDGE restricted distribution program; pts, prescribers, pharmacies, and distributors must enroll. **Uses:** *Severe nodular acne resistant to other Tx* **Action:** Inhib sebaceous gland Fxn & keratinization **Dose:** *Adults and Peds ≥ 12 y.* 0.5–1 mg/kg/d 2 ÷ doses × 15–20 wk, do NOT take only 1 ×/d; PRG test prior to RX each mo, end of Tx, and 1 mo after D/C **Caution:** [X, −] Microdosed progesterone BCPs NOT acceptable method of birth control; depression; suicidal thoughts and behaviors, psychosis/aggressive/violent behavior; pseudotumor cerebri; TEN, SJS; ↓ hearing, corneal opacities, ↓ night vision, IBD, pancreatitis, hepatic toxicity **CI:** PRG, hypersens **Disp:** Caps 10, 20, 30, 40 mg **SE:** Dry/chapped lips, cheilitis, dry skin, dermatitis, dry eye, ↓ vision, HA, epistaxis, nasopharyngitis, URI, back pain **Interactions:** ↑ Effects W/ corticosteroids, phenytoin, vit A; ↑ risk of pseudotumor cerebri W/ tetracyclines; ↑ triglyceride levels W/ EtOH; ↓ effects OF carbamazepine **Labs:** ↑ LFTs, triglycerides; ✓ LFTs & lipids before using drug & regularly while using drug; vit A may ↑ adverse events **NIPE:** ↑ Risk of photosensitivity—use sunblock, take w/ food, ⊘ PRG; ⊘ drugs that may interfere w/BCP effectiveness; risk-management program required

Isradipine (DynaCirc) [Antihypertensive/CCB] **Uses:** *HTN* **Action:** CCB **Dose:** *Adults.* 2.5–5 mg PO bid **Caution:** [C, ?/–] **CI:** Severe heart block, sinus bradycardia, CHF, dosing w/in several h of IV BBs; Hypotension < 90 mm HG systolic **Disp:** Caps 2.5, 5 mg; tabs CR 5, 10 mg **SE:** HA, edema, flushing, fatigue, dizziness, palpitations **Interactions:** ↑ Effects W/ antihypertensives, azole antifungals, BBs, cimetidine; fentanyl, nitrates, quinidine, EtOH, grapefruit juice; ↑ effects OF carbamazepine, cyclosporine, digitalis glycosides, prazosin, quinidine; ↑ risk of bradycardia/conduction defects/AV W/ BB, digoxin, disopyramide, phenytoin; ↓ effects W/ Ca, NSAIDs, rifampin; ↓ effects OF lovastatin **Labs:** ↑ LFTs; ↓ K+, ↓ Cr, K+, LFT **NIPE:** ⊘ D/C abruptly

Itraconazole (Onmel, Sporanox, Generic) [Antifungal] **WARNING:** CI w/ cisapride, pimozide, quinidine, dofetilide, or levacetylmethadol. Serious CV events (eg, ↑ QT, torsades de pointes, VT, cardiac arrest, and/or sudden death) reported w/ these meds & other CYP3A4 Inhibs. Do not use for onychomycosis w/ ventricular dysfunction; negative inotropic effects have been observed following IV administration D/C/reassess use if S/sx of HF occur during Tx **Uses:** *Fungal Infxns (aspergillosis, blastomycosis, histoplasmosis, candidiasis, onychomycosis)* **Action:** Azole antifungal, ↓ ergosterol synth **Dose:** Dose based on indication. 200 mg PO daily–tid (caps w/ meals or cola/grapefruit juice). PO soln on empty stomach; avoid antacids **Caution:** [C, ?] Numerous interactions **CI:** See Warning; PRG or considering PRG; ventricular dysfunction CHF **Disp:** Caps 100 mg; soln 10 mg/mL **SE:** N/V, rash, hepatotoxic, CHF, ↑ BP, neuropathy **Interactions:** ↑ Effects W/ clarithromycin, erythromycin; ↑ effects OF alprazolam, anticoagulants, atevirdine, atorvastatin, buspirone, cerivastatin, chlordiazepoxide, cyclosporine, diazepam, digoxin, felodipine, fluvastatin, indinavir, lovastatin, methadone, methylprednisolone, midazolam, nelfinavir, pravastatin, ritonavir, saquinavir, simvastatin, tacrolimus, tolbutamide, triazolam, warfarin; ↑ QT prolongation W/ astemizole, cisapride, pimozide, quinidine, terfenadine; ↓ effects W/ antacids, Ca, cimetidine, didanosine, famotidine, lansoprazole, Mg, nizatidine, omeprazole, phenytoin, rifampin, sucralfate, grapefruit juice **Labs:** ↑ LFTs, BUN, SCr; ↓ K+; monitor LFTs **NIPE:** Take caps w/ food & soln w/o food; ⊘ PRG or breast-feeding; ↑ risk of disulfiram-like response w/ EtOH; PO soln & caps not interchangeable; useful in pts who cannot take amphotericin B, can cause ↑ QTc in combo w/ other drugs—monitor ECG

Ivacaftor (Kalydeco) [Cystic Fibrosis Transmembrane Conductance Regulator (CFTR) Potentiator] Uses: *Cystic fibrosis w/G551D mutation transmembrane conductance regulator (CFTR) gene* **Action:** ↑ Chloride transport, **Dose:** *Adult & Peds > 6 y.* 150 mg bid; w/ fatty meal; ↓ hepatic impair or w CYP3A inhib **Caution:** [B, ?/–) w/ hepatic impair Child-Pugh Class C; severe renal impair **CI:** None **Disp:** Tabs 150 mg **SE:** HA, URI, oropharyngeal pain, Abd pain, N/D; **Interactions:** ↑ Effects **W/** CYP3A inhibitors (ketoconazole, itraconazole, posaconazole, voriconazole, clarithromycin), erythromycin, grapefruit; ↑ effects **OF** digoxin, cyclosporin, tacrolimus, benzodiazepine levels **Labs:** ✓ LFTs q3mo × 4, then yearly; D/C if AST/ALT 5 × ULN **NIPE:** May restart drug once AST/ALT returns to normal

Ivermectin, Oral (Stromectol) [Avemeclin] Uses: *Strongyloidiasis (intestinal), onchocerciasis* **Action:** Binds glutamate-gated chloride channels in nerve and muscle cells, paralysis and death of nematodes **Dose:** *Adult and Peds.* Based on wgt and condition. *Intestinal strongyloidiasis* 1 tab 15–24 kg, 2 tabs 25–35 kg, 3 tabs 36–50 kg, 4 tabs 51–65 kg, 5 tabs 66–79 kg, 80 or > 200 mcg/kg *Onchocerciasis* Repeat dose × 1 in 2 wk, 1 tab 15–25 kg, 2 tabs 26–44 kg, 3 tabs 45–64 kg, 4 tabs 65–84 kg; 85 or > 150 mcg/kg **Caution:** [C, ?/–) Potential severe allergic/inflammatory reactions Tx of onchocerciasis **CI:** Hypersensitivity **Disp:** Tabs 3 mg **SE:** N/V/D, dizziness, pruritus **Labs:** ↑ AST/ALT; ↓ WBC, RBC **NIPE:** From fermented *Streptomyces avermitilis*; does not kill adult onchocerca, requires re-dosing; take with H$_2$O; take on empty stomach

Ivermectin, Topical (Sklice) [Pediculicide] Uses: *Head lice* **Acts:** Binds to glutamate-gated chloride channels in nerve and muscle cells, paralysis and death of lice **Dose:** *Adult & Peds > 6 mo.* Coat hair/scalp **Caution:** [C, ?/–) **CI:** None **Disp:** Lotion 0.5%, 4 oz tube **SE:** Conjunctivitis, red eye, dry skin **NIPE:** From fermented *Streptomyces avermitilis*; coat dry hair and scalp thoroughly for 10 min, then rinse; avoid contact w/ eyes; use w/ lice management plan; not for oral, ophthalmic or intravaginal use; apply to dry hair and scalp and leave on for 10 min, then rinse w/ H$_2$O

Ixabepilone Kit (Ixempra) [Epothilone Microtubule Inhibitor] **WARNING:** CI in combo w/ capecitabine w/ AST/ALT > 2.5 × ULN or bilirubin > 1 × ULN d/t ↑ tox & neutropenia-related death Uses: *Met/locally advanced breast CA after failure of an anthracycline, a taxane, & capecitabine* **Action:** Microtubule Inhib **Dose:** 40 mg/m^2 IV over 3 h q3wk, 88 mg max **Caution:** [D, ?/–] **CI:** Hypersensitivity to Cremophor EL; baseline ANC < 1500 cells/mm^3 or plt < 100,000 cells/mm^3; AST/ALT > 2.5 × UNL, bilirubin > 1 × ULN capecitabine **Disp:** Inj 15, 45 mg (use supplied diluent) **SE:** Neutropenia, leukopenia, anemia, thrombocytopenia peripheral sensory neuropathy, fatigue/asthenia, myalgia/arthralgia, alopecia, N/V/D, stomatitis/mucositis **Interactions:** ↑ Effects **W/** strong CYP3A4 Inhibs (azole antifungals, protease Inhibs, certain macrolides, nefazodone) grapefruit juice; ↓ effects **W/** CYP3A4 inducers (phenytoin, carbamazepine, rifampin, phenobarbital); St. John's wort **Labs:** Monitor LFTs, ↓ plt, neutropenia **NIPE:** Monitor for neuropathy, S/Sx infection & sore throat; D/C if cardiac ischemia or cardiac dysfunction occurs

Japanese Encephalitis Vaccine, Inactivated, Adsorbed [Vaccine] (Ixiaro, Je-Vax)
Uses: *Prevent Japanese encephalitis* **Action:** Inactivated vaccine **Dose:** *Adults.* 0.5 mL IM, repeat 28 d later given at least 1 wk prior to exposure **Peds.** Use Je-Vax *1–3 y:* Three 0.5 mL SQ doses on d 0, 7, 30; *> 3 y:* Three 1 mL SQ doses on d 0, 7, 30 **Caution:** [B (Ixiaro)/C (Je-Vax),?] Severe urticaria or angioedema may occur up to 10 d after vaccination **SE:** HA, fatigue, Inj site pain, flu-like synd, hypersensitivity Rxn **Interactions:** ↓ Response *W/* other vaccines, immunosuppressants (eg, radiation, chemotherapy, high-dose steroids) **NIPE:** Complete immunizations ≤ 1 wk prior to potential exposure to JEV; booster dose recommended after 2 y; ⊘ EtOH 48 h after dose

Ketamine (Ketalar) [C-III] [Anesthetic]
Uses: *Induction/maintenance of anesthesia* (in combo w/ sedatives), sedation, analgesia **Action:** Dissociative anesthesia; IV onset 30 s, duration 5–10 min **Dose:** *Adults.* 1–4.5 mg/kg IV, typical 2 mg/kg; 3–8 mg/kg IM **Peds.** 0.5–2 mg/kg IV; 0.5–1 mg/kg for minor procedures (also IM/PO regimens) **Caution:** w/ CAD, ↑ BP, tachycardia, EtOH use/abuse [C, ?/–] **CI:** When ↑ BP hazardous **Disp:** Soln 10, 50, 100 mg/mL **SE:** Arrhythmia, bradycardia, ↑/↓ HR, ↓ BP, N/V, resp depression, emergence Rxns, ↑ CSF pressure **Interactions:** CYP2B6 Inhibs ↓ metabolism (see Table 10) **NIPE:** Used in RSI protocols; street drug of abuse—known as Special K, K, Cat Valium, super acid; used as date rape drug

Ketoconazole (Nizoral) [Antifungal/Imidazole]
WARNING: (Oral use) Risk of fatal hepatotox. Concomitant terfenadine, astemizole, and cisapride are CI d/t serious CV adverse events **Uses:** *Systemic fungal Infxns (Candida, blastomycosis, histoplasmosis, etc); refractory topical dermatophyte Infxn*; PCa when rapid ↑ testosterone needed or hormone refractory **Action:** Azole, ↓ fungal cell wall synth; high dose blocks P450 to ↓ testosterone production **Dose:** *PO:* 200 mg PO daily; ↑ to 400 mg PO daily for serious Infxn *PCa:* 400 mg PO tid; best on empty stomach **Caution:** [C, ?/–] w/ Any agent that ↑ gastric pH (↓ absorption); may enhance anticoagulants; w/ EtOH (disulfiram-like Rxn); numerous interactions including statins, niacin; do not use w/ clopidogrel (↓ effect) **CI:** CNS fungal Infxns, w/ astemizole, triazolam **Disp:** Tabs 200 mg **SE:** N, rashes, hair loss, HA, ↑ wgt gain, dizziness, disorientation, fatigue, impotence, hepatox, adrenal suppression, acquired cutaneous adherence ("sticky skin synd") **Interactions:** ↑ Effects *OF* alprazolam, anticoagulants, atevirdine, atorvastatin, buspirone, chlordiazepoxide, cyclosporine, diazepam, felodipine, fluvastatin, indinavir, lovastatin, methadone, methylprednisolone, midazolam, nelfinavir, pravastatin, ritonavir, saquinavir, simvastatin, tacrolimus, tolbutamide, triazolam, warfarin; ↑ QT prolongation *W/* astemizole, cisapride, quinidine, terfenadine; ↓ effects *W/* antacids, Ca, cimetidine, didanosine, famotidine, lansoprazole, Mg, nizatidine, omeprazole, phenytoin,

rifampin, sucralfate **Labs:** ↑ LFTs; monitor LFTs w/ systemic use; can rapidly ↓ testosterone levels **NIPE:** Take tabs w/ citrus juice, take w/ food; take ≥ 2 h before taking an antacid; ⊘ EtOH; ⊘ PRG or breast-feeding

Ketoconazole, Topical (Extina, Nizoral A-D Shampoo, Xolegel) [Antifungal/Imidazole] [Shampoo–OTC] Uses: *Topical for seborrheic dermatitis, shampoo for dandruff*; local fungal Infxns d/t dermatophytes & yeast **Action:** Azole, ↓ fungal cell wall synth **Dose:** *Topical:* Apply qd–bid **Cream:** [C, +/−] **Disp:** Topical cream 2%; (*Xolegel*) gel 2%, (*Extina*) foam 2%, shampoo 2% **SE:** Irritation, pruritus, stinging **NIPE:** Do not dispense foam into hands; shampoo wet hair 1 min, rinse, repeat for 3 min

Ketoprofen (Orudis, Oruvail) [Analgesic/NSAID] WARNING: May ↑ risk of fatal CV events & GI bleeding; CI for perioperative pain in CABG surgery **Uses:** *Arthritis (RA/OA), pain* **Action:** NSAID; ↓ prostaglandins **Dose:** 25–75 mg PO tid–qid, 300 mg/d/max; SR 200 mg/d; w/ food; ↓ w/ hepatic/renal impair, elderly **Caution:** [C (D 3rd tri), −] w/ ACE, diuretics, ↑ warfarin, Li, MTX, avoid EtOH **CI:** NSAID/ASA sensitivity **Disp:** Caps 50, 75 mg; caps, SR 200 mg **SE:** GI upset, peptic ulcers, dizziness, edema, rash, ↑ BP, ↑ LFTs, renal dysfunction **Interactions:** ↑ Effects *W/* ASA, corticosteroids, NSAIDs, probenecid, EtOH; ↑ effects *OF* antineoplastics, hypoglycemics, insulin, Li, MTX, warfarin; ↑ risk of nephrotox *W/* aminoglycosides, cyclosporines; ↑ risk of bleeding *W/* anticoagulants, defamandole, cefotetan, cefoperazone, clopidogrel, eptifibatide, plicamycin, thrombolytics, tirofiban, valproic acid, dong quai, feverfew, garlic, ginkgo, ginger, horse chestnut, red clover; ↓ effects *OF* antihypertensives, diuretics **Labs:** ↑ LFTs, BUN, Cr, PT; ↓ plts, WBCs **NIPE:** ↑ Risk of photosensitivity—use sunblock, take w/ food & 8 oz H₂O; ⊘ lie down for ≥ 10 min after taking

Ketorolac (Toradol) [Analgesic/NSAID] WARNING: For short-term (≤ 5 d) Rx of mod–severe acute pain; CI w/ PUD, GI bleed, post CBG, anticipated major surgery, severe renal Insuff, bleeding diathesis, L&D, nursing, & w/ ASA/ NSAIDs. NSAIDs may cause ↑ risk of CV thrombotic events (MI, stroke). PO CI in peds < 16 y, dose adjustments for < 50 kg; **Uses:** *Pain* **Action:** NSAID; ↓ prostaglandins **Dose:** *Adults.* 15–30 mg IV/IM q6h; 10 mg PO qid only as continuation of IM/IV; max IV/IM 120 mg/d, max PO 40 mg/d *Peds 2–16 y.* 1 mg/kg IM × 1 dose; 30 mg max *IV:* 0.5 mg/kg, 15 mg max; do not use for > 5 d; ↓ if > 65 y, elderly, w/ renal impair, < 50 kg **Caution:** [C (D 3rd tri), −] w/ ACE inhib, diuretics, BP meds, warfarin **CI:** See Warning **Disp:** Tabs 10 mg; Inj 15 mg/mL, 30 mg/ mL **SE:** Bleeding, peptic ulcer Dz, ↑ CR & LFTs, ↑ BP, edema, dizziness, allergy **Interactions:** ↑ Effects *W/* ASA, corticosteroids, NSAIDs, probenecid, EtOH; ↑ effects *OF* antineoplastics, hypoglycemics, insulin, Li, MTX; ↑ risk of nephrotox *W/* aminoglycosides, cyclosporines; ↑ risk of bleeding *W/* anticoagulants, defamandole, cefotetan, cefoperazone, clopidogrel, eptifibatide, plicamycin, thrombolytics, tirofiban, valproic acid, dong quai, feverfew, garlic, ginkgo, ginger, horse chestnut, red clover; ↓ effects of antihypertensives, diuretics **Labs:** ↑ LFTs, Cr,

PT; ↓ HMG, Hct **NIPE:** 30-mg dose equals comparative analgesia of meperidine 100 mg or morphine 12 mg; PO only as continuation of IM/IV therapy; take w/8 oz H₂O; ⊘ lie down for ≥ 10 min after taking; may take w/ food

Ketorolac Nasal (Sprix) [NSAID] **WARNING:** For short-term (< 5 d) use; CI w/ PUD, GI bleed, suspected bleeding risk, post-op CABG, advanced renal Dz or risk of renal failure w/ vol depletion; severe CV thrombotic events (MI, stroke; not indicated for use in children **Uses:** *Short-term (< 5 d) Rx pain requiring opioid level analgesia* **Action:** NSAID; ↓ prostaglandins **Dose:** < *65 y:* 31.5 mg (one 15.75 mg spray each nostril) q6–8h; max 126 mg/d ≥ *65 y w/ renal impair or < 50 kg:* 15.75 mg (one 15.75 mg spray in only 1 nostril) q6–8 h; max 63 mg/d **Caution:** [C (D 3rd tri), –] Do not use w/ other NSAIDs; can cause severe skin Rxns; do not use w/ critical bleeding risk; w/ CHF **CI:** See Warning; prophylactic to major surgery/L&D; w/ Hx allergy to aspirin or NSAIDs recent or Hx of GI bleed or perforation **Disp:** Nasal spray 15.75 mg ketorolac/100 mcL spray (8 sprays/bottle) **SE:** Nasal discomfort/rhinitis, ↑ lacrimation, throat irritation, oliguria, rash, ↓ HR, ↓ urine output, ↑ ALT/AST, ↑ BP **Interactions:** ↑ Effects **W/** ASA, corticosteroids, NSAIDs; ↑ risk of hallucinations **W/** fluoxetine, thiothixene, alprazolam; ↓ effects **OF** furosemide, thiazides, ACE Inhibs, angiotensin II receptor antagonists **LABS:** ↑ ALT/ AST **NIPE:** Not for peds; discard open bottle after 24 h; ↑ fluids

Ketorolac Ophthalmic (Acular, Acular LS, Acular PF, Acuvail) [Analgesic, Anti-Inflammatory/NSAID] **Uses:** *Ocular itching w/ seasonal allergies; inflammation w/ cataract extraction*; pain/photophobia w/ incisional refractive surgery (Acular PF); pain w/ corneal refractive surgery (*Acular LS*) **Action:** NSAID **Dose:** 1 gtt qid **Caution:** [C, +] Possible cross-sensitivity to NSAIDs, ASA **CI:** Hypersens **Disp:** *Acular LS:* 0.4% 5 mL; *Acular:* 0.5% 3, 5, 10 mL; *Acular PF:* Soln 0.5%, Acuvail soln 0.45% **SE:** Local irritation, ↑ bleeding ocular tissues, hyphemas, slow healing, keratitis **NIPE:** Do not use w/ contacts; teach use of eye drops

Ketotifen (Alaway, Claritin Eye, Zaditor, Zyrtec Itchy Eye) [Ophthalmic Antihistamine/Histamine Antagonist & Mast Cell Stabilizer] [OTC] **Uses:** *Allergic conjunctivitis* **Action:** Antihistamine H₁-receptor antagonist, mast cell stabilizer **Dose:** *Adults & Peds > 3 y.* 1 gtt in eye(s) q8–12h **Caution:** [C, ?/–] **Disp:** Soln 0.025%/5 & 10 mL **SE:** Local irritation, HA, rhinitis, keratitis, mydriasis **NIPE:** Wait 10 min before inserting contacts; ⊘ wear contact lenses if eyes red; teach use of eye drops

Kunecatechins [Sinecatechins] (Veregen) [Botanical] **Uses:** *External genital/perianal warts* **Action:** Unknown; green tea extract **Dose:** Apply 0.5-cm ribbon to each wart 3 ×/d until all warts clear; not > 16 wk **Caution:** [C, ?] **Disp:** Oint 15% **SE:** Erythema, pruritus, burning, pain, erosion/ulceration, edema, induration, rash, phimosis **NIPE:** Wash hands before/after use; not necessary to wipe off prior to next use; avoid on open wounds; may weaken condoms & Vag diaphragms

Labetalol (Trandate) [Antihypertensive/Alpha Blocker & BB]
Uses: *HTN* & hypertensive emergencies (IV) Action: α- & β-adrenergic blocker Dose: *Adults. HTN:* Initial, 100 mg PO bid, then 200–400 mg PO bid. *Hypertensive emergency:* 20–80 mg IV bolus, then 2 mg/min IV Inf, titrate up to 300 mg *ECC 2010:* 10 mg IV over 1–2 min; repeat or double dose q10min (150 mg max); or initial bolus, then 2–8 mg/min *Peds.* PO: 1–3 mg/kg/d in ÷ doses, 1200 mg/d max. *Hypertensive emergency:* 0.4–1.5 mg/kg/h IV cont Inf Caution: [C (D in 2nd or 3rd tri), +] CI: Asthma/COPD, cardiogenic shock, uncompensated CHF, heart block, sinus brady Disp: Tabs 100, 200, 300 mg; Inj 5 mg/mL SE: Dizziness, N, ↓ BP, fatigue, CV effects Interactions: ↑ Effects *W/* cimetidine, diltiazem, nitroglycerine, quinidine, paroxetine, verapamil; ↑ tremors *W/* TCAs; ↓ effects *W/* glutethimide, NSAIDs, salicylates; ↓ effects *OF* antihypertensives, β-adrenergic bronchodilators, sulfonylureas Labs: False(+) amphetamines in urine drug screen; ↑ LFTS NIPE: May have transient tingling of scalp; ⊘ abrupt cessation; caution driving; change positions slowly, esp. in elderly

Lacosamide (Vimpat) [Antiepileptic] Uses: *Adjunct in partial-onset Szs* Action: Anticonvulsant Dose: *Initial:* 50 mg IV or PO bid, ↑ weekly Maint: 200–400 mg/d; 300 mg/d max if CrCl < 30 mL/min or mild–mod hepatic Dz Caution: [C, ?] DRESS ↑ PR [C-V] Antieplieptics associated w ↑ risk of suicide ideation CI: None Disp: *IV:* 200 mg/20 mL; Tabs: 50, 100, 150, 200 mg; oral soln 10 mg/mL SE: Dizziness, N/V, ataxia NIPE: ⊘ Abrupt cessation—withdraw over 1 wk, ✓ ECG before dosing & periodically—may ↑ PR interval; contains aspartame—⊘ PKU; caution driving

Lactic Acid & Ammonium Hydroxide [Ammonium Lactate] (Lac-Hydrin) [Emollient] Uses: *Severe xerosis & ichthyosis* Action: Emollient moisturizer, humectant Dose: Apply bid Caution: [B, ?] Disp: Cream, lotion, lactic acid 12% w/ ammonium hydroxide SE: Local irritation, photosensitivity NIPE: ⊘ Children < 2 y; ⊘ sun exposure—use sunblock; risk of hyperpigmentation; may need to shake well before use—check label

Lactobacillus (Lactinex Granules) [Antidiarrheal] [OTC] Uses: *Control of D*, especially after antibiotic Rx Action: Replaces nl intestinal flora, lactase production; *Lactobacillus acidophilus & L helveticus* Dose: *Adults & Peds > 3 y.* 1 packet, 1–2 caps, or 4 tabs qd–qid Caution: [A, +] Some products may contain whey CI: Milk/lactose allergy Disp: Tabs, caps; granules in packets (all OTC) SE: Flatulence NIPE: May take granules on food; take 2 h after antibiotic

Lactulose (Constulose, Generlac, Enulose, Others) [Laxative/Osmotic] Uses: *Hepatic encephalopathy; constipation* Action: Acidifies the colon, allows ammonia to diffuse into colon; osmotic effect to ↑ peristalsis Dose: *Acute hepatic encephalopathy:* 30–45 mL PO q1h until soft stools, then tid–qid, adjust 2–3 stool/d *Constipation:* 15–30 mL/d, ↑ to 60 mL/d 1–2 ÷ doses, adjust to 2–3 stools *Rectally:* 200 g in 700 mL of water PR, retain 30–60 min q4–6h *Peds. Infants.* 2.5–10 mL/24 h ÷ tid–qid *Other Peds.* 40–90 mL/24 h ÷ tid–qid *Peds* *constipation:* 1–3 mL/kg/d ÷ doses (max 60 mL/d) PO after breakfast **Caution:** [B, ?] **CI:** Galactosemia **Disp:** Syrup 10 g/15 mL, soln 10 g/15 mL, 10, 20 g/packet **SE:** Severe D, N/V, cramping, flatulence; life-threatening lyte abnormalities **Interactions:** ↓ Effects W/ antacids, antibiotics, neomycin **Labs:** ↓ Serum ammonia **NIPE:** May take 24–48 h for results; mix w/ fruit juice, water, carb citrus bev; ⊘ food

Lamivudine (Epivir, Epivir-HBV, 3TC [Many Combo Regimens]) [Antiretroviral/NRTI] **WARNING:** Lactic acidosis & severe hepatomegaly w/ steatosis reported w/ nucleoside analogues; do not use Epivir-HBV for Tx of HIV, monitor pts closely following D/C of therapy for hep B **Uses:** *HIV Infxn, chronic hep B* **Action:** NRTI, ↓ HIV RT & hep B viral polymerase, causes viral DNA chain termination **Dose:** *HIV: Adults & Peds > 16 y.* 150 mg PO bid or 300 mg PO daily *Peds able to swallow pills. 14–21 kg.* 75 mg bid; *22–29 kg.* 75 mg qAM, 150 mg qPM *> 30 kg.* 150 mg bid. *Neonates < 30 d.* 2 mg/kg bid *Infants 1–3 mo.* 4 mg/kg/dose *> 3 mo Child < 16 y.* 4 mg/kg/dose bid (max 150 mg bid) *Epivir-HBV: Adults.* 100 mg/d PO *Peds 2–17 y.* 3 mg/kg/d PO, 100 mg max; ↓ w/ CrCl < 50 mL/min **Caution:** [C, ?] w/ Interferon-α & ribavirin may cause liver failure; do not use w/ zalcitabine or w/ ganciclovir/valganciclovir **Disp:** Tabs 100 mg (*Epivir-HBV*) 150, 300 mg; soln 5 mg/mL (*Epivir-HBV*), 10 mg/mL **SE:** Malaise, fatigue, N/V/D, HA, pancreatitis, lactic acidosis, peripheral neuropathy, fat redistribution, rhabdomyolysis hyperglycemia, nasal Sxs **Interactions:** ↑ Effects W/ cotrimoxazole, TMP/SMX; ↑ risk of lactic acidosis W/ antiretrovirals, RT Inhibs **Labs:** ↑ LFTs; ↓ HMG, Hct, plts **NIPE:** Take w/ food to < GI upset; differences in formulations; ⊘ use Epivir-HBV for hep in pt w/ unrecognized HIV d/t rapid emergence of HIV resistance; not a cure for HIV—continue transmission precautions

Lamotrigine (Lamictal) [Anticonvulsant/Phenyltriazine] **WARNING:** Life-threatening rashes, including Stevens-Johnson synd and toxic epidermal necrolysis, and/or organ-related death reported; D/C at first sign of rash **Uses:** *Epilepsy adjunct ≥ 2 y or mono Rx ≥ 16 y old; bipolar disorder ≥ 18 y old* **Action:** Phenyltriazine antiepileptic, ↓ glutamate, stabilize neuronal membrane **Dose:** *Adults. Szs:* Initial 50 mg/d PO, then 50 mg PO bid for × 1–2 wk, maint 300–500 mg/d in 2 ÷ doses *Bipolar.* Initial 25 mg/d PO × 1–2 wk, 50 mg PO daily for 2 wk, 100 mg PO daily for 1 wk, maint 200 mg/d *Peds.* 0.6 mg/kg in 2 ÷ doses for wk 1 & 2, then 1.2 mg/kg for wk 3 & 4, q1–2wk to maint 5–15 mg/kg/d (max 400 mg/d) in 2 ÷ doses; ↓ in hepatic Dz or w/ enzyme inducers or valproic acid **Caution:** [C, –] ↑ Suicide risk, higher for those w/ epilepsy vs. psych use. Interact w/ other antiepileptics, estrogen, rifampin **Disp:** (Color-coded for those w/interacting meds) Starter titrate kits; tabs 25, 100, 150, 200 mg; chew tabs 2, 5, 25 mg; ODT 25, 50, 100, 200 mg **SE:** Photosensitivity, HA, GI upset, dizziness, diplopia, blurred vision, blood dyscrasias, ataxia, rash (more life-threatening in peds vs. adults) **Interactions:** ↑ Effects *OF* valproic acid; ↑ effects *OF* carbamazepine; ↓ effects W/ APAP, OCPs, phenobarbital, phenytoin, primidone **NIPE:** Report any skin rash immed; ↑ risk of photosensitivity—use sunblock; taper w/ D/C

Lamotrigine Extended-Release (Lamictal XR) [Anticonvulsant/ Phenyltriazine] WARNING: Life-threatening rashes, including Stevens-Johnson synd and toxic epidermal necrolysis, and/or rash-related death reported; D/C at first sign of rash Uses: *Adjunct primary generalized tonic–clonic Sz, conversion to monoRx in pt > 13 y w/ partial Szs* **Action:** Phenyltriazine antiepileptic, ↓ glutamate, stabilize neuronal membrane Dose: Adjunct target 200–600 mg/d; monoRx conversion target dose 250–300 mg/d **Adults:** w/ Valproate: wk 1–2: 25 mg qod; wk 3–4: 25 mg qd; wk 5: 50 mg qd; wk 6: 100 mg qd; wk 7: 150 mg qd; then maint 200–250 mg qd w/o Carbamazepine, phenytoin, phenobarbital, primidone or valproate: wk 1–2: 25 mg qd; wk 3–4: 50 mg qd, wk 5: 100 mg qd, wk 6: 150 mg qd, wk 7: 200 mg qd, then maint 300–400 mg qd Convert IR to ER tabs: Initial dose = total daily dose of IR. Convert adjunctive to monoRx: Maint: 250–300 mg qd. See label. w/ OCP: See insert Peds > 13 y. See Adult Caution: [C, –] Interacts w/ other antiepileptics, estrogen (OCP), rifampin; valproic acid ↑ levels at least 2 ×; ↑ suicidal ideation; withdrawal Szs CI: Component hypersensitivity (see Warning) Disp: Tabs 25, 100, 150, 200 mg SE: Dizziness, tremor/intention tremor, V, diplopia, rash (more life-threatening in peds than adults), aseptic meningitis, blood dyscrasias Interactions: w/ Other antiepileptics, estrogen (OCP), rifampin; valproic acid ↑ levels at least 2 ×; ↑ suicidal ideation Labs: Monitor CBC NIPE: Taper over 2 wk w/ D/C; can have withdrawal Szs; report any skin rash immed

Lansoprazole (Prevacid, Prevacid 24HR [OTC]) [Antisecretory/ Proton Pump Inhibitor] Uses: *Duodenal ulcers, prevent & Rx NSAID gastric ulcers, active gastric ulcers, H pylori Infxn, erosive esophagitis, & hypersecretory conditions, GERD* **Action:** Proton pump inhib Dose: 15–30 mg/d PO; NSAID ulcer prevention: 15 mg/d PO = 12 wk NSAID ulcers: 30 mg/d PO × 8 wk Hypersecretory condition: 60 mg/d PO before food, doses of 90 mg bid have been used; ↓ w/ severe hepatic impair Caution: [B, ?/–] w/ Clopidogrel Disp: Prevacid: DR caps 15, 30 mg; Prevacid 24HR [OTC] 15 mg; Prevacid SoluTab (ODT) 15 mg, (contains phenylalanine) SE: N/V Abd pain HA, fatigue Interactions: ↓ Effects W/ sucralfate; ↓ effects OF ampicillin, digoxin, Fe, ketoconazole, atazanavir Labs: Monitor theophylline & warfarin levels if taking these drugs NIPE: Take ac; do not crush/chew; DR caps/granules can be given w/ applesauce/yogurt/pudding; for NG tube mix granules w/ apple juice only; ODT w/ NG tube mix in syringe w/ 4 mL H₂O for 15 mg/10 mL for 30 mg, adm ≤ 15 min, rinse w/ 2 mL water; ? ↑ risk of fxs w/ all PPI; risk of hypomagnesemia w/ long-term use, monitor; may give antacids concomitantly; OTC preparation—take whole

Lanthanum Carbonate (Fosrenol) [Renal & GU Agent/Phosphate Binder] Uses: *Hyperphosphatemia in end-stage renal Dz* **Action:** Phosphate binder Dose: 750–1500 mg PO qd ÷ doses, w/ or immediately after meal; titrate q2–3wk based on PO₄²⁻ levels Caution: [C, ?/–] No data in GI Dz; not for peds CI: Bowel obstruction, fecal impaction, ileus Disp: Chew tabs 500,

750, 1000 mg **SE:** N/V, graft occlusion, HA, ↓ BP **Labs:** ↑ Serum Ca level; monitor serum phosphate levels **NIPE:** Use cautiously w/ GI Dz; monitor for bone pain or deformity; chew tabs before swallowing; separate from meds that interact w/ antacids by 2 h

Lapatinib (Tykerb) [Tyrosine Kinase Inhibitor]   WARNING: Hepatotox has been reported (severe or fatal) **Uses:** *Advanced breast CA w/ capecitabine w/ tumors that overexpress HER2 & failed w/ anthracycline, taxane, & trastuzumab* and in combo w/ letrozole in postmenopausal women **Action:** TKI **Dose:** Per protocol, 1250 mg PO d 1–21 w/ capecitabine 2000 mg/m²/d ÷ 2 doses/d on d 1–14; 1500 mg PO daily in combo w/ letrozole; ↓ w/ severe cardiac or hepatic impair **Caution:** [D, ?/+] Avoid CYP3A4 Inhib/inducers **CI:** Component hypersensitivity **Disp:** Tabs 250 mg **SE:** N/V/D, anemia, ↓ plt, neutropenia ,↑ QT interval, hand–foot synd, ↑ LFTs, rash, ↓ left ventricular ejection fraction, interstitial lung Dz and pneumonitis **Interactions:** ↑ Effects *W/* potent CYP3A4 Inhibs (eg, ketoconazole), grapefruit; ↓ effects *W/* potent CYP3A4 inducers (eg, carbamazepine) **Labs:** ↑ LFTs; ↓ plt, neutropenia **NIPE:** Consider baseline LVEF & periodic ECG; take 1 h before or 1 h after a meal; ⊘ consume grapefruit/juice; LFTs at baseline and during Tx; photosensitivity—use sunscreen

Latanoprost (Xalatan) [Glaucoma Agent/Prostaglandin]   Uses: *Open-angle glaucoma, ocular HTN* **Action:** Prostaglandin, ↑ outflow of aqueous humor **Dose:** 1 gtt eye(s) hs **Caution:** [C, M] **Disp:** 0.005% soln **SE:** May darken light irides; blurred vision, ocular stinging, & itching, ↑ number & length of eyelashes **Interactions:** ↑ Risk *OF* precipitation if mixed w/ eye drops w/ thimerosal **NIPE:** Wait 15 min before using contacts; separate from other eye products by 5 min; teach use of eye drops

Leflunomide (Arava) [Antirheumatic DMARDs/Immunomodulator]   WARNING: PRG must be excluded prior to start of Rx; hepatotox; Tx should not be initiated in pts w/ acute or chronic liver Dz **Uses:** *Active RA, orphan drug for organ rejection* **Action:** DMARD, ↓ pyrimidine synth **Dose:** Initial 100 mg/d PO for 3 d, then 10–20 mg/d **Caution:** [X, –] w/ Bile acid sequestrants, warfarin, rifampin, MTX; not rec in pts w/ preexisting liver Dz **CI:** PRG **Disp:** Tabs 10, 20, mg **SE:** D, Infxn, HTN, alopecia, rash, N, Jt pain, hep, interstitial lung Dz, immunosuppression peripheral neuropathy **Interactions:** ↑ Effects *W/* rifampin; ↑ risk of hepatotox *W/* hepatotoxic drugs, MTX; ↑ effects *OF* NSAIDs; ↓ effects *W/* activated charcoal, cholestyramine **Labs:** ↑ LFTs; monitor LFTs, CBC, PO₄ during initial therapy and monthly; D/C therapy if ALT > 3 × ULN & begin drug elimination procedure **NIPE:** ⊘ PRG, ⊘ breast-feeding, ⊘ live virus vaccines; immunizations should be up to date; take w/ or w/o food; may cause dizziness—caution driving

Lenalidomide (Revlimid) [Immunomodulator]   WARNING: Significant teratogen; pt must be enrolled in RevAssist risk-reduction program; hematologic tox, DVT & PE risk **Uses:** *MDS, combo w/ dexamethasone in multiple myeloma in pt failing one prior Rx **Action:** Thalidomide analog, immune modula-tor **Dose:** *Adults.* 10 mg PO daily; swallow whole w/ H₂O; multiple myeloma 25 mg/d d 1–21 of 28-d cycle w/ protocol dose of dexamethasone **Caution:** [X, −] w/ Renal impair **CI:** PRG **Disp:** Caps 5, 10, 15, 25 mg **SE:** D, pruritus, rash, fatigue, night sweats, edema, nasopharyngitis, ↓ BM (plt, WBC), ↑ K⁺, ↑ LFTs, thrombo-embolism **Interactions:** Monitor digoxin **Labs:** ↓ BM (plt, WBC)—monitor CBC, ↑ K⁺, ↑ LFTs; routine PRG tests required **NIPE:** Monitor for myelosuppression, thromboembolism, hepatotox; Rx only in 1-mo increments; limited distribution network; males must use condom & not donate sperm; use at least 2 forms of con-traception > 4 wk beyond D/C; see pkg insert for dose adjustments based on non-hematologic & hematologic tox; take w/ or w/o food; ↑ fluids

Lepirudin (Refludan) [Anticoagulant/Thrombin Inhibitor] Uses: *HIT* **Action:** Direct thrombin inhib **Dose:** *Bolus:* 0.4 mg/kg IV push, then 0.15 mg/kg/h Inf; if > 110 kg 44 mg of Inf 16.5 mg/h max; ↓ dose & Inf rate w/ CrCl < 60 mL/min or if used w/ thrombolytics **Caution:** [B, ?/−] Hemorrhagic event or severe HTN **CI:** Active bleeding **Disp:** Inj 50 mg **SE:** Bleeding, anemia, hema-toma, anaphylaxis **Interactions:** ↑ Risk of bleeding **W/** antiplt drugs, cephalospo-rins, NSAIDs, thrombolytics, salicylates, feverfew, ginkgo, ginger, valerian **Labs:** Adjust based on aPTT ratio, maint aPTT 1.5–2.5 × control **NIPE:** Monitor for bleeding: bleeding gums, nosebleed, unusual bruising, tarry stools, hematuria, guaiac + stool

Letrozole (Femara) [Antineoplastic/Aromatase Inhibitor] Uses: *Breast CA:* Adjuvant w/ postmenopausal hormone receptor positive early Dz; adjuvant in postmenopausal women w/ early breast CA w/ prior adjuvant tamoxi-fen therapy; 1st/2nd line in postmenopausal w/ hormone receptor positive or unknown Dz* **Action:** Nonsteroidal aromatase inhib **Dose:** 2.5 mg/d PO; qod w/ severe liver Dz or cirrhosis **Caution:** [D, ?] [X, ?/−] **CI:** PRG, women who may become pregnant **Disp:** Tabs 2.5 mg **SE:** Anemia, N, hot flashes, arthralgia, hyper-cholesterolemia, decreased BMD, CNS depression **Interactions:** ↑ Risk of interference **W/** action of drug **W/** estrogens & OCPs **Labs:** ↑ LFTs, cholesterol; monitor CBC, thyroid Fxn, lytes, cholesterol, LFT, & SCr; **NIPE:** Take w/ or w/o food; monitor BP, bone density; teach how to reduce risk of bone loss—wgt-bearing exercises, adequate intake Ca/vit D, ↓ EtOH, ⊘ smoking

Leucovorin (Generic) [Folic Acid Derivative/Vitamin] Uses: *OD of folic acid antagonist; megaloblastic anemia, augment 5-FU impaired MTX elim-ination; w/ 5-FU in colon CA* **Action:** Reduced folate source; circumvents action of folate reductase inhib (eg, MTX) **Dose:** *Leucovorin rescue:* 10 mg/m² PO/IM/IV q6h; start w/in 24 h after dose or 15 mg PO/IM/IV q6h, for 10 doses until MTX level < 0.05 micromole/L *Folate antagonist OD (eg, Pemetrexed)* 100 mg/m² IM/ IV × 1, then 50 mg/m² IM/IV q6h × 8 d *5-FU adjuvant Tx, colon CA per protocol; low dose* 20 mg/m²/d IV × 5 d w/ 5-FU 425 mg/m²/d IV × 5 d, repeat q4–5wk × 6 *High dose:* 200 mg/m² in combo w/ 5-FU 370 mg/m² *Megaloblastic anemia:* 1 mg

IM/IV qd **Caution:** [C, ?/–] **CI:** Pernicious anemia or vit B$_{12}$ deficient megaloblastic anemias **Disp:** Tabs 5, 10, 15, 25 mg; Inj 50, 100, 200, 350, 500 mg **SE:** Allergic Rxn, N/V/D, fatigue, wheezing ↑ plt **Interactions:** ↑ Effects *OF* 5-FU; ↓ effects *OF* MTX, phenobarbital, phenytoin, primidone, TMP/SMX **Labs:** ↑ Plt; monitor Cr, methotrexate levels q24h w/ leucovorin rescue; w/ 5-FU monitor CBC w/ different plt, LFTs, lytes **NIPE:** ↑ Fluids to 3 L/d; do not use intrathecally/intraventricularly

Leuprolide (Eligard, Lupron, Lupron DEPOT, Lupron DEPOT-Ped, Generic) [Antineoplastic/GnRH Analogue]

Uses: *Advanced PCa (all except DEPOT-Ped), endometriosis (Lupron), uterine fibroids (Lupron), & precocious puberty (Lupron-Ped)* **Action:** LHRH agonist; paradoxically ↓ release of GnRH w/ ↓ LH from anterior pituitary; in men ↓ testosterone, in women ↓ estrogen **Dose: Adults.** PCa: *Lupron DEPOT:* 7.5 mg IM q28d or 22.5 mg IM q3mo or 30 mg IM q4mo or 45 mg IM q6 mo *Eligard:* 7.5 mg SQ q28d or 22.5 mg SQ q3mo or 30 mg SQ q4mo or 45 mg SQ 6 mo *Endometriosis (Lupron DEPOT):* 3.75 mg IM qmo × 6 or 11.25 IM q3mo × 2 *Fibroids:* 3.75 mg IM qmo × 3 or 11.25 mg IM × 1 **Peds.** *CPP (Lupron DEPOT-Ped):* 50 mcg/kg/d SQ Inj; ↑ by 10 mcg/kg/d until total downregulation achieved *Lupron DEPOT: < 25 kg.* 7.5 mg IM q4wk *> 25–37.5 kg.* 11.25 mg IM q4wk *> 37.5 kg.* 15 mg IM q4wk, ↑ by 3.75 mg q4wk until response **Caution:** [X, –] w/ Impending cord compression in PCa, ↑ QT w/ meds or preexisting CV Dz **CI:** AUB, implant in women/peds; PRG **Disp:** Inj 5 mg/mL *Lupron DEPOT* 3.75 (1 mo for fibroids, endometriosis) *Lupron DEPOT for PCa:* 7.5 mg (1 mo), 11.25 mg (3 mo), 22.5 mg (3 mo), 30 mg (4 mo), 45 mg (6 mo) *Eligard depot for PCa:* 7.5 mg (1 mo), 22.5 mg (3 mo), 30 mg (4 mo), 45 mg (6 mo) *Lupron DEPOT-Ped:* 7.5, 11.25, 15, 30 mg **SE:** Hot flashes, gynecomastia, N/V, alopecia, anorexia, dizziness, HA, insomnia, paresthesias, depression exacerbation, peripheral edema, & bone pain (transient "flare Rxn" at 7–14 d after the 1st dose [LH/testosterone surge before suppression]); ↓ BMD w/ > 6 mo use, bone loss possible, abnormal menses, hyperglycemia **Interactions:** ↓ Effects *W/* androgens, estrogens **Labs:** ↑ LFTs, BUN, Cr, uric acid, lipids, WBC; ↓ PT, PTT, plts **NIPE:** Nonsteroidal antiandrogen (eg, bicalutamide) may block flare in men w/ PCa; teach SQ Inj technique

Leuprolide Acetate/Norethindrone Acetate Kit (Lupaneta Pack)

Uses: *Painful endometriosis* **Action:** GnRH agonist w/ a progestin **Dose:** Leuprolide 11.25 mg IM q3mo × 2 w/ norethindrone 5 mg PO daily, 6 mo total; if symptoms recur, consider another 6 mo Tx **Caution:** [B, ?/–] Assess BMD before; monitor for depression; D/C w/ vision loss/changes **CI:** Component sensitivity; AUB, PRG, breast-feeding, Hx breast/hormonally sensitive CA, thrombosis, liver tumor or Dz **Disp:** Copackaged leuprolide 11.25 mg depot w/ 90 norethindrone 5 mg tabs **SE:** *Leuprolide:* Hot flashes/sweats, HA/migraine, depression/emotional lability, N/V, nervousness/anxiety, insomnia, pain, acne, asthenia, vaginitis, ↑ wgt, constipation/diarrhea *Norethindrone:* Breakthrough bleeding/spotting **NIPE:** Use nonhormonal methods of contraception; Rx limited to two 6-mo courses; ↑ risk for ↓ BMD; see Leuprolide and Norethindrone

Levalbuterol (Xopenex, Xopenex HFA) [Bronchodilator/Beta-2 Agonist] **Uses:** *Asthma (Rx & prevention of bronchospasm)* **Action:** Sympathomimetic bronchodilator; *R*-isomer of albuterol, β₂-agonist **Dose:** Based on NIH Guidelines 2007 *Adults.* Acute-severe exacerbation Xopenex HFA 4–8 puffs q20min up to 4 h, then q1–4h PRN or nebulizer 1.25–2.5 mg q20min × 3, then 1.25–5 mg q1–4h PRN *Peds < 5 y.* Quick relief 0.31–1.25 mg q4–6h PRN, severe 1.25 mg q20min × 3, then 0.075–0.15 mg/kg q1–4h PRN, 5 mg max *5–11 y.* Acute-severe exacerbation 1.25 mg q20min × 3, then 0.075–0.15 mg/kg q1–4h PRN, 5 mg max, quick relief: 0.31–0.63 q8h PRN *> 12 y.* 0.63–1.25 mg nebulizer q8h **Caution:** [C, M] w/ Non–K⁺-sparing diuretics, CAD, HTN, arrhythmias, ↓ K⁺, hyperthyroidism, glaucoma, diabetes **CI:** Component hypersensitivity **Disp:** Multidose inhaler (Xopenex HFA) 45 mcg/puff (15 g); soln nebulizer Inh 0.31, 0.63, 1.25 mg/3 mL; concentrate 1.25 mg/0.5 mL **SE:** Paradox bronchospasm, anaphylaxis, angioedema, tachycardia, nervousness, V, ↓ K⁺ **Interactions:** ↑ Effects W/ MAOIs, TCAs; ↑ risk of hypokalemia W/ loop & thiazide diuretics; ↓ effects W/ BBs; ↓ effects *OF* digoxin **Labs:** ↑ Serum glucose, ↓ serum K⁺ **NIPE:** May ↓ CV SE compared w/ albuterol; do not mix w/ other nebulizers or dilute; use only with nebulizer; use other inhalants 5 min after this drug; monitor ECG for hypokalemia (flattened T waves); do not give within 14 d of MAOI; teach use of peak flow meter—monitoring of Sx

Levetiracetam (Keppra, Keppra XR) [Anticonvulsant/Pyrrolidine Agent] **Uses:** *Adjunctive PO Rx in partial-onset Sz (adults & peds ≥ 4 y), myoclonic Szs (adults & peds ≥ 12 y) w/ juvenile myoclonic epilepsy (JME), primary generalized tonic–clonic (PGTC) Szs (adults & peds ≥ 6 y) w/ idiopathic generalized epilepsy. Adjunctive Inj PO Rx partial-onset Szs in adults w/ epilepsy; myoclonic Szs in adults w/ JME. Inj alternative for adults (≥ 16 y) when PO not possible* **Action:** Unknown **Dose:** *Adults & Peds > 16 y.* 500 mg PO bid, titrate q2wk, may ↑ 3000 mg/d max *Peds 4–15 y.* 10 mg/kg/d ÷ in 2 doses, 60 mg/kg/d max (↓ in renal Insuff) **Caution:** [C, ?/–] Elderly, w/ renal impair, psychological disorders; ↑ suicidality risk for antiepileptic drugs, higher for those w/ epilepsy vs those using drug for psychological indications; Inj not for < 16 y **CI:** Component allergy **Disp:** Tabs 250, 500, 750, 1000 mg, ER 500, 750 mg soln 100 mg/mL; Inj 100 mg/mL **SE:** Dizziness, somnolence, HA, N/V hostility, aggression, hallucinations, hematologic abnormalities, impaired coordination **Interactions:** ↑ Effects W/ antihistamines, TCAs, benzodiazepines, narcotics, phenytoin; EtOH **NIPE:** May take w/ or w/o food; ⊘ crush/chew; do not D/C abruptly—may cause Szs; post-market hepatic failure & pancytopenia reported

Levobunolol (A-K Beta, Betagan) [Glaucoma Agent/Beta-Adrenergic Blocker] **Uses:** *Open-angle glaucoma, ocular HTN* **Action:** β-Adrenergic blocker **Dose:** 1 gtt daily–bid **Caution:** [C, M] w/ Verapamil or systemic β-blockers **CI:** Asthma, COPD sinus bradycardia, heart block (2nd-, 3rd-degree) CHF **Disp:** Soln 0.25%, 0.5% **SE:** Ocular stinging/burning, ↓ HR, ↓ BP **Interactions:** ↑ Effects **W/** BBs; ↑ risk of hypotension & bradycardia **W/** quinidine, verapamil; ↓ IOP **W/** carbonic anhydrase Inhibs, epinephrine, pilocarpine **NIPE:** Night vision & acuity may be ↓; possible systemic effects if absorbed; wait ≥ 15 min before inserting contact lenses; may cause dizziness—caution driving

Levocetirizine (Xyzal) [Antihistamine] Uses: *Perennial/seasonal allergic rhinitis, chronic urticaria* **Action:** Antihistamine **Dose:** *Adults.* 5 mg qd *Peds 6 mo–5 y.* 1.25 mg qd *6–11 y.* 2.5 mg qd **Caution:** [B, ?/–] ↓ Adult dose w/ renal impair, CrCl 50–80 mL/min 2.5 mg qd, 30–50 mL/min 2.5 mg qod; 10–30 mL/min 2.5 mg 2 ×/wk **CI:** Peds 6–11 y, w/ renal impair, adults w/ ESRD **Disp:** Tab 5 mg, soln 0.5 mL/mL (150 mL) **SE:** CNS depression, drowsiness, fatigue, xerostomia **Interactions:** ↑ Effects **W/** theophylline, ritonavir **NIPE:** Take in evening; caution driving; avoid EtOH, CNS depressants

Levofloxacin (Levaquin) [Antibiotic/Fluoroquinolone]
WARNING: ↑ Risk Achilles tendon rupture and tendonitis, may exacerbate muscle weakness related to myasthenia gravis **Uses:** *Skin/skin structure Infxn (SSSI), UTI, chronic bacterial prostatitis, acute pyelo, acute bacterial sinusitis, acute bacterial exacerbation of chronic bronchitis, CAP, including multidrug-resistant S pneumoniae, nosocomial pneumonia; Rx inhalational anthrax in adults & peds ≥ 6 mo* **Action:** Quinolone. ↓ DNA gyrase. *Spectrum:* Excellent gram(+) except MRSA & E faecium;* excellent gram(–) except *Stenotrophomonas maltophilia* & *Acinetobacter* sp; poor anaerobic **Dose:** *Adults ≥ 18 y.* IV/PO: *Bronchitis:* 500 mg qd × 7 d *CAP:* 500 mg qd × 7–14 d or 750 mg qd × 5 d *Sinusitis:* 500 mg qd × 10–14 d or 750 mg qd × 5 d *Prostatitis:* 500 mg qd × 28 d *Uncomp SSSI:* 500 mg qd × 7–10 d *Comp SSSI/ nosocomial pneumonia:* 750 mg qd × 7–14 d *Anthrax:* 500 mg qd × 60 d *Uncomp UTI:* 250 mg qd × 3 d *Comp UTI/acute pyelo:* 250 mg qd × 10 d or 750 mg qd × 5 d, CrCl 10–19 mL/min; 500 mg then 250 mg qod or 750 mg, then 500 mg q48h *Hemodialysis:* 750 mg, then 500 mg q48h *Peds ≥ 6 mo.* Anthrax: > 50 kg: 500 mg q24h × 60 d, < 50 kg 8 mg/kg (250 mg/dose max) q12h for 60 d ↓ w/ renal impair, avoid antacids w/ PO; oral soln 1 h before, 2 h after meals; Cap: ≥ 6 mo–≤ 4 y. 8 mg/kg/dose q12h (max 750 mg/d) *5–16 y.* 8 mg/kg/dose qd (750 mg/d) **Caution:** [C, –] w/ Cation-containing products (eg, antacids), w/ drugs that ↑ QT interval **CI:** Quinolone sensitivity **Disp:** Tabs 250, 500, 750 mg; premixed IV 250, 500, 750 mg, Inj 25 mg/mL; Leva-Pak 750 mg × 5 d **SE:** N/D, dizziness, rash, GI upset, photosens, CNS stimulant w/ IV use, *C difficile* enterocolitis; rare fatal hepatox, peripheral neuropathy risk **Interactions:** ↑ Effects *OF* cyclosporine, digoxin, theophylline, warfarin, caffeine; ↑ risk of Szs **W/** foscarnet, NSAIDs; ↑ risk of hyper-/hypoglycemia **W/** hypoglycemic drugs; ↓ effects **W/** antacids, antineoplastics, Ca, cimetidine, didanosine, famotidine, Fe, lansoprazole, Mg, nizatidine, omeprazole, phenytoin, ranitidine, NaHCO₃, sucralfate, zinc **NIPE:** Risk of tendon rupture & tendonitis—D/C if pain or inflammation; use w/ steroids ↑ tendon risk;

take on empty stomach; ↑ fluids, use sunscreen, antacids 2 h before or after this drug; only for anthrax in peds

Levofloxacin Ophthalmic (Quixin, Iquix) [Antibiotic/Fluoroquinolone] Uses: *Bacterial conjunctivitis* Action: See Levofloxacin Dose: *Ophthal:* 1–2 gtt in eye(s) q2h while awake up to 8 ×/d × 2 d then q4h while awake × 5 d Caution: [C, –] CI: Quinolone sensitivity Disp: 25 mg/mL ophthal soln 0.5% (Quixin), 1.5% (Iquix) SE: Ocular burning/pain, ↓ vision, fever, foreign body sensation, HA, pharyngitis, photophobia NIPE: Teach use of eye drops

Levomilnacipran (Fetzima) WARNING: Risk of suicidal thoughts/behavior in children, adolescents, and young adults; monitor for worsening depression and emergence of suicidal thoughts/behaviors Uses: *Depression in adults* Action: SNRI Dose: *Adults.* 20 mg 1 ×/d for 2 d, then 40 mg 1 ×/d, may ↑ by 40 mg every 2 d to 120 mg max; usual 40–120 mg/d; ↓ w/ CrCl < 60 mL/min Peds. Not approved Caution: [C, ?/–] CDC rec: HIV-infected mothers not breast-feed (transmission risk); see Warning; serotonin synd w/ certain meds: tricyclics, Li, triptans, fentanyl, tramadol, buspirone St. John's wort; SSRIs & SNIRs may cause ↓ Na+; ↑ BP, ↑ HR; ↑ risk of bleeding w/ ASA, NSAIDs, warfarin; urinary retention/hesitancy; may elicit mania in bipolar patients presenting w/ depression Disp: ER caps, 20, 40, 80, 120 mg CI: Hypersensitivity; do not use w/ MAOI, linezolid, or methylene blue (serotonin synd risk); uncontrolled NAG, ESRD SE: N, V, ED, testicular pain, ejaculation disorder, hyperhidrosis Notes: 80 mg/d max w/ strong CYP3A4 Inhib; with abrupt D/C confusion, dysphoria, irritability, agitation, anxiety, insomnia, paresthesias, HA & insomnia can occur; EtOH may accelerate drug release NIPE: Take w/o regard to food; swallow whole; taper dose and monitor w/ D/C; ⊘ EtOH; may ↑ BP—check regularly; caution driving

Levonorgestrel (Next Choice, Plan B One Step) [Progestin/Hormone] Uses: *Emergency contraceptive ("morning-after pill")* Action: Prevents PRG if taken < 72 h after unprotected sex/contraceptive failure; progestin, alters tubal transport & endometrium to implantation Dose: *Adults & Peds (postmenarche ♂).* w/in 72 h of unprotected intercourse: *Next Choice* 0.75 mg q12h × 2; *Plan B One Step* 1.5 mg × 1 Caution: [X, M] w/ AUB; may ↑ ectopic PRG risk CI: Known/suspected PRG Disp: *Next Choice* tab, 0.75 mg, 2 blister packs; *Plan B One Step* tab, 1.5 mg, 1 blister pack SE: N/V/D, Abd pain, fatigue, HA, menstrual changes, dizziness, breast changes Interactions: ↓ Effects W/ barbiturates, carbamazepine, modafinil, phenobarbital, phenytoin, pioglitazone, rifabutin, rifampin, ritonavir, topiramate, St. John's wort NIPE: Most effective if taken as soon as possible after unprotected intercourse; will not induce abortion; OTC ("behind the counter") if > 17 y, Rx if < 17 y but varies by state; if V occurs w/in 2 h of ingesting drug—may consider repeating dose

Levonorgestrel IUD (Mirena) [Progestin/Hormone] Uses: *Contraception, long term* Action: Progestin, alters endometrium, thicken cervical mucus, inhibits ovulation & implantation Dose: Up to 5 y, insert w/in 7 d menses onset or immediately after 1st-tri Ab; wait 6 wk if postpartum; replace any time during menstrual cycle **Caution:** [X, M] **CI:** PRG, w/ active hepatic Dz or tumor, uterine anomaly, breast CA, acute/Hx of PID, postpartum endometriosis, infected Ab last 3 mo, gynecological neoplasia, abnormal Pap, AUB, untreated cervicitis/vaginitis, multiple sex partners, ↑ susceptibility to Infxn **Disp:** 52 mg IUD **SE:** Failed insertion, ectopic PRG, sepsis, PID, infertility, PRG comps w/ IUD left in place, Ab, embedment, ovarian cysts, perforation uterus/cervix, intestinal obst/perforation, peritonitis, N, Abd pain, ↑ BP, acne, HA **NIPE:** Inform pt does not protect against STD/HIV; see package insert for insertion instructions; reexamine placement after 1st menses; 80% PRG w/in 12 mo of removal; teach how to check placement after each menses

Levorphanol (Levo-Dromoran) [C-II] [Narcotic Analgesic] Uses: *Mod–severe pain; chronic pain* **Action:** Narcotic analgesic, morphine derivative **Dose:** 2–4 mg PO PRN q6–8h; ↓ in hepatic impair **Caution:** [B/D (prolonged use/ high doses at term), ?/–] w/ ↑ ICP, head trauma, adrenal Insuff **CI:** Component allergy **Disp:** Tabs 2 mg **SE:** Tachycardia, ↓ BP, drowsiness, GI upset, constipation, resp depression, pruritus **Interactions:** ↑ CNS effects W/ antihistamines, cimetidine, CNS depressants, glutethimide, methocarbamol, EtOH, St. John's wort **Labs:** ↑ Amylase, lipase **NIPE:** ↑ Fluids & fiber, take w/ food; caution driving

Levothyroxine (Synthroid, Levoxyl, Others) [Thyroid Hormone] WARNING: Not for obesity or wgt loss; tox w/ high doses, especially when combined w/ sympathomimetic amines **Uses:** *Hypothyroidism, pituitary thyroid-stimulating hormone (TSH) suppression, myxedema coma* **Action:** T_4 supl L-thyroxine **Dose: *Adults.*** *Hypothyroid* titrate until euthyroid > 50 y w/ heart Dz or < 50 w/ heart Dz 25–50 mcg/d, ↑ q6–8wk; > 50 y w/ heart Dz 12.5–25 mcg/d, ↑ q6–8wk; usual 100–200 mcg/d *Myxedema:* 200–500 mcg IV, then 100–300 mcg/d **Peds.** *Hypothyroid:* **1–3 mo:** 10–15 mcg/kg/24 h PO **3–6 mo:** 8–10 mcg/kg/d PO **6–12 mo.:** 6–8 mcg/kg/d PO **1–5 y:** 5–6 mcg/kg/d PO **6–12 y:** 4–5 mcg/kg/d PO **>12 y:** 2–3 mcg/kg/d PO; if growth and puberty complete 1.7 mcg/kg/d; ↓ dose by 50% if IV; titrate based on response & thyroid tests; dose can ↑ rapid in young/middle-aged; best on empty stomach **Caution:** [A, M] Many drug interactions; in elderly w/ CV Dz; thyrotoxicosis; w/ warfarin monitor **INR CI:** Recent MI, uncorrected adrenal Insuff **Disp:** Tabs 25, 50, 75, 88, 100, 112, 125, 137, 150, 175, 200, 300 mcg; Inj 200, 500 mcg **SE:** Insomnia, wgt loss, N/V/D, ↑ LFTs, irregular periods, ↓ BMD, alopecia, arrhythmia **Interactions:** ↑ Effects *OF* anticoagulants, sympathomimetics, TCAs, warfarin; ↓ effects *W/* antacids, BBs, carbamazepine, cholestyramine, estrogens, Fe salts, phenytoin, phenobarbital, rifampin, simethicone, sucralfate, ↓ effects *OF* digoxin, hypoglycemics, theophylline **Labs:** ↑ LFTs—Monitor: ↓ thyroid Fxn tests; drug alters thyroid uptake of radioactive I—D/C drug 4 wk before studies NIPE: ⊘ Switch brands d/t different bioavailabilities; take in AM, 30–60 min before breakfast; take w/ full glass of H_2O (prevents choking); PRG may ↑ need for higher doses; takes 6 wk to see effect on TSH; wait 6 wk before checking TSH after dose change; w/ warfarin monitor INR

Lidocaine, Systemic (Xylocaine, Others) [Antiarrhythmic]
Uses: *Rx cardiac arrhythmias* **Action:** Class IB antiarrhythmic **Dose:** *Adults.*
Antiarrhythmic, ET: 5 mg/kg; follow w/ 0.5 mg/kg in 10 min if effective. *IV load:*
1 mg/kg/dose bolus over 2–3 min; repeat in 5–10 min; 200–300 mg max; cont
Inf 20–50 mcg/kg/min or 1–4 mg/min *ECC 2010:* **Cardiac arrest from VF/VT
refractory VF:** *Initial:* 1–1.5 mg/kg IV/IO, additional 0.5–0.75 mg/kg IV push,
repeat in 5–10 min, max total 3 mg/kg *ET:* 2–4 mg/kg as last resort **Reperfusing
stable VT, wide complex tachycardia or ectopy:** Doses of 0.5–0.75 mg/kg to
1–1.5 mg/kg may be used initially; repeat 0.5–0.75 mg/kg q5–10min; max dose
3 mg/kg *Peds. ECC 2010:* **VF/pulseless VT, wide-complex tach (w/ pulses):**
1 mg/kg IV/IO, then maint 20–50 mcg/kg/min (repeat bolus if Inf started > 15 min
after initial dose) **RSI:** 1–2 mg/kg IV/IO **Caution:** [B, M] ↓ Dose in severe hepatic
impairment **CI:** Adams–Stokes synd; heart block; corn allergy **Disp:** Inj IV: 1%
(10 mg/mL), 2% (20 mg/mL); admixture 4, 10, 20% *IV Inf:* 0.2, 0.4% **SE:** Dizziness, paresthesias, & convulsions associated w/ tox **Interactions:** ↑ Effects *W/*
amprenavir, BBs, cimetidine; ↑ neuromuscular blockade *W/* aminoglycosides,
tubocurarine; ↑ cardiac depression *W/* procainamide, phenytoin, propranolol, quinidine, tocainide; ↑ effects *OF* succinylcholine **Labs:** ↑ SCr, ↑ CPK for 48 h after
IM Inj **NIPE:** 2nd line to amiodarone in ECC; dilute ET dose 1–2 mL w/ NS; for
IV forms, ↓ w/ liver Dz or CHF *Systemic levels:* Steady state 6–12 h *Therapeutic:*
1.2–5 mcg/mL *Toxic:* > 6 mcg/mL *1/2-life:* 1.5 h; monitor ECG

Lidocaine; Lidocaine with Epinephrine (Anestacon Topical, Xylocaine, Xylocaine Viscous, Xylocaine MPF, Others) [Anesthetic]
Uses: *Local anesthetic, epidural/caudal anesthesia, regional nerve blocks, topical on
mucous membranes (mouth/pharynx/urethra)* **Action:** Anesthetic; stabilizes neuronal
membranes; inhibits ionic fluxes required for initiation and conduction **Dose:** *Adults.*
Local Inj anesthetic: 4.5 mg/kg max total dose or 300 mg; w/ epi 7 mg/kg or total
500 mg max dose *Oral:* 15 mL viscous swish and spit or *pharyngeal* gargle and
swallow, do not use < 3-h intervals or > 8 × in 24 h. *Urethra:* Jelly 5–30 mL (200–
300 mg) jelly in men, 5 mL female urethra; 600 mg/24 h max *Peds.* *Topical:* Apply
max 3 mg/kg/dose *Local Inj anesthetic:* Max 4.5 mg/kg (Table 1) **Caution:** [B, +]
Epi-containing soln may interact w/ TCA or MAOI & cause severe ↑ BP **CI:** Do
not use lidocaine w/ epi on digits, ears, or nose (vasoconstriction & necrosis) **Disp:**
Inj local: 0.5, 1, 1.5, 2, 4, 10, 20%; Inj w/ epi 0.5%/1:200,000, 1%/1:100,000,
2%/1:100,000; (MPF) 1%/1:200,000, 1.5%/1:200,000, 2%/1:200,000; (*Dental formulations*) 2%/1:50,000, 2%/1:100,000; cream 2,3, 4%; lotion 30%, jelly 2%, gel
2, 2.5, 4, 5%; oint 5%; Liq 2.5%; soln 2, 4%; viscous 2% **SE:** Dizziness, paresthesias, & convulsions associated w/ tox **Notes:** See Table 1 **NIPE:** Oral spray/soln
may impair swallowing; epi may be added for local anesthesia to ↑ effect & ↓
bleeding

Lidocaine/Prilocaine (EMLA, Oraq IX) [Topical Anesthetic]
Uses: *Topical anesthetic for intact skin or genital mucous membranes*; adjunct to phlebotomy or dermal procedures Action: Amide local anesthetics Dose: **Adults.** *EMLA cream,* thick layer 2–2.5 g to intact skin over 20–25 cm², cover w/ occlusive dressing (eg, Tegaderm) for at least 1 h *Anesthetic disc:* 1 g/10 cm² for at least 1 h Peds. **Max Dose: < 3 mo or < 5 kg.** 1 g/10 cm² for 1 h *3–12 mo & > 5 kg.* 2 g/20 cm² for 4 h *1–6 y & > 10 kg.* 10 g/100 cm² for 4 h *7–12 y & > 20 kg.* 20 g/200 cm² for 4 h Caution: [B, +] CI: Methemoglobinemia use on mucous membranes, broken skin, eyes; allergy to amide-type anesthetics Disp: Cream 2.5% lidocaine/2.5% prilocaine; periodontal gel 2.5/2.5% SE: Burning, stinging, methemoglobinemia NIPE: Longer contact time ↑ effect; low risk of systemic adverse effects; apply disc 1 h prior to procedure

Lidocaine/Tetracaine, Patch (Synera) Cream (Pliaglis) Uses: *Topical anesthesia for venipuncture and dermatologic procedures (*Synera*); dermatologic procedures (*Pliaglis*)* Action: Combo amide and ester local anesthetic Dose: **Adults and Peds.** *Synera:* Apply patch 20–30 min before procedure. **Adults.** *Pliaglis:* Apply cream 20–60 min before procedure, volume based on site surface (see label) Caution: [B, ?/–] Use on intact skin only; avoid eyes; not for mucous membranes; do not use w/Hx methemoglobinemia anaphylaxis reported; caution w/Class I antiarrhythmic drugs; remove before MRI CI: Component sensitivity (PABA or local anesthetics) Disp: *Synera* 70 mg lidocaine/70 mg tetracaine in 50 cm² patch *Pliaglis* 70 mg lidocaine/70 mg tetracaine/g (7%/7%) cream 30, 60, 100 g tube SE: Erythema, blanching, and edema NIPE: ⊘ Cut patch/remove top cover—may cause thermal injury; low risk of systemic adverse effects; ⊘ use multiple patches simultaneously or sequentially

Linaclotide (Linzess) **WARNING:** CI peds < 6 y; avoid in peds 6–17 y; death in juvenile mice Uses: *IBS w/ constipation, chronic idiopathic constipation* Action: Guanylate cyclase-C agonist Dose: *IBS-C:* 290 mcg PO qd *CIC:* 145 mcg PO qd Caution: [C, ?/–] CI: Pts < 6 y; GI obst Disp: Caps 145, 290 mcg SE: D, Abd pain/distention, flatulence NIPE: Take on empty stomach 30 min prior to 1st meal of the day; swallow whole; may cause diarrhea ≥ 2 wk after starting

Linagliptin (Tradjenta) Uses: *Type 2 DM* Action: Dipeptidyl peptidase-4 (DPP-4) inhibitor; ↑ active incretin hormones (↑ insulin release, ↓ glucagon) Dose: **Adults.** 5 mg qd Caution: [B, ?/–] CI: Hypersensitivity Disp: Tabs 5 mg SE: Hypoglycemia w/ sulfonylurea; nasopharyngitis, pancreatitis Notes: Inhibitor of CYP3A4 NIPE: Take w/ or w/o food; monitor s/s pancreatitis, hypoglycemia; not for use in type 1 DM

Linagliptin/Metformin (Jentadueto) **WARNING:** Lactic acidosis w/ metformin accumulation; ↑ risk w/ sepsis, vol depletion, CHF, renal/hepatic impair, excess alcohol; w/ lactic acidosis suspected D/C and hospitalize Uses: *Combo type 2 DM* Actions: DDP-4 Inhib; ↑ insulin synth/release w/ biguanide; ↓ hepatic glucose prod & absorption; ↑ insulin sensitivity Dose: Titrate as needed;

give bid w/meals, gradual ↑ do due to GI SE (metformin) max 2.5/1000 mg bid **Caution:** [X, –] May cause lactic acidosis, pancreatitis, hepatic failure, hypersensitivity Rxn; vit B$_{12}$ def **CI:** Component hypersensitivity, renal impair, metabolic acidosis **Disp:** Tabs (linagliptin mg/metformin mg): 2.5/500, 2.5/850, 2.5/1000 **SE:** ↓ Glucose, nasopharyngitis, D **Notes:** May ↑ metformin lactate effect; temp D/C w/ surgery or w/ iodinated contrast studies **NIPE:** Limit EtOH intake; maintain adequate hydration; see Linagliptin and Metformin

Lindane (Generic) [Scabicide/Pediculicide] **WARNING:** Only for pts intolerant/failed 1st-line Rx w/ safer agents. Szs and deaths reported w/ repeat/prolonged use. Caution d/t increased risk of neurotox in infants, children, elderly, w/ other skin conditions, & if < 50 kg. Instruct pts on proper use & inform that itching occurs after successful killing of scabies or lice **Uses:** *Head lice, pubic "crab" lice, body lice, scabies* **Action:** Ectoparasiticide & ovicide **Dose: Adults & Peds.** *Cream or lotion:* Thin layer to dry skin after bathing, leave for 8–12 h, rinse; also use on laundry *Shampoo:* Apply 30 mL to dry hair, develop a lather w/ warm water for 4 min, comb out nits **Caution:** [C, –] **CI:** Premature infants, uncontrolled Sz disorders norwedian scabies open wounds **Disp:** Lotion 1%; shampoo 1% **SE:** Arrhythmias, Szs, local irritation, GI upset, ataxia, alopecia, N/V, aplastic anemia **Interactions:** Oil-based hair creams ↑ drug absorption **NIPE:** Apply to dry hair/ dry, cool skin; scabies—use toothbrush to apply under nails; caution w/ overuse (may be absorbed); may repeat Rx in 7 d; try OTC 1st w/ pyrethrins (Pronto, Rid, others)

Linezolid (Zyvox) [Antibiotic/Oxazolidinones] **Uses:** *Infxns caused by gram(+) bacteria (including VRE), pneumonia, skin Infxns* **Action:** Unique, binds ribosomal bacterial RNA; bacteriocidal for streptococci, bacteriostatic for enterococci & staphylococci *Spectrum:* Excellent gram(+) including VRE & MRSA **Dose: Adults.** 600 mg IV or PO q12h *Peds ≤ 11 y.* 10 mg/kg IV or PO q8h (q12h in preterm neonates) **Caution:** [C, ?/–] **CI:** Concurrent MAOI use or w/in 2 wk, uncontrolled HTN, thyrotoxicosis, vasopressive agents, carcinoid tumor, SSRIs, tricyclics, w/ MAOI (may cause serotonin syndrome when used w/ these psych meds), w/ ↓ BM **Disp:** Inj 200, 600 mg; tabs 600 mg; susp 100 mg/5 mL **SE:** Lactic acidosis, peripheral/optic neuropathy, HTN, N/D, HA, insomnia, GI upset, ↓ BM, tongue discoloration prolonged use—*C difficile* Infxn **Interactions:** ↑ Risk of serotonin synd *W/* SSRIs, sibutramine, trazodone, venlafaxine; ↑ HTN *W/* amphetamines, dextromethorphan, DA, epinephrine, levodopa, MAOIs, meperidine, metaraminol, phenylephrine, phenylpropanolamine, pseudoephedrine, tyramine, ginseng, ephedra, ma huang, tyramine-containing foods; ↑ risk of bleeding *W/* antiplts **Labs:** Follow weekly CBC **NIPE:** Take w/o regard to food; avoid foods w/ tyramine (aged, smoked, pickled, fermented meats/dairy) & cough/cold products w/ pseudoephedrine; not for gram(−) Infxn, ↑ deaths in catheter-related Infxns

Liothyronine (Cytomel, Triostat, T$_3$) [Thyroid Hormone] **WARNING:** Not for obesity or wgt loss **Uses:** *Hypothyroidism, nontoxic goiter, myxedema coma* **Action:** T_3 replacement **Dose:** *Adults.* Initial 25 mcg/24 h, titrate q1–2wk to response & TFT; maint of 25–100 mcg/d PO *Myxedema coma:* 25–50 mcg IV *Myxedema:* 5 mcg/d, PO ↑ 5–10 mcg/d q1–2wk; maint 50–100 mcg/d *Nontoxic goiter:* 5 mcg/d PO, ↑ 5–10 mcg/d q1–2wk, usual dose 75 mcg/d *T_3 suppression test:* 75–100 mcg/d × 7 d; ↓ in elderly & CV Dz *Peds.* Initial 5 mcg/24 h, titrate by 50-mcg/24 h increments at q3–md intervals; maint *Infants–12 mo.* 20 mcg/d *Peds 1–3 y.* 50 mcg/d; *> 3 y.* Adult dose **Caution:** [A, +] **CI:** Recent MI, uncorrected adrenal Insuff, uncontrolled HTN, thyrotoxicosis, artificial rewarming **Disp:** Tabs 5, 25, 50 mcg; Inj 10 mcg/mL **SE:** Alopecia, arrhythmias, CP, HA, sweating, twitching, ↑ HR, ↑ BP, MI, CHF, fever **Interactions:** ↑ Effects *OF* anti-coagulants; ↓ effects *W/* bile acid sequestrants, carbamazepine, estrogens, phenytoin, rifampin; ↓ effects *OF* hypoglycemics, theophylline **Labs:** Monitor TFT; monitor glucose w/ DM meds **NIPE:** Monitor cardiac status, take in AM; separate antacids by 4 h; when switching from IV to PO, taper IV slowly

Liraglutide Recombinant (Victoza) [Glucagon-Like Peptide-1 (GLP-1) Receptor Agonist] **WARNING:** CI w/ personal or fam Hx of medullary thyroid Ca (MCT) or w/ multiple endocrine neoplasia synd type 2 (MEN 2) **Uses:** *Type 2 DM* **Action:** Glucagon-like peptide-1 receptor agonist **Dose:** 1.8 mg/d; begin 0.6 mg/d any time of d SQ (Abd/thigh/upper arm), ↑ to 1.2 mg after 1 wk, may ↑ to 1.8 mg after **Caution:** [C; ?/–] **CI:** See Warning **Disp:** Multidose pens, 0.6, 1.2, 1.8 mg/dose, 6 mg/mL **SE:** Pancreatitis, MTC, HA, N/D **Interactions:** ↓ Glucose w/ sulfonylurea **NIPE:** Delays gastric emptying; ⊘ Type 1 DM; teach SQ Inj technique

Lisdexamfetamine Dimesylate (Vyvanse) [Stimulant] [C-II] **WARNING:** Amphetamines have ↑ potential for abuse; prolonged administration may lead to dependence; may cause sudden death and serious CV events in pts w/ pre-existing structure cardiac abnormalities **Uses:** *ADHD* **Action:** CNS stimulant **Dose:** *Adults & Peds 6–12 y.* 30 mg daily, ↑ qwk 10–20 mg/d, 70 mg/d max **Caution:** [C, ?/–] w/ Potential for drug dependency in pt w/ psychological or Sz disorder, Tourette synd, HTN **CI:** Severe arteriosclerotic CV Dz, mod–severe ↑ BP, ↑ thyroid, sensitivity to sympathomimetic amines, NAG, agitated states, Hx drug abuse, w/ or w/in 14 d of MAOI **Disp:** Caps 20, 30, 40, 50, 60, 70 mg **SE:** HA, insomnia, decreased appetite **Interactions:** Risk of HTN crisis *W/* MAOIs, furazolidone; ↑ effects *W/* TCA, propoxyphene; ↑ effects *OF* meperidine, norepinephrine, phenobarbital, TCA; ↓ effects *W/* haloperidol, chlorpromazine, Li; ↓ effects *OF* adrenergic blockers, antihistamines, antihypertensives **Labs:** Monitor phenytoin levels; may interfere w/ urinary steroid tests **NIPE:** OK to open & dissolve in H_2O; AHA statement April 2008: All children diagnosed w/ ADHD who are candidates for stimulant meds should undergo CV assessment prior to use; may be inappropriate for geriatric use

Lisinopril (Prinivil, Zestril) [Antihypertensive/ACEI] **WARNING:** ACE Inhib can cause fetal injury/death in 2nd/3rd tri; D/C w/ PRG **Uses:** *HTN,

CHF, prevent DN & AMI* **Action:** ACE Inhib **Dose:** 5–40 mg/24 h PO daily–bid, CHF target 40 mg/d *AMI:* 5 mg w/in 24 h of MI, then 5 mg after 24 h, 10 mg after 48 h, then 10 mg/d; ↓ in renal Insuff; use low dose, ↑ slowly in elderly **Caution:** [C (1st tri) D (2nd/3rd tri), –] w/ Aortic stenosis/cardiomyopathy **CI:** PRG, ACE Inhib sensitivity, idiopathic or hereditary angioedema **Disp:** Tabs 2.5, 5, 10, 20, 30, 40 mg **SE:** Dizziness, HA, cough, ↓ BP, angioedema, ↑ K⁺, ↑ Cr, rare, ↓ BM **Interactions:** ↑ Effects **W/** α-blockers, diuretics ↑ risk of hyperkalemia **W/** K⁺-sparing diuretics, TMP, salt substitutes; ↑ risk of cough **W/** capsaicin; ↑ effects **OF** insulin, Li; ↓ effects **W/** ASA, indomethacin, NSAIDs **Labs:** ↑ LFTs, serum K⁺, Cr, BUN, monitor levels; rare ↓ BM-monitor WBC **NIPE:** Take w/o regard to food; max effect may take several wk; to prevent DN, start when urinary microalbuminemia begins; monitor ECG for hyperkalemia (peaked T waves); monitor BP for hypotension

Lisinopril & Hydrochlorothiazide (Prinzide, Zestoretic, Generic) [Antihypertensive/ACEI/HCTZ] **WARNING:** ACE Inhib can cause fetal injury/death in 2nd/3rd tri; D/C w/ PRG **Uses:** *HTN* **Action:** ACE Inhib w/ diuretic (HCTZ) **Dose:** Initial 10 mg lisinopril/12.5 mg HCTZ, titrate upward to effect; > 80 mg/d lisinopril or > 50 mg/d HCTZ are not recommended; ↓ in renal Insuff; use low dose, ↑ slowly in elderly **Caution:** [C 1st tri; D after, –] w/ Aortic stenosis/cardiomyopathy, bilateral RAS **CI:** PRG, ACE Inhib idiopathic or hereditary, angioedema, sensitivity (angioedema) **Disp:** Tabs (mg lisinopril/mg HCTZ) 10/12.5, 20/12.5; Zestoretic also available as 20/25 **SE:** Anaphylactoid Rxn (rare), dizziness, HA, cough, fatigue, ↓ BP, angioedema, ↑/↓ K⁺, ↑ Cr, rare ↓ BM/cholestatic jaundice **Interactions:** ↑ Effects **W/** α-blockers, diuretics ↑ risk of hyperkalemia **W/** K⁺-sparing diuretics, TMP, salt substitutes; ↑ risk of cough **W/** capsaicin; ↑ effects **OF** insulin, Li; ↓ effects **W/** ASA, indomethacin, NSAIDs **Labs:** ↑/↓ K⁺, ↑ Cr; ✓ K⁺, BUN, Cr, K⁺, WBC **NIPE:** Use only when monotherapy fails; monitor ECG for hyperkalemia (peaked T waves); see Lisinopril, Hydrochlorothiazide

Lithium Carbonate, Citrate (Generic) [Antipsychotic] **WARNING:** Li tox related to serum levels and can be seen at close to therapeutic levels **Uses:** *Manic episodes of bipolar Dz*, augment antidepressants, aggression, PTSD **Action:** Effects shift toward intraneuronal metabolism of catecholamines **Dose:** *Adults. Bipolar, acute mania:* 1800 mg/d PO in 2–3 ÷ doses (target serum 1–1.5 mEq/L (2 ×/wk until stable) *Bipolar maint:* 900–1800 /d PO in 2–3 ÷ doses (target serum 0.6–1.2 mEq/L) *Peds ≥ 12 y.* See Adults; ↓ in renal Insuff, elderly **Caution:** [D, –] Many drug interactions; avoid ACE Inhib or diuretics; thyroid Dz, caution in pts at risk of suicide **CI:** Severe renal impair or CV Dz, severe debilitation, dehydration, PRG, sodium depletion **Disp:** *Carbonate:* Caps 150, 300, 600 mg; tabs 300, 600 mg; SR tabs 300 mg, CR tabs 450 mg; *citrate:* syrup 300 mg/5 mL **SE:** Polyuria, polydipsia, nephrogenic DI, long-term may affect renal conc ability and cause fibrosis; tremor; Na⁺ retention or diuretic use may ↑ tox; arrhythmias, dizziness, alopecia, goiter ↓ thyroid, N/V/D, ataxia, nystagmus, ↓ BP **Notes:** Levels: *Trough:* Just before next dose *Therapeutic:* 0.8–1.2 mEq/mL *Toxic:* > 1.5 mEq/mL *1/2-life:*

18–20 h. Follow levels q1–2mo on maint **Interactions:** ↑ Effects *OF* TCA; ↑ effects W/ ACEIs, bumetanide, carbamazepine, ethacrynic acid, fluoxetine, furosemide, methyldopa, NSAIDs, phenytoin, phenothiazine, probenecid, tetracyclines, thiazide diuretics, dandelion, juniper; ↓ effects W/ acetazolamide, antacids, mannitol, theophylline, urea, verapamil, caffeine **Labs:** ↑ Serum glucose, I-131 uptake, WBC; ↓ uric acid, T_3, T_4 **NIPE:** Several wk before full effects of med, ↑ fluid intake to 2–3 L/d; take w/ or immediately after meals; do not change amt of salt in diet—consume normal amt of salt

Lodoxamide (Alomide) [Antihistamine] Uses: *Vernal conjunctivitis/keratitis* **Action:** Stabilizes mast cells **Dose:** *Adults & Peds > 2 y*. 1–2 gtt in eye(s) qid = 3 mo **Caution:** [B, ?] **Disp:** Soln 0.1% **SE:** Ocular burning, stinging, HA **NIPE:** Best not to use contact lenses during use; teach use of eye drops

Lomitapide (Juxtapid) WARNING: May cause ↑ transaminases and/or hepatic steatosis. Monitor ALT/AST & bili at baseline & regularly; adjust dose if ALT/ AST > 3× ULN (see label); D/C w/ significant liver tox **Uses:** *Homozygous familial hypercholesterolemia* **Action:** Microsomal triglyceride transfer protein Inhib **Dose:** *Adults*. 5 mg PO daily; ↑ to 10 mg after 2 wk, then at 4-wk intervals to 20, 40 mg; 60 mg max based on safety/tolerability; 40 mg max w/ ESRD on dialysis or mild hepatic impair; 30 mg max w/ weak CYP3A4 Inhib (see label) **Caution:** [X, –] Avoid grapefruit; adjust w/ warfarin, P-glycoprotein substrates, simvastatin, lovastatin **CI:** PRG, w/ strong–mod CYP3A4 inhibitors, mod–severe hepatic impair **Disp:** Caps 5, 10, 20 mg **SE:** N/V/D, hepatotox, dyspepsia, Abd pain, flatulence, CP, influenza, fatigue, ↓ wgt, ↓ Abs fat-soluble vits **Notes:** Limited distribution JUXTAPID REMS Program; PRG test before **NIPE:** Swallow whole w/ $H_2O > 2$ h after evening meal; low-fat diet to ↓ GI SEs; risk of fat sol vit def—take daily vit E, linoleic acid, ALA, EPA, DHA supl

Loperamide   (Diamode,   Imodium)   [Antidiarrheal]   [OTC] Uses: *D* **Action:** Slows intestinal motility **Dose:** *Adults*. Initial 4 mg PO, then 2 mg after each loose stool, up to 16 mg/d *Peds*. *2–5 y*, *13–20 kg*. 1 mg PO tid *6–8 y*, *20–30 kg*. 2 mg PO bid *8–12 y*, *> 30 kg*. 2 mg PO tid **Caution:** [C, –] Not for acute D caused by *Salmonella, Shigella,* or *C difficile*; w/ HIV may cause toxic megacolon **CI:** Pseudomembranous colitis, bloody D, Abd pain w/o D, < 2 y **Disp:** Caps 2 mg; tabs 2 mg; Liq 1 mg/5 mL, 1 mg/7.5 mL (OTC) **SE:** Constipation, sedation, dizziness, Abd cramp, N **Interactions:** ↑ Effects W/ antihistamines, CNS depressants, phenothiazines, TCAs, EtOH **NIPE:** Maintain adequate fluid intake; report to MD if no relief w/ OTC after 10 d

Lopinavir/Ritonavir (Kaletra) [Antiretroviral/Protease Inhibitor] Uses: *HIV Infxn* **Action:** Protease inhib **Dose:** *Adults*. TX naïve: 800/200 mg PO daily or 400/100 mg PO bid TX Tx-experienced pt: 400/100 mg PO bid (↑ dose if w/ amprenavir, efavirenz, fosamprenavir, nelfinavir, nevirapine); do not use qd dosing w/ concomitant Rx *Peds*. *7–15 kg*. 12/3 mg/kg PO bid *15–40 kg*. 10/2.5 mg/ kg PO bid *> 40 kg*: Adult dose; w/ food **Caution:** [C, ?/–] Numerous interactions, w/ hepatic impair, do not use w/ salmeterol, colchicine (w/ renal/hepatic failure); adjust dose w bosentan, tadalafil for PAH, ↑ QT w/ QT-prolonging drugs, hypokalemia, congenital long QT syndrome, immune reconstitution syndrome CI: w/ Drugs dependent on CYP3A/CYP2D6 (Table 10), lovastatin, rifampin, statins, St. John's wort, fluconazole; w/ α_1-adrenoreceptor antagonist (alfuzosin); w/ PDE5 Inhib sildenafil **Disp:** (mg lopinavir/mg ritonavir) Tab 100/25, 200/50, soln 400/100/5 mL **SE:** Avoid disulfiram (soln has EtOH), metronidazole; GI upset, asthenia, ↑ cholesterol/triglycerides, pancreatitis; protease metabolic synd **Interactions:** ↑ Effects **W/** clarithromycin, erythromycin; ↑ effects **OF** amiodarone, amprenavir, azole antifungals, bepridil, cisapride, cyclosporine, CCBs, ergot alkaloids, flecainide, flurazepam, HMG-CoA reductase Inhibs, indinavir, lidocaine, meperidine, midazolam, pimozide, propafenone, propoxyphene, quinidine, rifabutin, saquinavir, sildenafil, tacrolimus, terfenadine, triazolam, zolpidem; ↓ effects **W/** barbiturates, carbamazepine, dexamethasone, didanosine, efavirenz, nevirapine, phenytoin, rifabutin, rifampin, St. John's wort; ↓ effects **OF** OCPs, warfarin **Labs:** ↑ LFTs, cholesterol, triglycerides **NIPE:** Take w/ food, do not crush/chew; use barrier contraception; not a cure for HIV—maintain transmission prec

Loratadine (Claritin, Alavert) [Antihistamine] Uses: *Allergic rhinitis, chronic idiopathic urticaria* **Action:** Nonsedating antihistamine **Dose:** *Adults.* 10 mg/d PO **Peds 2–5 y.** 5 mg PO daily **> 6 y.** Adult dose; on empty stomach; ↓ in hepatic Insuff; qod dose w/ CrCl < 30 mL/min **Caution:** [B, +/–] **CI:** Component allergy **Disp:** Tabs 10 mg (OTC); rapidly disintegrating RediTabs 10 mg; chew tabs 5 mg; syrup 1 mg/mL **SE:** HA, somnolence, xerostomia, hyperkinesis in peds **Interactions:** ↑ Effects **W/** CNS depressants, erythromycin, ketoconazole, MAOIs, protease Inhibs, procarbazine, ETOH **NIPE:** Take w/o food; licorice consumption may prolong QT interval; not a sub for epinephrine—carry epi injector if prescribed

Lorazepam (Ativan, Others) [C-IV] [Anxiolytic, Sedative/Hypnotic/Benzodiazepine] Uses: *Anxiety & anxiety w/ depression; sedation; control status epilepticus*; EtOH withdrawal; antiemetic **Action:** Benzodiazepine; antianxiety agent; works via postsynaptic GABA receptors **Dose:** *Adults. Anxiety:* 1–10 mg/d PO in 2–3 ÷ doses *Pre-op:* 0.05 mg/kg-4 mg max IM 2 h before or 0.044 mg/ kg–2 mg dose max IV 15–20 min before surgery *Insomnia:* 2–4 mg PO hs *Status epilepticus:* 4 mg/dose slow over 2–5 min IV PRN q10–15min; usual total dose 8 mg *Antiemetic:* 0.5–2 mg IV or PO q4–6h PRN *EtOH withdrawal:* 1–4 mg IV or 2 mg PO initial depending on severity; titrate **Peds.** *Status epilepticus:* 0.05–0.1 mg/kg/dose IV over 2–5 min, max 4 mg/dose repeat at 10- to 15-min intervals × 2 PRN *Antiemetic, 2–15 y:* 0.05 mg/kg (to 2 mg/dose) prechemotherapy; ↓ in elderly; do not administer IV > 2 mg/min or 0.05 mg/kg/dose **Caution:** [D, –] w/ Hepatic impair, other CNS depression, COPD; ↓ dose by 50% w/ valproic acid and probenecid **CI:** Severe pain, severe ↓ BP, sleep apnea, NAG, allergy to propylene glycol or benzyl alcohol, severe resp Insuff (except mechanically ventilated) **Disp:** Tabs 0.5, 1, 2 mg; soln, PO conc 2 mg/mL; Inj 2, 4 mg/mL

SE: Sedation, memory impair, EPS, dizziness, ataxia, tachycardia, ↓ BP, constipation, resp depression, paradoxical reactions, fall risk, abuse potential, rebound/withdrawal after abrupt D/C **Interactions:** ↑ Effects W/ cimetidine, disulfiram, probenecid, calendula, catnip, hops, lady's slipper, passion-flower, kava kava, valerian; ↑ effects OF phenytoin; ↑ CNS depression W/ anticonvulsants, antihistamines, CNS depressants, MAOIs, scopolamine, EtOH; ↓ effects W/ caffeine, tobacco; ↓ effects OF levodopa **Labs:** ↑ LFTs **NIPE:** ⊘ D/C abruptly; ~ 10 min for effect if IV; IV Inf requires in-line filter; dilute oral soln in H_2O, juice, semi-solid food; ⊘ EtOH intake; caution driving

Lorcaserin (Belviq) **Uses:** *Manage Wt w/ BMI > 30 kg/m^2 or > 27 kg/m^2 w/ wgt-related comorbidity* **Action:** Serotonin 2C receptor agonist **Dose:** *Adults.* 10 mg PO bid; D/C if not 5% wgt loss by wk 12 **Caution:** [X, –] Check glucose w/ diabetic meds; monitor for depression/ suicidal thoughts, serotonin or neuroleptic malignant synd, cognitive impair, psych disorders, valvular disease Dz, priapism; risk of serotonin synd when used w/ other serotonergic drugs; caution w/ drugs that are CYP2D6 substrates **CI:** PRG **Disp:** Tabs 10 mg **SE:** HA, N, dizziness, fatigue, dry mouth, constipation, back pain, cough, hypoglycemia, euphoria, hallucination, dissociation, ↓ HR, ↑ prolactin **NIPE:** Take w/o regard to food; teach healthy diet, exercise

Losartan (Cozaar) [Antihypertensive/ARB] **WARNING:** Can cause fetal injury and death if used in 2nd & 3rd tri. D/C Rx if PRG detected **Uses:** *HTN, DN, prevent CVA in HTN & LVH* **Action:** Angiotensin II receptor antagonist **Dose:** *Adults.* 25–50 mg PO qd/bid, max 100 mg; ↓ in elderly/hepatic impair *Peds ≥ 6 y. HTN:* Initial 0.7 mg/kg qd, ↑ to 50 mg/d PRN; 1.4 mg/kg/d or 100 mg/d max **Caution:** [C (1st tri, D 2nd & 3rd tri), ?/–] w/ NSAIDs; w/ K^+-sparing diuretics, supl may cause ↑ K^+; w/ RAS, hepatic impair **CI:** PRG, component sensitivity **Disp:** Tabs 25, 50, 100 mg **SE:** ↓ BP in pts on diuretics; ↑ K^+, GI upset, facial/ angioedema, dizziness, cough, weakness, ↓ renal Fxn **Interactions:** ↑ Risk of hyperkalemia W/ K^+-sparing diuretics, K^+ supls, TMP; ↑ effects OF Li; ↓ effects W/ diltiazem, fluconazole, phenobarbital, rifampin **Labs:** ↑ K^+ **NIPE:** ⊘ PRG, breast-feeding; caution driving; monitor for hypotension

Loteprednol (Alrex, Lotemax) **Uses:** *Lotemax:* Steroid responsive inflammatory disorders of conjunctiva/cornea/anterior globe (keratitis, iritis, post-op); *Alrex:* seasonal allergic conjunctivitis* **Action:** Anti-inflammatory/steroid **Dose:** *Adults. Lotemax:* 1 drop conjunctival sac qid up to every h initially; *Alrex:* 1 drop qid **Caution:** [C, ?/–] glaucoma **CI:** Viral dz corneal and conjunctiva, varicella, mycobacterial and fungal Infxns; hypersensitivity **Disp:** *Lotemax* 0.5% susp, 2.5, 5, 10, 15 mL; *Alrex* 0.2% susp, 2.5, 5, 10 mL **SE:** Glaucoma; ↑ risk infection; cornea/sclera thinning; HA, rhinitis **NIPE:** May delay cataract surg healing; avoid use > 10 d; shake before use; may need to avoid using contact lenses during Rx; teach use of eye drops

Lovastatin (Altoprev, Mevacor) [Antilipemic/HMG-CoA Reductase Inhibitor] **Uses:** *Hypercholesterolemia to ↓ risk of MI, angina*

Action: HMG-CoA reductase Inhib **Dose:** *Adults.* 20 mg/d PO w/ PM meal; may ↑ at 4-wk intervals to 80 mg/d max or 60 mg ER tab; take w/ meals *Peds 10–18 y (at least 1-y postmenarchal).* *Familial* ↑ *cholesterol:* 10 mg PO qd, ↑ q4wk PRN to 40 mg/d max (immediate release w/ PM meal) **Caution:** [X, −] Avoid w/ grapefruit juice, gemfibrozil; use caution, carefully consider doses > 20 mg/d w/ renal impair **CI:** Active liver Dz, PRG, lactation **Disp:** Tabs generic 10, 20, 40 mg; Mevacor 20, 40 mg; Altoprev ER tabs 20, 40, 60 mg **SE:** HA & GI intolerance common; promptly report any unexplained muscle pain, tenderness, or weakness (myopathy) **Interactions:** ↑ Effects *W/* grapefruit juice; ↑ risk of severe myopathy *W/* azole antifungals, cyclosporine, erythromycin, gemfibrozil, HMG-CoA Inhbs, niacin; ↑ effects *OF* warfarin; ↓ effects *W/* isradipine, pectin **Labs:** ↑ LFTs; monitor LFT q12wk × 1 y, then q6mo; may alter TFT **NIPE:** ⊘ PRG; take drug PM; periodic eye exams; maint cholesterol-lowering diet, regular exercise; ⊘ grapefruit/grapefruit juice; ↓ EtOH intake

Lubiprostone (Amitiza) [Laxative] **Uses:** *Chronic idiopathic constipation in adults, IBS w/ constipation in females > 18 y* **Action:** Selective Cl⁻ channel activator; ↑ intestinal motility **Dose:** *Adults. Constipation:* 24 mcg PO bid w/ food H₂O *IBS:* 8 mcg bid; w/ food water **CI:** Mechanical GI obst **Caution:** [C, ?/−] Severe D, ↓ dose mod–severe hepatic impair **Disp:** Gelcaps 8, 24 mcg **SE:** N/D, may adjust dose based on (N), HA, GI distention, Abd pain **Labs:** Monitor LFTs & BUN/Cr; requires (−) PRG test before Tx **NIPE:** Utilize contraception; periodically reassess drug need; not for chronic use; suspend drug if D; ⊘ breast-feeding; may experience severe dyspnea w/in 1 h of dose, usually resolves w/in 3 h

Lucinactant (Surfaxin) **Uses:** *Prevention of RDS* **Action:** Pulmonary surfactant **Dose:** *Peds.* 5.8 mL/kg birth wgt intratracheally no more often than q6h; max 4 doses in first 48 h of life **Caution:** [N/A, N/A] Frequent clinical assessments; interrupt w/ adverse Rxns and assess/stabilize infant; not for ARDS **CI:** None **Disp:** Susp 8.5 mL/vial **SE:** ET tube reflux/obstruction, pallor, bradycardia, oxygen desaturation, anemia, jaundice, metabolic/resp acidosis, hyperglycemia, ↓ Na, pneumonia, ↓ BP **Notes:** Warm vial for 15 min; shake prior to use; discard if not used w/in 2 h of warming **NIPE:** Monitor for changes in O₂ & vent support; not for use in adults

Lurasidone (Latuda) [Atypical Antipsychotic/Serotonin Receptor Antagonist] **WARNING:** Elderly w/ dementia-related psychosis at ↑ death risk. Not approved for dementia-related psychosis **Uses:** *Schizophrenia* **Action:** Atypical antipsychotic: central DA type 2 (D2) and serotonin type 2 (5HT2A) receptor antagonist **Dose:** 40–80 mg/d PO w/ food; 40 mg max w/ CrCl 10–49 mL/min OR mod–severe hepatic impair **Caution:** [B, −] **CI:** w/ Strong CYP3A4 inhib/inducer **Disp:** Tabs 20, 40, 80, 120 mg **SE:** Somnolence, agitation, tardive dyskinesia, akathisia, parkinsonism, stroke, TIAs, Sz, orthostatic hypotension, syncope, dysphagia, neuroleptic malignant syndrome, body temp dysregulation, N, ↑ wgt, type 2 DM, ↑ lipids, hyperprolactinemia, ↓ WBC **Interactions:** Do not use w/ concomitant strong CYP3A4 Inhibs (eg, ketoconazole) & inducers (eg, rifampin); ↑ CNS effects *W/* EtOH & other CNS depressants **Labs:** ↓ WBC; ↑ lipids; monitor CBC, during first few mo of therapy; monitor FBS **NIPE:** w/ DM risk ✓ glucose; take w/ food (≥ 350 kcal)

Luliconazole (Luzu) Uses: *Tinea pedis, tinea cruris, tinea corporis* **Action:** azole antigungal, inhibits ergosterol synthesis **Dose:** *Tinea pedis:* Apply 1 ×/d for 2 wk *Tinea corporis, tinea cruris:* Apply 1 ×/d for 1 wk **Caution:** [C, ?/–] **CI:** None **Disp:** Cream, 1%; 30/60 g **SE:** Site reaction, rare **NIPE:** Apply to skin only—do not cover, wrap, bandage area; continue use as prescribed even if Sx disappear earlier

Lymphocyte Immune Globulin [Antithymocyte Globulin, ATG] (Atgam) [Immunosuppressant] **WARNING:** Should only be used by physician experienced in immunosuppressive therapy or management of solid-organ and/or BM transplant pts. Adequate lab and supportive resources must be readily available **Uses:** *Allograft rejection in renal transplant pts; aplastic anemia if not candidates for BMT*, prevent rejection of other solid-organ transplants, GVHD after BMT **Action:** ↓ Circulating antigen-reactive T lymphocytes; human & equine product **Dose:** *Adults. Prevent rejection:* 15 mg/kg/d IV × 14 d, then qod × 7 d for total 21 doses in 28 d; initial w/in 24 h before/after transplant *Rx rejection:* Same but use 10–15 mg/kg/d × 8–14 d; max 21 doses in 28 d, qd first 14 d *Aplastic anemia:* 10–20 mg/kg/d × 8–14 d, then qod × 7 doses for total 21 doses in 28 d *Peds. Prevent renal allograft rejection:* 5–25 mg/kg/d IV; aplastic anemia 10–20 mg/kg/d IV 8–14 d then qod for 7 more doses **Caution:** [C, ?/–] D/C if severe unremitting thrombocytopenia, leukopenia **CI:** Hx Previous Rxn or Rxn to other equine γ-globulin prep, w/ plt and WBC **Disp:** Inj 50 mg/mL **SE:** D/C w/ severe ↓ plt and WBC; rash, fever, chills, ↓ BP, HA, CP, edema, N/V/D, lightheadedness **Notes:** *Test Dose:* 0.1 mL 1:1000 dilution in NS **Interactions:** ↑ Immunosuppression *W/* azathioprine, corticosteroids, immunosuppressants **Labs:** ↑ LFTs, ↑ K⁺, ↓ plt & WBC; monitor WBC, plt; plt counts usually return to nl w/o D/C Rx therapy **NIPE:** A systemic Rxn precludes use; give via central line; consider pre-Tx w/ antipyretic, antihistamine, and/or steroids; may cause dizziness—caution driving

Macitentan (Opsumit) **WARNING:** Do not use w/ PRG, may cause fetal harm; exclude PRG before and 1 mo after stopping; use contraception during and 1 mo past stopping; for females, only available through a restricted distribution program **Uses:** *Pulm hypertension to prevent progression* **Action:** Endothelin receptor antag **Dose:** 10 mg 1 ×/d **Caution:** [X, –] may cause hepatic failure/toxicity; ↓ Hct; pulm edema w PE, ↓ sperm count **CI:** PRG **Disp:** Tab 10 mg **SE:** ↓ Hct; HA, UTI, influenza, bronchitis, nasopharyngitis, pharyngitis **Notes:** ✓ LFTs before and monitor; w/ PE D/C, may cause pulm edema; avoid w/ CYP3A4 inducers/inhibitors **NIPE:** ⊘ PRG; female pts must enroll in restricted program, OPSUMIT REMS; must have neg PRG test 1 mo before/after Rx; use 2 forms BC; take w/ or w/o food; ⊘ chew/crush/split tabs

Magaldrate & Simethicone (Riopan-Plus) [Antacid/Aluminum & Magnesium Salt] [OTC] Uses: *Hyperacidity associated w/ peptic ulcer, gastritis, & hiatal hernia* **Action:** Low-Na+ antacid **Dose:** 5–10 mL PO between meals & hs, on empty stomach **Caution:** [C, ?/+] **CI:** UC, diverticulitis, appendicitis, ileostomy/colostomy, renal Insuff (d/t Mg^{2+} content) **Disp:** Susp magaldrate/simethicone 540/20 mg/5 mL (OTC) **SE:** ↑ Mg^{2+}, ↓ PO_4 white flecked feces, constipation, N/V/D **Notes:** < 0.3 mg $Na1^{1+}$/tab or tsp **Interactions:** ↑ Effects *OF* levodopa, quinidine; ↓ effects *OF* allopurinol, anticoagulants, cefpodoxime, ciprofloxacin, clindamycin, digoxin, indomethacin, INH, ketoconazole, lincomycin, phenothiazine, quinolones, tetracyclines **Labs:** ↑ Mg^{2+}, ↓ PO_4 **NIPE:** ⊘ Other meds w/in 1–2 h

Magnesium Citrate (Citroma, Others) [Laxative/Magnesium Salt] [OTC] Uses: *Vigorous bowel prep*; constipation **Action:** Cathartic laxative **Dose:** *Adults.* 150–300 mL PO PRN *Peds.* *< 6 years:* 2–4 mL/kg × /or in ÷ dose ≥ *12 y.* 150–300 mL ×1 /or in ÷ doses **Caution:** [B, +] w/ Neuromuscular Dz & renal impairment **CI:** Severe renal Dz, heart block, N/V, rectal bleeding, intestinal obst/perforation/impaction, colostomy, ileostomy, UC, diverticulitis **Disp:** Soln 290 mg/5 mL (300 mL); 100 mg tabs **SE:** Abd cramps, gas, ↓ BP, ↑ Mg^{2+}, resp depression **Interactions:** ↓ Effects *OF* anticoagulants, digoxin, fluoroquinolones, ketoconazole, nitrofurantoin, phenothiazine, tetracyclines **Labs:** ↑ Mg^{2+}, ↓ protein, Ca^{2+}, K^+ **NIPE:** ⊘ Other meds w/in 1–2 h; only for occasional use w/ constipation; take w/ 8 oz H_2O

Magnesium Hydroxide (Milk of Magnesia) [OTC] [Laxative/Magnesium Salt] Uses: *Constipation*, hyperacidity, Mg^{2+} replacement **Action:** NS laxative **Dose:** *Adults.* *Antacid:* 5–15 mL (400 mg/5 mL) or 2–4 tabs (311 mg) PO PRN qid. *Laxative:* 30–60 mL (400 mg/5 mL) or 15–30 mL (800 mg/5 mL) or 8 tabs (311 mg) PO qhs or ÷ doses *Peds.* Antacid and *< 12 y* not recommended *Laxative:* *< 2 y* not OK *2–5 y.* 5–15 mL (400 mg/5 mL) PO qhs or ÷ doses *6–11 y.* 15–30 mL (400 mg/5 mL) or 7.5–15 mL (800 mg/5 mL) PO qhs or ÷ doses *3–5 y.* 2 (311 mg) tabs PO qhs or ÷ doses *6–11 y.* 4 mL (311 mg) tabs PO qhs or ÷ doses **Caution:** [B, +] w/ Neuromuscular Dz or renal impair **CI:** Component hypersens **Disp:** Chew tabs 311, 400 mg; Liq 400, 800 mg/5 mL (OTC) **SE:** D, Abd cramps **Interactions:** ↓ Effects *OF* chlordiazepoxide, dicumarol, digoxin, indomethacin, INH, quinolones, tetracyclines **Labs:** ↑ Mg^{2+}, ↓ protein, Ca^{2+}, K^+ **NIPE:** ⊘ Other meds w/in 1–2 h; for occasional use in constipation

Magnesium Oxide (Mag-Ox 400, Others) [OTC] [Antacid, Magnesium Supplement/Magnesium Salt] Uses: *Replace low Mg^{2+} levels* **Action:** Mg^{2+} supl **Dose:** 400–800 mg/d or ÷ w/ food in full glass of H_2O; ↓ w/ renal impair **Caution:** [B, +] w/ Neuromuscular Dz & renal impair, w/ bisphosphonates, calcitriol, CCBs, neuromuscular blockers, tetracyclines, quinolones **CI:** Component hypersensitivity **Disp:** Caps 140, 250, 500, 600 mg; tabs 400 mg (OTC) **SE:** D, N **Interactions:** ↓ Effects *OF* chlordiazepoxide, dicumarol, digoxin, indomethacin, INH, quinolones, tetracyclines **Labs:** ↑ Mg^{2+}, ↓ protein, Ca^{2+}, K^+ **NIPE:** ⊘ Other meds w/in 1–2 h

Magnesium Sulfate (Various) [Magnesium Supplement/Magnesium Salt]

Uses: *Replace low Mg^{2+}; preeclampsia, eclampsia, & premature labor, cardiac arrest, AMI arrhythmias, cerebral edema, barium poisoning, Szs, pediatric acute nephritis*; refractory *↓ K^+ & ↓ Ca^{2+}* **Action:** Mg^{2+} supl, bowel evacuation, ↓ acetylcholine in nerve terminals, ↓ rate of sinoatrial node firing **Dose:** **Adults.** 1 g q6h IM × 4 doses & PRN 1–2 g q3–6h IV then PRN to correct deficiency *Preeclampsia/premature labor:* 4-g load, then 1–2 g/h IV Inf *ECC 2010:* **VF/pulseless VT arrest w/ torsades de pointes:** 1–2 g IV push (2–4 mL 50% soln) in 10 mL D_5W. If pulse present, then 1–2 g in 50–100 mL D_5W over 5–60 min *Peds & Neonates.* 25–50 mg/kg/dose IV repeat PRN; max 2 g single dose *ECC 2010:* **Pulseless VT w/ torsades:** 25–50 mg/kg IV/IO over 10–20 min; max dose 2 g **Pulseless VT w/ torsades or hypomagnesemia:** 25–50 mg/kg IV/IO over 10–20 min; max dose 2 g **Status asthmaticus:** 25–50 mg/kg IV/IO over 15–30 min **Caution:** [A/C (manufacturer specific), +] w/ Neuromuscular Dz; interactions see Magnesium Oxide & Aminoglycosides **CI:** Heart block, myocardial damage **Disp:** Premix Inj: 10, 20, 40, 80 mg/mL; Inj 125, 500 mg/mL; oral/topical powder 227, 454, 480, 1810, 2720 g **SE:** CNS depression, D, flushing, heart block, ↓ BP, vasodilation **Interactions:** ↑ CNS depression *W/* antidepressants, antipsychotics, anxiolytics, barbiturates, hypnotics, narcotics; EtOH; ↑ neuromuscular blockade *W/* aminoglycosides, atracurium, gallamine, pancuronium, tubocurarine, vecuronium **Labs:** ↑ Mg^{2+}; ↓ protein, Ca^{2+}, K^+ **NIPE:** Check for absent patellar reflexes, respiratory depression; different formulation may contain Al^{2+}; have calcium gluconate Inj available as antidote for Mg toxicity

Mannitol, Inhalation (Aridol)

WARNING: Powder for Inh; use may result in severe bronchospasm, testing only done by trained professionals **Uses:** *Assess bronchial hyperresponsiveness in pts w/o clinically apparent asthma* **Action:** Bronchoconstrictor, ? mechanism **Dose:** *Adults, Peds > 6 y.* Inhal caps ↑ dose (see disp) until + test (15% ↓ FEV_1 or 10% ↓ FEV_1 between consecutive doses) or all caps inhaled **Caution:** [C, ?/M] Pt w/ comorbid condition that may ↑ effects **CI:** Mannitol/gelatin hypersensitivity **Disp:** Dry powder caps graduated doses: 0, 5, 10, 20, 40 mg **SE:** HA, pharyngeal pain, irritation, N, cough, rhinorrhea, dyspnea, chest discomfort, wheezing, retching, dizziness **Notes:** Not a stand-alone test or screening test for asthma **NIPE:** Have meds for Rx of severe bronchospasm (short-acting inhaled beta-agonist) in testing area

Mannitol, Intravenous (Generic) [Osmotic Diuretic]

Uses: *Cerebral edema, ↑ IOP, renal impair, poisonings* **Action:** Osmotic diuretic **Dose:** Test dose: 0.2 g/kg/dose IV over 3–5 min; if no diuresis w/in 2 h, D/C. *Oliguria:* 50–100 g IV over 90 min *↑ IOP:* 0.25–2 g/kg IV over 30 min *Cerebral edema:* 0.25–1.5 g/kg/dose IV q6–8h PRN, maintain serum osmolarity < 300–320 mOsm/kg **Caution:** [C, ?/M] w/ CHF or vol overload, w/ nephrotoxic drugs & Li **CI:** Anuria, dehydration, heart failure, PE intracranial bleeding **Disp:** Inj 5, 10, 15, 20, 25% **SE:** May exacerbate CHF, N/V/D, ↓/↑ BP, ↑ HR **Interactions:** ↑ Effects *OF* cardiac glycosides; ↓ effects *OF* barbiturates, imipramine, Li, salicylates **Labs:** ↑/↓ Lytes **NIPE:** Monitor for vol depletion, Na and K

Maraviroc (Selzentry) [CCR5 Coreceptor Antagonist] WARNING: Possible drug-induced hepatotox **Uses:** *Tx of CCR5-tropic HIV Infxn* **Action:** Antiretroviral, CCR5 coreceptor antagonist **Dose:** 300 mg bid **Caution:** [B, –] w/ Concomitant CYP3A inducers/Inhib and ↓ renal Fxn, caution in mild–mod hepatic impair **CI:** Pts w/ severe renal impairment/ ESRD taking potent CXP3A4 Inhib/ inducer **Disp:** Tab 150, 300 mg **SE:** Fever, URI, cough, rash; HIV attaches to the CCR5 receptor to infect CD4+ T cells **Interactions:** ↑ Effects *W/* CYP3A Inhibts (most protease Inhibs, delavirdine, ketoconazole, itraconazole, clarithromycin, nefazodone, telithromycin) & ↓ effects *W/* CYP3A inducers (efavirenz, rifampin, carbamazepine, phenobarbital, phenytoin); substantial ↓ effect *W/* St. John's wort **Labs:** ↑ LFTs **NIPE:** Swallow whole; monitor for immune reconstitution synd, Infxns, malignancies; ⊘ breast-feeding; ⊘ for < 16 y; take w/ or w/o food; must be given w/ another antiretroviral

Measles, Mumps, & Rubella Vaccine Live [MMR] (M-M-R II) [Live Attenuated Vaccine] Uses: *Vaccination against measles, mumps, & rubella 12 mo and older* **Action:** Active immunization, live attenuated viruses **Dose:** 1 (0.5-mL) SQ Inj, 1st dose 12 mo, 2nd dose 4–6 y, at least 3 mo between doses (28 d if > 12 y), adults born after 1957 unless CI, Hx measles & mumps or documented immunity & childbearing age women w/ rubella immunity documented **Caution:** [C, ?/M] Hx of cerebral injury, Szs, family Hx Szs (febrile Rxn), ↓ plt **CI:** Component and gelatin sensitivity, Hx anaphylaxis to neomycin, blood dyscrasia, lymphoma, leukemia, malignant neoplasias affecting BM, immunosuppression, fever, PRG, Hx of active untreated TB **Disp:** Inj, single dose **SE:** Fever, febrile Szs (5–12 d after vaccination), Inj site Rxn, rash, ↓ plt **Interactions:** ↑ Immunosuppression w/ other immunosuppresents **Labs:** ↓ Plt; may interfere w/ tuberculin test **NIPE:** Per FDA, CDC of febrile Sz (2 ×) w/ MMRV vs MMR & varicella separately; preferable to use 2 separate vaccines; allow 1 mo between Inj & any other measles vaccine or 3 mo between any other varicella vaccine; limited availability of MMRV; avoid those who have not been exposed to varicella for 6 wk post-Inj; may contain albumin or trace egg antigen; avoid salicylates for 6 wk postvaccination; avoid PRG for 3 mo following vaccination; do not give w/in 3 mo of transfusion or immune globulin

Measles, Mumps, Rubella, & Varicella Virus Vaccine Live [MMRV] (ProQuad) [Vaccine/Live Attenuated] Uses: *Vaccination against measles, mumps, rubella, & varicella* **Action:** Active immunization, live attenuated viruses **Dose:** 1 (0.5-mL) vial SQ Inj 12 mo–12 y or for 2nd dose of measles, mumps, & rubella (MMR), at least 3 mo between doses (28 d if > 12 y) **Caution:** [C, ?/M] Hx of cerebral injury or Szs & fam Hx Szs (febrile Rxn), w/ ↓

plt **CI:** Component and gelatin sensitivity, Hx anaphylaxis to neomycin, blood dyscrasia, lymphoma, leukemia, malignant neoplasias affecting BM, immunosuppression, fever, active untreated TB, PRG **Disp:** Inj **SE:** Fever, febrile Szs, (5–12 d after vaccination, Inj site Rxn, rash, ↓ plt **LABs:** ↓ plt **NIPE:** Per FDA, CDC ↑ of febrile Sz (2 ×) w/ combo vaccine (MMRV) vs MMR & varicella separately; preferable to use 2 separate vaccines; allow 1 mo between Inj & any other measles vaccine or 3 mo between any other varicella vaccine; limited availability of MMRV; substitute MMR II or Varivax; avoid those who have not been exposed to varicella for 6 wk post-Inj; may contain albumin or trace egg antigen; avoid salicylates

Mecasermin (Increlex, Iplex) [Human IGF-1] Uses: *Growth failure in severe primary IGF-1 deficiency or human growth hormone (HGH) antibodies* **Action:** Human IGF-1 (recombinant DNA origin) **Dose:** *Peds. Increlex ≥ 2 y.* 0.04–0.08 mg/kg SQ bid; may ↑ by 0.04 mg/kg per dose to 0.12 mg/kg bid; take w/ in 20 min of meal d/t insulin-like hypoglycemic effect; Iplex ≥ 3 y 0.5 mg/kg once daily ↑ to 1–2 mg/kg/d hold if hypoglycemia **Caution:** [C, ?/M] Contains benzyl alcohol **CI:** Closed epiphysis, neoplasia, not for IV **Disp:** Vial 10 mg/mL (40 mL) **SE:** Tonsillar hypertrophy, ↑ AST, ↑ LDH, HA, Inj site Rxn, V, hypoglycemia **Labs:** Rapid dose ↑ may cause hypoglycemia; consider monitoring glucose until dose stable **NIPE:** Administer 20 min before or after meal/snack; initial funduscopic exam & during Tx; limited distribution; teach SQ Inj technique

Mechlorethamine (Mustargen) [Antineoplastic/Alkylating Agent] **WARNING:** Highly toxic, handle w/ care, limit use to experienced physicians; avoid exposure during PRG; vesicant **Uses:** *Hodgkin Dz (stages III, IV), cutaneous T-cell lymphoma (mycosis fungoides), lung CA, CML, malignant pleural effusions, CLL, polycythemia vera*, psoriasis **Action:** Alkylating agent, nitrogen analog of sulfur mustard **Dose:** Per protocol; 0.4 mg/kg single dose or 0.1 mg/kg/d for 4 d, or 0.2 mg/kg/d for 2 d, repeat at 4-to-6-wk intervals *MOPP:* 6 mg/ m^2 IV on d 1 & 8 of 28-d cycle *Intracavitary* 0.2–0.4 mg/kg ×, may repeat PRN *Topical:* 0.01–0.02% soln, lotion, oint **Caution:** [D, ?/–] Severe myleosuppression **CI:** PRG, known infect Dz **Disp:** Inj 10 mg; topical soln, lotion, oint **SE:** ↓ BM, thrombosis, thrombophlebitis at site; tissue damage w/ extrav (Na thiosulfate used topically to Rx); N/V/D, skin rash/allergic dermatitis w/ contact, amenorrhea, sterility (especially in men), secondary leukemia if treated for Hodgkin Dz, chromosomal alterations, hepatotox, peripheral neuropathy **Interactions:** ↑ Risk of blood dyscrasias **W/** amphotericin B; ↑ risk of bleeding **W/** anticoagulants, NSAIDs, plt Inhibs, salicylates; ↑ myelosuppression **W/** antineoplastic drugs, radiation therapy; ↓ effects of IV live virus vaccines **Labs:** ↑ Serum uric acid **NIPE:** Highly volatile & emetogenic; give w/in 30–60 min of prep; ↑ fluids to 2–3 L/d; ⊘ PRG, breast-feeding, vaccines, exposure to Infxn; ↑ risk of tinnitus

Mechlorethamine Gel (Valchlor) **Uses:** *Stage 1A and 1B mycosis fungoides-type cutaneous T-cell lymphoma* **Action:** Alkylating agent **Dose:** Apply thin film daily, if skin ulceration/blistering or mod dermatitis, D/C; w/ improvement, restart w/ ↓ dose to q3d; must be refrigerated, apply w/in 30 min, apply to dry skin and no shower for 4 h or wait 30 min after shower to apply **Caution:** [D, –] Mucosal injury may be severe; w/ eye contact irrigate immediately × 15 min and seek consultation, may cause blindness; dermatitis including blisters, swelling, pruritus, redness, ulceration; caregivers/others must avoid skin contact w/ pt; nonmelanoma skin CA risk; flammable **CI:** Hypersensitivity **Disp:** Gel, 60 g tube **SE:** Dermatitis, pruritus, skin/ulceration/blistering/hyperpigmentation/skin Infxn **NIPE:** Caregivers must wear disposable nitrile gloves and wash hands thoroughly; alcohol based—avoid fire, flame, smoking until dry

Meclizine (Antivert) (Bonine, Dramamine [OTC]) [Antiemetic/ Antivertigo/Anticholinergic] Uses: *Motion sickness, vertigo* **Action:** Antiemetic, anticholinergic, & antihistaminic properties **Dose:** *Adults & Peds > 12 y. Motion sickness:* 12.5–25 mg PO 1 h before travel, repeat PRN q12–24h *Vertigo:* 25–100 mg/d ÷ doses **Caution:** [B, ?/–] NAG, BPH, BOO, elderly, asthma **Disp:** Tabs 12.5, 25, 50 mg; chew tabs 25 mg; caps 12.5 mg (OTC) **SE:** Drowsiness, xerostomia, blurred vision, thickens bronchial secretions **Interactions:** ↑ Sedation W/ antihistamines, CNS depressants, neuroleptics, EtOH; ↑ anticholinergic effects W/ anticholinergics, atropine, disopyramide, haloperidol, phenothiazine, quinidine **NIPE:** Use prophylactically; ↑ risk of heat exhaustion; may cause drowsiness—caution driving; avoid EtOH

Medroxyprogesterone (Provera, Depo-Provera, Depo-Sub Q Provera) [Antineoplastic/Progestin] WARNING: Do not use in the prevention of CV Dz or dementia; ↑ risk MI, stroke, breast CA, PE, & DVT in postmenopausal women (50–79 y). ↑ Dementia risk in postmenopausal women (≥ 65 y). Risk of sig bone loss; does not prevent STD or HIV, long-term use > 2 y should be limited to situations where other birth control methods are inadequate Uses: *Contraception; secondary amenorrhea; endometrial CA; ↓ endometrial hyperplasia*; AUB caused by hormonal imbalance **Action:** Progestin supl **Dose:** *Contraception:* 150 mg IM q3mo depo or 104 mg SQ q3mo (depo SQ) *Secondary amenorrhea:* 5–10 mg/d PO for 5–10 d *AUB:* 5–10 mg/d PO for 5–10 d beginning on the 16th or 21st d of menstrual cycle *Endometrial CA:* 400–1000 mg/wk IM *Endometrial hyperplasia:* 5–10 mg/d × 12–14 d on d 1 or 16 of cycle; ↓ in hepatic Insuff **Caution:** *Provera* [X, –] *Depo Provera* [X, +] **CI:** Thrombophlebitis/ embolic disorders, cerebral apoplexy, severe hepatic dysfunction, CA breast/genital organs, undiagnosed Vag bleeding, missed Ab, PRG, as a diagnostic test for PRG **Disp:** *Provera* tabs 2.5, 5, 10 mg; depot Inj 150, 400 mg/mL; depo SQ Inj 104 mg/0.65 mL **SE:** Breakthrough bleeding, spotting, altered menstrual flow, breast tenderness, galactorrhea, depression, insomnia, jaundice, N, wgt gain, acne, hirsutism, vision changes **Interactions:** ↓ Effects W/ aminoglutethimide, phenytoin, carbamazepine, phenobarbital, rifampin, rifabutin **Labs:** ↑ LFTs **NIPE:** Sunlight exposure may cause melasma; if GI upset take w/ food; perform breast exam & Pap smear before contraceptive therapy; obtain PRG test if last Inj > 3 mo

Megestrol Acetate (Megace, Megace-ES) [Antineoplastic/Progestin] Uses: *Breast/endometrial CAs; appetite stimulant in cachexia (CA & HIV)* **Action:** Hormone; antileuteinizing; progesterone analog **Dose:** *CA:* 40–320 mg/d PO in ÷ doses *Appetite* 800 mg/d PO ÷ dose or *Megace ES* 625 mg/d PO **Caution:** PRG CI [D (tablet)/ X (suspension), Breast fdg] Thromboembolism; handle w/ care **CI:** PRG **Disp:** Tabs 20, 40 mg; susp 40 mg/mL, *Megace-ES* 125 mg/mL **SE:** DVT, edema, menstrual bleeding, photosens, N/V/D, HA, mastodynia, ↑ CA, ↑ glucose, insomnia, rash, ↓ BM, ↑ BP, CP, palpitations **Interactions:** ↑ Effects *OF* warfarin **Labs:** ↑ CA, glucose; ↓ BM **NIPE:** ↑ Risk of photosensitivity—use sunblock; do not D/C abruptly; Megace ES not equivalent to others mg/mg; Megace ES approved only for anorexia; caution in the elderly

Meloxicam (Mobic) [Analgesic/Anti-Inflammatory/NSAIDs] WARNING: May ↑ risk of CV events & GI bleeding; CI in post-op CABG Uses: *OA, RA, JRA* **Action:** NSAID w/ ↑ COX-2 activity **Dose:** *Adults.* 7.5–15 mg/d PO *Peds ≥ 2 y.* 0.125 mg/kg/d, max 7.5 mg; ↓ in renal Insuff; take w/ food **Caution:** [C, D (3rd tri) ?/–) w/ Severe renal Insuff, CHF, ACE Inhib, diuretics, Li²⁺, MTX, warfarin **CI:** Peptic ulcer, NSAID, or ASA sensitivity, PRG, post-op CABG **Disp:** Tabs 7.5, 15 mg; susp 7.5 mg/5 mL **SE:** HA, dizziness, GI upset, GI bleeding, edema, ↑ BP, renal impair, rash (SJS), **Interactions:** ↑ Effects *OF* ASA, anticoagulants, corticosteroids, Li, NSAIDs, ↑ LFTs EtOH, tobacco; ↓ effects *W/* cholestyramine; ↓ effects *OF* antihypertensives **Labs:** ↑ LFTs, BUN, Cr; ↓ HMG, WBCs, plt **NIPE:** Take w/ food, may take several d for full effect; ↑ risk of GI bleed in the elderly and w/ concurrent use of EtOH & tobacco; avoid other NSAIDs

Melphalan [L-PAM] (Alkeran) [Antineoplastic/Alkylating Agent] WARNING: Administer under the supervision of a qualified physician experienced in the use of chemotherapy; severe BM depression, leukemogenic, & mutagenic hypersens Uses: *Multiple myeloma, ovarian CAs*, breast & testicular CA, melanoma; allogenic & ABMT (high dose), neuroblastoma, rhabdomyosarcoma **Action:** Alkylating agent, nitrogen mustard **Dose:** *Adults. Multiple myeloma:* 16 mg/m² IV q2wk × 4 doses then at 4-wk intervals after tox resolves; w/ renal impair ↓ IV dose 50% or 6 mg PO qd × 2–3 wk, then D/C up to 4 wk, follow counts then 2 mg qd *Ovarian CA:* 0.2 mg/kg qd × 5 d, repeat q4–5wk based on counts, ↓ in renal Insuff **Caution:** [D, ?/–) w/ Cisplatin, digitalis, live vaccines extravasation, need central line **CI:** Allergy or resistance **Disp:** Tabs 2 mg; Inj 50 mg **SE:** N/V, secondary malignancy, AF, ↓ LVEF, ↓ BM, secondary leukemia, alopecia, dermatitis, stomatitis, pulm fibrosis, rare allergic Rxns, thrombocytopenia **Interactions:** ↑ Risk of nephrotox *W/* cisplatin, cyclosporine; ↓ effects *W/* cimetidine, interferon-α **Labs:** ↓ HMG, RBCs, WBCs, plt; false(+) direct Coombs test **NIPE:** ↑ Fluids, ⊘ PRG, breast-feeding; take PO on empty stomach; ↑ risk infxn; ⊘ live vaccines

Memantine (Namenda) [N-Methyl-D-Aspartate (NMDA) Receptor Antagonist] Uses: *Mod–severe Alzheimer Dz*, mild–mod vascular dementia, mild cognitive impair **Actions:** *N*-methyl-D-aspartate (NMDA) receptor antagonist **Dose:** *Namenda:* Target 20 mg/d, start 5 mg/d, ↑ 5–20 mg/d, wait > 1 wk before ↑ dose; use bid if > 5 mg/dose; *Vascular dementia:* 10 mg PO bid *Namenda XR* (Alzheimer) 7 mg inital 1 × qd, ↑ by 7 mg/wk each wk to maint 28 mg/d × 1; ↓ to 14 mg w/ severe renal impair **Caution:** [B, ?/–] Hepatic/mod renal impair; Sx disorders, cardiac Dz **Disp:** *Namenda* Tabs 5, 10 mg, combo pack: 5 mg × 28 + 10 mg × 21; soln 2 mg/mL. **CI:** Component hypersens **SE:** Dizziness, HA, D **Interactions:** ↑ Effects *W/* amantadine, carbonic anhydrase Inhibits, dextromethorphan, ketamine, NaHCO₃; ↑ effects *W/* any drug, herb, food that alkalinizes urine **Labs:** Monitor BUN, SCr **NIPE:** Take w/o regard to food; EtOH ↑ adverse effects & ↓ effectiveness; renal clearance ↓ by alkaline urine (↓ 80% at pH 8)

Meningococcal Conjugate Vaccine [Quadrivalent, MCV4] (Menactra, Menveo) [Vaccine/Live] **Uses:** *Immunize against *N meningitidis* (meningococcus) high-risk 2–10 & 19–55 y and everyone 11–18* high-risk (college freshman, military recruits, travel to endemic areas, terminal complement deficiencies, asplenia); if given age 11–12, give booster at 16, should have booster w/in 5 y of college **Action:** Active immunization; *N meningitidis* A, C, Y, W-135 polysaccharide conjugated to diphtheria toxoid (*Menactra*) or lyophilized conjugate component (*Menveo*) **Dose:** *Adults.* *18–55 y Peds > 2 y* 0.5 mL IM × 1 **Caution:** [B/C (manufacturer dependent) ?/–] w/ Immunosuppression (↓ response) and bleeding disorders, Hx Guillain-Barré **CI:** Allergy to class/diphtheria toxoid/compound/latex; Hx Guillain-Barré **Disp:** Inj **SE:** Inj site Rxns, HA, N/V/D, anorexia, fatigue, irritability, arthralgia, Guillain-Barré **Interactions:** ↓ Effects *W/* Ig if administer w/in 1 mo **NIPE:** IM only, reported accidental SQ ; keep epi available for Rxns; use polysaccharide *Menomune* (MPSV4) if > 55 y; do not confuse w/ *Menactra, Menveo*; ACIP rec: MCV4 for 2–55 y, ↑ local Rxn compared to *Menomune* (MPSV4) but ↑ Ab titers; peds 2–10, Ab levels ↓ 3 y w/ MPSV4, revaccinate in 2–3 y, use MCV4 for revaccination

Meningococcal Groups C and Y and Haemophilus b Tetanus Toxoid Conjugate Vaccine (Menhibrix) **Uses:** *Prevent meningococcal Dz and *Haemophilus influenzae* type b (Hib) in infants/young children* **Action:** Active immunization; antibodies specific to organisms **Dose:** *Peds 6 wk–18 mo.* 4 doses 0.5 mL IM at 2, 4, 6, and 12–15 mo **Caution:** [C, N/A] Apnea in some infants reported; w/ Hx Guillain Barré; fainting may occur **CI:** Severe allergy to similar vaccines **Disp:** Inj 40 mg/mL/vial **SE:** Inj pain, redness; irritability; drowsiness; ↓ appetite; fever **Notes:** New in 2012 **NIPE:** Used cautiously in infants born prematurely

Meningococcal Polysaccharide Vaccine [MPSV4] (Menomune A/C/Y/W-135) [Immunization] **Uses:** *Immunize against *N meningitidis* (meningococcus)* in high risk (college freshman, military recruits, travel to endemic areas, terminal complement deficiencies, asplenia) **Action:** Active immunization

Dose: *Adults & Peds > 2 y.* 0.5 mL SQ only; children < 2 y not recommended; 2 doses 3 mo apart may repeat 3–5 y if high risk; repeat in 2–3 y if 1st dose given 2–4 y **Caution:** [C, ?/M] If immunocompromised (↓ response) **CI:** Thimerosal/latex sensitivity; w/ pertussis or typhoid vaccine, < 2 y **Disp:** Inj SE: *Peds 2–10 y:* Inj site Rxns, drowsiness, irritability *11–55 y:* Inj site Rxns, HA, fatigue, malaise, fever, D **NIPE:** Keep epi (1:1000) available for Rxns. Recommended > 55 y, but also alternative to MCV4 in 2–55 y if no MCV4 available (MCV4 is preferred). Active against serotypes A, C, Y, & W-135 but not group B; Ab levels ↓ 3 y, high-risk revaccination q3–5 y (use MCV4)

Meperidine (Demerol, Meperitab) [C-II] [Opioid Analgesic]
Uses: *Mod–severe pain*, post-op shivering, rigors from amphotericin B **Action:** Narcotic analgesic **Dose:** *Adults.* 50–150 mg PO or IV/IM/SQ q3–4h PRN *Peds.* 1–1.5 mg/kg/dose PO or IM /SQ q3–4h PRN, up to 100 mg/dose; hepatic impair, avoid in renal impair, avoid use in elderly **Caution:** [C /–] ↓ Sz threshold, adrenal Insuff, head injury, ↑ ICP, hepatic impair, not OK in sickle cell Dz **CI:** w/ MAOIs **Disp:** Tabs 50, 100 mg; syrup/soln 50 mg/5 mL; Inj 25, 50, 75, 100 mg/mL **SE:** Resp/CNS depression, Szs, sedation, constipation, ↓ BP, rash N/V, biliary & urethral spasms, dyspnea **Interactions:** ↑ Effects *W/* antihistamines, barbiturates, cimetidine, MAOIs, neuroleptics, selegiline, TCAs, St. John's wort, EtOH; ↑ effects *OF* INH; ↓ effects *W/* phenytoin **Labs:** ↑ Serum amylase, lipase **NIPE:** Analgesic effects potentiated w/ hydroxyzine; 75 mg IM = 10 mg morphine IM; not best in elderly; do not use oral for acute pain; not recommended for repetitive use in ICU setting; ⊘ EtOH

Meprobamate (Generic) [C-IV] [Antianxiety]
Uses: *Short-term relief of anxiety* muscle spasm, TMJ relief **Action:** Mild tranquilizer; antianxiety **Dose:** *Adults.* 400 mg PO tid-qid, max 2400 mg/d *Peds 6–12 y.* 100–200 mg PO bid–tid; ↓ in renal/liver impair **Caution:** [D, +/–] Elderly, Sz Dz, caution with depression or suicidal tendencies **CI:** Acute intermittent porphyria **Disp:** Tabs 200, 400 mg **SE:** Drowsiness, syncope, tachycardia, edema, rash (SJS), N/V/D, ↓ WBC, agranulocytosis **Interactions:** ↑ Effects *W/* antihistamines, barbiturates, CNS depressants, narcotics, EtOH; **Labs:** ↓ WBC—monitor **NIPE:** Do not abruptly D/C; avoid EtOH

Mercaptopurine [6-MP] (Purinethol) [Antineoplastic/Antimetabolite]
Uses: *ALL* 2nd-line Rx for CML & NHL, maint ALL in children, immunosuppressant w/ autoimmune Dzs (Crohn Dz, UC) **Action:** Antimetabolite, mimics hypoxanthine **Dose:** *Adults. ALL induction:* 1.5–2.5 mg/kg/d *Maint:* 60 mg/m²/d w/ allopurinol use 67–75% ↓ dose of 6-MP (interference w/ xanthine oxidase metabolism) *Peds. ALL induction:* 1.5–2.5 mg/kg/d *Maint:* 1.5–2.5 mg/kg/d PO or 60 mg/m²/d w/ renal/hepatic Insuff; take on empty stomach; **Caution:** [D, ?] w/ Allopurinol, immunosuppression, TMP–SMX, warfarin, salicylates, severe BM Dz, PRG **CI:** Prior resistance, PRG **Disp:** Tabs 50 mg **SE:** Mild hematotoxicity, mucositis, stomatitis, D, rash, fever, eosinophilia, jaundice, hep, hyperuricemia,

hyperpigmentation, alopecia **Interactions:** ↑ Effects *W*/ allopurinol; ↑ risk of BM suppression *W*/ TMP–SMX; ↓ effects *OF* warfarin **Labs:** False ↑ serum glucose, uric acid; ↑ LFTs; ↑ HMG, RBCs, WBC, plt **NIPE:** ↑ Fluid intake to 2–3 L/d, may take 4+ wk for improvement; handle properly; limit use to experienced healthcare providers; for ALL, evening dosing may ↓ risk of relapse; low emetogenicity; ↑ risk infxn; ⊘ PRG

Meropenem (Merrem) [Antibiotic/Carbapenem] Uses: *Intra-Abd Infxns, bacterial meningitis, skin Infxn* **Action:** Carbapenem; ↓ cell wall synth *Spectrum:* Excellent gram(+) (except MRSA, methicillin-resistant *S epidermidis* [MRSE], & *E faecium*); excellent gram(−) including extended-spectrum β-lactamase producers; good anaerobic **Dose:** *Adults. Abd Infxn:* 1–2 g IV q8h *Skin Infxn:* 500 mg IV q8h *Meningitis:* 2 g IV q8h *Peds > 3 mo, < 50 kg. Abd Infxn:* 20 mg/kg IV q8h *Skin Infxn:* 10 mg/kg IV q8h *Meningitis:* 40 mg/kg IV q8h *Peds > 50 kg.* Use adult dose; max 2 g IV q8h; ↓ in renal Insuff (see PI) **Caution:** [B, ?/M] w/ Probenecid, VPA **CI:** β-Lactam anaphylaxis **Disp:** Inj 1 g, 500 mg **SE:** Less Sz potential than imipenem; *C difficile* enterocolitis, D, ↓ plt **Interactions:** ↑ Effects *W*/ probenecid **Labs:** ↑ LFTs, BUN, Cr, eosinophils ↓ HMG, Hct, WBCs, plt **NIPE:** Monitor for super Infxn; overuse ↑ bacterial resistance

Mesalamine (Asacol, Asacol, Asacol HD, Canasa, Lialda, Pentasa, Rowasa) [Anti-Inflammatory/Salicylate] Uses: *Rectal: mild–mod distal UC, proctosigmoiditis, proctitis; oral: Tx/maint of mild–mod ulcerative colitis* **Action:** 5-ASA derivative, may inhibit prostaglandins, may ↓ leukotrienes & TNF-α **Dose:** *Rectal:* 60 mL qhs, retain 8 h (enema) *PO: Caps:* 1 g PO qid *Tab:* 1.6–2.4 g/d ÷ doses (tid–qid) × 6 wk; DR 2.4–4.8 g PO daily 8 wk max, do not cut/crush/chew w/ food; ↓ initial dose in elderly **Maint:** Depends on formulation **Caution:** [B/C (product specific), M] w/ Digitalis, PUD, pyloric stenosis, renal Insuff, elderly **CI:** Salicylate sensitivity **Disp:** Tabs ER (*Asacol*) 400, (*Ascarol HD*) 800 mg; ER caps (*Pentasa*) 250, 500 mg, (*Apriso*) 375 mg; DR tab (*Lialda*) 1.2 g; supp (*Canasa*) 1000 mg; (*Rowasa*) rectal susp 4 g/60 mL **SE:** Yellow-brown urine, HA, malaise, Abd pain, flatulence, rash, pancreatitis, pericarditis, dizziness, rectal pain, hair loss, intolerance synd (bloody D) **Interactions:** ↓ Effect *OF* digoxin **Labs:** ✓ CBC, Cr, BUN **NIPE:** May discolor urine yellow-brown; best used after BM; retain rectally 3 h; Sx may ↑ when starting

Mesna (Mesnex) [Uroprotectant/Antidote] Uses: *Prevent hemorrhagic cystitis d/t ifosfamide or cyclophosphamide* **Action:** Antidote, reacts w/ acrolein and other metabolites to form stable compounds **Dose:** Per protocol; dose as % of ifosfamide or cyclophosphamide dose *IV bolus:* 20% (eg, 10–12 mg/kg) IV at 0, 4, & 8 h *IV Inf:* 20% prechemotherapy, 40% w/ chemotherapy, for 12–24 h *Oral:* 100% ifosfamide dose given as 20% IV at 0 h, then 40% PO at 4 & 8 h; if PO dose vomited repeat or give dose IV; mix PO w/ juice **Caution:** [B; ?/–] **CI:** Thiol sensitivity **Disp:** Inj 100 mg/mL; (Mesnex) tabs 400 mg **SE:** ↓ BP, ↓ plt, ↑ HR, ↑ RR allergic Rxns, HA, GI upset, taste perversion **Labs:** ↑ LFTs, ↓ plt

NIPE: Hydration helps ↓ hemorrhagic cystitis; higher dose for BMT; IV contains benzyl alcohol

Metaproterenol (Generic) [Bronchodilator/Beta-Adrenergic Agonist] Uses: *Asthma & reversible bronchospasm, COPD* **Action:** Sympathomimetic bronchodilator **Dose:** *Adults. Nebulized:* 5% 2.5 mL q4–6h or PRN *MDI:* 1–3 Inh q3–4h, 12 Inh max/24 h; wait 2 min between Inh *PO:* 20 mg q6–8h *Peds ≥ 12 y. MDI:* 2–3 Inh q3–4h, 12 Inh/d max *Nebulizer:* 2.5 mL (soln 0.4, 0.6%) tid–qid, up to q4h *Peds > 9 y or ≥ 27 kg.* 20 mg PO tid–qid *6–9 y or < 27 kg.* 10 mg PO tid–qid; ↓ in elderly **Caution:** [C, ?/–] w/ MAOI, TCA, sympathomimetics; avoid w/ β-blockers **CI:** Tachycardia, other arrhythmias **Disp:** Aerosol 0.65 mg/Inh; soln for Inh 0.4%, 0.6%; tabs 10, 20 mg; syrup 10 mg/5 mL **SE:** Nervousness, tremor, tachycardia, HTN, ↑ glucose, ↓ K⁺, ↑ IOP **Interactions:** ↑ Effects W/ sympathomimetic drugs, xanthines; ↑ risk of arrhythmias W/ cardiac glycosides, halothane, levodopa, theophylline, thyroid hormones; ↑ HTN W/ MAOIs; ↓ effects W/ BBs **Labs:** ↑ Glucose, ↓ K⁺ **NIPE:** Separate additional aerosol use by 5 min; fewer β₁ effects than isoproterenol & longer acting, but not a 1st-line β-agonist. Use w/ face mask < 4 y; oral ↑ ADR (Alupent has been removed from US market)

Metaxalone (Skelaxin) [Skeletal Muscle Relaxant] Uses: *Painful musculoskeletal conditions* **Action:** Centrally acting skeletal muscle relaxant **Dose:** 800 mg PO tid–qid **Caution:** [C, ?/–] Elderly & CNS depression, anemia **CI:** Severe hepatic/renal impair; drug-induced, hemolytic, or other anemias **Disp:** Tabs 800 mg **SE:** N/V, HA, drowsiness, hep **Interactions:** ↑ Sedating effects W/ CNS depressants, antihistamines, opioid analgesics, sedative/hypnotics, chamomile, kava kava, valerian, EtOH **Labs:** False(+) urine glucose using Benedict test **NIPE:** Monitor elderly for sedation & weakness; ⊘ EtOH; high-fat meals may ↑ risk of SEs

Metformin (Fortmet, Glucophage, Glucophage XR, Glumetza, Riomet) [Hypoglycemic/Biguanide] WARNING: Associated w/ lactic acidosis, risk ↑ w/ sepsis, dehydration, renal/hepatic impair, ↑ alcohol, acute CHF; Sxs include myalgias, malaise, resp distress, Abd pain, somnolence Uses: *Type 2 DM*, polycystic ovary synd (PCOS) HIV lipodystrophy **Action:** Biguanide; ↓ hepatic glucose production & intestinal absorption of glucose; ↑ insulin sensitivity **Dose:** *Adults. Initial:* 500 mg PO bid; or 850 mg daily, titrate 1- to 2-wk intervals may ↑ to 2550 mg/d max; take w/ AM & PM meals; can convert total daily dose to daily dose of XR *Peds 10–16 y.* 500 mg PO bid, ↑ 500 mg/wk to 2000 mg/d max in ÷ doses; do not use XR formulation in peds **Caution:** [B, +/–] Avoid EtOH; hold dose before & 48 h after ionic contrast; hepatic impair, elderly **CI:** SCr ≥ 1.4 mg/dL in females or ≥ 1.5 mg/dL in males; hypoxemic conditions (eg, acute CHF/sepsis); metabolic acidosis, abnormal CrCl from any cause (AMI, shock) **Disp:** Tabs 500, 850, 1000 mg; XR tabs 500, 750, 1000 mg; (Riomet) soln 100 mg/mL **SE:** Anorexia, N/V/D, flatulence, weakness, myalgia, rash **Interactions:** ↑ Effects W/ amiloride, cimetidine, digoxin, furosemide, MAOIs, morphine, procainamide, quinidine, quinine, ranitidine, triamterene, TMP, vancomycin; ↓ effects *W/* corticosteroids, CCBs, diuretics, estrogens, INH, OCPs, phenothiazine, phenytoin, sympathomimetics, thyroid drugs, tobacco **Labs:** Monitor LFTs, BUN/Cr, serum vit B_{12} **NIPE:** Take w/ food; avoid dehydration—↑ fluids, EtOH, before surgery; ↓ pH, ↑ anion gap, ↑ blood lactate; D/C immediately & hospitalize if suspected

Methadone (Dolophine, Methadose) [C-II] [Opioid Analgesic]

WARNING: Deaths reported during initiation and conversion of pain pts to methadone Rx from Rx w/ other opioids. For PO only; tabs contain excipient. Resp depression and QT prolongation, arrhythmias observed. Only dispensed by certified opioid Tx programs for addiction. Analgesic use must outweigh risks **Uses:** *Severe pain not responsive to non-narcotics; detox w/ maint of narcotic addiction* **Action:** Narcotic analgesic **Dose:** *Adults.* 2.5–10 mg IM/IV/SQ q8–12h or PO q8h; titrate as needed; see PI for conversion from other opioids **Peds.** (Not FDA approved) 0.1 mg/kg q4–12h IV; ↑ slowly to avoid resp depression; ↓ in renal impair **Caution:** [C, –] Avoid w/ severe liver Dz **CI:** Resp depression, acute asthma, ileus w/ selegiline **Disp:** Tabs 5, 10 mg; tab dispersible 40 mg; PO soln 5, 10 mg/5 mL; PO conc 10 mg/mL; Inj 10 mg/mL **SE:** Resp depression, sedation, constipation, urinary retention, ↑ QT interval, arrhythmias, ↓ HR, syncope **Interactions:** ↑ Effects *W/* cimetidine, CNS depressants, protease Inhibs, EtOH; ↑ effects *OF* anticoagulants, EtOH, antihistamines, barbiturates, glutethimide, methocarbamol; ↓ effects *W/* carbamazepine, nelfinavir, phenobarbital, phenytoin, primidone, rifampin, ritonavir **Labs:** ↓ K^+, ↓ Mg^{2+} **NIPE:** ⊘ Chew or swallow whole—dissolve in 4 oz H_2O or acidic fruit juice; parenteral-to-PO ratio, 1:2 (5 mg parenteral = 10 mg PO); longer 1/2-life; resp depression occurs later & lasts longer than analgesic effect; use w/ caution to avoid iatrogenic OD; ↑ risk for abuse

Methenamine Hippurate (Hiprex), Methenamine Mandelate (UROQUID-Acid No. 2) [Urinary Anti-Infective]

Uses: *Suppress recurrent UTI long-term. Use only after Infxn cleared by antibiotics* **Action:** Converted to formaldehyde & ammonia in acidic urine; nonspecific bactericidal action **Dose:** *Adults. Hippurate:* 1 g PO bid *Mandelate:* Initial 1 g qid PO pc & hs, maint 1–2 g/d **Peds** *6–12 y. Hippurate:* 0.5–1 g PO bid PO ÷ bid. *> 2 y. Mandelate:* 50–75 mg/kg/d PO ÷ qid; take w/ food, ascorbic acid w/ hydration **Caution:** [C, +] **CI:** Renal Insuff, severe hepatic Dz, & severe dehydration w/ sulfonamides (may precipitate urine) **Disp:** *Methenamine hippurate:* Tabs 1 g *Methenamine mandelate:* 500 mg, 1 g EC tabs **SE:** Rash, GI upset, dysuria, ↑ LFTs , super Infxn w/ prolonged use, *C difficile*–associated diarrhea **Interactions:** ↓ Effects *W/* acetazolamide, antacids **Labs:** ↑ LFTs **NIPE:** ↑ Fluids to 2–3 L/d; take w/ food; use w/ sulfonamides may precipitate in urine; hippurate not indicated in peds < 6 y; not for pts w/ indwelling catheters as dwell time in bladder required for action; ⊘ citrus, dairy, antacids may ↑ effectiveness

Methenamine, Phenyl Salicylate, Methylene Blue, Benzoic Acid, Hyoscyamine (Prosed)

Uses: *Lower urinary tract discomfort*

Action: Methenamine in acid urine releases formaldehyde (antiseptic), phenyl salicylate (mild analgesic), methylene blue/benzoic acid (mild antiseptic), hyoscyamine (parasympatholytic), ↓ muscle spasm **Dose:** *Adults Peds > 12 y.* 1 tab PO qid w/ liberal fluid intake **Caution:** [C, ?/–] Avoid w/ sulfonamides, NAG, pyloric/duodenal obst, BOO, coronary artery spasm **CI:** Component hypersensitivity **Disp:** Tabs **SE:** Rash, dry mouth, flushing, ↑ pulse, dizziness, blurred vision, urine/feces discoloration, voiding difficulty/retention **NIPE:** Take whole w/ plenty of fluid, can cause crystalluria; not indicated in peds < 6 y; may cause urine/stool to appear blue or green; space antacids 1 h before or after taking this med

Methimazole (Tapazole) [Antithyroid Agent]
Uses: *Hyperthyroidism, thyrotoxicosis*, prep for thyroid surgery or radiation **Action:** Blocks T_3 & T_4 formation, but does not inactivate circulating T_3, T_4 **Dose:** *Adults.* Initial based on severity: 15–60 mg/d PO q8h *Maint:* 5–15 mg PO daily *Peds.* Initial: 0.4–0.7 mg/kg/24 h PO q8h *Maint:* 5–15 mg PO daily; take w/ food **Caution:** [D, –] w/ Other meds **CI:** Breast-feeding **Disp:** Tabs 5, 10, mg **SE:** GI upset, dizziness, blood dyscrasias, dermatitis, fever, hepatic Rxns, lupus-like synd **Interactions:** ↑ Effects *OF* digitalis glycosides, metoprolol, propranolol; ↓ effects *OF* anticoagulants, theophylline; ↓ effects *W/* amiodarone **Labs:** ↓ LFTs, PT; follow clinically & w/ TFT, CBC w/ diff **NIPE:** Take w/ food; ⊘ PRG; ↑ risk of infxn—⊘ live vaccines

Methocarbamol (Robaxin) [Skeletal Muscle Relaxant/Centrally Acting]
Uses: *Relief of discomfort associated w/ painful musculoskeletal conditions* **Action:** Centrally acting skeletal muscle relaxant **Dose:** *Adults & Peds ≥ 16 y.* 1.5 g PO qid for 2–3 d, then 1-g PO qid maint *Tetanus:* 1–2 g IV q6h × 3 d, then use PO, max dose 24g/d < *16 y.* 15 mg/kg/dose or 500 mg/m²/dose IV, may repeat PRN (tetanus only), max 1.8 g/m²/d × 3 d **Caution:** Sz disorders, hepatic & renal impair [C, ?/M] **CI:** MyG, renal impair w/ IV **Disp:** Tabs 500, 750 mg; Inj 100 mg/mL **SE:** Can discolor urine, lightheadedness, drowsiness, GI upset, ↓ HR, ↓ BP **Interactions:** ↑ Effects *W/* CNS depressant, EtOH **Labs:** ↑ Urine 5-HIAA **NIPE:** Monitor for blurred vision, orthostatic hypotension; tabs can be crushed & added to NG; do not operate heavy machinery;

Methotrexate (Rheumatrex Dose Pack, Trexall) [Antineoplastic, Antirheumatic (DMARDs), Immunosuppressant/Antimetabolite]
WARNING: Administration only by experienced healthcare physician; do not use in women of childbearing age unless absolutely necessary (teratogenic); impaired elimination w/ impaired renal Fxn, ascites, pleural effusion; severe ↓ BM w/ NSAIDs; hepatotox, occasionally fatal; can induce life-threatening pneumonitis; D and ulcerative stomatitis require D/C; lymphoma risk; may cause tumor lysis synd; can cause severe skin Rxn, opportunistic Infxns; w/ RT can ↑ tissue necrosis risk. Preservatives make this agent unsuitable for IT or higher dose use **Uses:** *ALL, AML, leukemic meningitis, trophoblastic tumors (choriocarcinoma, hydatidiform mole), breast, lung, head, & neck CAs, Burkitt lymphoma, mycosis fungoides, osteosarcoma, Hodgkin Dz & NHL, psoriasis; RA, JRA, SLE*, chronic Dz

Action: ↓ Dihydrofolate reductase-mediated product of tetrahydrofolate, causes ↓ DNA synth **Dose:** *Adults. CA:* Per protocol *RA:* 7.5 mg/wk PO 1/wk or 2.5 mg q12h PO for 3 doses/wk *Psoriasis:* 2.5–5 mg PO q12h × 3 d/wk or 10–25 mg PO/IM qwk *Chronic:* 15–25 mg IM/SQ qwk, then 15 mg/wk *Peds. JIA:* 10 mg/m² PO/IM qwk, then 5–14 mg/m² × 1 or as 3 ÷ doses 12 h apart; ↓ elderly, w/ renal/hepatic impair **Caution:** [X, −] w/ Other nephro-/hepatotox meds, multiple interactions, w/ Sz, profound ↓ BM other than CA related **CI:** Severe renal/hepatic impair, PRG/lactation **Disp:** Dose pack 2.5 mg in 8, 12, 16, 20, or 24 doses; tabs 2.5, 5, 7.5, 10, 15 mg; Inj 25 mg/mL; Inj powder 20 mg, 1 g **SE:** ↓ BM, N/V/D, anorexia, mucositis, hepatotox (transient & reversible; may progress to atrophy, necrosis, fibrosis, cirrhosis), rashes, dizziness, malaise, blurred vision, alopecia, photosens, renal failure, pneumonitis; rare pulm fibrosis; chemical arachnoiditis & HA w/ IT delivery **Notes:** *Systemic levels: Therapeutic:* > 0.01 mcmol *Toxic:* > 10 mcmol over 24 h **Interactions:** ↑ Effects *W/* chloramphenicol, cyclosporine, etretinate, NSAIDs, phenylbutazone, phenytoin, PCN, probenecid, salicylates, sulfonamides, sulfonylureas, EtOH; ↑ effects *OF* cyclosporine, tetracycline, theophylline; ↑ effects *W/* antimalarials, aminoglycosides, binding resins, cholestyramine, folic acid; ↓ effects *OF* digoxin **Labs:** Monitor CBC, LFTs, Cr, MTX levels & CXR **NIPE:** "High dose" > 500 mg/m² requires leucovorin rescue to ↓ tox; w/ IT, use preservative-free/alcohol-free soln; ↑ risk of photosensitivity—use sunscreen, ↑ fluids 2–3 L/d; ⊘ PRG

Methyldopa (Generic) [Antihypertensive/Centrally Acting Anti-adrenergic]

Uses: *HTN* **Action:** Centrally acting antihypertensive, ↓ sympathetic outflow **Dose:** *Adults.* 250–500 mg PO bid–tid (max 2–3 g/d) or 250 mg–1 g IV q6–8h *Peds Neonates.* 2.5–5 mg/kg PO/IV q8h *Other peds.* 10 mg/kg/24 h PO in 2–3 ÷ doses or 5–10 mg/kg/dose IV q6–8h to max 65 mg/kg/24 h; ↓ in renal Insuff/ elderly **Caution:** [B, +] **CI:** Liver Dz, w/ MAOIs, bisulfate allergy **Disp:** Tabs 250, 500 mg; Inj 50 mg/mL **SE:** Initial transient sedation/drowsiness, edema, hemolytic anemia, hepatic disorders, fevers, nightmares **Interactions:** ↑ Effects *W/* anesthetics, diuretics, levodopa, Li, methotrimeprazine, thioxanthenes, vasodilators, verapamil; ↑ effects *OF* haloperidol, Li, tolbutamide; ↓ effects *W/* amphetamines, Fe, phenothiazine, TCAs; ↓ effects *OF* ephedrine **Labs:** ↑ BUN, Cr; ↓ LFTs, HMG, RBC, WBC, plt; false(+) Coombs test **NIPE:** Tolerance may occur; may ↓ reaction time—caution driving; caution with EtOH

Methylene Blue (Urolene Blue, Various)

Uses: *Methemoglobinemia, vasoplegic synd, ifosfamide-induced encephalopathy, cyanide poisoning, dye in therapeutics/dx* **Action:** Low IV dose converts methemoglobin to hemoglobin; excreted, appears in urine as green/green-blue color; MAOI activity **Dose:** 1–2 mg/kg or 25–50 mg/m² IV over 5–10 min, repeat q1h; direct instillation into fistulous tract **Caution:** [X, −] w/ Severe renal impair w/ psych meds such as SSRI, SNRI, TCAs (may cause serotonin synd), w/ G6PD deficiency **CI:** Intraspinal Inj, severe renal Insuff **Disp:** 1, 10 mL Inj **SE:** IV use: N, Abd, CP, sweating, fecal/urine discoloration, hemolytic anemia **Notes:** Component of other meds; stains tissue blue, limits repeat use in surgical visualization **NIPE:** May cause urine/stool to turn blue or green; ↑ fluids

Methylergonovine (Methergine) [Oxytocic/Ergot Alkaloid]
Uses: *Postpartum bleeding (atony, hemorrhage)* **Action:** Ergotamine derivative, rapid and sustained uterotonic effect **Dose:** 0.2 mg IM after anterior shoulder delivery or puerperium, may repeat in 2–4-h intervals or 0.2–0.4 mg PO q6–12h for 2–7 d **Caution:** [C, ?] w/ Sepsis, obliterative vascular Dz, hepatic/renal impair, w/ CYP3A4 Inhib (Table 10) **CI:** HTN, PRG, toxemia **Disp:** Inj 0.2 mg/mL; tabs 0.2 mg **SE:** HTN, N/V, CP, ↓ BP, Sz **Interactions:** ↑ Vasoconstriction **W/** ergot alkaloids, sympathomimetics, tobacco **NIPE:** ⊘ Smoking; give IV only if absolutely necessary over > 1 min w/ BP monitoring; ⊘ breast-feeding w/in 12 h after end of Rx; grapefruit/grapefruit juice may ↑ risk of SEs

Methylnaltrexone Bromide (Relistor) [Opioid Antagonist] Uses:
Opioid-induced constipation in pt w/ advanced illness such as CA **Action:**
Peripheral opioid antagonist **Dose:** *Adults. Wgt-based < 38 kg:* 0.15 mg/kg SQ *38–61 kg:* 8 mg SQ *62–114 kg:* 12 mg SQ *> 114 kg:* 0.15 mg/kg, round to nearest 0.1 mL, dose qod PRN, max 1 dose q24h **Caution:** [B, ?/M] w/ CrCl < 30 mL/min ↓ dose 50% **Disp:** Inj 12 mg/0.6 mL **SE:** N/D, Abd pain, dizziness **NIPE:** Does not change opioid analgesic effects or induce withdrawal; not recommended for children; usually produces BM w/in 30 min of Inj

Methylphenidate, Oral (Concerta, Metadate CD, Metadate SR, Methylin Ritalin, Ritalin LA, Ritalin SR, Quillivant XR) [C-II] [CNS Stimulant/Piperidine Derivative] WARNING: w/ Hx of drug or alcohol dependence, avoid abrupt D/C; chronic use can lead to dependence or psychotic behavior; observe closely during withdrawal of drug **Uses:** *ADHD, narcolepsy*, depression* **Action:** CNS stimulant, blocks reuptake of norepinephrine and DA **Dose:** *Adults. Narcolepsy:* 10 mg PO 2–3 ×/d, 60 mg/d max *Depression:* 2.5 mg qAM; ↑ slowly, 20 mg/d max, ÷ bid 7 AM & 12 PM; use regular-release only *Adults & Peds > 6 y. ADHD: IR:* 5 mg PO bid, ↑ 5–10 mg/d to 60 mg/d, max 2 mg/kg/d *ER/SR* use total IR dose qd *CD/LA* 20 mg PO qd, ↑ 10–20 mg qwk to 60 mg/d max *Concerta:* 18 mg PO qAM, Rx naïve or already on 20 mg/d, 36 mg PO qAM if on 30–45 mg/d, 54 mg PO qAM if on 40–60 mg/d, 72 mg PO AM max **Caution:** [C, M] w/ Hx EtOH/drug abuse, CV Dz, HTN, bipolar Dz, Sz; separate from MAOIs by 14 d **Disp:** Chew tabs 2.5, 5, 10 mg; tabs scored IR (*Ritalin*) 5, 10, 20 mg; caps ER (*Ritalin LA*) 10, 20, 30, 40 mg; caps ER (*Metadate CD*) 10, 20, 30, 40, 50, 60 mg (*Methylin ER*) 10, 20 mg; tabs SR (*Metadate, Ritalin SR*) 20 mg; ER tabs (*Concerta*) 18, 27, 36, 54 mg; oral soln 5, 10 mg/5 mL (*QuilliVant XR*) ER susp 5 mg/mL **SE:** CV/CNS stimulation, growth retard, GI upset, pancytopenia, ↑ LFTs **CI:** Marked anxiety, tension, agitation, NAG, motor tics, family Hx or diagnosis of Tourette synd, severe HTN, angina, arrhythmias, CHF, recent MI, ↑ thyroid; w/ or w/in 14 d of MAOI **Interactions:**
↑ Risk of hypertensive crisis **W/** MAOIs; ↑ effects **OF** anticonvulsants, anticoagulants,

TCA, SSRIs; ↓ effects **OF** guanethidine, antihypertensives **Labs:** ↑ LFTs; monitor CBC, plts, LFTs **NIPE:** See also transdermal form; titrate dose; take 30–45 min ac; do not chew or crush; Concerta "ghost tab" may appear in stool—avoid w/ GI narrowing; abuse & diversion concerns; D/C if Sz or agitation occurs; Metadate contains sucrose, avoid w/ lactose/galactose problems; do not use these meds w/ halogenated anesthetics; AHA rec all ADHD peds need CV assessment & consideration for ECG before Rx

Methylphenidate, Transdermal (Daytrana) [CNS Stimulant] [C-II]   WARNING: w/ Hx of drug or alcohol dependence; chronic use can lead to dependence or psychotic behavior; observe closely during withdrawal of drug

Uses: *ADHD in children 6–17 y* **Action:** CNS stimulant, blocks reuptake of norepinephrine and DA **Dose:** *Adults & Peds 6–17 y.* Apply to hip in AM (2 h before desired effect), remove 9 h later; titrate 1st wk 10 mg/9 h, 2nd wk 15 mg/9 h, 3rd wk 20 mg/9 h, 4th wk 30 mg/9 h **Caution:** [C, +/–] See Methylphenidate, Oral; sensitization may preclude subsequent use of oral forms; abuse & diversion concerns **CI:** Significant anxiety, agitation; component allergy; glaucoma; w/ or w/in 14 d of MAOI; tics, or family Hx Tourette syndrome **Disp:** Patches 10, 15, 20, 30 mg **SE:** Local Rxns, N/V, nasopharyngitis, ↓ wgt, ↓ appetite, lability, insomnia, tic **Interactions:** ↑ Effects **OF** oral anticoagulants, phenobarbital, phenytoin, primidone, SSRIs, TCAs; ↑ risk **OF** hypertensive crisis **W/** MAOIs; caution **W/** pressor drugs **NIPE:** Titrate dose weekly; effects last h after removal; eval BP, HR at baseline & periodically; avoid heat exposure to patch, may cause OD, AHA rec all ADHD peds need CV assessment & consideration for ECG before Rx

Methylprednisolone (A-Methapred, Depo-Medrol, Medrol, Medrol Dosepak, Solu-Medrol) [See Steroids Table 2] Uses:

Steroid responsive conditions (endocrine, rheumatic, collagen, dermatologic, allergic, ophthalmic, respiratory, hematologic, neoplastic, edematous, GI, CNS, others) **Action:** Glucocorticoid **Dose:** See Steroids **Peds. ECC 2010.** Status asthmaticus, anaphylactic shock: 2 mg/kg IV/IO/IM (max 60 mg). Maint: 0.5 mg/kg IV q6h or 1 mg/kg q12h to 120 mg/d **Caution:** [C, ?/M] may mask Infx, cataract w/ prolonged use; avoid vaccines **CI:** Fungal Infx, component allergy **Disp:** Oral (*Medrol*) 4, 8, 16, 32 mg; (*Medrol Dosepak*) 21 4-mg tabs taken over 6 d; Inj acetate (*Depo-Medrol*) 20, 40, 80 mg/mL; Inj succinate (*Solu-Medrol*) 40, 125, 500 mg, 1, 2 g **SE:** Fluid and electrolyte disturbances, muscle weakness/loss, ulcers, impaired wound healing, others (see label) **Notes:** Taper dose to avoid adrenal Insuff **Interactions:** ↑ Risk of serotonin synd **W/** sertraline, venlafaxine; ↑ effects **OF** APAP, ASA, CNS depressants, cyclosporine, levodopa, Li, succinylcholine, tetracyclines, EtOH; ↓ effects **W/** anticholinergics, narcotics; ↓ effects **OF** cimetidine, digoxin **Labs:** ↑ Serum ALT, AST, amylase; ✓ baseline Cr **NIPE:** Monitor for extrapyramidal effects; ↓ w/ renal impair/elderly; ↑ risk of infxn; ⊘ live vaccines; grapefruit/grapefruit juice may ↑ SEs; wear or carry medical alert tag

Metoclopramide (Metozolv, Reglan, Generic)   WARNING: Chronic use may cause tardive dyskinesia; D/C if Sxs develop; avoid prolonged use (> 12 wk) **Uses:** *Diabetic gastroparesis, symptomatic GERD; chemo & post-op N/V, facilitate small-bowel intubation & upper GI radiologic exam*, *GERD, diabetic gastroparesis *(Metozolv)* stimulate gut in prolonged post-op ileus* **Action:** ↑ Upper GI motility; blocks dopamine in chemoreceptor trigger zone, sensitized tissues to ACH **Dose:** *Adults. Gastroparesis (Reglan):* 10 mg PO 30 min ac & hs for 2–8 wk PRN or same dose IM/IV for 10 d, then PO. *Reflux:* 10–15 mg PO 30 min ac & hs *Chemo antiemetic:* 1–2 mg/kg/dose IV 30 min before chemo, then q2h × 2 doses, then q3h × 3 doses *Post-op:* 10–20 mg IV/IM q4–6h PRN *Adults & Peds > 14 y. Intestinal intubation:* 10 mg IV × 1 over 1–2 min *Peds. Reflux:* 0.1–0.2 mg/kg/dose PO 30 min ac & hs *Chemo antiemetic:* 1–2 mg/kg/dose IV as adults *Post-op:* 0.25 mg/kg IV q6–8h PRN *Peds. Intestinal intubation:* *6–14 y:* 2.5–5 mg IV × 1 over 1–2 min *< 6 y:* Use 0.1 mg/kg IV × 1 **Caution:** [B, M] Drugs w/ extrapyramidal ADRs, MAOIs, TCAs, sympathomimetics **CI:** w/ EPS meds, GI bleeding, pheochromocytoma, Sz disorders, GI obst **Disp:** Tabs 5, 10 mg; syrup 5 mg/5 mL; ODT *(Metozolv)* 5, 10 mg; Inj 5 mg/mL **SE:** Dystonic Rxns common w/ high doses (Rx w/ IV diphenhydramine), fluid retention, restlessness, D, drowsiness **Notes:** ↓ w/ Renal impair/elderly; ✓ baseline Cr **NIPE:** May cause drowsiness—caution driving; ⊘ EtOH; elderly at ↑ risk for tardive dyskinesia; take 30 min ac; monitor BS in DM—may need insulin adjustment

Metolazone   (Zaroxolyn)   [Antihypertensive/Thiazide Diuretic] Uses: *Mild–mod essential HTN & edema of renal Dz or cardiac failure* **Action:** Thiazide-like diuretic; ↓ distal tubule Na reabsorption **Dose:** *HTN:* 2.5–5 mg/d PO qd *Edema:* 2.5–20 mg/d PO **Caution:** [B, –] Avoid w/ Li, gout, digitalis, SLE, many interactions **CI:** Anuria, hepatic coma or precoma **Disp:** Tabs 2.5, 5, 10 mg **SE:** Monitor fluid/lytes; dizziness, ↓ BP, ↓ K⁺, ↑ HR, ↑ uric acid, CP, photosensitivity **Interactions:** ↑ Effects *W/* antihypertensives, barbiturates, narcotics, nitrates, EtOH, food; ↑ effects *OF* digoxin, Li; ↑ hyperglycemia *W/* BBs, diazoxide; ↑ hypokalemia *W/* amphotericin B, corticosteroids, mezlocillin, piperacillin, ticarcillin; ↓ effects *W/* cholestyramine, colestipol, hypoglycemics, insulin, NSAIDs, salicylates; ↓ effects *OF* methenamine **Labs:** ↑ Uric acid; ↓ K⁺, NA⁺, Mg⁺, monitor lytes **NIPE:** ↑ Risk of photosensitivity—use sunblock; ↑ risk of gout; monitor ECG for hypokalemia (flattened T waves); ⊘ EtOH; maintain adequate hydration

Metoprolol Succinate (Toprol XL), Metoprolol Tartrate (Lopressor) [Antihypertensive/BB]   WARNING: Do not acutely stop Rx as marked worsening of angina can result; taper over 1–2 wk **Uses:** *HTN, angina, AMI, CHF (XL form)* **Action:** β₁-Adrenergic receptor blocker **Dose:** *Adults. Angina:* 50–200 mg PO bid max 400 mg/d; ER form dose qd *HTN:* 50–200 mg PO bid max 450 mg/d, ER form dose qd *AMI:* 5 mg IV q2min × 3 doses, then 50 mg PO q6h × 48 h, then 100 mg PO bid *CHF (XL form preferred)* 12.5–25 mg/d PO × 2 wk, ↑

2-wk intervals target: 200 mg max, use low dose w/ greatest severity *ECC 2010:* **AMI:** 5 mg slow IV q5min, total 15 mg; then 50 mg PO, titrate to effect *Peds.* *1–17 y.* *HTN* IR form 1–2 mg/kg/d PO, max 6 mg/kg/d (200 mg/d) ≥ *6 y.* *HTN* ER form 1 mg/kg/d PO, initial max 50 mg/d, ↑ PRN to 2 mg/kg/d max; ↓ w/ hepatic failure; take w/ meals **Caution:** [C, M] Uncompensated CHF, ↓ HR, heart block, hepatic impair, MyG, PVD, Raynaud, thyrotoxicosis **CI:** For HTN/angina SSS (unless paced), severe PVD, cardiogenic shock, severe PAD, 2nd-, 3rd-H block pheochromocytoma. For MI sinus brady < 45 BPM, 1st-degree block (PR > 0.24 s), 2nd-, 3rd-degree block, SBP < 100 mm Hg, severe CHF, cardiogenic shock **Disp:** Tabs 25, 50, 100 mg; ER tabs 25, 50, 100, 200 mg; Inj 1 mg/mL **SE:** Drowsiness, insomnia, ED, ↓ HR, bronchospasm **Interactions:** ↑ Effects *W/* cimetidine, dihydropyridine, diltiazem, fluoxetine, hydralazine, methimazole, OCPs, propylthiouracil, quinidine, quinolones; ↑ effects *OF* hydralazine; ↑ bradycardia *W/* digoxin, dipyridamole, verapamil; ↓ effects *W/* barbiturates, NSAIDs, rifampin; ↓ effects *OF* isoproterenol, theophylline **Labs:** ↑ BUN, SCr, LFTs, uric acid **NIPE:** IR: ER 1:1 daily dose but ER/XL is qd. OK to split XL tabs but do not crush/chew; take w/ food, ⊘ D/C abruptly—withdraw over 2 wk

Metronidazole (Flagyl, Flagyl ER, MetroCream, MetroGel, MetroLotion) [Antibacterial, Antiprotozoals] WARNING: Carcinogenic in rats Uses: *Bone/Jt, endocarditis, intra-Abd, meningitis, & skin Infxns; amebiasis & amebic liver abscess; trichomoniasis in pt & partner; bacterial vaginosis; PID; giardiasis; antibiotic associated pseudomembranous colitis (*C difficile*), eradicate *H pylori* w/ combo Rx, rosacea, prophylactic in post-op colorectal surgery* **Action:** Interferes w/ DNA synth **Spectrum:** Excellent anaerobic, *C difficile* **Dose:** *Adults.* *Anaerobic Infxns:* 500 mg IV q6–8h *Amebic dysentery:* 500–750 mg/d PO q8h × 5–10 d *Trichomonas:* 250 mg PO tid for 7 d or 2 g PO × 1 (Rx partner) *C difficile:* 500 mg PO or IV q8h for 7–10 d (PO preferred; IV only if pt NPO), if no response, change to PO vancomycin *Vaginosis:* 1 applicator intravag qd or bid × 5 d, or 500 mg PO bid × 7 d or 750 mg PO qd × 7 d *Acne rosacea/skin:* Apply bid *Giardia:* 500 mg PO bid × 5–7 d *H pylori:* 250–500 mg PO w/ meals & hs × 14 d, combine w/ other antibiotic & a PPI or H₂ antagonist *Peds.* *Anaerobic Infxns:* PO: 15–35 mg/kg/d ÷ q8h *IV:* 30 mg/kg IV/d ÷ q6h, 4 g/d max ÷ dose *Amebic dysentery:* 35–50 mg/kg/24 h PO in 3 ÷ doses for 5–10 d *Trichomonas:* 15–30 mg/kg/d PO ÷ q8h × 7 d *C difficile:* 30 mg/kg/d PO ÷ q6h × 10 d, max 2 g/d; ↓ w/ severe hepatic/renal impair **Caution:** [B, –] Avoid EtOH, w/ warfarin, CYP3A4 substrates (Table 10), ↑ Li levels **CI:** 1st tri of PRG **Disp:** Tabs 250, 500 mg; ER tabs 750 mg; caps 375 mg; IV 500 mg/100 mL; lotion 0.75%; gel 0.75%, 1%; intravag gel 0.75% (5 g/applicator 37.5 mg in 70-g tube); cream 0.75%,1% **SE:** Disulfiram-like Rxn; dizziness, HA, GI upset, anorexia, urine discoloration, flushing, metallic taste **Interactions:** ↑ Effects *W/* cimetidine; ↑ effects *OF* carbamazepine, 5-FU, Li, warfarin; ↓ effects *W/* barbiturates, cholestyramine, colestipol, phenytoin **Labs:** May cause ↓ values for LFTs, triglycerides, glucose

NIPE: Take w/ food; take ER on empty stomach; for trichomoniasis-Rx pt's partner; no aerobic bacteria activity; use in combo w/ serious mixed Infxns; wait 24 h after 1st dose to breast-feed or 48 h if extended therapy; ⊘ EtOH during and 3 d after Rx

Mexiletine (Generic) [Antiarrhythmic/Lidocaine Analogue]
WARNING: Mortality risks noted for flecainide and/or encainide (Class I antiarrhythmics). Reserve for use in pts w/ life-threatening ventricular arrhythmias **Uses:** *Suppress symptomatic vent arrhythmias* **DN Action:** Class Ib antiarrhythmic (Table 9) **Dose:** *Adults.* 200–300 mg PO q8h. Initial 200 mg q8h, can load w/ 400 mg if needed, ↑ q2–3d, 1200 mg/d max, ↓ dose w/ hepatic impairment or CHF, administer ATC & w/ food **Caution:** [C, +] CHF, may worsen severe arrhythmias; interacts w/ hepatic inducers & suppressors **CI:** Cardiogenic shock or 2nd-/3rd-degree AV block w/o pacemaker **Disp:** Caps 150, 200, 250 mg **SE:** Lightheadedness, dizziness, anxiety, incoordination, GI upset, ataxia, hepatic damage, blood dyscrasias, PVCs, N/V, tremor **Interactions:** ↑ Effects *W/* fluvoxamine, quinidine, caffeine; ↑ effects *OF* theophylline; ↓ effects *W/* atropine, hydantoins, phenytoin, phenobarbital, rifampin, tobacco **Labs:** ↑ LFTs; ↓ plts; monitor LFTs & CBC; false(+) ANA **NIPE:** Take w/ food or antacid ↓ GI upset; may cause drowsiness—caution driving

Micafungin (Mycamine) Uses: *Candidemia, acute disseminated, and esophageal candidiasis, Candida peritonitis & abscesses; prophylaxis Candida Infxn w/ HSCT* **Acts:** Echinocandin; ↓ fungal cell wall synth **Dose:** *Candidemia, acute disseminated candidiasis, Candida peritonitis & abscesses:* 100 mg IV qd *Esophageal candidiasis:* 150 mg IV daily *Prophylaxis of Candida Infxn:* 50 mg IV qd over 1 h **W/P:** [C, ?/–] Sirolimus, nifedipine, itraconazole dosage adj may be necessary **CI:** Component or other echinocandin allergy **Disp:** Inj 50, 100 mg vials **SE:** N/V/D, HA, pyrexia, Abd pain, ↓ K⁺, ↓ plt, histamine Sxs (rash, pruritus, facial swelling, vasodilatation), anaphylaxis, anaphylactoid Rxn, hemolysis, hemolytic anemia, ↑ LFTs, hepatotox, renal impair **NIPE:** Infuse over 1 h—rapid infusion ↑ risk of histamine-mediated reactions

Miconazole (Monistat 1 Combo, Monistat 3, Monistat 7) [OTC] (Monistat-Derm) [Antifungal] Uses: *Candidal Infxns, dermatomycoses (tinea pedis/tinea cruris/tinea corporis/tinea versicolor/candidiasis)* **Action:** Azole antifungal, alters fungal membrane permeability **Dose:** *Intravag:* 100 mg supp or 2% cream intravag qhs × 7 d or 200 mg supp or 4% cream intravag qhs × 3 d *Derm:* Apply bid, AM/PM *Tinea versicolor:* Apply qd. Treat tinea pedis and tinea corporis for 1 mo and other Infxns for 2 wk *Peds* ≥ *12 y.* 100 mg supp or 2% cream intravag qhs × 7 d or 200 mg supp or 4% cream intravag qhs × 3 d. Not for OTC use in children < 2 y **Caution:** [C, ?] Azole sensitivity **Disp:** *Monistat-Derm:* (Rx) Cream 2%; *Monistat 1 combo:* 2% cream w/ 1200 mg supp, *Monistat 3:* Vag cream 4%, supp 200 mg; *Monistat 7:* cream 2%, supp 100 mg; lotion 2%; powder 2%; effervescent tab 2%, oint 2%, spray 2%; Vag supp 100, 200, 1200 mg; Vag cream 2%, 4% [OTC] **SE:** Vag burning; on skin contact dermatitis, irritation, burning **Interactions:** ↑ Effects *OF* anticoagulants, cisapride, loratadine, phenytoin, quinidine; ↓ effects **W/** amphotericin B; ↓ effects **OF** amphotericin B **Labs:** ↑ Protein **NIPE:** Antagonistic to amphotericin B in vivo; may interfere w/ condom & diaphragm, do not use w/ tampons; avoid tight-fitting clothing

Miconazole/Zinc Oxide/Petrolatum (Vusion) [Antifungal] Uses:
Candidal diaper rash **Action:** Combo antifungal **Dose:** *Peds ≥ 4 wk.* Apply at each diaper change × 7 d **Caution:** [C, ?] **CI:** None **Disp:** Miconazole/zinc oxide/petrolatum oint 0.25/15/81.35%; 50-, 90-g tube **SE:** None **NIPE:** Keep diaper dry, not for prevention

Midazolam   (Generic)   [C-IV]   [Sedative/Benzodiazepine]
WARNING: Associated w/ resp depression and resp arrest especially when used for sedation in noncritical care settings. Reports of airway obst, desaturation, hypoxia, and apnea w/ other CNS depressants. Cont monitoring required; initial doses in elderly & debilitated should be conservative **Uses:** *Pre-op sedation, conscious sedation for short procedures & mechanically ventilated pts, induction of general anesthesia* **Action:** Short-acting benzodiazepine **Dose:** *Adults.* 1–5 mg IV or IM or 0.02–0.35 mg/kg based on indication; titrate to effect **Peds.** *Pre-op:* > 6 mo. 0.5–0.75 mg/kg PO, 20 mg max *> 6 mo.* 0.1–0.15 mg/kg IM × 1 max 10 mg *General anesthesia:* 0.025–0.1 mg/kg IV q2min for 1–3 doses PRN to induce anesthesia (↓ in elderly, w/ narcotics or CNS depressants) **Caution:** [D, M] w/ CYP3A4 substrate (Table 10), multiple drug interactions **CI:** NAG; w/ fosamprenavir, atazanavir, nelfinavir, ritonavir, intrathecal/epidural Inf of parenteral forms **Disp:** Inj 1, 5 mg/mL; syrup 2 mg/mL **SE:** Resp depression; ↓ BP w/ conscious sedation, N **Interactions:** ↑ Effects **W/** azole antifungals, antihistamines, cimetidine, CCBs, CNS depressants, erythromycin, INH, phenytoin, protease Inhibs, grapefruit juice, EtOH; ↓ effects **W/** rifampin, tobacco; ↓ effects **OF** levodopa **NIPE:** Monitor for resp depression; reversal w/ flumazenil; not for epidural/IT use; ⊘ EtOH after taking

Midodrine (Proamatine) [Antihypotensive/Vasopressor/Alpha-1 Agonist]
WARNING: Indicated for pts for whom orthohypotension significantly impairs daily life despite standard care **Uses:** *Tx orthostatic hypotension* **Action:** Vasopressor/antihypotensive; α₁-agonist **Dose:** 10 mg PO tid when pt plans to be upright **Caution:** [C, ?] **CI:** Pheochromocytoma, renal Dz, thyrotoxicosis, severe heart Dz, urinary retention, supine **Disp:** Tabs 2.5, 5, 10 mg **SE:** Supine HTN, paresthesia, urinary retention **Interactions:** ↑ Risk of bradycardia/AV block/ arrhythmias **W/** cardiac glycosides, BB, CNS drugs; ↑ effects **W/** pseudoephedrine, ergots, other α-agonists, & fludrocortisone; ↓ effects **W/** prazosin & other α-antagonists **NIPE:** SBP > 200 mm Hg in ~13% pts given 10 mg; may need to sleep with HOB ↑—monitor BP; ⊘ take ≤ 3 h hs

Mifepristone (Korlym)
WARNING: Antiprogestational; can cause termination of PRG. Exclude PRG before use or Rx is interrupted for > 14 d in ♀ of reproductive potential **Uses:** *Control hyperglycemia w/ Cushing synd and type 2 DM in nonsurgical or failed surgical candidates* **Acts:** Antiprogestin;

glucocorticoid receptor blocker **Dose:** Start 300 mg PO qd w/ meal, ↑ PRN 1200 mg/d max (20 mg/kg/d); mod renal hepatic impair 600 mg/d max **W/P:** [X, –] Do not use w/ severe hepatic impair or w/ OCP; avoid w/ ↑ QT or drugs that ↑ QT; ✓ for adrenal Insuff, ✓ K+; ✓ Vag bleed or w/ anticoagulants; caution w/ drugs metabolized by CYP3A, CYP2C8/2C9, CYP2B6 (eg, bupropion, efavirenz) **CI:** PRG, w/ simvastatin, lovastatin, CYP3A substrates, long-term steroids, unexplained uterine bleed, endometrial hyperplasia/CA **Disp:** 300 mg tab **SE:** N/V, fatigue, HA, ↓ K+, arthralgia, edema, ↑ BP, dizziness, ↓ appetite, endometrial hypertrophy **Notes:** RU486 discontinued NIPE: Take w/ meals; can ↓ effectiveness of BC pills—use non-hormone method of BC during and 1 mo after Rx ends; ⊘ PRG—will need a neg PRG test before starting; not for use in DM 2 not related to Cushing synd

Miglitol (Glyset) [Hypoglycemic/Alpha-Glucosidase Inhibitor]

Uses: *Type 2 DM* **Action:** α-Glucosidase Inhib; delays carbohydrate digestion **Dose:** Initial 25 mg PO tid; maint 50–100 mg tid (w/ 1st bite of each meal), titrate over 4–8 wk **Caution:** [B, –] w/ Digitalis & digestive enzymes, not rec w/SCr > 2 mg/dL **CI:** DKA, obstructive/inflammatory GI disorders; colonic ulceration **Disp:** Tabs 25, 50, 100 mg **SE:** Flatulence, D, Abd pain **Interactions:** ↑ Effects *W/* celery, coriander, juniper berries, ginseng, garlic; ↓ effects w/ INH, niacin, intestinal absorbents, amylase, pancreatin; ↓ effects *OF* digoxin, propranolol, ranitidine **Labs:** N Use w/ SCr > 2 mg/dL NIPE: Use alone or w/ sulfonylureas; ⊘ sugar for mild hypoglycemia—use gel or glucose tabs

Milnacipran (Savella) [Antidepressant/Serotonin & Norepinephrine Reuptake Inhibitor]

WARNING: Antidepressants associated w/ ↑ risk of suicide ideation in children and young adults **Uses:** *Fibromyalgia* **Action:** Antidepressant, SNRI **Dose:** 50 mg PO bid, max 200 mg/d; ↓ to 25 mg bid w/ CrCl < 30 mL/min **Caution:** [C, /?] Caution w/ hepatic impair, hepatox, serotonin syndrome, ↑ bleeding risk **CI:** NAG, w/ recent MAOI **Disp:** Tabs 12.5, 25, 50, 100 mg **SE:** HA, N/V, constipation, dizziness, ↑ HR, ↑ BP **Interactions:** ↑ Effects *OF* anticoagulants ↑ risk of serotonin synd *W/* Li, tramadol, triptans; ↓ effects *OF* clonidine **Labs:** ↑ LFTs NIPE: Monitor HR & BP; withdraw gradually; wait 14 d > D/C MAOI to start this drug. Wait 5 d > D/C this drug to start MAOI; ⊘ EtOH; may impair reaction time—caution driving

Milrinone (Primacor) [Vasodilator/Bipyridine Phosphodiesterase Inhibitor]

Uses: *CHF acutely decompensated* **Action:** Phosphodiesterase Inhib + inotrope & vasodilator; little chronotropic activity **Dose:** 50 mcg/kg, IV over 10 min, then 0.375–0.75 mcg/kg/min IV Inf; ↓ w/ renal impair **Caution:** [C, ?] **CI:** Allergy to drug; w/ inamrinone **Disp:** Inj 200 mcg/mL **SE:** Arrhythmias, ↓ BP, HA **Interactions:** ↑ Hypotension *W/* nesiritide **Labs:** Lytes, CBC, Mg2+ NIPE: Monitor fluids, BP, HR; not for long-term use; given in medical setting

Mineral Oil [OTC] [Emollient Laxative] Uses: *Constipation, bowel irrigation, fecal impaction* **Action:** Lubricant laxative **Dose:** *Adults. Constipation:* 15–45 mL PO/d PRN *Fecal impaction or after barium:* 118 mL rectally × 1 *Peds. > 6 y. Constipation:* 5–25 mL PO qd *2–12 y. Fecal impaction:* 59 mL rectally × 1 **Caution:** [?, ?] w/ N/V, difficulty swallowing, bedridden pts; may ↓ absorption of vits A, D, E, K, warfarin **CI:** Colostomy/ileostomy, appendicitis, diverticulitis, UC **Disp:** All [OTC] Liq, PO microemulsion 2.5 mL/5 mL, rectal enema 118 mL **SE:** Lipid pneumonia (aspiration of PO), N/V, temporary anal incontinence **Interactions:** ↑ Effects *W/* stool softeners; ↓ effects *OF* cardiac glycosides, OCPs, sulfonamides, vits, warfarin **NIPE:** Rectal incontinence; take PO upright; do not use PO in peds < 6 y; ☺ use > 1 wk

Mineral Oil-Pramoxine HCl/Zinc Oxide (Tucks Ointment [OTC]) [Topical Anesthetic] Uses: *Temporary relief of anorectal disorders (itching, etc)* **Action:** Topical anesthetic **Dose:** *Adults & Peds ≥ 12 y.* Cleanse, rinse, & dry, apply externally or into anal canal w/ tip 5 ×/d × 7 d max **Caution:** [? /?] Do not place into rectal tube **CI:** None **Disp:** Oint 30-g tube **SE:** Local irritation **NIPE:** D/C w/ or if rectal bleeding occurs or if condition worsens or does not improve w/in 7 d

Minocycline (Arestin, Dynacin, Minocin, Solodyn) [Antibiotic/Tetracycline] Uses: *Mod–severe nonnodular acne (Solodyn),* anthrax, rickettsiae, skin Infxn, URI, UTI, nongonoccocal urethritis, amebic dysentery, asymptomatic meningococcal carrier, *Mycobacterium marinum,* adjunct to dental scaling for periodontitis *(Arestin)*∗ **Action:** Tetracycline, bacteriostatic, ↓ protein synth **Dose:** *Adults & Peds > 12 y. Usual:* then 100 mg q12h or 100–200 mg IV or PO, then 50 mg qid *Gonococcal urethritis, men:* 100 mg q12h × 5 d *Syphilis:* Usual dose × 10–15 d *Meningococcal carrier:* 100 mg q12h × 5 d *M marinum:* 100 mg q12h × 6–8 wk *Uncomp urethral, endocervical, or rectal Infxn:* 100 mg q12h × 7 d minimum *Adults & Peds > 12 y. Acne: (Solodyn)* 1 mg/kg PO qd × 12 wk *> 8 y.* 4 mg/kg initially then 2 mg/kg q12h w/ food to ↓ irritation, hydrate well, ↓ dose or extend interval w/ renal impair **Caution:** [D, −] Associated w/ pseudomembranous colitis, w/ renal impair, may ↑ OCP, or w/ warfarin may ↑ INR **CI:** Allergy, children < 8 y **Disp:** Tabs 50, 75, 100 mg; tabs ER *(Solodyn)* 45, 65, 90, 115, 135 mg, caps *(Minocin)* 50, 100 mg, susp 50 mg/mL *(Arestin)* **SE:** D, HA, fever, rash, joint pain, fatigue, dizziness, photosensitivity, hyperpigmentation, SLE synd, pseudotumor cerebri **Interactions:** ↑ Effects *OF* digoxin, oral anticoagulants; ↑ risk of nephrotox *W/* methoxyflurane; ↓ effects *W/* antacids, cholestyramine, colestipol, laxatives, cimetidine, Fe products; ↓ effects *OF* hormonal contraceptives **Labs:** ↑ LFTs, BUN; ↓ HMG, plts, WBCs **NIPE:** Do not cut/crush/chew; keep away from children; risk of photosensitivity—use sunblock; may take *W/* food to < GI upset; ↑ fluids; tooth discoloration in < 8 y or w/ use last half of PRG; may ↓ effectiveness of hormonal BC

Minoxidil, Oral [Antihypertensive/Vasodilator] WARNING: May cause pericardial effusion, occasional tamponade, and angina pectoris may be exacerbated. Only for nonresponders to max doses of 2 other antihypertensives and a diuretic. Administer under supervision w/ a β-blocker and diuretic. Monitor for ↓ BP in those receiving guanethidine w/ malignant HTN **Uses:** *Severe HTN* **Action:** Peripheral vasodilator **Dose:** *Adults & Peds > 12 y.* 5 mg PO qd, titrate q3d, 100 mg/d max usual range 2.5–80 mg/d in 1–2 ÷ doses *Peds.* 0.2–1 mg/kg/24 h ÷ PO q12–24h, titrate q3d, max 50 mg/d; ↓ w/ elderly, renal Insuff **Caution:** [C,] Caution in renal impairment, CHF **CI:** Pheochromocytoma, component allergy **Disp:** Tabs 2.5, 10 mg **SE:** Pericardial effusion & vol overload w/ PO use; hypertrichosis w/ chronic use, edema, ECG changes, wgt gain **Interactions:** ↑ Hypotension **W/** guanethidine **Labs:** ↑ Alk phos, BUN, Cr, ↓ HMG, Hct **NIPE:** Take PO drug w/ food to < GI upset; avoid for 1 mo after MI

Minoxidil, Topical (Theroxidil, Rogaine) [OTC] [Topical Hair Growth]
Uses: *Male & female pattern baldness* **Action:** Stimulates vertex hair growth **Dose:** Apply 1 mL bid to area, D/C if no growth in 4 mo **Caution:** [?, ?] **CI:** Component allergy **Disp:** Soln & aerosol foam 2, 5% **SE:** Changes in hair color/texture **NIPE:** Hypertrichosis w/ chronic use; may take 4 mo to see results; requires chronic use to maintain hair; ⊘ to irritated/sunburned scalp

Mipomersen (Kynamro)
WARNING: May cause hepatotoxicity; ✓ AST, ALT , bili, alk phos before and during; hold if ALT/AST > 3 × ULN; D/C w/hepatotoxicity; may cause ↑ hepatic fat w or w/o ↑ ALT/AST (see label; D/C w/ significant liver tox; restricted KNAMRO REMS distribution) **Uses:** *Adjunct to lipid- lowering meds to ↓ LDL* **Action:** Inhib apolipoprotein B-100 synth **Dose:** *Adults* 200 mg SQ, 1 × wk **Caution:** [B, –] Inj site Rxns (pain, redness, etc); flu-like symptoms w/in 48 h **CI:** Mod/severe liver Dz, unexplained ↑ ALT/AST **Disp:** Single-use vial or prefilled syringe, 1 mL, 200 mg/mL **SE:** HA, palpitations, N, V, pain in ext, ↑ ALT/AST **NIPE:** Available only from certified pharm—Kynamro REMS program; teach SQ Inj tech; monitor LFTs; limit EtOH

Mirabegron (Myrbetriq)
Uses: *OAB* **Action:** β₃-adrenergic agonist; relaxes smooth muscle **Dose:** *Adults.* 25 mg PO daily; ↑ to 50 mg daily after 8 wk PRN; 25 mg max daily w/ severe renal or mod hepatic impair; swallow whole **Caution:** [C, –] w/ Severe uncontrolled HTN; urinary retention w/ BOO & antimuscarinic drugs; w/ drugs metabolized by CYP2D6; do not use w/ ESRD or severe hepatic impair **CI:** None **Disp:** Tabs ER 25, 50⁻mg **SE:** HTN, HA, UTI, nasopharyngitis, N/D, constipation, Abd pain, dizziness, tachycardia, URI, arthralgia, fatigue **NIPE:** Take w/out regard to food; swallow whole w/ H₂O—⊘ chew/crush/split; may take up to 8 wk to see + effects; check BP often

Mirtazapine (Remeron, Remeron SolTab) [Tetracyclic Antidepressant]
WARNING: ↑ Risk of suicidal thinking and behavior in children, adolescents, and young adults w/ major depression and other psychological disorders. Not for peds **Uses:** *Depression* **Action:** α₂-Antagonist antidepressant, ↑ norepinephrine & 5-HT **Dose:** 15 mg PO hs, up to 45 mg/d hs **Caution:** [C, M] Has anticholergic effects, w/ Sz, clonidine, CNS depressant use, CYP1A2,

CYP3A4 inducers/Inhib w/ hepatic & renal impairment **CI:** MAOIs w/in 14 d **Disp:** Tabs 7.5, 15, 30, 45 mg; rapid dispersion tabs (SolTab) 15, 30, 45 mg **SE:** Somnolence, ↑ cholesterol, constipation, xerostomia, wgt gain, agranulocytosis, ↓ BP, edema, musculoskeletal pain **Interactions:** ↑ Effects W/ CNS depressants, fluvoxamine; ↑ risk of HTN crisis W/ MAOIs **Labs:** ↑ ALT, cholesterol, triglycerides **NIPE:** Handle rapid tabs w/ dry hands, do not cut or chew; do not ↑ dose at intervals < q1–2wk; ⊘ rapid withdrawal; may cause dizziness/drowsiness—caution driving; limit EtOH

Misoprostol (Cytotec) [Mucosal Protective Agent/Prostaglandin] **WARNING:** Use in PRG can cause Ab, premature birth, or birth defects; do not use to ↓ ulcer risk in women of childbearing age; must comply w/ birth control measures **Uses:** *Prevent NSAID-induced gastric ulcers; medical termination of PRG < 49 d w/ mifepristone*; induce labor (cervical ripening); incomplete & therapeutic Ab **Action:** Prostaglandin (PGE-1), antisecretory & mucosal protection; induces uterine contractions **Dose:** *Ulcer prevention:* 100-200 mcg PO qid w/ meals; in females, start 2nd/3rd d of next nl period *Induction of labor (term):* 25–50 mcg intravag *PRG termination:* 400 mcg PO on d 3 of mifepristone; take w/ food **Caution:** [X, –] **CI:** PRG, component allergy **Disp:** Tabs 100, 200 mcg **SE:** Miscarriage w/ severe bleeding; HA, D, Abd pain, constipation **Interactions:** ↑ HA & GI Sxs W/ phenylbutazone **NIPE:** Not used for induction of labor w/ previous C-section or major uterine surgery

Mitomycin (Mitosol) [Antineoplastic/Alkylating Agent] **WARNING:** Administration only by physician experienced in chemotherapy; myelosuppressive; can induce hemolytic-uremic synd w/ irreversible renal failure **Uses:** *Stomach, pancreas*, breast, colon CA; squamous cell CA of the anus; NSCLC, head & neck, cervical; bladder CA (intravesically), *Mitosol* for glaucoma surgery **Action:** Alkylating agent; generates oxygen-free radicals w/ DNA strand breaks **Dose:** (Per protocol) 20 mg/m² q6–8wk IV or 10 mg/m² combo w/ other myelosuppressive drugs q6–8wk *Bladder CA:* 20–40 mg in 40 mL NS via a urethral catheter once/wk; ↓ in renal/hepatic impair **Caution:** [D, –] w/ Cr > 1.7 mg/dL/ ↑ cardiac tox w/ vinca alkaloids/doxorubicin **CI:** ↓ Plt, coagulation disorders, ↑ bleeding tendency PRG **Disp:** Inj 5, 20, 40 mg; *Mitosol* 0.2 mg/vial **SE:** ↓ BM (persists for 3–8 wk, may be cumulative; minimize w/ lifetime dose < 50–60 mg/m²), N/V, anorexia, stomatitis, renal tox, microangiopathic hemolytic anemia w/ renal failure (hemolytic–uremic synd), venoocclusive liver Dz, interstitial pneumonia, alopecia, extrav Rxns, contact dermatitis; CHF w/ doses > 30 mg/m² **Interactions:** ↑ Bronchospasm W/ vinca alkaloids; ↑ BM suppression W/ antineoplastics **Labs:** ↓ Plt, ↓ WBC, monitor plts, WBCs, differential, Hgb repeatedly during & for at least 8 wk after therapy **NIPE:** Monitor fluid balance & avoid overhydration; ⊘ PRG or breast-feeding

Mitoxantrone (Generic) [Antineoplastic/Antibiotic] **WARNING:** Administer only by physician experienced in chemotherapy; except for acute leukemia, do not use w/ ANC of < 1500 cells/mm³; severe neutropenia can result in Infxn, follow CBC; cardiotox (CHF), secondary AML reported **Uses:** *AML w/ (cytarabine), ALL, CML, PCA, MS, lung CA,* breast CA, & NHL **Action:** DNA-intercalating agent; ↓ DNA synth by interacting w/ topoisomerase II **Dose:** Per protocol; ↓ w/ hepatic impair, leukopenia, thrombocytopenia **Caution:** [D, −] Reports of secondary AML, w/ MS ↑ CV risk, do not treat MS pt w/ low LVEF **CI:** PRG, sig ↓ in LVEF **Disp:** Inj 2 mg/mL **SE:** ↓ BM, N/V, stomatitis, alopecia (infrequent), cardiotox, urine discoloration, secretions & scleras may be blue-green **Interactions:** ↑ BM suppression *W/* antineoplastics; ↓ effects *OF* live virus vaccines **Labs:** ↑ AST, ALT, uric acid **NIPE:** ↑ Fluids to 2–3 L/d, maint hydration, ⊘ vaccines, Infxn; baseline CV eval w/ ECG & LVEF; cardiac monitoring prior to each dose; not for IT use; may cause urine to turn blue-green color

Modafinil (Provigil) [C-IV] [Analeptic/CNS Stimulant] **Uses:**
Improve wakefulness in pts w/ excess daytime sleepiness (narcolepsy, sleep apnea, shift work sleep disorder)* **Action:** Alters dopamine & norepinephrine release, ↓ GABA-mediated neurotransmission **Dose:** 200 mg PO qAM; ↓ dose 50% w/ elderly/hepatic impair **Caution:** [C, M] CV Dz; ↑ effects of warfarin, diazepam, phenytoin; ↓ OCP, cyclosporine, & theophylline effects **CI:** Component allergy **Disp:** Tabs 100, 200 mg **SE:** Serious rash including SJS, HA, N, D, paresthesias, rhinitis, agitation, psychological Sx **Interactions:** ↑ Effects *OF* CNS stimulants, diazepam, phenytoin, propranolol, TCAs, warfarin; ↓ effect *OF* cyclosporine, OCPs, theophylline **Labs:** ↑ Glucose, AST, GTT **NIPE:** Take w/o regard to food; monitor BP; use barrier contraception; CV assessment before using; avoid large amts beverages w/ caffeine

Moexipril (Univasc) [Antihypertensive/ACEI] **WARNING:** ACE
Inhib can cause fatal injury/death in 2nd/3rd tri; D/C w/ PRG **Uses:** *HTN, post-MI*, DN* **Action:** ACE Inhib **Dose:** 7.5–30 mg in 1–2 ÷ doses 1 h ac ↓ in renal impair **Caution:** [C (1st tri, D 2nd & 3rd tri), ?] **CI:** ACE Inhib sensitivity **Disp:** Tabs 7.5, 15 mg **SE:** ↓ BP, edema, angioedema, HA, dizziness, cough, ↑ K⁺ **Interactions:** ↑ Effects *W/* diuretics, antihypertensives, EtOH, probenecid, garlic; ↑ effects *OF* insulin, Li; ↑ risk of hyperkalemia *W/* K⁺ supl, K⁺-sparing diuretics; ↓ effects *W/* antacids, ASA, NSAIDs, ephedra, yohimbe, ginseng **Labs:** ↑ BUN, Cr, K⁺; ↓ Na⁺ **NIPE:** May alter sense of taste, may cause cough, ⊘ salt substitutes, ⊘ PRG, use barrier contraception; take 1 h ac

Mometasone and Formoterol (Dulera) **WARNING:** Increased risk of
worsening wheezing or asthma-related death in pediatric/adolescent pts w/ long-acting Beta₂-adrenergic agonists; use only if asthma not controlled on agent such as inhaled steroid **Uses:** *Maint Rx for asthma* **Action:** Corticosteroid (mometasone) w/ LA bronchodilator Beta₂ agonist (formoterol) **Dose:** Adults & Peds > 12 y. 2 Inh q12h Caution: [C, ?/M] w/ P450 3A4 Inhib (eg, ritonavir), adrenergic/beta blockers, meds that ↑ QT interval; candida Infxn of mouth/throat, immunosuppression, adrenal suppression, ↓ bone density, w/ glaucoma/cataracts, may ↑ glucose, ↓

K; other LABA should not be used **CI:** Acute asthma attack; component hypersensitivity **Disp:** MDI 120 Inh/canister **SE:** mometasone/mcg formoterol) 100/5, 200/5 **SE:** Nasopharyngitis, sinusitis, HA, palpitations, CP, rapid heart rate, tremor or nervousness, oral candidiasis **Notes:** For pts not controlled on other meds (eg, low-medium dose Inh steroids) or whose Dz severity warrants 2 maint therapies **NIPE:** ⊘ asthma attack; may take up to 1 wk before Sx improve; ↑ risk of Infxn; rinse mouth with H_2O after inhalation;⊘ swallow rinse H_2O; ↑ risk bone loss in adults

Mometasone, Inhaled (Asmanex Twisthaler) [Corticosteroid]
Uses: *Maint Rx for asthma* **Action:** Corticosteroid **Dose:** *Adults & Peds > 11 y. On bronchodilators alone or inhaled steroids:* 220 mcg × 1 qPM (max 440 mcg/d) *On oral steroids:* 440 mcg bid (max 880 mcg/d) w/ slow oral taper *Peds 4–11 y.* 110 mcg × 1 qPM (max 110 mcg/d) **Caution:** [C, ?/M] *Candida* Infxn of mouth/ throat; hypersens Rxns possible; may worsen certain Infxn (TB, fungal, etc); monitor for ↑ / ↓ cortisol Sxs; ↓ bone density; ↓ growth in peds; monitor for NAG or cataracts; may ↑ glucose **CI:** Acute asthma attack; component hypersensitivity/ milk proteins **Disp:** MDI Inhal mometasone 110 mcg Twisthaler delivers 100 mcg/ actuation; 220 mcg Twisthaler delivers 200 mcg/actuation **SE:** HA, allergic rhinitis, pharyngitis, URI, sinusitis, oral candidiasis, dysmenorrhea, musculoskeletal/ back pain, dyspepsia **Labs:** Monitor for ↑/↓ cortisol; may ↑ glucose **NIPE:** Rinse mouth after use—⊘ swallow rinse H_2O; treat paradoxical bronchospasm w/ inhaled bronchodilator

Mometasone, Nasal (Nasonex) [Corticosteroid] **Uses:** *Nasal Sx allergic/seasonal rhinitis; prophylaxis of seasonal allergic rhinitis; nasal polyps in adults* **Action:** Corticosteroid **Dose:** *Adults & Peds ≥12 y. Rhinitis:* 2 sprays/each nostril qd *Adults. Nasal polyps:* 2 sprays/each nostril bid *Peds 2–11 y.* 1 spray/each nostril qd **Caution:** [C, M] Monitor for adverse effects on nasal mucosa (bleeding candidal Infxn, ulceration, perf); may worsen existing Infxns; monitor for NAG, cataracts; monitor for ↑/↓ cortisol Sxs ↓ growth in peds **CI:** Component hypersens **Disp:** 50 mg mometasone/spray **SE:** Viral Infxn, pharyngitis, epistaxis, HA **Labs:** Monitor for ↑/↓ cortisol Sxs **NIPE:** May take up to 2 wk to see + results; avoid exposure to Infxn

Montelukast (Singulair) [Bronchodilator/Leukotriene Receptor Antagonist] **Uses:** *Prevent/chronic Rx asthma ≥ 12 mo; seasonal allergic rhinitis ≥ 2 y; perennial allergic rhinitis ≥ 6 mo; prevent exercise bronchoconstriction (EIB) ≥ 15 y; prophylaxis & Rx of chronic asthma, seasonal allergic rhinitis* **Action:** Leukotriene receptor antagonist **Dose:** *Asthma: Adults & Peds > 15 y.* 10 mg/d PO in PM *6–23 mo:* 4-mg pack granules qd *2–5 y.* 4 mg/d PO qPM *6–14 y.* 5 mg/d PO qPM **Caution:** [B, M] **CI:** Component allergy **Disp:** Tabs 10 mg; chew tabs 4, 5 mg; granules 4 mg/pack **SE:** HA, dizziness, fatigue, rash, GI upset, Churg–Strauss synd, flu, cough, neuropsych events (agitation, restlessness, suicidal ideation) **Interactions:** ↑/↓ Effects W/ phenobarbital, rifampin **Labs:** ↑ AST, ALT

NIPE: Not for acute asthma; do not dose w/in 24 h of previous; granules can be mixed only with applesauce, mashed carrots, rice, or ice cream, breast milk or formula—⊘ mix with H_2O

Morphine (Avinza XR, Astramorph/PF, Duramorph, Infumorph, MS Contin, Kadian SR, Oramorph SR, Roxanol) [C-II] [Analgesic/Opioid Agonist] WARNING: Do not crush/chew SR/CR forms; swallow whole or sprinkle on applesauce. 100 or 200 mg for opioid-tolerant pt only for mod–severe pain when pain control needed for an extended period and not PRN. Be aware of misuse, abuse, diversion. No alcoholic beverages while on therapy.

Uses: *Rx severe pain*AMI, acute pulmonary edema **Action:** Narcotic analgesic; SR/CR forms for chronic use **Dose:** *Adults. Short-term use PO:* 5–30 mg q4h PRN *IV/IM:* 2.5–15 mg q2–6h *Supp:* 10–30 mg q4h *SR formulations* 15–60 mg q8–12h (do not chew/crush) *IT/epidural* (Duramorph, Infumorph, Astramorph/PF): Per protocol in Inf device *ECC 2010:* **STEMI:** 2–4 mg IV (over 1–5 min), then give 2–8 mg IV q5–15min PRN **NSTEMI:** 1–5 mg slow IV if Sxs unrelieved by nitrates or recur; use w/ caution; can be reversed w/ 0.4–2 mg IV naloxone *Peds > 6 mo.* 0.1–0.2 mg/kg/dose IM/IV q2–4h PRN; 0.15–0.2 mg/kg PO q3–4h PRN **Caution:** [C, +/–] Severe resp depression possible, w/ head injury; chewing delayed release forms can cause severe rapid release of morphine. Administer *Duramorph* in staffed environment d/t cardiopulmonary effects. IT doses 1/10 of epidural dose **CI: (many product specific)** Severe asthma, resp depression, GI obst/ileus *Oral soln:* CHF d/t lung Dz, head injury, arrhythmias, brain tumor, acute alchoholism, DTs, Sz disorders *MS Contin and Kadian* CI include hypercarbia **Disp:** IR tabs 15, 30 mg; soln 10, 20, 100 mg/5 mL; supp 5, 10, 20, 30 mg; Inj 2, 4, 5, 8, 10, 15, 25, 50 mg/mL *MS Contin CR* tabs 15, 30, 60, 100, 200 mg *Oramorph SR* tabs 15, 30, 60, 100 mg *Kadian SR* caps 10, 20, 30, 40, 50, 60, 70, 80, 100, 130, 150, 200 mg; *Avinza XR* caps 30, 60, 90, 120 mg *Duramorph/Astramorph PF* Inj 0.5, 1 mg/mL *Infumorph* 10, 25 mg/mL **SE:** Narcotic SE (resp depression, sedation, constipation, N/V, pruritus, diaphoresis, urinary retention, biliary colic), granulomas w/ IT **Interactions:** ↑ Effects *W/* cimetidine, CNS depressants, dextroamphetamine, TCAs, EtOH, kava kava, valerian, St. John's wort; ↑ effects *OF* warfarin; ↑ risk of HTN crisis *W/* MAOIs; ↓ effects *W/* opioids, phenothiazines **Labs:** ↑ Serum amylase, lipase **NIPE:** May require scheduled dosing to relieve severe chronic pain; do not crush/chew SR/CR forms; ⊘ EtOH; ensure Rx to prevent constipation is available; ⊘ abrupt withdrawal

Morphine & Naltrexone (Embeda) [C-II] [Opioid Receptor Agonist/Antagonist] WARNING: For mod–severe chronic pain; do not use as PRN analgesic; swallow whole or sprinkle contents of cap on applesauce; do not crush/dissolve, chew caps—rapid release & absorption of morphine may be fatal & of naltrexone may lead to withdrawal in opioid-tolerant pts; do not consume EtOH or EtOH-containing products; 100/4 mg caps for opioid-tolerant pts only, may cause fatal resp depression; high potential for abuse **Uses:** *Chronic mod–severe

pain* **Action:** Mu-Opioid receptor agonist & antagonist **Dose:** *Adult.* Individualize PO q12–24h; if opioid naive start 20/0.8 mg q24h; titrate q48h; ↓ start dose in elderly, w/ hepatic/renal Insuff; taper to D/C **Caution:** [C, –] w/ EtOH, CNS depress, muscle relaxants, use w/in 14 d of D/C of MAOI **CI:** Resp depression, acute/severe asthma/hypercarbia, ileus, hypersensitivity **Disp:** Caps ER (morphine mg/naltrexone mg) 20/0.8, 30/1.2, 50/2, 60/2.4, 80/3.2, 100/4 **SE:** N/V/D, constipation, somnolence, dizziness, HA, ↓ BP, pruritus, insomnia, anxiety, resp depression, Sz, MI, apnea, withdrawal w/ abrupt D/C, anaphylaxis, biliary spasm **Interactions:** ↑ Morphine absorption *W/* EtOH; ↑ CNS depression *W/* antiemetics, phenothiazines, sedatives, hypnotics, muscle relaxants; ↓ effects *OF* diuretics **NIPE:** Withdrawal w/ abrupt D/C, do not give via NG tube; do not use during or w/in 14 d of MAOIs; see Morphine

Moxifloxacin (Avelox) [Antibiotic/Fluoroquinolone] WARNING: ↑ Risk of tendon rupture & tendonitis; ↑ risk w/ age > 60, transplant pts; may ↑ Sx of MG **Uses:** *Acute sinusitis & bronchitis, skin/soft-tissue/intra-Abd Infxns, conjunctivitis, CAP,* TB, anthrax, endocarditis **Action:** 4th-gen quinolone; ↓ DNA gyrase **Spectrum:** Excellent gram(+) except MRSA & *E faecium*; good gram(−) except *P aeruginosa, Stenotrophomonas maltophilia,* & *Acinetobacter* sp; good anaerobic **Dose:** 400 mg/d PO/IV daily; avoid cation products, antacids tid **Caution:** [C, –] Quinolone sensitivity; interactions w/ Mg^{2+}, Ca^{2+}, Al^{2+}, Fe^{2+}-containing products, & Class IA & III antiarrhythmic agents (Table 9) **CI:** Quinolone/component sensitivity **Disp:** Tabs 400 mg, *ABC Pak* 5 tabs, Inj **SE:** Dizziness, N, QT prolongation, Szs, photosensitivity, peripheral neuropathy risk **Interactions:** ↑ Effects *W/* probenecid; ↑ effects *OF* diazepam, theophylline, caffeine, metoprolol, propranolol, phenytoin, warfarin; ↓ effects *W/* antacids, didanosine, Fe salts, Mg, sucralfate, $NaHCO_3$, Zinc **Labs:** ↑ LFTs, BUN, SCr, amylase, PT, triglycerides, cholesterol; ↓ HMG, Hct **NIPE:** ⊘ Give to children < 18 y; ↑ fluids to 2–3 L/d; take w/ or w/o food; ↑ risk photosensitivity—use sunscreen

Moxifloxacin Ophthalmic (Moxeza, Vigamox) [Antibiotic/Fluoroquinolone] Uses: *Bacterial conjunctivitis* **Action:** See Moxifloxacin Instill into affected eye/s: *Moxeza:* 1 gtt bid × 7 d *Vigamox* 1 gtt tid × 7 d **Caution:** [C, M] Not well studied in Peds < 12 mo **CI:** Quinolone/component sensitivity **Disp:** Ophthal soln 0.5% **SE:** ↓ Visual acuity, ocular pain, itching, tearing, conjunctivitis; prolonged use may result in fungal overgrowth, do not wear contacts w/ conjunctivitis **NIPE:** Prolonged use may result in fungal overgrowth, do not wear contacts w/ conjunctivitis; teach use of eye drops

Multivitamins, Oral [OTC] (Table 12)

Mupirocin (Bactroban, Bactroban Nasal) [Topical Anti-Infective] Uses: *Impetigo (oint); skin lesion infect w/ *S aureus* or *S pyogenes*; eradicate MRSA in nasal carriers* **Action:** ↓ Bacterial protein synth **Dose:** *Topical:* Apply small amount 3 ×/d × 5–14 d *Nasal:* Apply 1/2 single-use tube bid in nostrils × 5 d **Caution:** [B, ?/M] **CI:** Do not use w/ other nasal products **Disp:** Oint 2%; cream

2%; nasal oint 2% 1-g single-use tubes **SE:** Local irritation, rash **Interactions:** ↓ Bacterial action **W/** chloramphenicol **NIPE:** Pt to contact healthcare provider if no improvement in 3–5 d

Mycophenolic Acid (Myfortic) [Immunosuppressant/Mycophenolic Acid Derivative]
WARNING: ↑ Risk of Infxns, lymphoma, other CAs, progressive multifocal leukoencephalopathy (PML), risk of PRG loss and malformation, female of childbearing potential must use contraception **Uses:** *Prevent rejection after renal transplant* **Action:** Cytostatic to lymphocytes **Dose:** **Adults.** 720 mg PO bid. Doses differ based on transplant. **Peds.** BSA 1.19–1.58 m^2: 540 mg bid BSA > 1.58 m^2: Adult dose; used w/ steroids or tacrolimus ↓ w/ renal Insuff/neutropenia; take on empty stomach **Caution:** [D, –] **CI:** Component allergy **Disp:** Delayed-release tabs 180, 360 mg **SE:** N/V/D, GI bleed, pain, fever, HA, anemia, leukopenia, HTN, anemia, leukopenia, pure red cell aplasia, edema **Interactions:** ↓ **OF** phenytoin, theophylline; ↓ **W/** antacids, cholestyramine, Fe **Labs:** ↑ Cholesterol; monitor CBC **NIPE:** Best if taken on empty stomach; if GI distress—take w/ food; ⊘ take w/ antacids; avoid crowds & people w/ Infxns

Mycophenolate Mofetil (CellCept) [Immunosuppressant/Mycophenolic Acid Derivative]
WARNING: ↑ Risk of Infxns, lymphoma, other CAs, progressive multifocal leukoencephalopathy (PML); risk of PRG loss and malformation; female of childbearing potential must use contraception **Uses:** *Prevent organ rejection after transplant* **Action:** Cytostatic to lymphocytes **Dose:** **Adults.** 1 g PO bid, doses based on transplant **Peds.** BSA 1.2–1.5 m^2: 750 mg PO bid. BSA > 1.5 m^2: 1 g PO bid; used w/ steroids & cyclosporine or tacrolimus; ↓ in renal Insuff or neutropenia **IV:** Infuse over > 2 h PO: Take on empty stomach, do not open caps **Caution:** [D, –] **CI:** Component allergy; IV use in polysorbate 80 allergy **Disp:** Caps 250, 500 mg; susp 200 mg/ mL, Inj 500 mg **SE:** N/V/D, pain, fever, HA, Infxn, anemia, leukopenia, edema **Interactions:** ↑ Effects **W/** acyclovir, ganciclovir, probenecid; ↑ effects **OF** acyclovir, ganciclovir; ↓ effects **W/** antacids, cholestyramine, cyclosporine, Fe, food; ↓ effects **OF** OCPs, phenytoin, theophylline **Labs:** ↑ Cholesterol; monitor CBC **NIPE:** Use barrier contraception during & 6 wk after drug therapy; ⊘ exposure to Infxn; take w/o food; ⊘ crush/chew/split tab or cap

Nabilone (Cesamet) [C-II] [Synthetic Cannabinoid]
Uses: *Refractory chemotherapy-induced emesis* **Action:** Synthetic cannabinoid **Dose:** **Adults.** 1–2 mg PO bid 1–3 h before chemotherapy, 6 mg/d max; may continue for 48 h beyond final chemotherapy dose **Peds:** ↑ Per protocol; < 18 kg 0.5 mg bid; 18–30 kg 1 mg bid; > 30 kg 1 mg tid **Caution:** [C, –] Elderly, HTN, heart failure, w/ psychological illness, substance abuse; high protein binding w/ 1st-pass metabolism may lead to drug interactions **Disp:** Caps 1 mg **SE:** Drowsiness, vertigo, xerostomia, euphoria, ataxia, HA, difficulty concentrating, tachycardia, ↓ BP **Interactions:** ↑ CNS depression **W/** benzodiazepines, barbiturates, CNS depressants, EtOH; ↑ effects **W/** opioids; ↑ effects **OF** opioids; cross-tolerance **W/** opioids

NIPE: May require initial dose evening before chemotherapy; Rx only quantity for single Tx cycle

Nabumetone (Relafen) [Analgesic, Anti-Inflammatory, Antipyretic/NSAID]
WARNING: May ↑ risk of CV events & GI bleeding, perforation; CI W/ postop CABG **Uses:** *OA & RA*, pain **Action:** NSAID; ↓ prostaglandins **Dose:** 1000–2000 mg/d ÷ daily–bid W/ food **Caution:** [C, –] Severe hepatic Dz, peptic ulcer Dz, anaphylaxis w/ "ASA triad" **CI:** NSAID sensitivity, perioperative pain, after CABG surgery **Disp:** Tabs 500, 750 mg **SE:** Dizziness, rash, GI upset, edema, peptic ulcer, ↑ BP, photosens **Interactions:** ↑ Effects W/ aminoglycosides; ↑ effects OF anticoagulants, hypoglycemics, Li, MTX, thrombolytics; ↑ GI effects W/ ASA, corticosteroids, K⁺ supls, NSAIDs, EtOH; ↓ effects OF antihypertensives, diuretics **NIPE:** Photosens—use sunblock; ↑ risk of GI bleed w/ concurrent use of EtOH & tobacco; take w/ 8 oz H₂O, remain in upright position for ≥ 15 min

Nadolol (Corgard) [Antihypertensive, Antianginal/Beta-Blocker]
Warning: Do not abruptly withdraw **Uses:** *HTN & angina migraine prophylaxis*, prophylaxis of variceal hemorrhage **Action:** Competitively blocks β-adrenergic receptors (β₁, β₂) **Dose:** 40–80 mg/d; ↑ to 240 mg/d (angina) or 320 mg/d (HTN) at 3–7-d intervals; ↓ in renal Insuff & elderly **Caution:** [C +M] **CI:** Uncompensated CHF, shock, heart block, asthma **Disp:** Tabs 20, 40, 80, mg **SE:** Nightmares, paresthesias, ↓ BP, ↓ HR, fatigue, ↓ sex Fxn **Interactions:** ↑ Effects W/ antihypertensives, diuretics, nitrates, EtOH; ↑ effects OF aminophylline, lidocaine; ↑ risk of HTN W/ clonidine, ephedrine, epinephrine, MAOIs, phenylephrine, pseudoephedrine; ↑ bradycardia W/ digitalis glycosides, ephedrine, epi, phenylephrine, pseudoephedrine; ↓ effects W/ ampicillin, antacids, clonidine, NSAIDs, thyroid meds; ↓ effects OF glucagon, theophylline **NIPE:** May ↑ cold sensitivity; ⊘ D/C abruptly; may impair Rxn time—caution driving

Nafarelin, Metered Spray (SYNAREL)
Uses: *Endometriosis, CPP* **Action:** GnRH agonist; ↓ gonadal steroids w/ use > 4 wk **Dose:** **Adults.** Endometriosis: 400 mcg/d (1 spray qAM/PM) alternate nostril; if no amenorrhea ↑ 2 sprays bid, start d 2–4 of menstrual cycle **Peds.** CPP: 1600 mcg/d (2 sprays each nostril qAM/PM), can ↑ to 1800 mcg/d **Caution:** [X, –] **CI:** Component hypersensitivity, undiagnosed uterine bleeding, PRG, breast-feeding **Disp:** 0.5-oz bottle 60 sprays (200 mcg/spray) **SE:** ♀: Hot flashes, headaches, emotional lability, ↓ libido, vaginal dryness, acne, myalgia, ↓ breast size, ↓ BMD *Peds:* Drug sensitivity Rxn, acne, transient ↑ breast enlargement/pubic hair, Vag bleed, emotional lability, body odor, seborrhea **Notes:** ✓ PRG test before use; for endometriosis only if > 18 y, and no more than 6 mo; no sig effect w/ rhinitis; if needed, use decongestant 2 h before dose **NIPE:** Teach use of nasal spray; may ↓ effectiveness of oral contraceptives—use nonhormonal method of BC

Nafcillin (Nallpen, Generic) [Antibiotic/Penicillinase-Resistant Penicillin]
Uses: *Infxns d/t susceptible strains of Staphylococcus & Streptococcus* **Action:** Bactericidal; antistaphylococcal PCN; ↓ cell wall synth *Spectrum:*

Good gram(+) except MRSA & enterococcus, no gram(−), poor anaerobe **Dose:** *Adults.* 1–2 g IV q4–6h *Peds.* 50–200 mg/kg/d ÷ q4–6h **Caution:** [B, ?] **CI:** PCN allergy, allergy to corn-related products **Disp:** Inj powder 1, 2 g **SE:** Interstitial nephritis, N/D, fever, rash, allergic Rxn **Interactions:** ↑ Effects *OF* MTX; ↓ effects *W/* chloramphenicol, macrolides, tetracyclines; ↓ effects *OF* cyclosporine, OCPs, tacrolimus, warfarin **Labs:** ↑ Serum protein; no adjustments for renal Fxn **NIPE:** Aminoglycosides not compatible; monitor for super Infxn; no adjustment for renal Fxn

Naftifine (Naftin) [Antifungal/Antibiotic] **Uses:** *Tinea pedis, cruris, & corporis* **Action:** Allylamine antifungal, ↓ cell membrane ergosterol synth **Dose:** Apply daily (cream) or bid (gel) **Caution:** [B, ?] **CI:** Component sensitivity **Disp:** 1% Cream; gel **SE:** Local irritation **NIPE:** D/C if irritation occurs; confirm diagnosis w/ KOH smear and/or culture; avoid occlusive dressings, mucous membranes; re-evaluate if no improvement in 4 wk

Nalbuphine (Generic) [Analgesic/Narcotic Agonist-Antagonist] **Uses:** *Mod–severe pain; pre-op & obstetric analgesia* **Action:** Narcotic agonist–antagonist; ↓ ascending pain pathways **Dose:** *Adults. Pain:* 10 mg/70 kg IV/IM/SQ q3–6h; adjust PRN; 20 mg/dose or 160 mg/d max. *Anesthesia: Induction:* 0.3–3 mg/kg IV over 10–15 min *Maint:* 0.25–0.5 mg/kg IV *Peds.* 0.2 mg/kg IV or IM, 20 mg/dose or 160 mg/d max; ↓ w/ renal/in hepatic impair **Caution:** [B, M] w/ Opiate use **CI:** Component sensitivity **Disp:** Inj 10, 20 mg/mL **SE:** CNS depression, drowsiness; caution, ↓ BP **Interactions:** ↑ CNS depression *W/* cimetidine, CNS depressants; EtOH ↑ effects *OF* digitoxin, phenytoin, rifampin **Labs:** ↑ Serum amylase, lipase **NIPE:** Monitor for resp depression—can occur at lower dosage

Naloxone (Generic) [Antidote/Opioid Antagonist] **Uses:** *Opioid addiction (diagnosis) & OD* **Action:** Competitive narcotic antagonist **Dose:** *Adults.* 0.4–2 mg IV, IM, or SQ q2–3min; total dose 10 mg max *Peds.* 0.01–0.1 mg/kg/dose IV, IM, or SQ; repeat IV q3min × 3 doses PRN **ECC 2010: Total reversal of narcotic effects:** 0.1 mg/kg q2min PRN; max dose 2 mg; smaller doses (1–5 mcg/kg may be used); cont Inf 2–160 mcg/kg/h **Caution:** [C, ?] May precipitate acute withdrawal in addicts **Disp:** Inj 0.4, 1 mg/mL **SE:** ↓ BP, tachycardia, irritability, GI upset, pulm edema **Interactions:** ↓ Effects *OF* opiates **NIPE:** If no response after 10 mg, suspect nonnarcotic cause

Naloxone (Generic, Evzio) Uses: *Opioid addiction (dx) & OD* **Action:** Competitive opioid antagonist **Dose:** *Adults.* 0.4–2 mg IV, IM, or SQ q2–3 min; via endotracheal tube, dilute in 1–2 mL NS; may be given intranasal; total dose 10 mg max *Evzio:* 0.4 mg IM or sub-Q *Peds.* 0.01–0.1 mg/kg/dose IV, IM, or SQ; repeat IV q3min × 3 doses PRN *ECC 2010. Reverse narcotic effects:* 0.1 mg/kg q2min PRN; max dose 2 mg; smaller doses (1–5 mcg/kg may be used); cont Inf 2–160 mcg/kg/h **Caution:** [C, ?] *Evzio:* [B, ?/–] May precipitate withdrawal in addicts **CI:** Component hypersensitivity **Disp:** Inj 0.4, 1 mg/mL *Evzio:* 0.4 mg/0.4 mL prefilled auto-injector, w/ electronic voice instructions **SE:** ↓ BP,

↑ BP, fever, tachycardia, VT, VF, irritability, agitation, coma, GI upset, pulm edema, tremor, piloerection, sweating **NIPE:** Auto injector can be stored at home and used by caregiver; if no response after 10 mg, suspect nonnarcotic cause; w/ *Evizo* use in the field, seek emergent care immediately; duration of action less than most opioids, may need repeat dosing; for bystander use, administer in anterolateral thigh

Naltrexone (ReVia, Vivitrol, Generic) [Opioid Antagonist]
WARNING: Can cause hepatic injury, CI w/ active liver Dz **Uses:** *EtOH/narcotic addiction* **Action:** Antagonizes opioid receptors **Dose:** *EtOH/narcotic addiction:* 50 mg/d PO; must be opioid-free for 7–10 d *EtOH dependence:* 380 mg IM q4wk (*Vivitrol*) **Caution:** [C, M] Monitor for Inj site Rxns (*Vivitrol*) **CI:** Acute hep, liver failure, opioid use **Disp:** Tabs 50 mg; Inj 380 mg (*Vivitrol*) **SE:** Hepatotx; insomnia, GI upset, Jt pain, HA, fatigue **Interactions:** ↑ Lethargy & somnolence *W/* thiorida-zine; ↓ effects *OF* opioids **Labs:** ↑ LFTs **NIPE:** Must have negative naloxone challenge test before starting Rx; give IM in gluteal muscle & rotate; should carry med ID card

Naphazoline (Albalon, Naphcon, Generic), Naphazoline & Phe-niramine Acetate (Naphcon A, Visine A) [Ophthalmic Antihista-mine] **Uses:** *Relieve ocular redness & itching caused by allergy* **Action:** Sympathomimetic (α-adrenergic vasoconstrictor) & antihistamine (pheniramine) **Dose:** 1–2 gtt up to q6h, 3 d max **Caution:** [C, +] **CI:** NAG, in children < 6 y, w/ contact lenses, component allergy **SE:** CV stimulation, dizziness, local irritation **Disp:** Ophthal 0.012%, 0.025%, 0.1%/15 mL; naphazoline & pheniramine 0.025%/0.3% soln **Interactions:** ↑ Risk of HTN crisis *W/* MAOIs, TCAs **NIPE:** Teach use of eye drops; wait 15 min before inserting contact lenses

Naproxen (Aleve [OTC], Anaprox, Anaprox DS, EC-Naprosyn, Naprelan, Naprosyn, Generic) [Analgesic, Anti-Inflammatory, Antipyretic/NSAID] **WARNING:** May ↑ risk of CV events & GI bleeding **Uses:** *Arthritis & pain* **Action:** NSAID; ↓ prostaglandins **Dose:** *Adults & Peds > 12 y.* 200–500 mg bid–tid to 1500 mg/d max *> 2 y:* JRA 5 mg/kg/dose bid; ↓ in hepatic impair **Caution:** [C, (D 3rd tri), –] **CI:** NSAID or ASA triad sensitivity, peptic ulcer, post-CABG pain, 3rd tri PRG **Disp:** *Tabs:* 250, 375, 500 mg *DR:* 375, 500, 750 mg *CR:* 375, 550 mg; *susp* 25 mg/5 mL (*Aleve*) 200 mg multiple OTC forms **SE:** Dizziness, pruritus, GI upset, peptic ulcer, edema **Interactions:** ↑ Effects *W/* aminoglycosides; ↑ effects *OF* anticoagulants, hypoglycemics, Li, MTX, thrombolytics; ↑ GI effects *W/* ASA, corticosteroids, K+ supls, NSAIDs, EtOH; ↓ effects *OF* antihypertensives, diuretics **Labs:** ↑ BUN, Cr, LFTs, PT **NIPE:** Take w/ food to ↓ GI upset; take with 8 oz H_2O, remain upright for ≥ 15 min

Naproxen & Esomeprazole (Vimovo) [NSAID + Proton Pump Inhibitor] **WARNING:** ↑ Risk MI, stroke, PE; CI, CABG surgery pain; ↑ risk GI bleed, gastric ulcer, gastric/duodenal perforation **Uses:** *Pain and/or swelling, RA, OA, ankylosing spondylitis, ↓ risk NSAID-associated gastric ulcers*

Action: NSAID; ↓ prostaglandins & PPI, ↓ gastric acid **Dose:** 375/20 mg (naproxen/esomeprazole) to 500/20 mg PO bid **Caution:** [C 1st, 2nd tri; D 3rd; −] **CI:** PRG 3rd tri; asthma, urticaria from ASA or NSAID; mod–severe hepatic/ renal **Disp:** Tabs (naproxen/esomeprazole) DR 375/20 mg; 500/20 mg **SE:** N/D, Abd pain, gastritis, ulcer, ↑ BP, CHF, edema, serious skin rash (eg, Stevens-Johnson synd, etc), ↓ renal Fxn, papillary necrosis **Interactions:** ↑ Effects *OF* saquinavir, hydantoins, sulfonamides, sulfonylureas; ↑ Li levels; ↑ risk of GI bleed *W/* oral corticosteroid, SSRIs, smoking, EtOH; ↓ effects *OF* diuretics, BB, ACEI **Labs:** May ↑ Li levels; may cause MTX tox; may ↑ INR on warfarin; monitor levels Li, MTX, INR **NIPE:** Swallow whole; ⊘ crush/chew/split; risk of GI adverse events elderly; atrophic gastritis w/ long-term PPI use; possible ↑ risk of fxs w/ all PPI; may ↓ effect BP meds; may ↓ absorption of drugs requiring acid environment

Naratriptan (Amerge, Generic) [Migraine Suppressant/5-HT Agonist] **Uses:** *Acute migraine* **Action:** Serotonin 5-HT$_1$ receptor agonist **Dose:** 1–2.5 mg PO once; repeat PRN in 4 h; 5 mg/24 h max; ↓ in mild renal/hepatic Insuff, take w/ fluids **Caution:** [C, M] **CI:** Severe renal/hepatic impair, avoid w/ angina, ischemic heart Dz, uncontrolled HTN, cerebrovascular synds, & ergot use **Disp:** Tabs 1, 2.5 mg **SE:** Dizziness, sedation, GI upset, paresthesias, ECG changes, coronary vasospasm, arrhythmias **Interactions:** ↑ Effects *W/* MAOIs, SSRIs; ↑ effects *OF* ergot drugs; ↓ effects *W/* nicotine **NIPE:** Take w/ food; monitor ECG for ↑ PR or QT interval; ✓ BP; if 2nd dose needed, wait ≥ 4 h before taking

Natalizumab (Tysabri) [Immunomodulator/Monoclonal Antibody] **WARNING:** PML reported **Uses:** *Relapsing MS to delay disability and* ↓ recurrences, Crohn Dz* **Action:** Integrin receptor antagonist **Dose:** *Adults.* 300 mg IV q4wk; 2nd-line Tx only **CI:** PML; immune compromise or w/ immunosuppressant **Caution:** [C, ?/−] Baseline MRI to rule out PML **Disp:** Vial 300 mg **SE:** Infxn, immunosuppression; Inf Rxn precluding subsequent use; HA, fatigue, arthralgia **Interactions:** ↑ Risk of Infxn *W/* corticosteroids, immunosuppressants **Labs:** ↑ LFTs **NIPE:** Give slowly (over 1 h) w/ ↑ Rxns; limited distribution (TOUCH Prescribing Program); D/C stat w/ signs of PML (weakness, paralysis, vision loss, impaired speech, cognitive ↓); eval at 3 & 6 mo, then q6mo thereafter

Nateglinide (Starlix, Generic) [Hypoglycemic/Amino Acid Derivative] **Uses:** *Type 2 DM* **Action:** ↑ Pancreatic insulin release **Dose:** 120 mg PO tid 1–30 min ac; ↓ to 60 mg tid if near target HbA$_{1c}$ **Caution:** [C, −] w/ CYP2C9 metabolized drug (Table 10) **CI:** DKA, type 1 DM **Disp:** Tabs 60, 120 mg **SE:** Hypoglycemia, URI; salicylates, nonselective BBs may enhance hypoglycemia **Interactions:** ↑ Effects of hypoglycemia *W/* nonselective BBs, MAOIs, NSAIDs, salicylates, ↓ effects *W/* corticosteroids, niacin, sympathomimetics, thiazide diuretics, thyroid meds **Labs:** ↓ Glucose **NIPE:** ⊘ Take med if meal skipped; avoid EtOH

Nebivolol (Bystolic) [Cardioselective Beta-Blocker] **Uses:** *HTN* **Action:** β$_1$-Selective blocker **Dose:** *Adults.* 5 mg PO daily, ↑ q2wk to 40 mg/d max, ↓ w/ CrCl < 30 mL/min **Caution:** [D, +/−] **W/** Bronchospastic Dz, DM, heart failure, pheochromocytoma, **W/** CYP2D6 Inhib **CI:** ↓ HR, cardiogenic shock, decompensated CHF, severe hepatic impair **Disp:** Tabs 2.5, 5, 10, 20 mg **SE:** HA, fatigue, dizziness **Interactions:** ↑ Effects **W/** CYP2D6 Inhibs: Quinidine, propafenone, paroxetine, fluoxetine; may block epinephrine; **NIPE:** ⊘ D/C abruptly—taper over 1–2 wk; may impair Rxn time—caution driving

Nefazodone [Antidepressant/Serotonin Modulator] WARNING: Fatal hep & liver failure possible, D/C if LFTs > 3 × ULN, do not retreat; closely monitor for worsening depression or suicidality, particularly in ped pts **Uses:** *Depression* **Action:** ↓ Neuronal uptake of serotonin & norepinephrine **Dose:** Initial 100 mg PO bid; usual 300–600 mg/d in 2 ÷ doses **Caution:** [C, M] **CI:** w/ MAOIs, pimozide, carbamazepine, alprazolam; active liver Dz **Disp:** Tabs 50, 100, 150, 200, 250 mg **SE:** Postural ↓ BP & allergic Rxns; HA, drowsiness, xerostomia, constipation, GI upset, liver failure **Interactions:** ↑ Risk of hypotension **W/** antihypertensives, nitrates; ↑ effects **OF** alprazolam, CCB, digoxin, HMG-CoA reductase Inhibs, triazolam; ↑ risk of QT prolongation **W/** astemizole, cisapride, pimozide; ↑ risk of serious and/or fatal Rxn **W/** MAOIs; ↓ effects **OF** propranolol **Labs:** ↑ LFTs, cholesterol; ↓ Hct **NIPE:** Take w or W/o food; may take 2–4 wk for full therapeutic effects; monitor HR, BP; may cause dizziness—caution changing positions; avoid EtOH

Nelarabine (Arranon) [Antineoplastic/Antimetabolite] WARNING: Fatal neurotox possible **Uses:** *T-cell ALL or T-cell lymphoblastic lymphoma unresponsive > 2 other regimens* **Action:** Nucleoside (deoxyguanosine) analog **Dose:** *Adults.* 1500 mg/m² IV over 2 h ds 1, 3, 5 of 21-d cycle *Peds.* 650 mg/m² IV over 1 h ds 1–5 of 21-d cycle **Caution:** [D, ?/−] **Disp:** Vial 250 mg **SE:** Neuropathy, ataxia, Szs, coma, hematologic tox, GI upset, TLS (tumor lysis syndrome), HA, blurred vision **Labs:** Monitor CBC, ↑ transaminase levels, bilirubin ↓ **NIPE:** Prehydration, urinary alkalinization, allopurinol before dose; D/C if = grade 2 neurotox occurs; ⊘ live vaccines – avoid exposure to Infxn; ↑ fluids

Nelfinavir (Viracept) [Antiretroviral/Protease Inhibitor] **Uses:** *HIV Infxn, other agents* **Action:** Protease Inhib causes immature, noninfectious virion production **Dose:** *Adults.* 750 mg PO tid or 1250 mg PO bid. *Peds.* 25–35 mg/kg PO tid or 45–55 mg/kg bid; take w/ food **Caution:** [B, −] Many drug interactions; do not use **W/** salmeterol, colchicine (w/ renal/hepatic failure); adjust dose w/ bosentan, tadalafil for PAH; do not use tid dose w/ PRG **CI:** Phenylketonuria, w/ triazolam/midazolam use or drug dependent on CYP3A4 (Table 10); w/ α₁-adrenoreceptor antagonist (alfuzosin), PDE5 Inhib sildenafil **Disp:** Tabs 250, 625 mg; powder 50 mg/g **SE:** Dyslipidemia, lipodystrophy, D, rash **Interactions:** ↑ Effects **W/** erythromycin, ketoconazole, indinavir, ritonavir; ↑ effects **OF** barbiturates, carbamazepine, cisapride, ergot alkaloids, erythromycin, lovastatin, midazolam, phenytoin, saquinavir, simvastatin, triazolam; ↓ effects **W/** barbiturates, carbamazepine, phenytoin, rifabutin, rifampin, St. John's wort; ↓ effects **OF** OCP

Labs: ↑ LFTs **NIPE:** Take w/ food ↑ absorption; ⊘ mix with acidic foods; tabs can be dissolved in H_2O; use barrier contraception; PRG registry; maintain transmission precautions

Neomycin (Neo-Fradin, Generic) [Antibiotic]

WARNING: Systemic absorption of oral route may cause neuro-/oto-/nephrotox; resp paralysis possible w/ any route of administration **Uses:** *Hepatic coma, bowel prep* **Action:** Aminoglycoside, poorly absorbed PO; ↓ GI bacterial flora **Dose:** *Adults.* 3–12 g/24 h PO in 3–4 ÷ doses *Peds.* 50–100 mg/kg/24 h PO in 3–4 ÷ doses **Caution:** [C, ?/–] Renal failure, neuromuscular disorders, hearing impair **CI:** Intestinal obst **Disp:** Tabs 500 mg; PO soln 125 mg/5 mL **SE:** Hearing loss w/ long-term use; rash, N/V **NIPE:** Do not use parenterally (↑ tox); part of the condon bowel prep; ⊘ use > 2 wk; ⊘ PRG

Neomycin, Bacitracin, & Polymyxin B (Neosporin Ointment) (See Bacitracin, Neomycin, & Polymyxin B Topical)

Neomycin, Colistin, & Hydrocortisone (Cortisporin-TC Otic Drops); Neomycin, Colistin, Hydrocortisone, & Thonzonium (Cortisporin-TC Otic Susp) [Antibiotic/Aminoglycoside]

Uses: *Otitis externa, Infxns of mastoid/fenestration cavities* **Action:** Antibiotic w/ anti-inflammatory **Dose:** *Adults.* 5 gtt in ear(s) q6–8h. *Peds.* 3–4 gtt in ear(s) q6–8h **CI:** Component allergy; HSV, vaccinia, varicella **Caution:** [B, ?] **Disp:** Otic gtt & susp **SE:** Local irritation, rash **NIPE:** Shake well, limit use to 10 d/t minimize hearing loss; re-evaluation if no improvement in 1 wk

Neomycin, Polymyxin, & Hydrocortisone Ophthalmic (Generic) [Antibiotic/Anti-Inflammatory]

Uses: *Ocular bacterial Infxns* **Action:** Antibiotic w/ anti-inflammatory **Dose:** Apply a thin layer to the eye(s) or 1 gtt 1–4 ×/d **Caution:** [C, ?] **Disp:** Ophthal soln; ophthal oint **SE:** Local irritation **NIPE:** ⊘ wear contact lenses

Neomycin, Polymyxin, & Hydrocortisone Otic (Cortisporin Otic Solution, Generic Susp) [Antibiotic/Anti-Inflammatory]

Uses: *Otitis externa and infected mastoidectomy and fenestration cavities* **Action:** Antibiotic w/ anti-inflammatory **Dose:** *Adults.* 3–4 gtt in the ear(s) q6–8h *Peds > 2 y.* 3 gtt in the ear(s) q6–8h **CI:** Viral Infxn, hypersens to components **Caution:** [C, ?] **Disp:** Otic susp (generic); otic soln (Cortisporin) **SE:** Local irritation

Neomycin, Polymyxin B, & Dexamethasone (Maxitrol) [Antibiotic/Corticosteroid]

Uses: *Steroid-responsive ocular conditions w/ bacterial Infxn* **Action:** Antibiotic w/ anti-inflammatory corticosteroid **Dose:** 1–2 gtt in eye(s) q3–4h; apply oint in eye(s) q6–8h **CI:** Component allergy; viral, fungal, TB eye Dz **Caution:** [C, ?] **Disp:** Oint neomycin sulfate 3.5 mg/ polymyxin B sulfate 10,000 units/dexamethasone 0.1%/g; susp: identical/1 mL, 5 mL bottle **SE:** Local irritation **NIPE:** Use under supervision of ophthalmologist; teach use of eye drops/ ointment

Neomycin, Polymyxin B, & Prednisolone (Poly-Pred Ophthalmic) [Antibiotic/Corticosteroid] Uses: *Steroid-responsive ocular conditions w/ bacterial Infxn* Action: Antibiotic & anti-inflammatory Dose: 1–2 gtt in eye(s) q4–6h; apply oint in eye(s) q6–8 h Caution: [C, ?] Disp: Susp neomycin/polymyxin B/prednisolone 0.5%/mL SE: Irritation NIPE: Use under supervision of ophthalmologist; teach use of eye drops/ointment

Neomycin & Dexamethasone (AK-Neo-Dex Ophthalmic, Neo-Decadron Ophthalmic) [Antibiotic/Corticosteroid] Uses: *Steroid-responsive inflammatory conditions of the cornea, conjunctiva, lid, & anterior segment* Action: Antibiotic w/ anti-inflammatory corticosteroid Dose: 1–2 gtt in eye(s) q3–4h or thin coat q6–8h until response, then ↓ to daily Caution: [C, ?] Disp: Cream neomycin 0.5%/dexamethasone 0.1%; oint neomycin 0.35%/dexamethasone 0.05%; soln: neomycin 0.35%/dexamethasone 0.1% SE: Local irritation NIPE: Use under ophthalmologist's supervision; teach use of eye drops/ointment

Neomycin & Polymyxin B (Neosporin Cream) [OTC] [Antibiotic] Uses: *Infxn in minor cuts, scrapes, & burns* Action: Bactericidal Dose: Apply 2–4 ×/d Caution: [C, ?] CI: Component allergy Disp: Cream neomycin 3.5 mg/polymyxin B 10,000 units/g SE: Local irritation NIPE: Available only as generic; different from *Neosporin oint*

Neomycin-Polymyxin Bladder Irrigant [Neosporin GU Irrigant] [Antibiotic] Uses: *Cont irrigant prevent bacteriuria & gram(−) bacteremia associated w/ indwelling catheter* Action: Bactericidal; not for *Serratia* sp or streptococci Dose: 1 mL irrigant in 1 L of 0.9% NaCl; cont bladder irrigation w/ 1 L of soln/ 24 h, 10 d max Caution: [D] CI: Component allergy Disp: Soln neomycin sulfate 40 mg & polymyxin B 200,000 units/mL; amp 1, 20 mL SE: Rash, neomycin ototox or nephrotox (rare) NIPE: Potential for bacterial/fungal super Infxn; not for Inj; use only 3-way catheter for irrigation; ⊘ use > 10 d

Nepafenac (Nevanac) [Analgesic, Anti-Inflammatory, Antipyretic/NSAID] Uses: *Inflammation postcataract surgery* Action: NSAID Dose: 1 gtt in eye(s) tid 1 d before, and continue 14 d after surgery CI: NSAID/ASA sensitivity Caution: [C, ?/–] May ↑ bleeding time, delay healing, causes keratitis Disp: Susp 0.1% 3 mL SE: Capsular opacity, visual changes, foreign-body sensation, ↑ IOP Interactions: ↑ Effects *OF* oral anticoagulants NIPE: Prolonged use ↑ risk of corneal damage; shake well before use; separate from other drops by > 5 min; teach use of eye drops; ⊘ insert contact lenses for ≥ 15 min

Nesiritide (Natrecor) [Vasodilator/Human B-Type Natriuretic Peptide] Uses: *Acutely decompensated CHF* Action: Human b-type natriuretic peptide Dose: 2 mcg/kg IV bolus, then 0.01 mcg/kg/min IV Caution: [C, ?/–] When vasodilators are not appropriate CI: SBP < 100 mm Hg, cardiogenic shock Disp: Vials 1.5 mg SE: ↓ BP, HA, GI upset, arrhythmias, ↑ Cr Interactions: ↑ hypotension *W/* ACEIs, nitrates Labs: ↑ Cr; NIPE: Must be administered in medical setting; requires cont BP monitoring; FDA—neutral effect on mortality

Nevirapine (Viramune, Viramune XR, Generic) [Antiretroviral/ NNRTI] **WARNING:** Reports of fatal hepatotox even W/ short-term use; severe life-threatening skin Rxns (SJS, toxic epidermal necrolysis, & allergic Rxns); monitor closely during 1st 18 wk of Rx **Uses:** *HIV Infxn* **Action:** Nonnucleoside RT Inhib **Dose:** *Adults.* Initial 200 mg/d PO × 14 d, then 200 mg bid, 400 mg daily (XR) *Peds. > 15.* 150 mg/m² PO daily × 14 d, then 150 mg/m² PO bid (w/o regard to food) **Caution:** [B, –] OCP **Disp:** Tabs 200 mg; *(Viramune XR)* tabs ER 100, 400 mg; susp 50 mg 5 mL **SE:** Life-threatening rash; HA, fever, D, neutropenia, hep **Interactions:** ↑ Effects W/ clarithromycin, erythromycin; ↓ effects W/ rifabutin, rifampin, St. John's wort; ↓ effects OF clarithromycin, indinavir, ketoconazole, methadone, OCPs, protease Inhibs, warfarin **NIPE:** Take w/ or w/o food; ER—⊘ chew/crush/split; use barrier contraception; HIV resistance when given as monotherapy; always use in combo w/ at least 2 additional antiretroviral agents; ⊘ women if CD4 > 250 mcL or men > 400 mcL unless benefit > risk of hepatotox

Niacin (Nicotinic Acid) (Niaspan, Slo-Niacin, Niacor, Nicolar) [Some OTC Forms] [Antilipemic/Vitamin B Complex] **Uses:** *Sig hyperlipidemia/hypercholesteremia, nutritional supl* **Action:** Vit B₃; ↓ lipolysis; ↓ esterification of triglycerides; ↑ lipoprotein lipase **Dose:** *Hypercholesterolemia:* Start 500 mg PO qhs, ↑ 500 mg q4wk, maint 1–2 g/d; 2 g/d max; qhs w/ low-fat snack; do not crush/chew; niacin supl 1 ER tab PO qd or 100 mg PO qd *Pellagra:* Up to 500 mg/d **Caution:** [C, +] **CI:** Liver Dz, peptic ulcer, arterial hemorrhage **Disp:** ER tabs *(Niaspan)* 500, 750, 1000 mg & *(Slo-Niacin)* 250, 500, 750 mg; tab 500 mg *(Niacor)*; many OTC: tabs 50, 100, 250, 500 mg, ER caps 125, 250, 400 mg, ER tabs 250, 500 mg, elixir 50 mg 5 mL **SE:** Upper body/facial flushing & warmth; hepatox, GI upset, flatulence, exacerbate peptic ulcer, HA, paresthesias, liver damage, gout, altered glucose control in DM **Interactions:** ↑ Effects OF antihypertensives, anticoagulants; ↓ effects OF hypoglycemics, probenecid, sulfinpyrazone **Labs:** ✓ Cholesterol, LFTs, if on statins (eg, Lipitor) ✓ CPK & K⁺ **NIPE:** EtOH, hot beverages & spicy foods ↑ flushing; flushing ↓ by taking ASA or NSAID; may cause dizziness—caution driving, changing positions 30–60 min prior to dose *RDA adults:* Male 16 mg/d, female 14 mg/d

Niacin & Lovastatin (Advicor) [Nicotinic Acid Derivative + HMG-CoA Reductase Inhibitor] **Uses:** *Hypercholesterolemia* **Action:** Combo antilipemic agent, w/ HMG-CoA reductase Inhib **Dose:** *Adults.* Niacin 500 mg/ lovastatin 20 mg, titrate q4wk, max niacin 2000 mg/lovastatin 40 mg **Caution:** [X, –] See individual agents, D/C w/ LFTs > 3 × ULN **CI:** PRG **Disp:** Niacin mg/ lovastatin mg: 500/20, 750/20, 750/20, 1000/20, 1000/40 tabs **SE:** Flushing, myopathy/ rhabdomyolysis, N, Abd pain, ↑ LFTs **Interactions:** ↑ Effects OF ganglionic blockers, vasoactive drugs; separate dosing of bile acid sequestrants by 4–6 h; ↑ risk of myopathy W/ cyclosporine; ↑ effects OF antihypertensives, anticoagulants **Labs:** ↑ LFTs; monitor CK, PT, plts **NIPE:** Take with low-fat meal/snack—⊘ take on empty stomach; ↓ flushing by taking ASA or NSAID 30 min before; ⊘ grapefruit/ grapefruit juice; ⊘ PRG/breast-feeding; also see Niacin

Niacin & Simvastatin (Simcor) [HMG-CoA Reductase Inhibitor & a Nicotinic Acid Derivative] **Uses:** *Hypercholesterolemia* **Action:** Combo antilipemic agent w/ HMG-CoA reductase Inhib **Dose:** *Adults.* Niacin 500 mg/simvastatin 20 mg, titrate q4wk not to exceed max niacin 2000 mg/simvastatin 40 mg; max 1000 mg/20 mg w/ amlodipine and ranolazine **Caution:** [X, −] See individual agents, discontinue Rx if LFTs > 3 × ULN **CI:** PRG, active liver Dz, PUD, arterial bleeding, w/ strong CYP3A4 Inhib, w/ gemfibrozil, cyclosporine, danazol, verapamil, or diliazem, hypersensitivity to components **Disp:** Niacin mg/ simvastatin mg: 500/20, 500/40, 750/20, 1000/40 tabs **SE:** Flushing, myopathy/ rhabdomyolysis, N, Abd pain, ↑ LFTs **Interactions:** ↑ Effects **W/** amiodarone, verapamil; ↑ risk of postural hypotension **W/** ganglionic blockers, vasoactive drugs **Labs:** ↑ LFTs; monitor blood glucose, PT, plts; D/C therapy if LFTs > 3 × nl **NIPE:** Take hs w/ low-fat snack; swallow whole; separate dosing of bile acid sequestrants by 4–6 h; ↓ flushing by taking ASA or NSAID 30 min before; also see Niacin

Nicardipine (Cardene) [Antianginal/Antihypertensive/CCB] **Uses:** *Chronic stable angina & HTN*; prophylaxis of migraine **Action:** CCB **Dose:** *Adults.* PO: 20–40 mg PO tid **IV:** 5 mg/h IV cont Inf; ↑ by 2.5 mg/h q15min to max 15 mg/h **Peds.** (Not established) PO: 20–30 mg PO q8h **IV:** 0.5–5 mcg/kg/min; ↓ in renal/hepatic impair **Caution:** [C, ?/−] Heart block, CAD **CI:** Cardiogenic shock, aortic stenosis **Disp:** Caps 20, 30 mg; SR caps 30, 45, 60 mg; Inj 2.5 mg/mL **SE:** Flushing, tachycardia, ↓ BP, edema, HA **Notes:** *PO-to-IV conversion:* 20 mg tid = 0.5 mg/h, 30 mg tid = 1.2 mg/h, 40 mg tid = 2.2 mg/h **Interactions:** ↑ Effects **W/** cimetidine, grapefruit juice; ↑ effects **OF** cyclosporine; ↓ hypotension **W/** antihypertensives, fentanyl, nitrates, quinidine, EtOH; ↑ dysrhythmias **W/** digoxin, disopyramide, phenytoin; ↓ effects **W/** NSAIDs, rifampin; high-fat food **Labs:** ↑ LFTs **NIPE:** ↑ Risk of photosens—use sunblock; take w/ food (not high fat); limit EtOH, grapefruit/grapefruit juice; ER preferred— may ↓ SEs; may cause dizziness—caution driving, changing positions

Nicotine Gum (Nicorette, Others) [OTC] [Smoking Deterrent/ Cholinergic] **Uses:** *Aid to smoking cessation, relieve nicotine withdrawal* **Action:** Systemic delivery of nicotine **Dose:** Wk 1–6 one piece q1–2h PRN; wk 7–9 one piece q2–4h PRN; wk 10–12 one piece q4–8h PRN; max 24 pieces/d **Caution:** [C, ?] **CI:** Life-threatening arrhythmias, unstable angina **Disp:** 2 mg, 4 mg/ piece; mint, orange, original flavors **SE:** Tachycardia, HA, GI upset, hiccups **Interactions:** ↑ Effects **W/** cimetidine; ↑ effects **OF** catecholamines, cortisol; ↑ hemo-dynamic & AV blocking effects **OF** adenosine; ↓ effects **W/** coffee, cola **NIPE:** ⊘ Eat or drink for 15 min before using; chew 30 min for full dose of nicotine; ↓ absorption **W/** coffee, soda, juices, wine w/in 15 min; must stop smoking & perform behavior modification for max effect; use at least 9 pieces 1st 6 wk;

> 25 cigarette/d use 4 mg; < 25 cigarette/d use 2 mg; may cause dizziness—caution driving

Nicotine Nasal Spray (Nicotrol NS) [Smoking Deterrent/Cholinergic] Uses: *Aid to smoking cessation, relieve nicotine withdrawal* Action: Systemic delivery of nicotine Dose: 0.5 mg/actuation; 1–2 doses/h, 5 doses/h max; 40 doses/d max Caution: [D, M] CI: Life-threatening arrhythmias, unstable angina Disp: Nasal inhaler 10 mg/mL SE: Local irritation, tachycardia, HA, taste perversion Interactions: ↑ Effects W/ cimetidine, blue cohash; ↑ effects OF catecholamines, cortisol; ↑ hemodynamic & AV blocking effects OF adenosine NIPE: ⊘ In pts w/ chronic nasal disorders or severe reactive airway Dz; ↑ incidence of cough; must stop smoking & perform behavior modification for max effect; 1 dose = 1 spray each nostril = 1 mg; ⊘ swallow

Nicotine Transdermal (Habitrol, Nicoderm CQ [OTC], Others) [Smoking Deterrent/Cholinergic] Uses: *Aid to smoking cessation; relief of nicotine withdrawal* Action: Systemic delivery of nicotine Dose: Individualized; 1 patch (14–21 mg/d) & taper over 6 wk Caution: [D, M] CI: Life-threatening arrhythmias, unstable angina, adhesive allergy Disp: Habitrol & Nicoderm CQ: 7, 14, 21 mg of nicotine/24 h SE: Insomnia, pruritus, erythema, local site Rxn, tachycardia, vivid dreams Interactions: ↑ Effects W/ cimetidine, blue cohash; ↑ effects OF catecholamines, cortisol; ↑ hemodynamic & AV blocking effects OF adenosine; ↑ HTN W/ bupropion NIPE: Change application site daily; wear patch 16–24 h; must stop smoking & perform behavior modification for max effect; > 10 cigarette/d start w/ 2-mg patch; < 10 cigarette/d 1-mg patch

Nifedipine (Adalat CC, Afeditab CR, Procardia, Procardia XL) [Antihypertensive, Antianginal/CCB] Uses: *Vasospastic or chronic stable angina & HTN*; tocolytic Action: CCB Dose: Adults. SR tabs 30–90 mg/d Tocolysis: Per local protocol Peds. 0.25–0.5 mg/kg/24 h ÷ 3–4/d Caution: [C, +] Heart block, aortic stenosis, cirrhosis CI: IR preparation for urgent or emergent HTN; acute AMI Disp: Caps 10, 20 mg; SR tabs 30, 60, 90 mg SE: HA common on initial Rx; reflex tachycardia may occur w/ regular-release dosage forms; peripheral edema, ↓ BP, flushing, dizziness Interactions: ↑ Effects W/ antihypertensives, azole antifungals, cimetidine, cisapride, CCBs, diltiazem, famotidine, nitrates, quinidine, ranitidine, EtOH, grapefruit juice; ↑ effects OF digitalis glycosides, phenytoin, vincristine; ↓ effects W/ barbiturates, nafcillin, NSAIDs, phenobarbital, rifampin, St. John's wort, tobacco; ↓ effects OF quinidine Labs: ↑ LFTs NIPE: Adalat CC & Procardia XL not interchangeable; SL administration not OK; ↑ risk of photosens—use sunblock; ⊘ EtOH; caution w/ consumption of grapefruit/grapefruit juice

Nilotinib (Tasigna) [Kinase Inhibitor] WARNING: May ↑ QT interval; sudden deaths reported, use w/ caution in hepatic failure; administer on empty stomach Uses: *Ph(+) CML, refractory or at 1st dx* Action: TKI Dose: Adults. 300 mg bid bid—newly diagnosed; 400 mg bid resistant/intolerant on empty stomach 1 h prior or 2 h post meal **Caution:** [D, ?/–] Avoid w/ CYP3A4 Inhib/inducers (Table 10), adjust w/ hepatic impair, heme tox, QT ↑, avoid QT-prolonging agents w/ Hx pancreatitis, ↓ absorption w/ gastrectomy **CI:** ↓ K⁺, ↓ Mg²⁺, long QT synd **Disp:** 200 mg caps **SE:** ↓ WBC, ↓ plt, anemia, N/V/D, rash, edema, ↑ lipase, tumor lysis synd **Interactions:** ↑ Effects *W/* strong Inhibs of CYP3A4 such as ketoconazole, itraconazole, clarithromycin, atazanavir, indinavir, nefazodone, nelfinavir, ritonavir, saquinavir, telithromycin, voriconazole; grapefruit; strong CYP3A4 inducers ↓ effects *W/* dexamethasone, phenytoin, carbamazepine, rifampin, phenobarbital, St. John's wort; this drug is an Inhib of CYP3A4, CYP2C8, CYP2C9, CYP2D6, UGT1A1 enzymes & ↑ conc of drugs metabolized by these enzymes **Labs:** ↓ WBCs, plts; monitor CBCs q2wk for 1st 2 mo, then once monthly; monitor ECG at baseline, after 7 d, then periodically & after dose changes; monitor serum lipase, LFTs **NIPE:** ⊘ Eat anything for 1 h prior or 2 h after taking; swallow whole; capsule contents may be mixed with 1 tsp applesauce; ⊘ stomach acid reducers 10 h before or 2 h after taking; ⊘ antacids 2 h before or after taking; avoid grapefruit products; use chemotherapy precautions when handling; ⊘ PRG or breast-feeding—use adequate contraception

Nilutamide (Nilandron) [Antineoplastic/Antiandrogen] WARNING: Interstitial pneumonitis possible; most cases in first 3 mo; check CXR before & during Rx **Uses:** *Combo w/ surgical castration for metastatic PCa* **Action:** Nonsteroidal antiandrogen **Dose:** 300 mg/d PO × 30 d, then 150 mg/d **Caution:** [Not used in females] **CI:** Severe hepatic impair, resp Insuff **Disp:** Tabs 150 mg **SE:** Interstitial pneumonitis, hot flashes, ↓ libido, impotence, N/V/D, gynecomastia, hepatic dysfunction **Interactions:** ↑ Effects *OF* phenytoin, theophylline, warfarin **Labs:** ↑ LFTs (monitor) **NIPE:** Take w/o regard to food; visual adaptation may be delayed; may cause Rxn when taken w/ EtOH

Nimodipine (Generic) [Cerebral Vasodilator/CCB] WARNING: Do not give IV or by other parenteral routes; can cause death **Uses:** *Prevent vasospasm following subarachnoid hemorrhage* **Action:** CCB **Dose:** 60 mg PO q4h for 21 d; start w/in 96 h of subarachnoid hemorrhage; ↓ in hepatic failure **Caution:** [C, ?] **CI:** Component allergy **Disp:** Caps 30 mg **SE:** ↓ BP, HA, constipation, rash **Interactions:** ↑ Effects *W/* other CCB; grapefruit juice, EtOH; ↓ effects *W/* ephedra, St. John's wort, any food **Labs:** ↑ LFTs **NIPE:** Give via NG tube if caps cannot be swallowed whole, PO administration only on empty stomach; ↑ risk of photosens—use sunblock; ⊘ abrupt D/C

Nisoldipine (Sular) [Antihypertensive/CCB] Uses: *HTN* **Action:** CCB **Dose:** 8.5–34 mg/d PO; take on empty stomach; ↓ start doses w/ elderly or hepatic impair **Caution:** [C, –] **Disp:** ER tabs 8.5, 17, 25.5, 34 mg **SE:** Edema, HA, flushing, ↓ BP **Interactions:** ↑ Effects *W/* antihypertensives, cimetidine, nitrates, EtOH, high-fat foods; ↓ effects *W/* phenytoin, St. John's wort **NIPE:** Do not take w/ grapefruit products or high-fat meal; ✓ BP reg

Nitazoxanide (Alinia) [Anti-Infective/Antiprotozoal] Uses: *Cryptosporidium* or *Giardia lamblia*, C difficile–associated D* Action: Antiprotozoal interferes w/ pyruvate ferredoxin oxidoreductase *Spectrum: Cryptosporidium, Giardia* Dose: *Adults.* 500 mg PO q12h × 3 d; for C difficile × 10 d *Peds. 1–3 y.* 100 mg PO q12h × 3 d *4–11 y.* 200 mg PO q12h × 3 d > *12 y.* 500 mg q12h × 3 d; take w/ food Caution: [B, ?] Not effective in HIV or immunocompromised Disp: 100 mg/5 mL PO susp, 500 tab SE: Abd pain Interactions: ↑ Effects W/ warfarin NIPE: Susp contains sucrose, interacts w/ highly protein-bound drugs

Nitrofurantoin (Furadantin, Macrobid, Macrodantin) [Urinary Anti-Infective] Uses: *Prophylaxis & Rx UTI* Action: Interferes w/ metabolism & cell wall synthesis. *Spectrum:* Some gram(+) & (−) bacteria; *Pseudomonas, Serratia,* & most *Proteus* resistant Dose: *Adults.* Prophylaxis: 50–100 mg PO Rx: 50–100 mg PO qid × 7 d; *Macrobid* 100 mg PO bid × 7 d *Peds.* Prophylaxis: 1–2 mg/kg/d ÷ in 1–2 doses, max 100 mg/d Rx: 5–7 mg/kg/24 h in 4 ÷ doses (w/ food/milk/antacid) Caution: [B, +/not OK if child < 1 mo] Avoid w/ CrCl < 60 mL/min CI: Renal failure, infants < 1 mo, PRG at term Disp: Caps 25, 50, 100 mg *Furadantin:* Susp 25 mg/5 mL SE: GI effects, dyspnea, various acute/chronic pulm Rxns, peripheral neuropathy, hemolytic anemia w/ G6PD deficiency, rare aplastic anemia Interactions: ↑ Effects W/ probenecid, sulfinpyrazone; ↓ effects W/ antacids, quinolones Labs: ↑ Serum bilirubin, alk phos NIPE: Take W/ food; may turn urine brown; macrocrystals (Macrodantin) cause < N than other forms; not for comp UTI

Nitroglycerin (Nitrostat, Nitrolingual, Nitro-Bid Ointment, Nitro-Bid IV, Nitrodisc, Transderm-Nitro, NitroMist, Others) [Antianginal, Vasodilator/Nitrate] Uses: *Angina pectoris, acute & prophylactic Rx, CHF, BP control* Action: Relaxes vascular smooth muscle, dilates coronary arteries Dose: *Adults. SL:* 1 tab q5min SL PRN × 3 doses *Translingual:* 1–2 metered-doses sprayed onto PO mucosa q3–5min, max 3 doses *PO:* 2.5–9 mg tid *IV:* 5–20 mcg/min, titrated to effect *Topical:* Apply 1/2 in of oint to chest wall tid, wipe off at night *Transdermal:* 0.2–0.4 mg/h/patch daily *Aerosol:* 1 spray at 5-min intervals, max 3 doses *ECC 2010.* IV bolus: 12.5–25 mcg (if no spray or SL dose given) Inf: Start 10 mcg/min, ↑ by 10 mcg/min q3–5min until desired effect; ceiling dose typically 200 mcg/min SL: 0.3–0.4 mg, repeat q5min **Aerosol spray:** Spray 0.5–1 s at 5-min intervals *Peds.* 0.25–0.5 mcg/kg/min IV, titrate *ECC 2010:* Heart failure, HTN emergency, pulm HTN: Cont Inf 0.25–0.5 mcg/kg/min initial, titrate 1 mcg/kg/min q15–20min (typical dose 1–5 mcg/kg/min) Caution: [B, ?] Restrictive cardiomyopathy CI: w/ Sildenafil, tadalafil, vardenafil, head trauma, NAG, pericardial tamponade, constrictive pericarditis Disp: SL tabs 0.3, 0.4, 0.6 mg; translingual spray 0.4 mg/dose; SR caps 2.5, 6.5, 9 mg; Inj 0.1, 0.2, 0.4 mg/mL (premixed); 5 mg/mL Inj soln; oint 2%; transdermal patches 0.1, 0.2, 0.4, 0.6 mg/h; aerosol (*NitroMist*) 0.4 mg/spray; (*Rectiv*) intra-anal 0.4% **SE:** HA, ↓ BP, lightheadedness, GI upset **Interactions:** ↑ Hypotensive effects *W/* antihypertensives, phenothiazine, sildenafil, tadalafil, vardenafil, EtOH; ↓ effects *W/* ergot alkaloids; ↓ effects *OF* SL tabs & spray *W/* antihistamines, phenothiazine, TCAs **Labs:** False ↑ cholesterol, triglycerides **NIPE:** Nitrate tolerance w/ chronic use after 1–2 wk; minimize by providing 10–12 h nitrate-free period daily, using shorter-acting nitrates tid, & removing LA patches & oint before sleep to ↓ tolerance

Nitroprusside (Nitropress) [Antihypertensive/Vasodilator] **WARNING:** Cyanide tox & excessive hypotension **Uses:** *Hypertensive crisis, acute decompensated heart failure, controlled ↓ BP perioperation (↓ bleeding)*, aortic dissection, pulm edema **Action:** ↓ Systemic vascular resistance **Dose:** *Adults & Peds.* 0.25–10 mcg/kg/min IV Inf, titrate; usual dose 3 mcg/kg/min *ECC 2010:* 0.1 mcg/kg/min start, titrate dose (max dose 5–10 mcg/kg/min) *Peds. ECC 2010: Cardiogenic shock, severe HTN:* 0.3–1 mcg/kg/min, then titrate to 8 mcg/kg/min PRN **Caution:** [C, ?] ↓ Cerebral perfusion **CI:** High output failure, compensatory HTN **Disp:** Inj 25 mg/mL **SE:** Excessive hypotensive effects, palpitations, HA **Interactions:** ↑ Effects *W/* antihypertensives, anesthetics, sildenafil, tadalafil, vardenafil; ↑ risk of arrhythmias *W/* TCA **Labs:** ↑ Cr **NIPE:** Thiocyanate (metabolite w/ renal excretion) w/ tox at 5–10 mg/dL, more likely if used for > 2–3 d; w/ aortic dissection use w/ BB; discard colored soln other than light brown; monitor HR, resp, BP, SaO₂

Nizatidine (Axid, Axid AR [OTC]) [Gastric Antisecretory/H₂-Receptor Antagonist] **Uses:** *Duodenal ulcers, GERD, heartburn* **Action:** H₂-receptor antagonist **Dose:** *Adults. Active ulcer:* 150 mg PO bid or 300 mg PO hs; maint 150 mg PO hs *GERD:* 150 mg PO bid *Heartburn:* 75 mg PO bid *Peds. GERD:* 10 mg/kg PO bid, 150 mg bid max; ↓ in renal impair **Caution:** [B, ?] **CI:** H₂-receptor antagonist sensitivity **Disp:** Tabs 75 mg [OTC]; caps 150, 300 mg; soln 15 mg/mL **SE:** Dizziness, HA, constipation, D **Interactions:** ↑ Effects *OF* salicylates, EtOH; ↓ effects *W/* antacids, tomato/mixed veg juice **Labs:** ↑ LFTs, uric acid **NIPE:** Take w/ or w/o food; smoking ↑ gastric acid secretion; ⊘ EtOH; may ↓ Rxn time—caution driving

Norepinephrine (Levophed) [Adrenergic Agonist/Vasopressor/Sympathomimetic] **Uses:** *Acute ↓ BP, cardiac arrest (adjunct)* **Action:** Peripheral vasoconstrictor of arterial/venous beds **Dose:** *Adults.* 8–30 mcg/min IV, titrate *Peds.* 0.05–0.1 mcg/kg/min IV, titrate **Caution:** [C, ?] **CI:** ↓ BP d/t hypovolemia, vascular thrombosis, do not use w/ cyclopropane/halothane anesthetics **Disp:** Inj 1 mg/mL **SE:** ↓ HR, arrhythmia **Interactions:** ↑ HTN *W/* antihistamines, BBs, ergot alkaloids, guanethidine, MAOIs, methyldopa, oxytocic meds; interaction w/ TCAs leads to severe HTN; ↑ risk of arrhythmias *W/* cyclopropane, halothane **Labs:** ↑ Glucose **NIPE:** Correct vol depletion as much as possible before vasopressors; use large vein to avoid extrav; phentolamine 5–10 mg/10 mL NS injected locally for extrav

Norethindrone Acetate/Ethinyl Estradiol Tablets (Femhrt) (See Estradiol/Norethindrone Acetate)

Norfloxacin (Noroxin, Chibroxin Ophthalmic) [Antibiotic/Fluoroquinolone] **WARNING:** Use associated w/ tendon rupture, tendonitis, & myasthenia gravis exacerbation **Uses:** *Comp & uncomp UTI d/t gram(–) bacteria, prostatitis, gonorrhea*, infectious D, conjunctivitis **Action:** Quinolone, ↓ DNA gyrase, bactericidal. *Spectrum:* Broad gram(+) & (–) E faecalis, E coli, K pneumoniae, P mirabilis, P aeruginosa, S epidermidis, & S saprophyticus **Dose:** *Uncomp UTI (E coli, K pneumoniae, P mirabilis):* 400 mg PO bid × 3 d; other uncomp UTI Rx × 7–10 d *Comp UTI:* 400 mg PO q12h for 10–21 d *Gonorrhea:* 800 mg × 1 dose *Prostatitis:* 400 mg PO bid × 28 d *Gastroenteritis, travelers D:* 400 mg PO bid × 1–3 d; take 1 h ac or 2 h pc *Adults & Peds > 1 y.* Ophthal: 1 gtt each eye q2h for 7 d; CrCl < 30 mL/min use 400 mg qd *Gonorrhea:* [C, –] Quinolone sensitivity, w/ some antiarrhythmics ↑ QT **CI:** Hx allergy or tendon problems **Disp:** Tabs 400 mg; ophthal 3 mg/mL **SE:** Photosens, HA, dizziness, asthenia, GI upset, pseudomembranous colitis; ocular burning w/ ophthal, peripheral neuropathy risk w/PO only **Interactions:** ↑ Effects *W/* probenecid; ↑ effects *OF* diazepam, theophylline, caffeine, metoprolol, propranolol, phenytoin, warfarin; ↓ effects *W/* antacids, didanosine, Fe salts, mg, sucralfate, NaHCO₃, zinc; ↓ effects *W/* food **Labs:** ↑ LFTs, BUN, SCr **NIPE:** ⊘ Give to children < 18 y except for opthal sol; ↑ fluids to 2–3 L/d; may cause photosens—use sunblock; good conc in the kidney & urine, poor blood levels; not for urosepsis; ↑ risk of developing fluoroquinolone-associated tendonitis & tendon rupture is higher in pts > 60 y, in those taking corticosteroids, & in kidney, heart, & lung transplant recipients; take 2 h before/after Ca-enriched juice, bismuth subsalicylate, sucralfate, iron, and zinc and antacids w/ Mg, Al, or Ca; avoid caffeine, dairy

Nortriptyline (Aventyl, Pamelor) [Antidepressant/TCA] **WARNING:** ↑ Suicide risk in pts < 24 y w/ major depressive/ other psychological disorders esp during 1st mo of Tx; risk ↓ pts > 65 y; observe all pts for clinical Sxs; not for ped use **Uses:** *Endogenous depression* **Action:** TCA; ↑ synaptic CNS levels of serotonin &/or norepinephrine **Dose:** *Adults.* 25 mg PO tid–qid; > 150 mg/d not OK *Elderly.* 10–25 mg hs *Peds 6–7 y.* 10 mg/d *8–11 y.* 10–20 mg/d *> 11 y.* 25–35 mg/d, ↓ w/ hepatic Insuff **Caution:** [D, –] NAG, CV Dz **CI:** TCA allergy, use w/ MAOI **Disp:** Caps 10, 25, 50, 75 mg; (*Aventyl*) soln 10 mg/5 mL **SE:** Anticholinergic (blurred vision, retention, xerostomia, sedation) **Interactions:** ↑ Effects *W/* antihistamines, CNS depressants, cimetidine, fluoxetine, OCP, phenothiazine, quinidine, EtOH; ↑ effects *OF* anticoagulants; ↑ risk of HTN *W/* clonidine, levodopa, sympathomimetics; ↓ effects *W/* barbiturates, carbamazepine, rifampin **Labs:** ↑ Serum bilirubin, alk phos **NIPE:** Concurrent use *W/* MAOIs have resulted in HTN, Szs, death; ↑ risk of photosens—use sunscreen; max effect may take > 2–3 wk; teach measures to prevent constipation; caution driving

Nystatin (Mycostatin, Nilstat, Nystop) [Anti-Infective/Antifungal] Uses: *Mucocutaneous *Candida* Infxns (oral, skin, Vag)* **Action:** Alters membrane permeability *Spectrum:* Susceptible *Candida* sp **Dose:** *Adults & Peds. PO:* 400,000–600,000 units PO "swish & swallow" qid *Vag:* 1 tab Vag hs × 2 wk *Topical:* Apply bid–tid to area **Peds Infants.** 200,000 units PO q6h **Caution:** [B (C PO), +] **Disp:** PO susp 100,000 units/mL; PO tabs 500,000 units; troches 200,000 units; Vag tabs 100,000 units; topical cream/oint 100,000 units/g, powder 100,000 units/g **SE:** GI upset, SJS **NIPE:** Retain in mouth as long as possible; ⊘ eat ≥ 10 min after administration; store susp up to 10 d in refrigerator; not absorbed PO

Obinutuzumab (Gazyva) **WARNING:** May reactivate Hep B and cause progressive multifocal leukoencephalopathy w/death **Uses:** *CLL* **Action:** Cytolytic anti-CD20 antibody **Dose:** *Adults.* Six 28-day cycles; 100 mg d 1, 900 mg d 2, 1000 mg on d 8 & 15, then 1000 mg d 1 cycle 2–6 **Caution:** [C, –] Tumor lysis synd, give fluids, premedicate for ↑ uric acid, monitor renal Fxn; infusion reactions, premedicate w/ glucocorticoid, acetaminophen, and antihistamine; ↓ WBC, ↓ plts; Do not give live vaccines before or during Tx **CI:** None **Disp:** 1000 mg/40 mL; Single-use vial **SE:** Fever; cough; ↑ Cr; ↑ ALT/AST, alk phos; ↓ alb, ↓ Ca⁺⁺, ↓ Na⁺ **Notes:** Do not use if CrCl < 30 mg/mL **NIPE:** Premedicate as above to ↓ risk of infusion reaction; ↑ risk of Infxn—avoid exposure; no live vaccines; monitor neuro/mental status changes

Octreotide (Sandostatin, Sandostatin LAR) [Antidiarrheal/Hormone] **Uses:** *↓ Severe D associated w/ carcinoid & neuroendocrine GI tumors (eg, vasoactive intestinal peptide-secreting tumor [VIPoma], ZE synd), acromegaly*; bleeding esophageal varices **Action:** LA peptide; mimics natural somatostatin **Dose:** *Adults.* 100–600 mcg/d SQ/IV in 2–4 ÷ doses; start 50 mcg daily–bid *Sandostatin LAR (depot):* 10–30 mg IM q4wk **Peds.** 1–10 mcg/kg/24 h SQ in 2–4 ÷ doses **Caution:** [B, +] Hepatic/renal impair **Disp:** Inj 0.05, 0.1, 0.2, 0.5, 1 mg/mL; 10, 20, 30 mg/5 mL LAR depot **SE:** N/V, Abd discomfort, flushing, edema, fatigue, cholelithiasis, hyper-/hypoglycemia, hep, hypothyroidism **Interactions:** ↓ Effects *OF* cyclosporine, vit B₁₂ **Labs:** Small ↑ LFTs, ↑ serum thyroxine, vit B₁₂ **NIPE:** May alter BG; stabilize for at least 2 wk before changing to LAR form; use smallest volume to deliver desired dose to ↓ pain at Inj site; may cause dizziness—caution driving

Ofatumumab (Arzerra) [MoAb] **Uses:** *Rx refractory CLL* **Action:** MoAb, binds CD20 molecule on nl & abnormal B-lymphocytes w/ cell lysis **Dose:** *Adults.* 300 mg (0.3 mg/mL) IV week 1, then 2000 mg (2 mg/mL) weekly × 7 doses, then 2000 mg q4wk × 4 doses. Titrate Inf; start 12 mL/h × 30 min, ↑ 25 mL/h for 30 min, ↑ to 50 mL/h × 30 min, ↑ to 100 mL/h × 30 min, then titrate to max Inf 200 mL/h **Caution:** [C, ?] ✔ WBC, screen high risk for hep B, can reactivate, D/C immediately **Disp:** Inj 20 mg/mL (5 mL) **Disp:** Inj 20 mg/mL (5 mL) **SE:** Infusion Rxns (bronchospasm, pulmonary edema, ↑/↓ BP, syncope, cardiac ischemia, angioedema), ↓ WBC, anemia, fever, fatigue, rash, N/D, pneumonia,

Infxns; PML **Labs:** ↓ WBC, HMG; monitor CBC **NIPE:** Premedicate w/ APAP, antihistamine, & IV steroid; avoid w/ live viral vaccines. Monitor for neurologic changes; ↑ risk of Infxn—avoid exposure

Ofloxacin (Floxin) [Antibiotic/Fluoroquinolone] **WARNING:** Use associated w/ tendon rupture & tendonitis **Uses:** *Lower resp tract, skin & skin structure, & UTI, prostatitis, uncomp GC, & *Chlamydia* Infxns* **Action:** Bactericidal; ↓ DNA gyrase. Broad-spectrum gram(+) & (−): S pneumoniae, S aureus, S pyogenes, H influenzae, P mirabilis, N gonorrhoeae, C trachomatis, E coli **Dose:** **Adults.** 200–400 mg PO bid or IV q12h ↓ in renal impair, take on empty stomach **Caution:** [C, −] ↓ Absorption w/ antacids, sucralfate, Al^{2+}-, Ca^{2+}-, Mg^{2+}-, Fe^{2+}-, Zn^{2+}- containing drugs, Hx Szs **CI:** Quinolone allergy **Disp:** Tabs 200, 300, 400 mg; Inj 20, 40 mg/mL; ophthal & otic 0.3% **SE:** N/V/D, photosensitivity, insomnia, HA, local irritation, ↑ QTC interval, peripheral neuropathy risk **Interactions:** ↑ Effects **W/** cimetidine, probenecid; ↑ effects **OF** procainamide, theophylline, warfarin; ↑ risk of tendon rupture **W/** corticosteroids; ↓ effects **W/** antacids, antineoplastics, Ca, didanosine, Fe, $NaHCO_3$, sucralfate, Zinc **NIPE:** Take w/o food; use sunscreen; ↑ fluids to 2–3 L/d; do not take vit/supp/antacids containing Mg, Ca, Al, Zn, or Fe w/in 2 h of administration

Ofloxacin, Ophthalmic (Ocuflox Ophthalmic) [Antibiotic/Fluoroquinolone] **Uses:** *Bacterial conjunctivitis, corneal ulcer* **Action:** See Ofloxacin **Dose:** *Adults & Peds > 1 y.* 1–2 gtt in eye(s) q2–4h × 2 d, then qid × 5 more d **Caution:** [C, +/−] **CI:** Quinolone allergy **Disp:** Ophthal 0.3% soln **SE:** Burning, hyperemia, bitter taste, chemosis, photophobia **NIPE:** Teach use of eye drops; may cause development of crystals on contact lenses

Ofloxacin Otic (Floxin Otic, Floxin Otic Singles) [Antibiotic/Fluoroquinolone] **Uses:** *Otitis externa; chronic suppurative otitis media w/ perf drums; otitis media in peds w/ tubes* **Action:** See Ofloxacin **Dose:** *Adults & Peds > 13 y. Otitis externa:* 10 gtt in ear(s) × 7 d *Peds 1–12 y. Otitis media:* 5 gtt in ear(s) bid × 10 d **Caution:** [C, −] **CI:** Quinolone allergy **Disp:** Otic 0.3% soln 5/10 mL bottles; singles 0.25 mL foil pack **SE:** Local irritation **NIPE:** OK w/ tubes/perforated drums; 10 gtt = 0.5 mL; to ↓ risk of dizziness, warm by holding bottle in hand for 1–2 min; teach use of ear drops

Olanzapine (Zyprexa, Zydis) [Antipsychotic/Thienobenzodiazepine] **WARNING:** ↑ Mortality in elderly w/ dementia-related psychosis **Uses:** *Bipolar mania, schizophrenia*, psychotic disorders, acute agitation in schizophrenia* **Action:** Dopamine & serotonin antagonist; atypical antipsychotic **Dose:** *Bipolar/schizophrenia:* 5–10 mg/d, weekly PRN, 20 mg/d max *Agitation: atypical antipsychotic* 5–10 mg IM q2–4h PRN, 30 mg/d/max **Caution:** [C, −] **Disp:** Tabs 2.5, 5, 7.5, 10, 15, 20 mg; ODT (Zyprexa, Zydis) 5, 10, 15, 20 mg; Inj 10 mg **SE:** HA, somnolence, orthostatic ↓ BP, tachycardia, dystonia, xerostomia, constipation, hyperglycemia; ↑ wgt, ↑ prolactin levels; and sedation may be ↑ in peds **Interactions:** ↑ Effects **W/** fluvoxamine; ↑ sedation **W/** CNS depressants, EtOH; ↑ Szs

W/ anticholinergics, CNS depressants; ↑ hypotension *W/* antihypertensives, diazepam; ↓ effects *W/* activated charcoal, carbamazepine, omeprazole, rifampin, St. John's wort, tobacco; ↓ effects *OF* DA agonists, levodopa **Labs:** ↑ LFTs, ↑ prolactin levels **NIPE:** ↑ Risk of tardive dyskinesia, photosensitivity—use sunscreen, body temperature impair—↑ risk of dehydration in hot weather, strenuous exercise; avoid EtOH—↑ sleepiness; takes 1 wk to titrate dose; do not confuse Zyprexa IM w/ Zyprexa Relprevv

Olanzapine, LA Parenteral (Zyprexa Relprevv) [Antipsychotic/Thienobenzodiazepine]

WARNING: ↑ Risk for severe sedation/coma following parenteral Inj, observe closely for 3 h in appropriate facility; restricted distribution; ↑ mortality in elderly w/ dementia-related psychosis; not approved for dementia-related psychosis **Uses:** *Schizophrenia* **Action:** See Olanzapine **Dose:** *IM:* 150 mg/2 wk, 300 mg/q4wk, 210 mg/q2wk, 405 mg/q4wk, or 300 mg/q2wk **Caution:** [C, –] IM only, do not confuse w/ *Zyprexa IM*; can cause neuroleptic malignant synd, ↑ glucose/lipids/prolactin, ↓ BP, tardive dyskinesia, cognitive impair, ↓ CBC **CI:** None **Disp:** Vials, 210, 300, 405 mg **SE:** HA, sedation, ↑ wgt, cough, N/V/D, ↑ appetite, dry mouth, nasopharyngitis, somnolence **Interactions:** ↑ Risk of hypotension *W/* antihypertensives, benzodiazepines, EtOH; ↓ effects *W/* rifampin, omeprazole, carbamazepine, others that induce CYP1A2; ↓ effects *OF* levodopa, DA agonists **Labs:** ✓ Glucose/lipids/CBC baseline & periodically **NIPE:** Must be given in medical setting w/ 3 h close monitoring after administration; Efficacy shown w/o need for oral supplementation for 2–4 wk depending on dose; do not confuse Zyprexa IM w/ Zyprexa Relprevv

Olmesartan, Olmesartan & Hydrochlorothiazide (Benicar, Benicar HCT) [Antihypertensive/ARB/ARB + HCTZ]

WARNING: Use in PRG 2nd/3rd tri can harm fetus; D/C when PRG detected **Uses:** *Hypertension, alone or in combo* **Action:** *Benicar* angiotensin II receptor blocker (ARB); *Benicar HCT* ARB w/ diuretic HCTZ **Dose:** *Adults. Benicar:* 20–40 mg qd *Benicar HCT:* 20–40 mg olmesartan w/ 12.5–25 mg *HCTZ* based on effect *Peds 6–16 y. Benicar:* < 35 kg start 10 mg PO, range 10–20 mg qd ≥ *35 kg.* Start 20 mg PO qd, target 20–40 mg qd **Caution:** [C (1st tri, D 2nd, 3rd, ?/–); ?/–] *Benicar HCT* not rec w/ CrCl < 30 mL/min; follow closely if volume depleted with start of med **CI:** Component allergy **Disp:** *Benicar* Tabs 5, 20, 40 mg; (*Benicar HCT*) mg olmesartan/mg HCTZ: 20/12.5, 40/12.5, 40/25 **SE:** Dizziness, ↓ K⁺ w/ HCTZ product (may require replacement) **Interactions:** ↑ Risk of digitalis, Li tox; ↑ risk of hypokalemia *W/* ACTH, amphotericin B, corticosteroids; ↑ risk of hyperkalemia *W/K⁺* supls, K⁺-sparing diuretics or K⁺-containing salt substitutes; ↓ effects *W/* NSAIDs; ↓ effect *OF* norepinephrine **Labs:** May interfere w/ parathyroid tests **NIPE:** ⊘ PRG; caution using K⁺ supp/salt subs; if *Benicar* does not control BP, a diuretic can be added or *Benicar HCT* used; titrate at 2–4-wk intervals

Olmesartan/Amlodipine/Hydrochlorothiazide (Tribenzor) [Anti-hypertensive/Angiotensin II Receptor Blocker + Calcium Channel Blocker + Hydrochlorothiazide] Uses: *Hypertension* Action: Combo angiotensin II receptor blocker, CCB, thiazide diuretic Dose: Begin w/ 20/5/12.5 olmesartan/amlodipine/HCTZ, ↑ to max 40/10/25 mg Caution: [C, (1st tri; D 2nd/3rd); –] CI: Anuria; sulfa allergy; PRG, neonate exposure, CrCl < 30 mg/min, age > 75 y, severe liver Dz Disp: Tabs: (olmesartan/amlodipine/HCTZ mg) 20/5/12.5; 40/5/12.5; 40/5/25; 40/10/12.5; 40/10/25 mg SE: Edema, HA, fatigue, N/D, muscle spasms, Jt swelling, URI, syncope Interactions: ↑ Risk of digitalis, Li tox; ↑ risk of hypokalemia W/ ACTH, amphotericin B, corticosteroids; ↑ risk of hyperkalemia W/ K⁺ supls, K⁺-sparing diuretics or K⁺-containing salt substitutes; ↓ effects W/ NSAIDs; ↓ effect OF norepinephrine Labs: Monitor lytes, uric acid Avoid w/ vol depletion; thiazide diuretics may exacerbate SLE, associated NA glaucoma; titrate at 2-wk intervals; caution w/ EtOH—may ↓ BP; use reliable BC; best taken 4 h prior hs

Olopatadine Nasal (Patanase) [Antihistamine (H₁-Blocker)] Uses: *Seasonal allergic rhinitis* Action: H₁-receptor antagonist Dose: 2 sprays each nostril bid Caution: [C, ?] Disp: 0.6% 240-spray bottle SE: Epistaxis, bitter taste somnolence, HA, rhinitis Interaction: ↑ Effects OF CNS depressants; ↑ CNS depression W/ EtOH NIPE: Avoid eyes; monitor for nasal changes; may ↓ mental alertness—caution driving; ⊘ EtOH

Olopatadine Ophthalmic (Patanol, Pataday) [Ophthalmic Antihistamine] Uses: *Allergic conjunctivitis* Action: H₁-receptor antagonist Dose: *Patanol:* 1 gtt in eye(s) bid *Pataday:* 1 gtt in eye(s) qd Caution: [C, ?] Disp: *Patanol:* soln 0.1% 5 mL *Pataday:* 0.2% 2.5 mL SE: Local irritation, HA, rhinitis NIPE: ⊘ In children < 3 y; may reinsert contacts 10 min later if eye not red

Olsalazine (Dipentum) [Anti-Inflammatory/Aminosalicylic Acid Derivative] Uses: *Maintain remission in UC* Action: Topical anti-inflammatory Dose: 500 mg PO bid (w/ food) Caution: [C, –] CI: Salicylate sensitivity Disp: Caps 250 mg SE: D, HA, blood dyscrasias, hep Interaction: ↑ Effects OF anticoagulants Labs: ↑ LFTs NIPE: Food ↓ GI upset

Omacetaxine (Synribo) Uses: *CML w/ resist &/or intol to > 2 TKI* Action: Inhib protein synthesis Dose: *Adults.* Induct: 1.25 mg/m² SQ bid × 14 consecutive d 28-d cycle, repeat until hematologic response achieved Maint: 1.25 mg/m² SQ twice daily ×7 consecutive d 28-d cycle, continue as long as beneficial; adjust based on toxicity (see label) Caution: [D, –] Severe myelosuppression (✓ CBC q 1–2 wk); severe bleeding (✓ plt); glucose intol (✓ glucose); embryofetal tox CI: None Disp: Inj powder 3.5 mg/vial SE: Anemia, neutropenia, ↓ plts/WBC, N/V/D, fatigue, asthenia, Inj site Rxn, pyrexia, Infxn, bleeding, ↑ glucose, constipation, Abd pain, edema, HA, arthralgia, insomnia, cough, epistaxis, alopecia, rash NIPE: Teach SC Inj tech; wear protective eyewear/gloves when preparing and administering; monitor CBCs; ⊘ PRG; may cause fatigue—caution driving

Omalizumab (Xolair) [Antiasthmatic/Monoclonal Antibody] **WARNING:** Reports of anaphylaxis 2–24 h after administration, even in previously treated pts **Uses:** *Mod–severe asthma in ≥ 12 y w/ reactivity to an allergen & when Sxs inadequately controlled w/ inhaled steroids* **Action:** Anti-IgE Ab **Dose:** 150–375 mg SQ q2–4wk (dose/frequency based on serum IgE level & body wgt; see PI) **Caution:** [B, ?/–] **CI:** Component allergy, acute bronchospasm **Disp:** 150-mg single-use 5-mL vial **SE:** Site Rxn, sinusitis, HA, anaphylaxis reported in 3 pts **Interactions:** No drug interaction studies done **NIPE:** Not for acute bronchospasm; administration w/in 8 h of reconstitution & store in refrigerator; continue other asthma meds as indicated; usually given in health care setting

Omega-3 Fatty Acid [Fish Oil] (Lovaza) [Lipid Regulator/Ethyl Ester] **Uses:** *Rx hypertriglyceridemia* **Action:** Omega-3 acid ethyl esters, ↓ thrombus inflammation & triglycerides **Dose:** *Hypertriglyceridemia:* 4 g/d ÷ in 1–2 doses **Caution:** [C, –] Fish hypersensitivity; PRG, risk factor, w/ anticoagulant use, w/ bleeding risk **CI:** Hypersensitivity to components **Disp:** 1000-mg gel caps **SE:** Dyspepsia, N, GI pain, rash, flu-like synd **Interactions:** ↑ Effects *OF* anticoagulants **Labs:** Monitor triglycerides, LDL, ALT **NIPE:** Only FDA-approved fish oil supl; not for exogenous hypertriglyceridemia (type 1 hyperchylomicronemia); many OTC products; follow low-fat, low-chol diet; avoid EtOH; D/C after 2 mo if triglyceride levels do not ↓

Omeprazole (Prilosec, Prilosec [OTC]) [Anti-Ulcer Agent/Proton Pump Inhibitor] **Uses:** *Duodenal/gastric ulcers (adults), GERD, and erosive gastritis (adults & children),* prevent NSAID ulcers, ZE synd, *H pylori* Infxns **Action:** PPI **Dose:** *Adults.* 20–40 mg PO daily–bid × 4–8 wk; *H pylori* 20 mg PO bid × 10 d w/ amoxicillin & clarithromycin or 40 mg PO × 14 d w/ clarithromycin; pathologic hypersecretory cond 60 mg/d (varies); 80 mg/d max *Peds (1–16 y) 5–10 kg.* 5 mg/d max *10–20 kg.* 10 mg PO qd *> 20 kg.* 20 mg/d max; 40 mg/d max **Caution:** [C, –/+] w/ Drugs that rely on gastric acid (eg, ampicillin); avoid w/ atazanavir and nelfinavir; caution w/ warfarin, diazepam, phenytoin; do not use w/ clopidogrel (controversial ↓ effect); response does not R/O malignancy **Disp:** OTC tabs 20 mg; Prilosec DR caps 10, 20, 40 mg; Prilosec DR susp 2.5, 10 mg **SE:** HA, Abd pain, N/V/D, flatulence **Interactions:** ↑ Effects *OF* clarithromycin, digoxin, phenytoin, warfarin; ↓ effects *W/* sucralfate; ↓ effects *OF* ampicillin, cyanocobalamin, ketoconazole **Labs:** ↑ LFTs; risk of hypomagnesemia w/ long-term use, monitor **NIPE:** Take w/ H$_2$O only, no other Liq; combo w/ antibiotic Rx for *H pylori*, ? ↑ risk of fxs w/ all PPIs; do not use OTC Prilosec > 14 days

Omeprazole, Sodium Bicarbonate (Zegerid, Zegerid OTC) [Anti-Ulcer Agent/Proton Pump Inhibitor] **Uses:** *Duodenal/gastric ulcers, GERD & erosive gastritis, (↓ GI bleed in critically ill pts)* prevent NSAID ulcers, ZE synd, *H pylori* Infxns **Action:** PPI w/ sodium bicarb **Dose:** *Duodenal ulcer:* 20 PO daily–bid × 4–8 wk *Gastric ulcer:* 40 PO daily–bid × 4–8 wk *GERD no erosions:*

20 mg PO daily × 4 wk *w/ erosions* treat 4–6 wk *UGI bleed prevention:* 40 mg q6–8h then 40 mg/d × 14 d **Caution:** [C, –/+] w/ drugs that rely on gastric acid (eg, ampicillin); avoid w/ atazanavir and nelfinavir; w/ warfarin, diazepam, phenytoin; do not use w/ clopidogrel (controversial ↓ effect); response does not R/O malignancy **Disp:** omeprazole mg/sodium bicarb mg: *Zegerid OTC* caps 20/1100; *Zegerid* 20/1100, 40/1100; *Zegerid powder packet* for oral susp 20/1680, 40/1680 **SE:** ↑ HA, Abd pain, N/V/D, flatulence **Interactions:** Avoid w/ atazanavir & nelfinavir; ↑ effects *OF* clarithromycin, digoxin, diazepam, phenytoin, warfarin; ↓ effects *W/* sucralfate; ↓ effects *OF* ampicillin, clopidogrel, cyanocobalamin, ketoconazole **Labs:** ↑ LFTs; risk of hypomagnesemia w/ long-term use, monitor **NIPE:** Not approved in Peds; take 1 h ac; mix powder in small cup w/ 2 tbsp H₂O (not food or other Liq) refill & drink; do not open caps; possible ↑ risk of fxs w/ all PPIs

Omeprazole, Sodium Bicarbonate, Magnesium Hydroxide (Zegerid w/ Magnesium Hydroxide) [Anti-Ulcer Agent/Proton Pump Inhibitor] Uses: *Duodenal or gastric ulcer, GERD, maintenance esophagitis* **Action:** PPI w/ acid buffering **Dose:** 20–40 mg omeprazole daily, empty stomach 1 h pc; *Duodenal ulcer, GERD:* 20 mg 4–8 wk *Gastric ulcer:* 20 mg 4–8 wk *Esophagitis maint:* 20 mg **Caution:** [C, ?/–] w/ Resp alkalosis; ↓ K⁺, ↓ Ca²⁺, ↑ drug levels metabolized by cytochrome P450; may ↑ INR w/ warfarin; may ↓ absorption drugs requiring acid environment **CI:** ↓ Renal Fxn **Disp:** Chew tabs, 20, 40 mg omeprazole; w/ 600 mg NaHCO₃; 700 mg MgOH₂ **SE:** N, V, D, Abd pain, HA **Interactions:** ↑ Drug levels metabolized by cytochrome P450; ↑ effects *OF* diazepam, phenytoin, warfarin tacrolimus, clarithromycin **Labs:** ↓ K⁺, ↓ Ca²⁺, monitor INR w/ warfarin **NIPE:** Do not swallow whole, chew tab, can use water only to swallow; atrophic gastritis w/ long-term PPI; ?; ↑ risk of fxs w/ all PPI; long-term use + Ca²⁺ → milk-alkali synd

Ondansetron (Zofran, Zofran ODT) [Antiemetic/5-HT Antagonist] Uses: *Prevent chemotherapy-associated & post-op N/V* **Action:** Serotonin receptor (5-HT₃) antagonist **Dose:** *Adults & Peds. Chemotherapy:* 0.15 mg/kg/dose IV prior to chemotherapy, then 4 & 8 h after 1st dose or 4–8 mg PO tid; 1st dose 30 min prior to therapy & give on schedule, not PRN *Adults. Post-op:* 4 mg IV immediately preanesthesia or post-op *Peds. Post-op:* < 40 kg. 0.1 mg/kg > 40 kg. 4 mg IV; ↓ w/ hepatic impair **Caution:** [B, +/–] Arrhythmia risk, may ↑ QT interval **Disp:** Tabs 4, 8, 24 mg, soln 4 mg/5 mL, Inj 2 mg/mL, Zofran ODT tabs 4, 8 mg **SE:** D, HA, constipation, dizziness **Interactions:** ↓ Effects W/ cimetidine, phenobarbital, rifampin **Labs:** ↑ LFTs **NIPE:** Food ↑ absorption; may cause drowsiness/dizziness—caution driving

Ondansetron, Oral Soluble Film (Zuplenz) [Antiemetic/5-HT Antagonist] Uses: *Prevent chemotherapy/ RT-associated & post-op N/V* **Action:** Serotonin receptor (5-HT₃) antagonist **Dose:** *Adults. Highly emetogenic chemotherapy:* 24 mg (8 mg film × 3) 30 min pre-chemotherapy *RT N & V:* 8 mg film tid *Adults & Peds > 12 y. Mod emetogenic chemotherapy:* 8 mg film 30 min pre-chemotherapy, then 8 mg in 8 h; 8 mg film bid × 1–2 d after chemotherapy *Adults. Post-op:* 16 mg (8 mg film × 2) 1 h pre-op; ↓ w/ hepatic impair **Caution:** [B, +/–] **CI:** w/ Apomorphine (↓ BP, LOC) **Disp:** Oral soluble film 4, 8 mg **SE:** HA, malaise/fatigue, constipation, D **Interactions:** ↓ Effects *W*/ potent CYP3A4 inducers (eg, phenytoin, carbamazepine, rifampicin); may ↓ analgesia of tramadol **NIPE:** Use w/ dry hands, do not chew/swallow; place on tongue, dissolves in 4–20 s

Oprelvekin (Neumega) [Thrombopoietic Growth Factor]
WARNING: Allergic Rxn w/ anaphylaxis reported; D/C w/ any allergic Rxn **Uses:** *Prevent ↓ plt w/ chemotherapy* **Action:** ↑ Proliferation & maturation of megakaryocytes (IL-11) **Dose:** *Adults.* 50 mcg/kg/d SQ for 10–21 d *Peds > 12 y.* 75–100 mcg *Oral contraceptives, biphasic, monophasic, triphasic, progestin-only:* 271 kg/d SQ for 10–21 d *< 12 y.* Use only in clinical trials; ↓ w/ CrCl < 30 mL/min 25 mcg/kg **Caution:** [C, ?/–] **Disp:** 5 mg powder for Inj **SE:** Tachycardia, palpitations, arrhythmias, edema, HA, dizziness, visual disturbances, papilledema, insomnia, fatigue, fever, N, anemia, dyspnea, allergic Rxns including anaphylaxis **Interactions:** None noted **Labs:** ↓ HMG, albumin; monitor lytes; obtain CBCs before & during therapy; monitor plt counts **NIPE:** Monitor for peripheral edema/fluid retention; use med w/in 3 h of reconstitution; initiate 6–24 h after chemotherapy completion; D/C at least ≥ 2 days before next chemo cycle

Oral Contraceptives (See Table 5) [Progestin/Hormone]
WARNING: Cigarette smoking ↑ risk of serious CV SEs; ↑ risk w/ > 15 cigarettes/d, > 35 y; strongly advise women on OCP to not smoke. Pts should be counseled that these products do not protect against HIV and other STD **Uses:** *Birth control; regulation of anovulatory bleeding; dysmenorrhea; endometriosis; polycystic ovaries; acne* (Note: FDA approvals vary widely, see PI) **Action:** *Birth control:* Suppresses LH surge, prevents ovulation; progestins thicken cervical mucus; ↓ fallopian tubule cilia, ↓ endometrial thickness to ↓ chances of fertilization *Anovulatory bleeding:* Cyclic hormones mimic body's natural cycle & regulate endometrial lining, results in regular bleeding q28d; may ↓ uterine bleeding & dysmenorrhea **Dose:** Start d 1 menstrual cycle or 1st Sunday after onset of menses; 28-d cycle pills take daily; 21-d cycle pills take daily, no pills during last 7 d of cycle (during menses); some available as transdermal patch; intrauterine ring **Caution:** [X, +] Migraine, HTN, DM, sickle cell Dz, gallbladder Dz; monitor for breast Dz, ; w/ drosperidone-containing OCP, ✓ K+ if taking drugs w/ ↑ K+ risk; drospirenone implicated in ↑ VTE risk **CI:** AUB, PRG, estrogen-dependent malignancy, ↑ hypercoagulation/liver Dz, hemiplegic migraine, smokers > 35 y; drosperinone has mineralocortocoid effect; do not use w/ renal/liver/adrenal problems **Disp:** See Table 5; 28-d cycle pills (21 active pills + 7 placebo or Fe or folate supl) 21-d cycle pills (21 active pills) **SE:** Intramenstrual bleeding, oligomenorrhea, amenorrhea, ↑ appetite/wgt gain, ↓ libido, fatigue, depression, mood swings, mastalgia, HA, melasma, ↑ Vag discharge, acne/greasy skin, corneal edema, N; drosperinone

containing pills have ↑ blood clots compared to other progestins **NIPE:** Taken correctly, up to 99.9% effective for contraception; no STDs prevention—instruct in use to reduce STDs, use additional barrier contraceptive; use back-up BC for missed dose; long term, can ↓ risk of ectopic PRG, benign breast Dz, ovarian & uterine CA. Suggestions for OCP prescribing and/or regimen changes are noted below. Listing of other forms of Rx birth control can be found in Table 5 Criteria for Specific OTC Choices:

- *Rx menstrual cycle control:* Start w/ monophasic × 3 mo before switching to another brand; w/ continued bleeding change to pill w/ ↑ estrogen
- *Rx birth control:* Choose pill w/ lowest SE profile for particular pt; SEs numerous; d/t estrogenic excess or progesterone deficiency; each pill's SE profile can be unique (see package insert); newer extended-cycle combos have shorter/fewer hormone-free intervals, ? ↓ PRG risk; OCP troubleshooting SE w/ suggested OCP
- *Absent menstrual flow:* ↑ Estrogen, ↓ progestin: Brevicon, Necon 1/35, Norinyl 1/35, Modicon, Necon 1/50, Norinyl 1/50, Ortho-Cyclen, Ortho-Novum 1/50, Ortho-Novum 1/35, Ovcon 35
- *Acne:* Use ↑ estrogen, ↓ androgenic: Brevicon, Ortho-Cyclen, Demulen 1/50, Estrostep, Ortho Tri-Cyclen, Mircette, Modicon, Necon, Ortho Evra, Yasmin, Yaz
- *Breakthrough bleed:* ↑ Estrogen, ↑ progestin, ↓ androgenic: Demulen 1/50, Desogen, Estrostep, Loestrin 1/20, Ortho-Cept, Ovcon 50, Yasmin, Zovia 1/50E
- *Breast tenderness or ↑ wgt:* ↑ Estrogen, ↓ progestin: Use ↓ estrogen pill rather than current; Alesse, Levlite, Loestrin 1/20 Fe, Ortho Evra, Yasmin, Yaz
- *Depression:* ↓ Progestin: Alesse, Brevicon, Levlite, Modicon, Necon, Ortho Evra, Ovcon 35, Ortho-Cyclen, Ortho Tri-Cyclen Tri-Levlen, Triphasil, Trivora
- *Endometriosis:* ↓ Estrogen, ↑ progestin: Demulen 1/35, Loestrin 1.5/30, Loestrin 1/20 Fe, Lo Ovral, Levlen, Levora, Nordette, Zovia 1/35; cont w/o placebo pills or w/ 4 d of placebo pills
- *HA:* ↓ Estrogen, ↓ progestin: Alesse, Levlite, Ortho Evra
- *Moodiness and/or irritability:* ↓ Progestin: Alesse, Brevicon, Levlite, Modicon, Necon 1/35, Ortho Evra, Ortho-Cyclen, Ortho Tri-Cyclen, Ovcon 35, Tri-Levlen, Triphasil, Trivora
- *Severe menstrual cramping:* ↑ Progestin: Demulen 1/50, Desogen, Loestrin 1.5/30, Mircette, Ortho-Cept, Yasmin, Yaz, Zovia 1/50E, Zovia 1/35E

Orphenadrine (Norflex) [Skeletal Muscle Relaxant] Uses: *Discomfort associated w/ painful musculoskeletal conditions* **Action:** Central atropine-like effect; indirect skeletal muscle relaxation, euphoria, analgesia **Dose:** 100 mg PO bid, 60 mg IM/IV q12h **Caution:** [C, +/–] **CI:** NAG, GI or bladder obst, cardiospasm, MyG **Disp:** SR tabs 100 mg; Inj 30 mg/mL **SE:** Drowsiness, dizziness, blurred vision, flushing, tachycardia, constipation **Interactions:** ↑ CNS depression **W/** anxiolytics, butorphanol, hypnotics, MAOIs, nalbuphine, opioids, pentazocine, phenothiazine, tramadol, TCAs, kava kava, valerian, EtOH; ↑ effects **W/** anticholinergics **NIPE:** Do not crush/chew/split ER; may impair reaction time—caution driving; caution w/ EtOH; impaired body temperature regulation

Oseltamivir (Tamiflu) [Antiviral/Neuraminidase Inhibitor]
Uses: *Prevention & Rx influenza A & B* **Action:** ↓ Viral neuraminidase **Dose:** *Adults.* Tx: 75 mg PO bid for 5 d w/in 48 h of Sx onset *Prophylaxis:* 75 mg PO daily × 10 d w/in 48 h on contact *Peds.* Tx: Dose bid × 5 d: < 15 kg: 30 mg 15–23 kg: 45 mg 23–40 kg: 60 mg > 40 kg: Adult dose. *Prophylaxis: Same dosing but once daily for 10 d* ↓ w/ renal impair **Caution:** [C, ?/–] **CI:** Component allergy **Disp:** Caps 30, 45, 75 mg, powder 6 mg/mL for suspension (**Note:** 12 mg/mL dose is being phased out due to dosing concerns) **SE:** N/V, insomnia, reports of neuropsychological events in children (self-injury, confusion, delirium) **Interactions:** ↑ Effects **W/** probenecid **NIPE:** Take w/o regard to food; cap contents may be mixed with sweetened liquid—see pkg insert; initiate w/in 48 h of Sx onset or exposure; ✓ CDC updates (*http://www.cdc.gov/h1n1flu/guidance/*)

Ospemifene (Osphena) WARNING: ↑ Risk endometrial CA; ↑ risk of CVA, DVT/PE
Uses: *Moderate to severe dyspareunia* **Acts:** Estrogen agonist/antagonist **Dose:** *Adults.* 1 tab 1 ×/d **Caution:** [X, –] DVT/PE, hemorrhagic or thrombotic stroke, arterial thromboembolic Dz; do NOT use if known, suspected or Hx of breast Ca; severe liver Dz **CI:** Undiagnosed abnormal genital bleeding; known or suspected estrogen sensitive cancer; PRG **Disp:** Tab 60 mg **SE:** Hot flashes; vaginal discharge; hyperhidrosis; muscle cramps **Notes:** Metabolized by CYP3A4, CYP2C9, and CYP2C9; highly protein bound, may be displaced by other highly protein-bound drugs **NIPE:** Take w/ food; may cause hot flashes; report unusual vaginal bleeding

Oxacillin (Generic) [Antibiotic/Penicillin]
Uses: *Infxns d/t susceptible S aureus, Streptococcus, & other organisms* **Action:** Bactericidal; ↓ cell wall synth **Spectrum:** Excellent gram(+), poor gram(−) **Dose:** *Adults.* 250–500 mg (2 g severe) IM/IV q4–6h *Peds.* 150–200 mg/kg/d IV ÷ q4–6h **Caution:** [B, M] **CI:** PCN sensitivity **Disp:** Powder for Inj 500 mg, 1, 2, 10 g **SE:** GI upset, interstitial nephritis, blood dyscrasias **Interactions:** ↑ Effects **W/** disulfiram, probenecid; ↑ effects **OF** anticoagulants, MTX; ↑ effects **W/** chloramphenicol, tetracyclines, carbonated drinks, fruit juice, beer; ↑ effects **OF** OCPs **NIPE:** Take w/o food; may ↓ effectiveness of BC pills—use additional BC

Oxaliplatin (Eloxatin) [Antineoplastic/Alkylating Agent]
WARNING: Administer w/ supervision of physician experienced in chemotherapy. Appropriate management is possible only w/ adequate diagnostic & Rx facilities. Anaphylactic-like Rxns reported **Uses:** *Adjuvant Rx stage III colon CA (primary resected) & metastatic colon CA w/ 5-FU* **Action:** Metabolized to platinum derivatives, crosslinks DNA **Dose:** Per protocol; see PI. *Premedicate:* Antiemetic w/ or w/o dexamethasone **Caution:** [D, –] See Warning **CI:** Allergy to components or

platinum **Disp:** Inj 50, 100 mg **SE:** Anaphylaxis, granulocytopenia, paresthesia, N/V/D, stomatitis, fatigue, neuropathy, hepatotox, pulm tox **Interactions:** ↑ Effects *OF* nephrotoxic drugs **Labs:** ↑ Bilirubin, Cr, LFTs; ↓ HMG, K⁺, neutrophils, plts, WBC; monitor CBC, plts, LFTs, BUN, & Cr before each chemotherapy cycle **NIPE:** ↑ Acute neurologic Sxs w/ cold exposure/cold Liq; avoid cold beverages, ice cubes, ice packs; epi, corticosteroids, & antihistamines alleviate severe Rxns; ↑ risk of Infxn – avoid exposure

Oxandrolone (Oxandrin) [C-III] [Anabolic Steroid] WARNING: Risk of peliosis hepatis, liver cell tumors, may ↑ risk atherosclerosis **Uses:** *Wgt ↑ after wgt ↓ from severe trauma, extensive surgery* **Action:** Anabolic steroid; ↑ lean body mass **Dose:** *Adults.* 2.5–20 mg/d PO ÷ bid-qid *Peds.* ≤ 0.1 mg/kg/d ÷ bid–qid **Caution:** [X; ?/–] ↑ INR w/ warfarin **CI:** PRG, prostate CA, breast CA, breast CA w/ hypercalcemia, nephrosis **Disp:** Tabs 2.5, 10 mg **SE:** Acne, hepatotox, dyslipidemia **Interactions:** ↑ Effects *OF* oral anticoagulants, oxyphenbutazone; ↑ risk of edema *W/* ACTH, corticosteroids **Labs:** ✓ Lipids & LFTS **NIPE:** Use intermittently, 2–4 wk typical; use barrier form of BC

Oxaprozin (Daypro, Generic) [Analgesic, Anti-Inflammatory, Antipyretic/NSAID] WARNING: May ↑ risk of CV events & GI bleeding **Uses:** *Arthritis & pain* **Action:** NSAID; ↓ prostaglandin synth **Dose:** *Adults.* 600–1200 mg/daily (÷ dose helps GI tolerance); ↓ w/ renal/hepatic impair *Peds. JRA (Daypro):* *22–31 kg.* 600 mg/d *32–54 kg.* 900 mg/d **Caution:** [C (D 3rd tri), ?] Peptic ulcer, bleeding disorders **CI:** ASA/NSAID sensitivity, perioperative pain w/ CABG **Disp:** Tabs 600 mg **SE:** CNS inhibition, sleep disturbance, rash, GI upset, peptic ulcer, edema, renal failure, anaphylactoid Rxn w/ "ASA triad" (asthmatic w/ rhinitis, nasal polyps, and bronchospasm w/NSAID use) **Interactions:** ↑ Effects *OF* aminoglycosides, anticoagulants, ASA, Li, MTX, ↓ effects *OF* antihypertensives, diuretics **NIPE:** ↑ Risk of photo-sensitivity—use sunblock; take w/ food, milk, or antacid to ↓ risk of GE SEs; do not lie down for ≤ 10 min

Oxazepam [C-IV] [Anxiolytic/Benzodiazepines] **Uses:** *Anxiety, acute EtOH withdrawal*, anxiety w/ depressive Sxs **Action:** Benzodiazepine; diazepam metabolite **Dose:** *Adults.* 10–15 mg PO tid–qid; severe anxiety & EtOH withdrawal may require up to 30 mg qid *Peds > 6 y.* 1 mg/kg/d ÷ doses **Caution:** [D, ?/–] **CI:** Component allergy, NAG **Disp:** Caps 10, 15, 30 mg; tabs 15 mg **SE:** Sedation, ataxia, dizziness, rash, blood dyscrasias, dependence **Interactions:** ↑ CNS effects *W/* anticonvulsants, antidepressants, antihistamines, barbiturates, MAOIs, opioids, phenothiazine, kava kava, lemon balm, sassafras, valerian, EtOH; ↑ effects *W/* cimetidine; ↓ effects *W/* OCPs, phenytoin, theophylline, tobacco; ↓ effects *OF* levodopa **Labs:** False ↑ serum glucose **NIPE:** Do not D/C abruptly; no EtOH; may cause dizziness/drowsiness—caution driving; ↑ risk of falling in the elderly; avoid PRG

Oxcarbazepine (Oxtellar XR, Trileptal) [Anticonvulsant/ Carbamazepine] **Uses:** *Partial Szs*, bipolar disorders **Action:** Blocks voltage-sensitive Na⁺ channels, stabilization of hyperexcited neural membranes **Dose: Adults.** 300 mg PO bid, ↑ weekly to target maint 1200–2400 mg/d **Peds.** 8–10 mg/kg bid, 600 mg/d max, ↑ weekly to target maint dose; ↓ w/ renal Insuff **Caution:** [C, –] Carbamazepine sensitivity **CI:** Components sensitivity **Disp:** Tabs 150, 300, 600 mg; (*Oxtellar XR*) ER tabs 150, 300, 600 mg; susp 300 mg/5 mL **SE:** ↓ Na⁺, HA, dizziness, fatigue, somnolence, GI upset, diplopia, coordination difficulties, fatal skin/multiorgan hypersensitivity Rxns **Interactions:** ↑ Effects **W/** benzodiazepines, EtOH; ↑ effects **OF** phenobarbital, phenytoin; ↓ effects **W/** barbiturates, carbamazepine, phenobarbital, valproic acid, verapamil; ↓ effects **OF** CCBs, OCPs **Labs:** ↓ Thyroid levels, serum Na; ✓ Na⁺ if fatigued **NIPE:** Take w/o regard to food; use barrier contraception; do not abruptly D/C; advise about SJS & topic epidermal necrolysis; may cause dizziness/drowsiness—caution driving; EtOH may ↑ risk of Sz

Oxiconazole (Oxistat) [Azole Antifungal] Uses: *Tinea cruris, tinea corporis, tinea pedis, tinea versicolor* **Action:** ? ↓ Ergosterols in fungal cell membrane *Spectrum:* Most *Epidermophyton floccosum, Trichophyton mentagrophytes, Trichophyton rubrum, Malassezia furfur* **Dose:** Apply thin layer daily–bid **Caution:** [B, M] **CI:** Component allergy **Disp:** Cream, lotion 1% **SE:** Local irritation **NIPE:** Avoid eyes, nose, mouth, mucous membranes; do not cover w/ occlusive dressing; wear loose-fitting cotton clothing

Oxybutynin (Ditropan, Ditropan XL) [GU Antispasmodic/ Anticholinergic] Uses: *Symptomatic relief of urgency, nocturia, incontinence w/ neurogenic or reflex neurogenic bladder* **Action:** Anticholinergic, relaxes bladder smooth muscle, ↑ bladder capacity **Dose: Adults.** 5 mg bid–tid, 5 mg 4 ×/d max. XL 5–10 mg/d, 30 mg/d max **Peds. > 5 y.** 5 mg PO bid–tid; 15 mg/d max **1–5 y.** 0.2 mg/kg/dose 2–4 ×/d (syrup 5 mg/5 mL); 15 mg/d max; ↓ in elderly; periodic drug holidays OK **Caution:** [B, ?] **CI:** NAG, MyG, GI/GU obst, UC, megacolon **Disp:** Tabs 5 mg; XL tabs 5, 10, 15 mg; syrup 5 mg/5 mL **SE:** Anticholinergic (drowsiness, xerostomia, constipation, tachycardia) **Interactions:** ↑ Effects **W/** CNS depressants, EtOH; ↑ effects **OF** atenolol, digoxin, nitrofurantoin; ↑ anticholinergic effects **W/** antihistamines, anticholinergics; ↓ effects **OF** haloperidol, levodopa **NIPE:** ↓ Temperature regulation; avoid becoming overheated or dehydrated during exercise and in hot weather; ↑ photosensitivity—use sunscreen; ER form empty shell expelled in stool; ↑ QT interval—monitor ECG; memory impair, dizziness—caution driving

Oxybutynin, Topical (Gelnique) [GU Antispasmodic/Anticholinergic] Uses: *OAB* **Action:** Anticholinergic, relaxes bladder smooth muscle, ↑ bladder capacity **Dose:** 1 g sachet qd to dry skin (Abd/shoulders/thighs/upper arms) **Caution:** [B, ?/–] **CI:** Gastric or urinary retention; NAG **Disp:** Gel 10%, 1-g sachets (100 mg oxybutynin) **SE:** Anticholinergic (lethargy, xerostomia, constipation, blurred vision, ↑ HR); rash, pruritus, redness, pain at site; UTI **Interactions:** CNS depression **W/** EtOH, other CNS depressants; additive effect **W/** other anticholinergics **NIPE:** Cover w/ clothing, skin-to-skin transfer can occur; gel is flammable; after applying wait 1 h before showering, bathing, exercising, swimming; avoid EtOH, may cause dizziness—caution driving; avoid becoming overheated in hot weather—maintain hydration

Oxybutynin Transdermal System (Oxytrol) [GU Antispasmodic/ Anticholinergic] Uses: *Rx OAB* **Action:** Anticholinergic, relaxes bladder smooth muscle, ↑ bladder capacity **Dose:** One 3.9 mg/d system apply 2 × /wk (q3–4d) to Abd, hip, or buttock **Caution:** [B, ?/–] **CI:** GI/GU obst, NAG **Disp:** 3.9-mg/d transdermal patch **SE:** Anticholinergic, itching/redness at site **Interactions:** ↑ Effects **W/** anticholinergics; CNS depression **W/** EtOH, other CNS depressants; metabolized by the cytochrome P450 CYP3A4 enzyme system **NIPE:** do not apply to same site w/in 7 d

Oxycodone [Dihydrohydroxycodeinone] (OxyContin, Roxicodone) [C-II] [Opioid Analgesic] WARNING: High abuse potential; controlled release only for extended chronic pain, not for PRN use; 60-, 80-mg tab for opioid-tolerant pts; do not crush, break, or chew Uses: *Mod–severe pain, usually in combo w/ nonnarcotic analgesics* **Action:** Narcotic analgesic **Dose:** *Adults.* 5 mg PO q6h PRN (IR). *Mod–severe chronic pain:* 10–160 mg PO q12h (ER); can give ER q8h if effect does not last 12 h *Peds 6–12 y.* 1.25 mg PO q6h PRN > *12 y:* 2.5 mg q6h PRN; ↓ w/ severe liver/renal Dz, elderly; w/ food **Caution:** [B (D if prolonged use/near term), M] **CI:** Allergy, resp depression, acute asthma, ileus w/ microsomal morphine **Disp:** IR caps (OxyIR) 5 mg; CR Roxicodone tabs 15, 30 mg; ER (OxyContin) 10, 15, 20, 30, 40, 60, 80 mg; Liq 5 mg/5 mL; soln conc 20 mg/mL **SE:** ↓ BP, sedation, resp depression, dizziness, GI upset, constipation, risk of abuse **Interactions:** ↑ CNS & resp depression **W/** amitriptyline, barbiturates, cimetidine, clomipramine, MAOIs, nortriptyline, protease Inhibs, TCAs **Labs:** ↑ Serum amylase, lipase **NIPE:** Take w/ food; ER OxyContin for chronic fracture pain; do not crush/ chew/cut ER product; may cause dizziness/drowsiness—caution driving; teach measures to prevent constipation; sought after as drug of abuse; reformulated product has abuse deterrent properties

Oxycodone/Acetaminophen (Percocet, Tylox) [C-II] [Opioid + Analgesic] Uses: *Mod–severe pain* **Action:** Narcotic analgesic **Dose:** *Adults.* 1–2 tabs/caps PO q4–6h PRN (acetaminophen max dose 4 g/d) *Peds.* Oxycodone 0.05–0.15 mg/kg/dose q4–6h PRN, 5 mg/dose max **Caution:** [C (D prolonged use or near term), M] **CI:** Allergy, paralytic ileus, resp depression **Disp:** Percocet tabs mg oxycodone/mg APAP: 2.5/325, 5/325, 7.5/325, 10/325, 7.5/500, 10/650; Tylox caps 5 mg oxycodone, 500 mg APAP; soln 5 mg oxycodone & 325 mg APAP/5 mL **SE:** ↓ BP, sedation, dizziness, GI upset, constipation **Interactions:** ↑ CNS & resp depression **W/** amitriptylline, barbiturates, cimetidine, clomipramine, MAOIs, nortriptylline, protease Inhibs, TCAs **Labs:** False ↑ serum amylase, lipase **NIPE:** Take w/ food; do not exceed ≥ 4 g acetaminophen/d from all sources; see Oxycodone

Oxycodone/Acetaminophen ER (Xartemis XR) [C-II] WARNING: Addiction risk, risk of resp depression. Accidental consumption, esp peds, can be fatal. Use during PRG can cause neonatal opioid withdrawal. Contains acetaminophen, associated w/ liver failure, transplant, and death **Uses:** *Acute pain that requires opiods where alternatives are inadequate* **Action:** Opioid agonist and acetaminophen **Dose:** 2 tabs q12h, w/ regard to food; do not crush/chew **Caution:** [C, –] Do not use before delivery; not equivalent to other combo products; caution w/ other CNS depressants, MAOI, neuromuscular blockers, elderly, debilitated, w/ hepatitic impair; may ↑ ICP (✔ pupils); assoc w/ skin reactions; may × BP; acetaminophen hepatotox > 4000 mg, avoid w/ other acetaminophen products; impairs mental/physical abilities; drugs that ↓ CYP3A4 may ↓ oxycodone clearance **CI:** Component hypersensitivity; resp depression, severe asthma/hypercarbia, ileus **Disp:** Tabs oxycodone/acetaminophen: 7.5/325 mg **SE:** ↓ Resp, ↓ BP, sedation, coma **NIPE:** Take w/ or w/o food; swallow whole with 8 oz H₂O—do not crush/chew/split; not interchangeable with other oxycodone/acetaminophen products; do not take other products containing acetaminophen; no EtOH; may cause sedation/dizziness—caution driving; high potential for abuse/addiction; for short-term use

Oxycodone/Aspirin (Percodan) [C-II] [Narcotic Analgesic/Nonsteroidal Analgesic] Uses: *Mod–severe pain* **Action:** Narcotic analgesic w/ NSAID **Dose:** *Adults.* 1–2 tabs/caps PO q4–6h PRN **Peds.** Oxycodone 0.05–0.15 mg/kg/dose q4–6h PRN, up to 5 mg/dose; ↓ in severe hepatic failure **Caution:** [D, –] w/ Peptic ulcer, CNS depression, elderly, Hx Szs **CI:** Component allergy, children (< 16 y) w/ viral Infxn (Reyes synd), resp depression, ileus, hemophilia **Disp:** *Generics:* 4.83 mg oxycodone hydrochloride, 0.38 mg oxycodone terephthalate, 325 mg ASA *Percodan* 4.83 mg oxycodone hydrochloride, 325 mg ASA **SE:** Sedation, dizziness, GI upset/ulcer, constipation, allergy **Interactions:** ↑ CNS & resp depression **W/** amitriptyline, barbiturates, cimetidine, clomipramine, MAOIs, nortriptyline, protease Inhibs, TCAs; ↑ effects **OF** anticoagulants **Labs:** ↑ Serum amylase, lipase **NIPE:** Take w/ food; do not lie down for ≥ 10 min; see Oxycodone

Oxycodone/Ibuprofen (Combunox) [C-II] [Narcotic Analgesic/NSAID] **WARNING:** May ↑ risk of serious CV events; CI in perioperative CABG pain; ↑ risk of GI events such as bleeding **Uses:** *Short-term (not > 7 d) management of acute mod–severe pain* **Action:** Narcotic w/ NSAID **Dose:** 1 tab q6h PRN 4 tabs max/24 h; 7 d max **Caution:** [C, –] w/ Impaired renal/hepatic Fxn; COPD, CNS depression, avoid in PRG **CI:** Paralytic ileus, 3rd-tri PRG, allergy to ASA or NSAIDs, where opioids are CI **Disp:** Tabs 5 mg oxycodone/400 mg ibuprofen **SE:** N/V, somnolence, dizziness, sweating, flatulence, ↑ LFTs **Interactions:** ↑ CNS & resp depression **W/** amitriptyline, barbiturates, cimetidine, clomipramine, MAOIs, nortriptyline, protease Inhibs, TCAs; ↑ effects **W/** ASA, corticosteroids, probenecid, EtOH; ↑ effects **OF** aminoglycosides, anticoagulants, digoxin, hypoglycemics, Li, MTX; ↑ risks of bleeding **W/** abciximab, cefotetan, valproic acid, thrombolytic drugs, warfarin, ticlopidine, garlic, ginger, ginkgo; ↓ effects *W/* feverfew; ↑ effects *OF* antihypertensives **Labs:** ↑ Serum amylase, lipase, LFTs, BUN, Cr; ✓ renal Fxn **NIPE:** Take w/ food, milk, or antacid to ↓ GI SEs; do not lie down for ≥ 10 min , see Oxycodone

Oxymorphone (Opana, Opana ER) [C-II] [Opioid Analgesic] WARNING: (Opana ER) Abuse potential, controlled release only for chronic pain; do not consume EtOH-containing beverages, may cause fatal OD
Uses: *Mod/severe pain, sedative* **Action:** Narcotic analgesic **Dose:** 10–20 mg PO q4–6h PRN if opioid-naïve or 1–1.5 mg SQ/IM q4–6h PRN or 0.5 mg IV q4–6h PRN; start 20 mg/dose max PO *Chronic pain:* ER 5 mg PO q12h; if opioid-naïve ↑ PRN 5–10 mg PO q12h q3–7d; take 1 h pc or 2 h ac; ↓ dose w/ elderly, renal/hepatic impair **Caution:** [B, ?] **CI:** ↑ ICP, severe resp depression, w/ EtOH or liposomal morphine, severe hepatic impair **Disp:** Tabs 5, 10 mg; ER 5, 10, 20, 30, 40 mg **SE:** ↓ BP, sedation, GI upset, constipation, histamine release **Interactions:** ↑ Effects *W/* CNS depressants, cimetidine, neuroleptics, EtOH; ↓ effects *W/* phenothiazines **Labs:** ↑ Amylase, lipase **NIPE:** See Hydromorphone

Oxytocin (Pitocin) [Oxytocic/Hormone] WARNING: Not rec for elective induction of labor
Uses: *Induce labor, control postpartum hemorrhage* **Action:** Stimulate muscular contractions of the uterus **Dose:** 0.0005–0.001 units/min IV Inf; titrate 0.001–0.002 units/min q30–60 min **Caution:** [Uncategorized, +/–] **CI:** Where Vag delivery not favorable, fetal distress **Disp:** Inj 10 units/mL **SE:** Uterine rupture, fetal death; arrhythmias, anaphylaxis, H$_2$O intoxication **Interactions:** ↑ Pressor effects *W/* sympathomimetics **NIPE:** Monitor vital signs, FHR; nasal form for breast-feeding use

Paclitaxel (Abraxane, Taxol) [Antineoplastic/Antimitotic] WARNING: Administration only by physician experienced in chemotherapy; fatal anaphylaxis & hypersensitivity possible; severe myelosuppression possible
Uses: *Ovarian & breast CA, PCa*, Kaposi sarcoma, NSCLC **Action:** Mitotic spindle poison; promotes microtubule assembly & stabilization against depolymerization **Dose:** Per protocols; use glass or polyolefin containers (eg, nitroglycerin tubing set); PVC sets leach plasticizer; ↓ in hepatic failure **Caution:** [D, –] **CI:** Neutropenia ANC <1500 cells/mm^3; < 1000 cells/mm^3 w/ AIDS-related Kaposi syndrome; solid tumors, component allergy **Disp:** Inj 6 mg/ mL, vial 5, 16.7, 25, 50 mL (Abraxane) 100 mg/vial **SE:** ↓ BM, peripheral neuropathy, transient ileus, myalgia, ↓ HR, ↓ BP, mucositis, N/V/D, fever, rash, HA, phlebitis; hematologic tox schedule-dependent; leukopenia dose-limiting by 24-h Inf; neurotox limited w/ short (1–3 h) Inf; allergic Rxns (dyspnea, ↓ BP, urticaria, rash) **Interactions:** ↑ Effects *W/* cyclosporine, dexamethasone, diazepam, ketoconazole, midazolam, quinidine, teniposide, verapamil, vincristine; ↑ risk of bleeding *W/* anticoagulants, plt Inhibs, thrombolytics; ↑ myelosuppression when cisplatin is administered before paclitaxel; ↓ effects *W/* carbamazepine, phenobarbital; ↓ effects of live virus vaccines **Labs:** ↑ AST, alk phos, triglycerides **NIPE:** Use effective barrier contraception;

males should not father a child during Tx; ⊘ PRG, breast-feeding, live virus vaccines; maint hydration; monitor for S/Sxs of Infx: if allergic Rxn occurs (rare), usually w/in 10 min of Inf; minimize/premedicate w/ corticosteroid, antihistamine; cimetidine pre-Tx; localized skin Rxns may occur up to 10 d after Inf; may cause profound BM suppression, mucous membrane irritation; ✓ S/Sxs peripheral neuropathy

Palifermin (Kepivance) Uses: *Oral mucositis w/ BMT* Action: Synthetic keratinocyte GF Dose: *Phase 1:* 60 mcg/kg IV daily × 3, 3rd dose 24–48 h before chemotherapy *Phase 2:* 60 mcg/kg IV daily × 3, after stem cell IV (at least 4 d from last dose) Caution: [C, ?/–] Hypersensitivity to palifermin, *E coli*–derived proteins, or any component & formulation Disp: Inj 6.25 mg SE: Unusual mouth sensations, tongue thickening, rash, ↑ amylase & lipase Notes: *E coli*–derived; separate phases by 4 d; safety unknown w/ nonhematologic malignancies NIPE: ⊘ Spicy foods/bland diet; ⊘ hot/cold fluids; assess oral mucosa for severity S/Sx of stomatitis; heparin can ↑ systemic exposure—avoid co-administration—rinse IV line w/ NS before & after palifermin

Paliperidone (Invega, Invega Sustenna) [Benzisoxazole] WARNING: Not for dementia-related psychosis Uses: *Schizophrenia* Action: Risperidone metabolite, antagonizes dopamine & serotonin receptors Dose: *Invega:* 6 mg PO qAM, 12 mg/d max; *CrCl 50–79 mL/min:* 6 mg/d max *CrCl 10–49 mL/min:* 3 mg/d max *Invega Sustenna:* 234 mg d 1, 156 mg 1 wk later IM (deltoid), then 117 mg monthly (deltoid or gluteal); range 39–234 mg/mo Caution: [C, ?/–] w/ ↓ HR, ↓ K^+/Mg^{2+}, renal/hepatic impair; w/ phenothiazines, ranolazine, ziprasidone, prolonged QT, Hx arrhythmia CI: Risperidone/paliperidone hypersensitivity Disp: *Invega* ER tabs 1.5, 3, 6, 9 mg; *Invega Sustenna* prefilled syringes 39, 78, 117, 156, 234 mg SE: Impaired temp regulation, ↑ QT & HR, HA, anxiety, dizziness, N, dry mouth, fatigue, EPS Interactions: ↑ Risk of prolongation of QT w/ Class Ia & Class III antiarrhythmics, chlorpromazine, thioridazine, gatifloxacin, moxifloxacin, EtOH; ↑ risk of orthostatic hypotension w/ CNS drugs; ↑ effects w/ divalproex Na; ↓ effects w/ carbamazepine; ↓ effects OF levodopa & other DA agonists Labs: Serum glucose, LFTs NIPE: ⊘ Chew/cut/crush pill determine tolerability to oral risperidone or paliperidone before using injectable; ✓ orthostatic effects & renal Fxn esp in elderly; ⊘ use in elderly w/ dementia-related psychosis

Palivizumab (Synagis) [Antiviral/Monoclonal Antibody] Uses: *Prevent RSV Infxn* Action: MoAb Dose: *Peds.* 15 mg/kg IM monthly, typically Nov–Apr; AAP rec max 3 doses for those born 32–34 6/7 wk w/o significant congenital heart/lung Dz Caution: [C, ?] Renal/hepatic dysfunction CI: Component allergy Disp: Vials 50, 100 mg SE: Hypersensitivity Rxn, URI, rhinitis, cough, ↑ LFTs, local irritation Labs: ↑ LFT NIPE: Infrequent nonfatal anaphylaxis has occurred w/subsequent doses; use drug w/in 6 h after reconstitution; give IM in anterolateral aspect of thigh; use only for RSV prophylaxis

Palonosetron (Aloxi) [Antiemetic/5-HT₃ Receptor Antagonist] WARNING: May ↑ QTc interval Uses: *Prevention acute & delayed N/V w/ emetogenic chemotherapy; prevent postoperative N/V* Action: 5-HT₃ receptor antagonist Dose: *Chemotherapy:* 0.25 mg IV 30 min prior to chemotherapy *Postoperative N/V:* 0.075 mg immediately before induction Caution: [B, ?] CI: Component allergy Disp: 0.05 mg/mL (1.5 & 5 mL vials) SE: HA, constipation, dizziness, Abd pain, anxiety Interactions: Potential for drug interactions low Labs: Monitor ECG NIPE: Not recommended for < 18 y; may ↑ QTc interval esp in pts taking diuretics & antiarrhythmics; ✓ for dehydration; report persistent V; ∅ ETOH, barbituates

Pamidronate (Generic) [Antihypercalcemic/Bisphosphonate] Uses: *Hypercalcemia of malignancy, Paget Dz, palliate symptomatic bone metastases* Action: Bisphosphonate; ↓ nl & abnormal bone resorption Dose: *Hypercalcemia:* 60–90 mg IV over 2–24 h or 90 mg IV over 24 h if severe; may repeat in 7 d *Paget Dz:* 30 mg/d IV slow Inf over 4 h × 3 d *Osteolytic bone mets in myeloma:* 90 mg IV over 4 h qmo *Osteolytic bone mets breast CA:* 90 mg IV over 2 h q3–4wk; 90 mg/max single dose Caution: [D, ?/–] Avoid invasive dental procedures w/ use CI: PRG, bisphosphonate sensitivity Disp: Inj 30, 60, 90 mg SE: Fever, malaise, convulsions, Inj site Rxn, uveitis, fluid overload, HTN, Abd pain, N/V, constipation, UTI, bone pain, ↓ K⁺, Ca²⁺, Mg²⁺, hypophosphatemia; jaw osteonecrosis (mostly CA pts; avoid dental work), renal tox Interactions: ↓ Serum Ca levels W/ foscarnet; ↓ effects W/ Ca, vit D Labs: ↓ K⁺, Ca²⁺, Mg²⁺; follow Cr, hold dose if Cr ↑ by 0.5 mg/dL w/ nl baseline or by 1 mg/dL w/ abnormal baseline; restart when Cr returns w/in 10% of baseline; may cause profound hypocalcemia—monitor Ca NIPE: ∅ Ingest food w/ Ca or vits w/ minerals before or 2–3 h after administration of drug; may cause fever 24 h post-Inj; perform dental exam preghnancy; ↑ risk of jaw fx; may ↑ atypical subtrochanteric femur fxs; ↑ risk GI bleed w/ 90 mg dose

Pancrelipase (Creon, Pancrease, Panakare Plus, Pertzye, Ultresa, Voikace, Zenpep) [Pancreatic Enzyme] Uses: *Exocrine pancreatic secretion deficiency (eg, CF, chronic pancreatitis, pancreatic Insuff), steatorrhea of malabsorption* Action: Pancreatic enzyme supl; amylase, lipase, protease Dose: 1–3 caps (tabs) w/ meals & snacks; ↑ to 8 caps (tabs); do not crush or chew EC products; dose dependent on digestive requirements of pt; avoid antacids Caution: [C, ?/–] CI: Pork product allergy, acute pancreatitis Disp: Caps, tabs SE: N/V, Abd cramps Interactions: ↓ Effects W/ antacids w/ Ca or Mg; ↓ effects OF Fe Labs: ↑ Serum & urine uric acid NIPE: Take w/ food/adequate hydration; stress adherence to diet (usually low fat, high protein, high calorie); monitor for GI obst; ∅ chew tabs

Pancuronium (Generic) [Skeletal Muscle Relaxant/Nondepolarizing Neuromuscular Blocking Agent] WARNING: Should only be administered by adequately trained individuals Uses: *Paralysis w/ mechanical ventilation* **Action:** Nondepolarizing neuromuscular blocker **Dose: *Adults & Peds > 1 mo.*** Initial 0.06–0.1 mg/kg; maint 0.01 mg/kg 60–100 min after, then 0.01 mg/kg q25–60min PRN; ↓ w/ renal/hepatic impair; intubate & maintain on controlled ventilation; use adequate sedation & analgesia **Caution:** [C, ?/–] **CI:** Component or bromide sensitivity **Disp:** Inj 1, 2 mg/mL **SE:** Tachycardia, HTN, pruritus, other histamine/hypersensitivity Rxns **Interactions:** ↑ Effects *W/* amikacin, clindamycin, Li, quinidine, succinylcholine, gentamicin, streptomycin, verapamil; ↓ effects *W/* carbamazepine, phenytoin, theophylline **NIPE:** Neuromuscular blocker does not alter pain threshold or level of consciousness, administer w/ adequate anesthesia/sedation

Panitumumab (Vectibix) [Human Epidermal Growth Factor Receptor (EGFR) Inhibitor] WARNING: Derm tox common (89%) and severe in 12%; can be associated w/ Infxn (sepsis, abscesses requiring I&D) w/ severe derm tox, hold or D/C and monitor for Infxn; severe Inf Rxns (anaphylactic Rxn, bronchospasm, fever, chills, hypotension) in 1%; w/ severe Rxns, immediately D/C Inf and possibly permanent D/C **Uses:** *Rx EGFR-expressing metastatic colon CA* **Action:** Anti-EGFR MoAb **Dose:** 6 mg/kg IV Inf over 60 min q14d; doses > 1000 mg over 90 min ↓ Inf rate by 50% w/ grade 1–2 Inf Rxn, D/C permanently w/ grade 3–4 Rxn. For derm tox, hold until < grade 2 tox. If improves < 1 mo, restart 50% original dose. If tox recurs or resolution > 1 mo permanently D/C. If ↓ dose tolerated, ↑ dose by 25% **Caution:** [C, –] D/C Nursing during, 2 mo after **Disp:** 20 mg/mL vial (5, 10 mL) **SE:** Rash, acneiform dermatitis, pruritus, paronychia, ↓ Mg^{2+}, Abd pain, N/V/D, constipation, fatigue, dehydration, photosens, conjunctivitis, ocular hyperemia, ↑ lacrimation, stomatitis, mucositis, pulm fibrosis, severe derm tox, Inf Rxns **Labs:** ✓ Lytes, ↓ Mg^{2+}, ✓ lytes **NIPE:** ⊘ PRG, breast-feeding; may impair female fertility; wear sunscreen/hats, limit sun exposure; ✓ for S/Sxs of Infxn/ sepsis; ✓ skin toxicities; ocular toxicities (keratitis)

Pantoprazole (Protonix) [Gastric Acid Suppressant/Proton Pump Inhibitor] Uses: *GERD, erosive gastritis*, ZE synd, PUD **Action:** Proton pump inhib **Dose: Adult:** 40 mg/d PO; do not crush/chew tabs; 40 mg IV/d (not > 3 mg/min) **Caution:** [B, ?/–] Do not use w/ clopidogrel (↓ effect) **Disp:** Tabs, DR 20, 40 mg; 40 mg powder for oral susp (mix in applesauce or juice, give immediately); Inj 40 mg **SE:** CP, anxiety, GI upset ↑ LFTs **Interactions:** ↑ Effects *OF* warfarin; ↑ effects of photosens *W/* St. John's wort; ↓ effects *OF* ketoconazole **Labs:** ↑ Serum glucose, lipids, LFTs; monitor PT, INR **NIPE:** ⊘ Sun exposure— use sunblock; take w/o regard to food; antacids will not affect drug absorption; ✓ risk of ↓ magnesemia w/ long-term use; ↑ risk of fxs

Paregoric [Camphorated Tincture of Opium] [C-III] [Narcotic Antidiarrheal] Uses: *D*, pain & neonatal opiate withdrawal synd **Action:** Narcotic **Dose: Adults.** 5–10 mL PO 1–4 ×/d PRN **Peds.** 0.25–0.5 mg/kg 1–4 ×/d **Caution:** [B (D w/ prolonged use/high dose near term, +] **CI:** Toxic D; convulsive disorder, morphine sensitivity **Disp:** Liq 2 mg morphine = 20 mg opium/5 mL

SE: ↓ BP, sedation, constipation **Interactions:** ↓ Effects *OF* ampicillin esters, azole antifungals, Fe salts **Labs:** ↑ LFTs, SCr **NIPE:** Take w/o regard to food; contains anhydrous morphine from opium; short-term use only; may cause constipation & CNS depression

Paroxetine (Brisdelle) **WARNING:** Potential for suicidal thinking/behavior; monitor closely **Uses:** *Mod–severe menopause vasomotor Sx (not for psych use)* **Action:** SSRI, nonhormonal Rx for condition **Dose:** 7.5 mg PO qhs **Caution:** [X, ?/M] Serotonin synd/ bleed w/ NSAID, ↓ Na⁺, ↓ tamoxifen effect, fxs, mania/hypomania activation, Szs, akathisia, NAG, cognitive/motor impair, w/ strong CYP2D6 Inhib **CI:** w/ or w/in 14 d of MAOI, w/ thioridazine/pimozide/ PRG **Disp:** Caps 7.5 mg **SE:** HA, fatigue, N/V **Notes:** See other paroxetine listings **NIPE:** ✓ for S/Sx ↑ suicidality, serotonin syndrome; allow 14 d of MAOI d/c before starting Brisdelle; ✓ S/Sx of ↓ Na⁺ (HA, weakness, confusion) (esp in elderly); ⊘ DC abruptly; ⊘ PRG

Paroxetine (Paxil, Paxil CR, Pexeva) [Antidepressant/ SSRI] **WARNING:** Closely monitor for worsening depression or emergence of suicidality, particularly in children, adolescents, and young adults; not for use in Peds **Uses:** *Depression, OCD, panic disorder, social anxiety disorder*, PMDD **Action:** SSRI **Dose:** 10–60 mg PO single daily dose in AM; CR 25 mg/d PO; ↑ 12.5 mg/wk (max range 26–62.5 mg/d) **Caution:** [D, ?/I] ↑ Bleeding risk **CI:** w/ MAOI, thioridazine, pimozide, linezolid, methylthioninium chloride (methylene blue) **Disp:** Tabs 10, 20, 30, 40 mg; susp 10 mg/5 mL; CR 12.5, 25, 37.5 mg **SE:** HA, somnolence, dizziness, GI upset, N/D, ↓ appetite, sweating, xerostomia, tachycardia, ↓ libido, ED, anorgasmia **Interactions:** ↑ Risk of QT prolongation *W/* pimozide, thioridazine; ↑ effects *W/* cimetidine; ↑ effects *OF* BBs, dexfenfluramine, dextromethorphan, fenfluramine, haloperidol, MAOIs, theophylline, TCAs, warfarin, St. John's wort, EtOH; ↓ effects *W/* cyproheptadine, phenobarbital, phenytoin; ↓ effects *OF* digoxin, phenytoin **Labs:** ↑ Alk phos, bilirubin, glucose **NIPE:** ✓ for S/Sx ↑ suicidality, serotonin syndrome; allow 14 d of MAOI d/c before starting paroxetine; ✓ S/Sx of ↓ Na⁺ (HA, weakness, confusion) (esp in elderly); ⊘ DC abruptly; swallow tab whole; ⊘ PRG

Pasireotide (Signifor) **Uses:** *Cushing Dz* **Action:** Somatostatin analogue Inhib ACTH secretion **Dose:** *Adults.* 0.6–0.9 mg SQ 2 ×/d; titrate on response/tolerability; hepatic impair (Child-Pugh B): 0.3–0.6 mg SQ bid, (Child-Pugh C): avoid **Caution:** [C, –] w/ Risk for ↓ HR or ↑ QT; w/ drugs that ↓ HR, ↑ QT, cyclosporine, bromocriptine **CI:** None **Disp:** Inj single-dose 0.3, 0.6, 0.9 mg/mL **SE:** N/V/D, hyperglycemia, HA, Abd pain, cholelithiasis, fatigue, ↓ DM, hypocortisolism, ↓ HR, QT prolongation, ↑ glucose, ↑ LFTs, ↓ pituitary hormones, Inj site Rxn, edema, alopecia, asthenia, myalgia, arthralgia **Notes:** Prior to and periodically (see label), ✓ FPG, HbA1c, LFTs, ECG, gallbladder US **NIPE:** Instruct pt on proper use/admin technique; rotate Inj sites; ⊘ reuse of unused portion of drug ampules—discard after use

Pazopanib (Votrient) [Kinase Inhibitor] **WARNING:** Administer only by physician experienced in chemotherapy. Severe and fatal hepatotox observed **Uses:** *Rx advanced RCC*, metastatic soft-tissue sarcoma after chemotherapy **Action:** TKI **Dose: Adults.** 800 mg PO once daily, ↓ to 200 mg daily if moderate hepatic impair, not rec in severe hepatic Dz (bilirubin > 3 × ULN) **Caution:** [D, –] Avoid w/ CYP3A4 inducers/Inhib & QTc prolonging drugs, all SSRI **CI:** Severe hepatic Dz **Disp:** 200-mg tablet **SE:** ↑ BP, N/V/D, GI perf, anorexia, hair depigmentation, ↓ WBC, ↓ plt, ↑ AST/ALT/bilirubin, ↓ Na, CP, ↑ QT **Interactions:** ↑ Effects W/ strong CYP3A4 Inhibs (eg, ketoconazole, ritonavir, clarithromycin), grapefruit juice; ↓ effects W/ strong CYP3A4 inducers (eg, rifampin) **Labs:** ↑ AST/ALT/bilirubin; ↓ WBC, ↓ Na, ↓ plt; monitor LFTs before starting drug & at least once q4wk for at least 1st 4 mo of Tx & then periodically **NIPE:** ⊘ Food 1 h before or 2 h after dose; ⊘ grapefruit products; hold for surgical procedures 7 d before; D/C w/ wound dehiscence; take on empty stomach; swallow whole; ✓ ECG

Pegfilgrastim (Neulasta) [Colony-Stimulating Factor] **Uses:** *↓ Frequency of Infxn in pts w/ nonmyeloid malignancies receiving myelosuppressive anti-CA drugs that cause febrile neutropenia* **Action:** Granulocyte & macrophage-stimulating factor **Dose: Adults.** 6 mg SQ × 1/chemotherapy cycle **Caution:** [C, M] w/ Sickle cell **CI:** Allergy to E coli–derived proteins or filgrastim **Disp:** Syringes: 6 mg/0.6 mL **SE:** Splenic rupture, HA, fever, weakness, fatigue, dizziness, insomnia, edema, N/V/D, stomatitis, anorexia, constipation, taste perversion, dyspepsia, Abd pain, granulocytopenia, neutropenic fever, ↑ LFTs & uric acid, arthralgia, myalgia, bone pain, ARDS, alopecia, worsen sickle cell Dz **Interactions:** ↑ Effects W/ Li **Labs:** ↑ LFTs, uric acid, alk phos, LDH **NIPE:** Avoid exposure to Infxn; never give between 14 d before & 24 h after dose of cytotoxic chemotherapy; ✓ for S/Sxs of Infxn; monitor for Kehr sign (LUQ Abd pain & referred left shoulder pain) associated w/ splenic rupture

Peginterferon Alfa-2a [Pegylated Interferon] (Pegasys) [Antiviral/Immunomodulator] **WARNING:** Can cause or aggravate fatal or life-threatening neuropsychological, autoimmune, ischemic, and infectious disorders. Monitor pts closely **Uses:** *Chronic hep C w/ compensated liver Dz* **Action:** Immune modulator **Dose:** 180 mcg (1 mL) SQ (see package insert); SQ dosing; ↓ in renal impair **Caution:** [C, /?–] **CI:** Autoimmune hep, decompensated liver Dz **Disp:** 180 mcg/mL Inj **SE:** Depression, insomnia, suicidal behavior, GI upset, ↓ WBC and plt, alopecia, pruritus; do not confuse w/ peginterferon alfa-2b **Interactions:** ↑ Effects OF methadone, theophylline **Labs:** ↑ ALTs; ↓ WBC & plt; monitor CBC, TFTs, LFTs, before & during Tx **NIPE:** CI in PRG or men w/ PRG partners; may have abortifacient effects; use 2 methods of contraception; refrigerate med; ✓ for depression, Abd pain, bloody diarrhea—indicative of colitis; takes 1–3 mo for clinical response

Peginterferon Alfa-2b (Pegylated Interferon) [Antiviral/Immunomodulator] WARNING: Can cause or aggravate fatal or life-threatening neuropsychological, autoimmune, ischemic, and infectious disorders; monitor pts closely Uses: *Rx hep C* Action: Immune modulator Dose: 1 mcg/kg/wk SQ; 1.5 mcg/kg/wk comb w/ ribavirin Caution: [C, ?/−] w/ Psychologicl disorder Hx CI: Autoimmune hep, decompensated liver Dz, hemoglobinopathy Disp: Vials 50, 80, 120, 150 mcg/0.5 mL; Redipen 50, 80, 120, 150 mcg/5 mL; reconstitute w/ 0.7 mL w/ sterile H_2O SE: Depression, insomnia, suicidal behavior, GI upset, neutropenia, thromboplastics, alopecia, pruritus Interactions: ↑ Myelosuppression W/ antineoplastics; ↑ effects OF doxorubicin, theophylline; ↑ neurotox W/ vinblastine Labs: ↑ ALT, ↓ neutrophils, plts; monitor CBC/plts NIPE: Maint hydration; ✓ for S/Sxs of Infxn; may exacerbate depression, autoimmune, ischemic & infectious disorder; use barrier contraception; give hs or w/APAP to ↓ flu-like Sxs; use stat or store in refrigerator × 24 h; do not freeze

Pegloticase (Krystexxa) [PEGylated Uric Acid–Specific Enzyme] WARNING: Anaphylaxis/Inf Rxn reported; admin in settings prepared to manage these Rxns; premed w/ antihistamines & corticosteroids Uses: *Refractory gout* Action: PEGylated recombinant urate–oxidase enzyme Dose: 8 mg IV q2wk (in 250 mL NS/1/2 NS over 120 min) premed w/ antihistamines and corticosteroids Caution: [C, −] CI: G6PD deficiency Disp: Inj 8 mg/mL in 1 ML vial SE: Inf Rxn (anaphylaxis, urticaria, pruritis, erythema, CP, dyspnea); may cause gout flare, N Labs: ✓ Uric acid level before each Inf, consider D/C if 2 consecutive levels > 6 mg/dL NIPE: ⊘ IV push/ ⊘ IV bolus—give via IV Inf only; monitor closely for anaphylaxis/Inf Rxns; pretreat w/ corticosteroids, antihistamines; observe at least 2 h post-Inf

Pemetrexed (Alimta) [Antineoplastic/Folate Antagonist] Uses: *w/ Cisplatin in nonresectable mesothelioma*, NSCLC Action: Antifolate antineoplastic Dose: 500 mg/m^2 IV over 10 min q3wk; hold if CrCl < 45 mL/min; give w/ vit B_{12} (1000 mcg IM q9wk) & folic acid (350–1000 mcg PO daily); start 1 wk before; dexamethasone 4 mg PO bid × 3, start 1 d before each Rx Caution: [D, −] w/ Renal/hepatic/BM impair CI: Component sensitivity Disp: 500-mg vial SE: Neutropenia, thrombocytopenia, N/V/D, anorexia, stomatitis, renal failure, neuropathy, fever, fatigue, mood changes, dyspnea, anaphylactic Rxns Interactions: ↑ Effects W/ NSAIDs, probenecid d/t ↓ pemetrexed clearance Labs: ↑ Cr, LFTs; ↓ HMG, Hct; monitor CBC/plts NIPE: ⊘ PRG/breast-feeding; pretreat w/ PO folic acid & IM B_{12} start 1 wk before Tx & continue × 21 d after last Tx (↓ severity of hematologic/GI toxicity); ↓ dose w/ grade 3–4 mucositis; may cause serious BM suppression & mucous membrane irritation

Pemirolast (Alamast) [Mast Cell Stabilizer] Uses: *Allergic conjunctivitis* Action: Mast cell stabilizer Dose: 1–2 gtt in each eye qid Caution: [C, ?/−] Disp: 0.1% (1 mg/mL) in 10-mL bottles SE: HA, rhinitis, cold/flu Sxs, local irritation **NIPE:** Wait 10 min before inserting contacts; ⊘ use contact lenses w/ eye reddness

Penbutolol (Levatol) [Antihypertensive/Beta-Blockers] Uses: *HTN* Action: β-Adrenergic receptor blocker, β₁, β₂ **Dose:** 20–40 mg/d; ↓ in hepatic Insuff **Caution:** [C 1st tri; D if 2nd/3rd tri, M] **CI:** Asthma, cardiogenic shock, cardiac failure, heart block, ↓ HR, COPD, pulm edema **Disp:** Tabs 20 mg **SE:** Flushing, ↓ BP, fatigue, hyperglycemia, GI upset, sexual dysfunction, bronchospasm **Interactions:** ↑ Effects *W/* CCBs, fluoroquinolones; ↑ bradycardia *W/* adenosine, amiodarone, digitalis, dipyridamole, epinephrine, neuroleptics, phenylephrine, physostigmine, tacrine; ↑ effects *OF* lidocaine, verapamil; ↓ effects *W/* antacids, NSAIDs; ↓ effects *OF* insulin, hypoglycemics, theophylline **Labs:** ↑ Serum glucose, BUN, K⁺, lipoprotein, triglycerides, uric acid **NIPE:** ↑ Cold sensitivity; ⊘ D/C abruptly—can lead to ↑ angina; may cause severe ↓ BP/↓ P

Penciclovir (Denavir) [Antiviral/Nucleoside Analogue] Uses: *Herpes simplex (herpes labialis/cold sores)* Action: Competitive Inhib of DNA polymerase **Dose:** Apply at 1st sign of lesions, then q2h while awake × 4 d **Caution:** [B, ?/−] **CI:** Allergy, previous Rxn to famciclovir **Disp:** Cream 1% **SE:** Erythema, HA **NIPE:** ⊘ Recommended in lactation or in children; apply at earliest S/Sx of cold sore

Penicillin G, Aqueous (Potassium or Sodium) (Pfizerpen, Pentids) [Antibiotic/Penicillin] Uses: *Bacteremia, endocarditis, pericarditis, resp tract Infxns, meningitis, neurosyphilis, skin/skin structure Infxns* Action: Bactericidal; ↓ cell wall synth *Spectrum:* Most gram(+) (not staphylococci), streptococci, *N meningitidis*, syphilis, clostridia, & anaerobes (not *Bacteroides*) **Dose:** *Adults.* Based on indication range 0.6–24/d in ÷ doses q4h *Peds. Newborns < 1 wk.* 25,000–50,000 units/kg/dose IV q12h *Infants 1 wk–< 1 mo.* 25,000–50,000 units/kg/dose IV q8h *Children.* 100,000–400,000 units/kg/24 h IV ÷ q4h; ↓ in renal impair **Caution:** [B, M] **CI:** Allergy **Disp:** Powder for Inj **SE:** Allergic Rxns; interstitial nephritis, D, Szs **Notes:** Contains 1.7 mEq of K⁺/MU **Interactions:** ↑ Effects *W/* probenecid; ↑ effects *OF* MTX; ↑ risk of bleeding *W/* anticoagulants; ↓ effects *W/* chloramphenicol, macrolides, tetracyclines; ↓ effects *OF* OCPs **Labs:** ↓ K⁺ (monitor ECG for peaked T waves), ↑ eosinophils; ↓ serum albumin **NIPE:** Monitor for super Infxn, & hypovolemia d/t D; caution w/ PRG; ✓ for rash

Penicillin V (Pen-Vee K, Veetids, Others) [Antibiotic/Penicillin] Uses: Susceptible streptococci Infxns, otitis media, URIs, skin/soft-tissue Infxns (PCN-sensitive staphylococci) **Action:** Bactericidal; ↓ cell wall synth *Spectrum:* Most gram(+), including streptococci **Dose:** *Adults.* 250–500 mg PO q6h, q8h, q12h *Peds.* 25–50 mg/kg/24 h PO in 3–4 ÷ doses above the age of 12 y, dose can be standardized vs wgt-based; ↓ in renal impair; take on empty stomach **Caution:** [B, M] **CI:** Allergy **Disp:** Tabs 125, 250, 500 mg; susp 125, 250 mg/5 mL **SE:** GI upset, interstitial nephritis, anaphylaxis, convulsions **Interactions:** ↓ Effects *W/* ASA, probenecid; ↑ effects *OF* MTX & anticoagulants; ↑ risk of anaphylaxis *W/*

BB; ↓ effects W/ chloramphenicol, macrolides, tetracyclines; ↓ effects OF OCPs **Labs:** ↓ Eosinophils; ↓ serum albumin, WBC **NIPE:** Monitor for super Infxn; monitor for signs hypovolemia d/t D; use barrier contraception; well-tolerated PO PCN; 250 mg = 400,000 units of PCN G; give 1 h ac or 2 h pc; space doses evenly

Penicillin G Benzathine (Bicillin) [Antibiotic/Penicillin] Uses: *Single-dose regimen for streptococcal pharyngitis, rheumatic fever, glomerulonephritis prophylaxis, & syphilis* Action: Bactericidal; ↓ cell wall synth Spectrum: See Penicillin G Dose: *Adults.* 1.2–2.4 MU deep IM Inj q2–4wk Peds. 50,000 units/kg/dose, 2.4 MU/dose max; deep IM Inj q2–4wk Caution: [B, M] CI: Allergy Disp: Inj 300,000,600,000 units/mL; Bicillin L-A benzathine salt only; Bicillin C-R combo of benzathine & procaine (300,000 units procaine w/ 300,000 units benzathine/mL or 900,000 units benzathine w/ 300,000 units procaine/2 mL) SE: Inj site pain, acute interstitial nephritis, anaphylaxis Interactions: ↑ Effects W/ probenecid; ↑ PCN 1/2-life W/ ASA, furosemide, indomethacin, sulfonamides, thiazide diuretics; ↑ risk of bleeding W/ anticoagulants; ↓ effects W/ chloramphenicol, macrolides, tetracyclines; ↓ effects OF OCPs Labs: ↑ Eosinophils; ↓ serum albumin NIPE: Monitor for super Infxn; use barrier contraception; IM use only; sustained action, w/ detectable levels up to 4 wk; drug of choice for noncongenital syphilis

Penicillin G Procaine (Wycillin, Others) [Antibiotic/Penicillin] Uses: *Infxns of resp tract, skin/soft tissue, scarlet fever, syphilis* Action: Bactericidal; ↓ cell wall synth Spectrum: PCN G-sensitive organisms that respond to low, persistent serum levels Dose: *Adults.* 0.6–4.8 MU/d in ÷ doses q12–24h; give probenecid at least 30 min prior to PCN to prolong action Peds. 25,000–50,000 units/kg/d IM ÷ daily–bid Caution: [B, M] CI: Allergy Disp: Inj 300,000, 500,000, 600,000 units/mL SE: Pain at Inj site, interstitial nephritis, anaphylaxis Interactions: ↑ Effects W/ probenecid; ↑ penicillin 1/2-life W/ ASA, furosemide, indomethacin, sulfonamides, thiazide diuretics; ↑ risk of bleeding W/ anticoagulants; ↓ effects W/ chloramphenicol, macrolides, tetracyclines; ↓ effects OF OCPs Labs: ↑ Eosinophils; ↓ serum albumin NIPE: Monitor for super Infxn; administer deep IM only in upper outer quadrant of buttock; ⊘ IV admin

Pentamidine (Pentam 300, NebuPent) [Antiprotozoal] Uses: *Rx & prevention of PCP* Action: ↓ DNA, RNA, phospholipid, & protein synth Dose: *Rx: Adults & Peds.* 4 mg/kg/24 h IV daily × 14–21 d Prevention: *Adults & Peds > 5 y.* 300 mg once q4wk, give via Respirgard II nebulizer; ↓ IV w/ renal impair Caution: [C, ?] CI: Component allergy, use w/ didanosine Disp: Inj 300 mg/vial; aerosol l300 mg SE: Pancreatic cell necrosis w/ hyperglycemia; pancreatitis, CP, fatigue, dizziness, rash, GI upset, renal impair, blood dyscrasias (leukopenia, thrombocytopenia) Interactions: ↑ Nephrotoxic effects W/ aminoglycosides, amphotericin B, capreomycin, cidofovir, cisplatin, cyclosporine, colistin, ganciclovir, methoxyflurane, polymyxin B, vancomycin; ↑ BM suppression W/ antineoplastics, radiation therapy Labs: ↑ LFTs, serum K⁺ (monitor ECG for peaked T waves), ↓ HMG, Hct, plts, WBCs; ↑/↓ glucose; monitor CBC, glucose, pancreatic Fxn monthly for 1st 3 mo **NIPE:** Reconstitute w/ sterile H_2O only for IM; Inh may cause metallic taste; ↑ fluids to 2–3 L/d; pt must be in a supine position only during IM or IV admin w/ ✓ freq BP during/following Tx (risk of severe hypotension); slow change in position post Tx

Pentazocine (Talwin, Talwin Compound, Talwin NX) [C-IV] [Narcotic Analgesic] **WARNING:** Oral use only; severe and potentially lethal Rxns from misuse by Inj **Uses:** *Mod–severe pain* **Action:** Partial narcotic agonist–antagonist **Dose:** *Adults.* 30 mg IM or IV; 50–100 mg PO q3–4h PRN *Peds 5–8 y.* 15 mg IM q4h PRN *9–14 y.* 30 mg IM q4h PRN; ↓ in renal/hepatic impair **Caution:** [C (1st tri, D w/ prolonged use/high dose near term), +/–] **CI:** Allergy, ↑ ICP (unless ventilated) **Disp:** *Talwin Compound* tab 12.5 mg + 325 mg ASA; *Talwin NX* 50 mg + 0.5 mg naloxone; Inj 30 mg/mL **SE:** Considerable dysphoria; drowsiness, GI upset, xerostomia, Szs **Notes:** 30–60 mg IM = 10 mg of morphine IM **Interactions:** ↑ CNS depression *W/* antihistamines, barbiturates, hypnotics, phenothiazine, EtOH; ↑ effects *W/* cimetidine; ↑ effects *OF* digitoxin, phenytoin, rifampin; ↓ effects *OF* opioids **Labs:** ↑ Serum amylase, lipase **NIPE:** May cause withdrawal in pts using opioids; Talwin NX has naloxone to curb abuse by nonoral route; ⊘ stop abruptly; ⊘ use w/ ETOH/CNS depressants

Pentobarbital (Nembutal) [C-II] [Anticonvulsant, Sedative/ Hypnotic/Barbiturate] **Uses:** *Insomnia (short-term), convulsions*, sedation, induce coma w/ severe head injury **Action:** Barbiturate **Dose:** *Adults. Sedative:* 150–200 mg IM, 100 mg IV, may repeat up to 500 mg/max *Hypnotic:* 100–200 mg PO or PR hs PRN *Induced coma:* Load 5–10 mg/kg IV, w/ maint 1–3 mg/kg/h IV *Peds. Induced coma:* As adult **Caution:** [D, +/–] Severe hepatic impair **CI:** Allergy **Disp:** Caps 50, 100 mg; elixir 18.2 mg/5 mL (= 20 mg pentobarbital); supp 30, 60, 120, 200 mg; Inj 50 mg/mL **SE:** Resp depression, ↓ BP w/ aggressive IV use for cerebral edema; ↓ HR, ↓ BP, sedation, lethargy, resp ↓, hangover, rash, SJS, blood dyscrasias **Interactions:** ↑ Effects *W/* MAOIs, narcotic analgesics, EtOH; ↓ effects *OF* anticoagulants, BBs, corticosteroids, cyclosporine, digoxin, doxycycline, griseofulvin, neuroleptics, OCPs, quinidine, theophylline, verapamil **NIPE:** Tolerance to sedative–hypnotic effect w/in 1–2 wk; ✓ for drowsiness, resp depression, hypotension

Pentosan Polysulfate Sodium (Elmiron) [Urinary Analgesic] **Uses:** *Relieve pain/discomfort w/ interstitial cystitis* **Action:** Bladder wall buffer **Dose:** 100 mg PO tid; on empty stomach w/ H_2O 1 h ac or 2 h pc **Caution:** [B, ?/–] **CI:** Hypersensitivity to pentosan or related compounds (LMWH, heparin) **Disp:** Caps 100 mg **SE:** Alopecia, N/D, HA, anticoagulant effects, ↓ plts, rectal bleed **Interactions:** Risk of ↑ anticoagulation *W/* anticoagulants, ASA, thrombolytics **Labs:** ↑ LFTs, ↓ plts **NIPE:** Reassess after 3 mo; take w/ H_2O 1h ac or 2 hrs pc

Pentoxifylline (Trental) [Hemorheologic/Xanthine Derivative] **Uses:** *Rx Sxs of peripheral vascular Dz* **Action:** ↓ Blood cell viscosity, restores RBC flexibility **Dose:** *Adults.* 400 mg PO tid pc; Rx min 8 wk for effect; ↓ to bid w/ GI/CNS SEs **Caution:** [C, +/−] **CI:** Cerebral/retinal hemorrhage, methylxanthine (caffeine) intolerance **Disp:** Tabs CR 400 mg; tabs ER 400 mg **SE:** Dizziness, HA, GI upset **Interactions:** ↑ Risk of bleeding *W/* anticoagulants, NSAIDs; ↑ effects *OF* antihypertensives, theophylline **NIPE:** Take w/ food; GI or CNS side effects are dose related, if present consider ↓ dosing

Perampanel (Fycompa) **WARNING:** Serious/life-threatening psychiatric & behavioral Rxns (aggression, hostility, irritability, anger, homicidal threats/ideation) reported; monitor; ↓ dose or D/C if Sxs are severe/worsen **Uses:** *Adjunct in partial-onset Sz w/ or w/o secondarily generalized Szs* **Action:** Noncompetitive AMPA glutamate receptor antagonist **Dose:** *Adults & Peds > 12 y.* 2 mg PO qhs if not on enzyme-inducing AEDs; 4 mg PO qhs if on enzyme-inducing AEDs; ↑ 2 mg qhs weekly; 12 mg qhs max; elderly, ↑ at 2-wk intervals; mild–mod hepatic impair 6 mg max & 4 mg w/ ↑ dose q2wk; severe hepatic/renal impair or dialysis: avoid **Caution:** [C, −] ✓ For suicidal behavior; avoid strong CYP3A inducers; monitor/dose adjust w/ CYP450 inducers; 12-mg daily dose may ↓ effect of OCP w/ levonorgestrel **CI:** None **Disp:** Tabs 2, 4, 6, 8, 10, 12 mg **SE:** N, dizziness, vertigo, ataxia, gait balance/disturb, falls, somnolence, fatigue, irritability, ↑, anxiety, aggression, anger, blurred vision **NIPE:** Immediately report change in mood or atypical behaviors (eg, irritability, aggression, anger, anxiety, paranoia, euphoria, mental status changes); ⊘ ETOH (can potentiate anger); educate pt/caregiver to ✓ monitor & report behavior changes asap

Perindopril Erbumine (Aceon) [Antihypertensive/ACEI] **WARNING:** ACE Inhib can cause death to developing fetus; D/C immediately w/ **PRG Uses:** *HTN*, CHF, DN, post-MI **Action:** ACE Inhib **Dose:** 2–8 mg/d ÷ dose; 16 mg/d max; avoid w/ food; ↓ w/ elderly/renal impair **Caution:** [C (1st tri, D 2nd & 3rd tri), ?/−] ACE-Inhib–induced angioedema **CI:** Bilateral RAS, primary hyperaldosteronism **Disp:** Tabs 2, 4, 8 mg **SE:** Weakness, HA, ↓ BP, dizziness, GI upset, cough **Interactions:** ↑ Effects *W/* antihypertensives, diuretics; ↑ effects *OF* cyclosporine, insulin, Li, sulfonylureas, tacrolimus; ↓ effects *W/* NSAIDs **Labs:** ↑ Serum K⁺, LFTs, uric acid, cholesterol, Cr **NIPE:** ✓ Effects if taken w/ food; risk of persistent cough; may need to ↓ diuretic before 1st dose; ✓ ECG for ↑ K⁺ (peaked T waves)

Permethrin (Nix, Elimite) [OTC] [Scabicides/Pediculicides] **Uses:** *Rx lice/scabies* **Action:** Pediculicide **Dose:** *Adults & Peds. Lice:* Saturate hair & scalp; allow 10 min before rinsing *Scabies:* Apply cream head to toe; leave for 8–14 h, wash w/ H₂O **Caution:** [B, ?/−] **CI:** Allergy > 2 mo **Disp:** Topical lotion 1%; cream 5% **SE:** Local irritation **NIPE:** Drug remains on hair up to 2 wk, reapply in 1 wk if live lice; sprays available (Rid, A200, Nix) to disinfect clothing, bedding, combs, & brushes; lotion not OK in Peds < 2 y; may repeat after 7 d

Perphenazine (Generic) [Antipsychotic, Antiemetic/Phenothiazine] **Uses:** *Psychotic disorders, severe N* **Action:** Phenothiazine, blocks brain dopaminergic receptors **Dose:** *Adults.* *Antipsychotic:* 4–16 mg PO tid; max 64 mg/d **Notes:** Starting doses for schizophrenia lower in nonhospitalized pts N/V: 8–16 mg/d in ÷ doses *Peds.* *1–6 y.* 4–6 mg/d PO in ÷ doses *6–12 y:* 6 mg/d PO in ÷ doses *>12 y.* 4–16 mg PO 2–4 ×/d; ↓ in hepatic Insuff **Caution:** [C. ?/–] NAG, severe ↑/↓ BP **CI:** Phenothiazine sensitivity, BM depression, severe liver or cardiac Dz **Disp:** Tabs 2, 4, 8, 16 mg; PO conc 16 mg/5 mL; Inj 5 mg/mL **SE:** ↓ BP, tachycardia, bradycardia, EPS, drowsiness, Szs, photosens, skin discoloration, blood dyscrasias, constipation **Interactions:** ↑ Effects *W/* antidepressants; ↑ effects *OF* anticholinergics, antidepressants, propranolol, phenytoin; ↑ CNS effects *W/* CNS depressants, EtOH; ↓ effects *W/* antacids, Li, phenobarbital, caffeine, tobacco; ↓ effects *OF* levodopa, Li **Labs:** ↑ Serum cholesterol, glucose, LFTs; ↓ HMG, plts, WBCs **NIPE:** Take oral dose w/ food; risk of photosens—use sunblock

Pertuzumab (Perjeta) **WARNING:** Embryo-fetal death & birth defects. Animal studies: oligohydramnios, delayed renal development, & death. Advise pt of risk & need for effective contraception **Uses:** *HER2-pos metastatic breast CA w/ trastuzumab & docetaxel in pts who have not received prior anti-HER2 therapy or chemo* **Action:** HER2 dimerization Inhib **Dose:** *Adults.* 840 mg 60 min IV Inf initially; then 420 mg 30–60 min IV Inf q3wk; see label tox dose adjust **Caution:** [D, –] LV dysfunction (monitor LVEF); Inf Rxn **CI:** None **Disp:** Inj vial 420 mg/14 mL **SE:** N/V/D, alopecia, ↑ RBC/WBC, fatigue, rash, peripheral neuropathy, hypersensitivity, anaphylaxis, pyrexia, asthenia, stomatitis, pruritus, dry skin, paronychia, HA, dysgeusia, dizziness, myalgia, arthralgia, URI, insomnia **NIPE:** ⊘ PRG/breast-feeding; use 2 methods of contraception to include barrier protection; admin via IV Inf only; ↓ LVEF; ✓ for Inf-associated Rxns—administer appropriate med Tx

Phenazopyridine (Pyridium, Azo-Standard, Urogesic, Many Others) [Urinary Analgesic] **Uses:** *Lower urinary tract irritation* **Action:** Anesthetic on urinary tract mucosa **Dose:** *Adults.* 100–200 mg PO tid; 2 d max w/ antibiotics for UTI; ↓ w/ renal Insuff **Caution:** [B, ?] Hepatic Dz **CI:** Renal failure, CrCl < 50 mL/min **Disp:** Tabs (Pyridium) 100, 200 mg [OTC] 45, 97.2, 97.5 mg **SE:** GI disturbances, red-orange urine color (can stain clothing, contacts), HA, dizziness, acute renal failure, methemoglobinemia, tinting of sclera/skin **Labs:** Interferes *W/* urinary tests for glucose, ketones, bilirubin, protein, steroids **NIPE:** Tinting of sclera/skin; urine may turn red-orange in color & can stain clothing & contacts; take w/ food; caution w/ elderly w/ renal impairment—avoid use if CrCl < 50 mL/min

Phenelzine (Nardil) [Antidepressant/MAOI] **WARNING:** Antidepressants ↑ risk of suicidal thinking and behavior in children and adolescents w/ major depressive disorder and other psychological disorders; not for Peds use **Uses:** *Depression*, bulimia **Action:** MAOI **Dose:** *Adults.* 15 mg PO tid, ↑ to 60–90 mg/d ÷ doses *Elderly:* 17.5–60 mg/d ÷ doses **Caution:** [C, –] Interacts w/ SSRI, ergots, triptans **CI:** CHF, Hx liver Dz, pheochromocytoma **Disp:** Tabs 15 mg **SE:** Postural ↓ BP; edema, dizziness, sedation, rash, sexual dysfunction, xerostomia, constipation, urinary retention **Interactions:** ↑ HTN Rxn **W/** amphetamines, fluoxetine, levodopa, metaraminol, phenylephrine, phenylpropanolamine, pseudoephedrine, reserpine, sertraline, tyramine, EtOH, foods **W/** tyramine, caffeine, tryptophan; ↑ effects **OF** barbiturates, narcotics, sedatives, sumatriptan, TCAs, ephedra, ginseng **Labs:** ↓ Glucose, false(+) ↑ in bilirubin & uric acid **NIPE:** 2–4 wk for effect; avoid tyramine-containing foods (eg, beer, red wine, aged cheeses/ meats, overripe & dried fruits) d/t risk of HTN; ✓ for ↑ suicidal ideations, ↑ depression; ✓ hypertensive crisis (occipital HA, neck stiffness/soreness)

Phenobarbital [C-IV] [Anticonvulsant, Sedative/Hypnotic/Barbiturate] Uses: *Sz disorders*, insomnia, anxiety Action: Barbiturate Dose:
Adults. *Sedative–hypnotic:* 30–120 mg/d PO or IM PRN *Anticonvulsant:* Load 10–20 mg/kg × 1 IV then 1–3 mg/kg/24 h PO, IM, or IV **Peds.** *Sedative–hypnotic:* 2–3 mg/kg/24 h PO or IM hs PRN *Anticonvulsant:* Load 15–20 mg/kg × 1 IV then 3–5 mg/kg/24 h PO ÷ in 2–3 doses / w/ CrCl < 10 mL/min **Caution:** [D, M] **CI:** Porphyria, hepatic impair, dyspnea, airway obst **Disp:** Tabs 15, 30, 60, 65, 100 mg; elixir 20 mg/5 mL; Inj 60, 65, 130 mg/mL **SE:** ↓ HR, ↓ BP, hangover, SJS, blood dyscrasias, resp depression **Notes:** Levels: *Trough:* Just before next dose *Therapeutic trough:* 15–40 mcg/mL *Toxic trough:* > 40 mcg/mL *1/2-life:* 40–120 h **Interactions:** ↑ CNS depression **W/** CNS depressants, anesthetics, antianxiety meds, antihistamines, narcotic analgesics, EtOH, Indian snakeroot, kava kava; ↑ effects **W/** chloramphenicol, MAOIs, procarbazine, valproic acid; ↓ effects **W/** rifampin; ↓ effects **OF** anticoagulants, BBs, carbamazepine, clozapine, corticosteroids, doxorubicin, doxycycline, estrogens, felodipine, griseofulvin, haloperidol, methadone, metronidazole, OCPs, phenothiazine, quinidine, TCAs, theophylline, verapamil **Labs:** ↓ Bilirubin **NIPE:** May take 2–3 wk for full effects; ◯ D/C abruptly; ◯ EtOH, caffeine; tolerance develops to sedation; paradoxic hyperactivity seen in Ped pts; long 1/2-life allows single daily dosing

Phentermine (Adipex-P, Suprenza) Uses: *Wgt loss in exogenous obesity* Action: anorectic/sympathomimetic amine Dose: Adults. 1 daily in AM, lowest dose possible; place on tongue, allow to dissolve, then swallow Caution: [X, –]
CI: CV Dz, hyperthyroidism, glaucoma, PRG, nursing, w/in 14 days of MOAI **Disp:** Tabs 15/30/37.5 mg (*Suprenza*) ODT 15, 30, 37.5 mg **SE:** Pulm hypertension; aortic/mitral/tricuspid regurg valve Dz; dependence, ↑ HR, ↑ BP, palpitations, insomnia, HA, psychosis, restlessness, mood change, impotence, dry mouth, taste disturbance **Notes:** Avoid use at night **NIPE:** Take w/o regard to food; ◯ EtOH; ◯ breast-feeding; short-term Tx only; risk of developing tolerance/dependence

Phentermine/Topiramate (Qsymia) [C-IV] Uses: *Wgt management w/ BMI > 30 kg/m² or > 27 kg/m² w/ wgt-related comorbidity* Acts: Anorectic
(sympathomimetic amine w/ anticonvulsant) **Dose:** *Adults.* 3.75/23 mg PO daily ×

14 d, then 7.5/46 mg PO daily; max dose 15/92 mg daily or 7.5/46 mg w/ mod/ severe renal impair or mod hepatic impair; D/C if not > 3% wgt loss on 7.5/46 mg dose or 5% wgt loss on 15/92 mg dose by week 12; D/C max dose gradually to prevent Szs **Caution:** [X, –] **CI:** PRG, glaucoma, hyperthyroidism, use w/ or w/in 14 d of MAOI **Disp:** Caps (phentermine/topiramate ER) 3.75/23, 7.5/46, 11.25/69, 15/92 mg **SE:** Paresthesia, dizziness, dysgeusia, insomnia, constipation, dry mouth, HR, BP, palpitations, HA, restlessness, mood change, memory impair, metabolic acidosis, kidney stones, Cr, acute myopia, glaucoma, depression, suicidal behavior/ideation: **NIPE:** ✓ PRG baseline & qmo; effective contraception necessary; take w/o regard to food; ✓ HR/BP/electrolytes REMS restricted distribution

Phenylephrine, Nasal (Neo-Synephrine Nasal) (OTC) [Vasopressor/Decongestant] **WARNING:** Not for use in Peds < 2 y **Uses:** *Nasal congestion* **Action:** α-Adrenergic agonist **Dose:** *Adults.* 0.25–1% 2–3 sprays/drops in each nostril q4h PRN *Peds. 2–6 y.* 0.125% 1 drop/nostril q2–4h *6–12 y.* 1–2 sprays/nostril q4h 0.25% 2–3 drops **Caution:** [C, +/–] HTN, acute pancreatitis, hep, coronary Dz, NAG, hyperthyroidism **CI:** ↓ HR, arrhythmias **Disp:** Nasal spray 0.25, 0.5, 1%; drops: 0.125, 0.25 mg/mL **SE:** Arrhythmias, HTN, nasal irritation, dryness, sneezing, rebound congestion w/ prolonged use, HA **NIPE:** Do not use > 3 d; use prior to nasal intubation & NG tube insertion to ↓ bleeding; rebound nasal congestion w/ excessive use

Phenylephrine, Ophthalmic (Neo-Synephrine Ophthalmic, AK-Dilate, Zincfrin [OTC]) [Vasopressor] **Uses:** *Mydriasis, ocular redness [OTC], perioperative mydriasis, posterior synechiae, uveitis w/ posterior synechiae* **Action:** α-Adrenergic agonist **Dose:** *Adults. Redness:* 1 gtt 0.12% q3–4h PRN up to qid *Exammydriasis:* 1 gtt 2.5% (15 min–1 h for effect) *Preop:* 1 gtt 2.5–10% 30–60 min pre-op *Peds.* As adult, only use 2.5% for exam, pre-op, and ocular conditions **Caution:** [C, May cause late-term fetal anoxia/↓ HR, +/–] HTN, w/ elderly w/ CAD **CI:** NAG **Disp:** Ophthal soln 0.12% (Zincfrin OTC), 2.5, 10% **SE:** Tearing, HA, irritation, eye pain, photophobia, arrhythmia, tremor **NIPE:** Wait 10 min before instilling other eye med

Phenylephrine, Oral (Sudafed, Others) (OTC) [Vasopressor/Decongestant] **WARNING:** Not for use in Peds < 2 y **Uses:** *Nasal congestion* **Action:** α-Adrenergic agonist **Dose:** *Adults.* 10–20 mg PO q4h PRN, max 60 mg/d *Peds. 4–5 y.* 2.5 mg q4h max 6 doses/d > *6–12.* 5 mg q4h, max 30 mg/d ≥ *12.* Adult dosing **Caution:** [C, +/–] HTN, acute pancreatitis, hep, coronary Dz, NAG, hyperthyroidism **CI:** MAOI w/in 14 d, NAG, severe ↑ BP or CAD, urinary retention **Disp:** Liq 7.5 mg/5 mL; drops: 1.25/0.8 mL, 2.5 mg/5 mL; tabs 5, 10 mg; chew tabs 10 mg; tabs once daily 10 mg; strips: 1.25, 2.5, 10 mg; many combo OTC products **SE:** Arrhythmias, HTN, HA, agitation, anxiety, tremor, palpitations; can be chemically processed into methamphetamine; products now sold behind pharmacy counter w/o prescription **Interactions:** ↑ Risk of HTN crisis *W /* MAOIs; ↑ risk of pressor effects *W/* BB; ↑ risk of arrhythmias *W/* epinephrine, isoproterenol;

↓ effects *OF* guanethidine, methyldopa, reserpine **NIPE:** Use w/ BB may cause severe HTN & cause intracranial bleed/arrhythmias; ⊘ concurrent use w/ MAOI

Phenylephrine, Systemic (Generic) [Vasopressor/Adrenergic]
WARNING: Prescribers should be aware of full prescribing info before use **Uses:** *Vascular failure in shock, allergy, or drug-induced ↓ BP* **Action:** α-Adrenergic agonist **Dose: Adults.** *Mild–mod* ↓ *BP:* 2–5 mg IM or SQ ↑ BP for 2 h; 0.1–0.5 mg IV elevates BP for 15 min *Severe* ↓ *BP shock:* Cont Inf at 100–180 mcg/min; after BP stable *Peds.* ↓ *BP:* 5–20 mcg/kg/dose IV q10–15min or 0.1–0.5 mcg/kg/min IV Inf, titrate to effect **Caution:** [C, +/–] HTN, acute pancreatitis, hep, coronary Dz, NAG, hyperthyroidism **CI:** ↑ HR, arrhythmias **Disp:** Inj 10 mg/mL **SE:** Arrhythmias, HTN, peripheral vasoconstriction ↑ w/ oxytocin, MAOIs, & TCAs; HA, weakness, necrosis, ↓ renal perfusion **Interactions:** ↑ HTN *W/* BBs, MAOIs; ↑ pressor response *W/* guanethidine, methyldopa, reserpine, TCAs **NIPE:** Restore blood vol if loss has occurred; use large veins to avoid extrav; phentolamine 10 mg in 10–15 mL of NS for local Inj to Rx extrav; ✓ ECG for arrhythmias

Phenytoin (Dilantin) [Anticonvulsant/Hydantoin] **Uses:** *Sz disorders* **Action:** ↓ Sz spread in the motor cortex **Dose: Adults & Peds.** *Load:* 15–20 mg/kg IV, 50 mg/min max or PO in 400-mg doses at 4-h intervals *Adults. Maint:* Initial 200 mg PO or IV bid or 300 mg hs then follow levels; alternately 5–7 mg/kg/d based on IBW *Peds. Maint:* 4–7 mg/kg/24 h PO or IV ÷ daily–bid; avoid PO susp (erratic absorption) **Caution:** [D, +] **CI:** Heart block, sinus bradycardia **Disp:** *Dilantin Infatab:* Chew tabs 50 mg *Dilantin/Phenytek:* caps 100 mg; caps ER 30, 100, 200, 300 mg; susp 125 mg/5 mL; Inj 50 mg/mL **SE:** Nystagmus/ataxia early signs of tox; gum hyperplasia w/ long-term use *IV:* ↓ BP, ↑ HR, arrhythmias, phlebitis; peripheral neuropathy, rash, blood dyscrasias, SJS **Notes:** *Levels: Trough:* Just before next dose *Therapeutic:* 10–20 mcg/mL *Toxic:* > 20 mcg/mL. Phenytoin albumin bound, levels = bound & free phenytoin; w/ ↓ albumin & azotemia, low levels may be therapeutic (nl free levels) **Interactions:** ↑ Effects *W/* amiodarone, allopurinol, chloramphenicol, disulfiram, INH, omeprazole, sulfonamides, quinolones, TMP; ↑ effects *OF* Li; ↓ effects *W/* cimetidine, cisplatin, diazoxide, folate, pyridoxine, rifampin; ↓ effects *OF* azole antifungals, benzodiazepines, carbamazepine, corticosteroids, cyclosporine, digitalis glycosides, doxycycline, furosemide, levodopa, OCPs, quinidine, tacrolimus, theophylline, thyroid meds, valproic acid **Labs:** ↑ Serum cholesterol, glucose, alk phos **NIPE:** Take w/ food; may alter urine color; use barrier contraception; ⊘ D/C abruptly; do not change dosage at intervals < 7–10 d; hold tube feeds 1 h before & after dose if using oral susp; avoid large dose ↑; ✓ bld levels w/ maintenance dose qmo × 1 y, then q3m ongoing

Physostigmine (Generic) [Antimuscarinic Antidote/Reversible Cholinesterase Inhibitor] Uses: *Reverse toxic CNS effects of atropine & scopolamine OD* **Action:** Reversible cholinesterase Inhib **Dose: Adults.** 0.5–2 mg IV or IM q20min **Peds.** 0.01–0.03 mg/kg/dose IV q5–10min up to 2 mg total PRN

Caution: [C, ?] **CI:** GI/GU obst, CV Dz, asthma **Disp:** Inj 1 mg/mL **SE:** Rapid IV administration associated w/ Szs; cholinergic SE; sweating, salivation, lacrimation, GI upset, asystole, changes in HR **Interactions:** ↑ Resp depression **W/** succinylcholine, ↑ effects **W/** cholinergics, jaborandi tree, pill-bearing spurge **Labs:** ↑ ALT, AST, serum amylase **NIPE:** Excessive readministration can result in cholinergic crisis; crisis reversed w/ atropine; ⊘ rapid IV admin can cause ↓ P, Sz, asystole

Phytonadione [Vitamin K] (Mephyton, Generic) [Blood Modifier/Vitamin K] **WARNING:** Hypersensitivity Rxns associated w/ or immediately following Inf Uses: *Coagulation disorders d/t faulty formation of factors II, VII, IX, X*; hyperalimentation **Action:** Cofactor for production of factors II, VII, IX, & X **Dose:** *Adults & Peds.* Anticoagulant-induced prothrombin deficiency: 1–10 mg PO or IV slowly *Hyperalimentation:* 10 mg IM or IV qwk *Infants.* 0.5–1 mg/dose IM w/in 1 h of birth or PO **Caution:** [C, +] **CI:** Allergy **Disp:** Tabs 5 mg; Inj 2, 10 mg/mL **SE:** Anaphylaxis from IV dosage; give IV slowly; GI upset (PO), Inj site Rxns **Interactions:** ↓ Effects **W/** antibiotics, cholestyramine, colestipol, salicylates, sucralfate; ↓ effects **OF** oral anticoagulants **Labs:** Falsely ↑ urine steroids **NIPE:** w/ Parenteral Rx, 1st change in PT/INR usually seen in 12–24 h; use makes rewarfarinization more difficult; may cause ↑ clotting risk

Pimecrolimus (Elidel) [Topical Immunomodulator] **WARNING:** Associated w/ rare skin malignancies and lymphoma, limit to area, not for age < 2 y Uses: *Atopic dermatitis* refractory, severe perianal itching **Action:** Inhibits Tlymphocytes **Dose:** *Adults & Peds > 2 y.* Apply bid **Caution:** [C, ?/–] w/ Local Infxn, lymphadenopathy; immunocompromised; avoid in pts < 2 y **CI:** Allergy component, < 2 y **Disp:** Cream 1% **SE:** Phototoxicity, local irritation/burning, flulike Sxs, may ↑ malignancy **NIPE:** Use on dry skin only; wash hands after; 2nd-line/artificial short-term use only; ⊘ natural/artificial sunlight

Pimozide (Orap) [Antipsychotic/Dopamine Antagonist] **WARNING:** ↑ Mortality in elderly w/ dementia-related psychosis Uses: *Tourette Dz* agitation, psychosis **Action:** Typical antipsychotic, dopamine antagonist **Dose:** Initial 1–2 mg/d to max of 10 mg/d (whichever is less); ↓ hepatic impair **Caution:** [C, –] NAG, elderly, hepatic impair, neurologic Dz **CI:** Compound hypersensitivity, CNS depression, coma, dysrhythmia, ↑ QT syndrome, w/ QT prolonging drugs, ↓ K, ↓ Mg, w/ CYP3A4 Inhib (Table 10) **Disp:** Tabs 1, 2 mg **SE:** CNS (somnolence, agitation, others), rash, xerostomia, weakness, rigidity, visual changes, constipation, ↑ salivation, akathisia, tardive dyskinesia, neuroleptic malignant syndrome, ↑ QT **Interactions:** ↑ Effects **OF** CYP1A2 Inhibs: eg, amiodarone, amprenavir, clarithromycin, diltiazem, ketoconazole, verapamil, grapefruit juice (Table 10); ↑ risk of CNS depression **W/** analgesics, other CNS depressants, EtOH **Labs:** ↓ K+, ↓ mg, monitor CBC—D/C w/ low WBCs **NIPE:** Monitor ECG for ↑ QT synd ✓ & hypokalemia (flattened T waves), ⊘ D/C abruptly; ⊘ use grapefruit products

Pindolol (Generic) [Antihypertensive/Beta-Blocker] Uses: **HTN** Action: β-Adrenergic receptor blocker, β₁, β₂, ISA Dose: 5–10 mg bid, 60 mg/d max; ↓ in hepatic/renal failure Caution: [B (1st tri, Dif 2nd/3rd tri), +/–] CI: Uncompensated CHF, cardiogenic shock, ↓ HR, heart block, asthma, COPD Disp: Tabs 5, 10 mg SE: Insomnia, dizziness, fatigue, edema, GI upset, dyspnea; fluid retention may exacerbate CHF Interactions: ↑ HTN & bradycardia W/ amphetamines, ephedrine, phenylephrine; ↑ effects W/ antihypertensives, diuretics; ↓ effects W/ NSAIDs; ↓ effect OF hypoglycemics Labs: ↑ LFTs, uric acid NIPE: ⊘ D/C abruptly—can cause angina; ↑ cold sensitivity; monitor for hyperglycemia; ⊘ breast-feeding, avoid use w/ PRG

Pioglitazone (Actos) [Hypoglycemic/Thiazolidinedione] WARNING: May cause or worsen CHF Uses: **Type 2 DM** Action: ↑ Insulin sensitivity, a thiazolidinedione Dose: 15–45 mg/d PO Caution: [C, –] w/ Hx bladder CA; do not use w/ active bladder CA CI: CHF, hepatic impair Disp: Tabs 15, 30, 45 mg SE: WGT gain, myalgia, URI, HA, hypoglycemia, edema, ↑ fx risk in women; may ↑ bladder CA risk Interactions: ↑ Effects W/ CYP2C8 Inhibs (eg, gemfibrozil); ↓ effects W/ CYP2C8 inducers (eg, rifampin); ↓ effects OF OC, midazolam; monitor for HF W/ insulin; control glycemic control W/ ketoconazole Labs: ↑ LFTs—monitor NIPE: Take w/o regard to food; use barrier contraception; ↑ fx risk in women; ↑ risk of fluid retention leading to CHF; ⊘ ETOH; assess/ instruct S/Sx ↓ glycemia; report wgt gain, edema

Pioglitazone/Metformin (ACTPplus Met, ACTPplus, MET XR) [Hypoglycemic/Thiazolidinedione & Biguanide] WARNING: Metformin can cause lactic acidosis, fatal in 50% of cases; pioglitazone may cause or worsen CHF Uses: **Type 2 DM as adjunct to diet an dexercise** Action: Combined ↑ insulin sensitivity w/ ↓ hepatic glucose release Dose: Initial 1 tab PO daily or bid, titrate; max daily pioglitazone 45 mg & metformin 2550 mg; XR: 1 tab PO daily w/ evening meal; max daily pioglitazone 45 mg & metformin 2550 mg; metformin IR 2550 mg, metformin ER 2000 mg; give w/ meals Caution: [C, –] Stop w/ radiologic IV contrast agents; w/ Hx bladder CA; do not use w/ active bladder CA CI: CHF; renal impair, Disp: Tabs (pioglitazone mg/metformin mg): 15/500, 15/850, tabs XR (pioglitazone mg/metformin ER mg): 15/1000, 30/1000 mg SE: Lactic acidosis, CHF, ↓ glucose, edema, wgt gain, myalgia, URI, HA, GI upset, liver damage Interactions: ↑ Effects of metformin on lactate W/ EtOH; ↑ Effects W/ amiloride, cimetidine, digoxin, furosemide, ketoconazole, MAOIs, morphine, procainamide, quinidine, quinine, ranitidine, triamterene, TMP, vancomycin; ↓ effects OF OCPs; ↓ effects W/ corticosteroids, CCBs, diuretics, estrogens, INH, OCPs, phenothiazine, phenytoin, sympathomimetics, thyroid drugs, tobacco; monitor for HF W/ insulin; BB may mask hypoglycemia Labs: ↑ LFTs, monitor serum glucose & LFTs NIPE: Take w/o regard to food; use barrier contraception; prevent dehydration; ⊘ EtOH; ↑ fx risk in women receiving pioglitazone; ✓ and instruct pt S/Sx HF, lactic acidosis

Piperacillin–Tazobactam (Zosyn) [Antibiotic/Extended-Spectrum Penicillin, Beta-Lactamase Inhibitor] Uses: *Infxns of skin, bone, resp & urinary tract, Abd, sepsis* **Action:** 4th-gen PCN plus β-lactamase Inhib; bactericidal; ↓ cell wall synth *Spectrum:* Good gram(+), excellent gram(−); anaerobes & β-lactamase producers **Dose:** *Adults.* 3.375–4.5 g IV q6h; ↓ in renal Insuff **Caution:** [B, M] **CI:** PCN or β-lactam sensitivity **Disp:** *Frozen & Powder for Inj:* 42.25, 3.375, 4.5 g **SE:** D, HA, insomnia, GI upset, serum sickness-like Rxn, pseudomembranous colitis **Interactions:** ↑ Effects *W/* probenecid; ↑ effects *OF* anticoagulants, MTX; ↓ effects *W/* macrolides, tetracyclines; ↓ effects *OF* OCPs **Labs:** ↑ LFTs, BUN, Cr, (+) direct Coombs test; ↓ K+ **NIPE:** Inactivation of aminoglycosides if drugs given together—administration at least 1 h apart; often used in combo w/ aminoglycoside; monitor for hypovolemia d/t D; ✓ S/sx super Infxn, ↑ GI effects d/t antibiotic-related colitis

Pirbuterol (Maxair, Autohaler) [Bronchodilator/Sympathomimetic] Uses: *Prevention & Rx reversible bronchospasm* **Action:** β₂-Adrenergic agonist **Dose:** 2 Inh q4–6h; max 12 Inh/d **Caution:** [C, ?/–] **Disp:** Aerosol 0.2 mg/actuation (contains ozone-depleting CFCs; will be gradually removed from US market) **SE:** Nervousness, restlessness, trembling, HA, taste changes, tachycardia **Interactions:** ↑ Effects *W/* epinephrine, sympathomimetics; ↑ vascular effects *W/* MAOIs, TCAs; ↓ effects *W/* BB **NIPE:** Rinse mouth after use; shake well before use; teach pt proper inhaler technique; monitor for hyperglycemia

Piroxicam (Feldene) [Bronchodilator/Beta-Adrenergic Agonist] WARNING: May ↑ risk of cardiovascular CV events & GI bleeding Uses: *Arthritis & pain* **Action:** NSAID; ↓ prostaglandins **Dose:** 10–20 mg/d **Caution:** [B 1st tri, D if 3rd tri or near term, +] GI bleeding **CI:** ASA/NSAID sensitivity **Disp:** Caps 10, 20 mg **SE:** Dizziness, rash, GI upset, edema, acute renal failure, peptic ulcer **Interactions:** ↑ Effects *W/* probenecid; ↑ effects *OF* aminoglycosides, anticoagulants, hypoglycemics, Li, MTX; ↑ risk of bleeding *W/* ASA, corticosteroids, NSAIDs, feverfew, garlic, ginger, ginkgo, EtOH; ↓ effect *W/* ASA, antacids, cholestyramine; ↓ effect *OF* BBs, diuretics **Labs:** ↑ BUN, Cr, LFTs **NIPE:** Take w/ food, full effect after 2 wk administration, ↑ risk of photosens—use sunblock; ⊘ ETOH, ASA during Tx; swallow tab whole

Pitavastatin (Livalo) [HMG-CoA Reductase Inhibitor] Uses: *Reduce elevated total cholesterol* **Action:** Statin, inhibits HMG-CoA reductase **Dose:** 1–4 mg once/d w/o regard to meals; CrCl < 60 mL/min start 1 mg/ 2 mg max **Caution:** [X, −] May cause myopathy & rhabdomyolysis **CI:** Active liver Dz, w/ lopinavir/ritonavir/cyclosporine, severe renal impair not on dialysis **Disp:** Tabs 1, 2, 4 mg **SE:** Muscle pain, backpain, Jt pain, & constipation, ↑ LFTs **Interactions:** ↑ Effects *W/* cyclosporine, erythromycin, lopinavir, rifampin, ritonavir; ↑ risk of myopathy *W/* fibrates, niacin; ↑ effects *OF* warfarin **Labs:** ↑ Glucose, LFTs—monitor < therapy & 12 wk > start of drug & periodically **NIPE:** ⊘ PRG, breast feeding; use nonhormonal contraception methods; ✓ hepatic function

Plasma Protein Fraction (Plasmanate) [Plasma Volume Expander] Uses: *Shock & ↓ BP* **Dose: Adults. Initial:** 250–500 mL IV (not > 10 mL/min); subsequent Inf based on response. **Peds.** 10–15 mL/kg/dose IV; subsequent Inf based on response; safety & efficacy in children not established **Caution:** [C, +] **CI:** Renal Insuff, CHF, cardiopulmonary bypass **Disp:** Inj 5% **SE:** ↓ BP w/ rapid Inf; hypocoagulability, metabolic acidosis, PE **NIPE:** ⊘ Rapid infusion→↑ risk of ↓ BP; 130–160 mEq Na^{2+}/L; not substitute for RBC

Plerixafor (Mozobil) [Hematopoietic Stem Cell Mobilizer] Uses: *Mobilize stem cells for ABMT in lymphoma & myeloma in combo w/ G-CSF* **Action:** Hematopoietic stem cell mobilizer **Dose:** 0.24 mg/kg SQ daily; max 40 mg/d; *CrCl < 50 mL/min:* 0.16 mg/kg, max 27 mg/d **Disp:** IV 20 mg/mL (1.2 mL) **SE:** HA, N/V, D, Inj site Rxns, ↑ WBC, ↓ plt **Interactions:** ↑ Effects w/ reduce renal Fxn or compete for active tubular secretion **Labs:** ↑ WBC, neutrophils ↓ plt **NIPE:** Initiate Tx after G-CSF has been given to pt qd × 4d; repeat mozobil dose up to 4 consecutive d; Give by SQ Inj approx 11 h before initiation of apheresis; ⊘ PRG; ✓ for splenic rupture (LUQ pain, left scapular or shoulder pain)

Pneumococcal 13-Valent Conjugate Vaccine (Prevnar 13) [Vaccine] Uses: *Immunization against pneumococcal Infxns in infants & children* **Action:** Active immunization **Dose:** 0.5 mL IM/dose; series of 4 doses; 1st dose age 2 mo; then 4 mo, 6 mo, and 12–15 mo; if previous *Prevnar* switch to *Prevnar 13*; if completed *Prevnar* series, supplemental dose *Prevnar 13* at least 8 wk after last *Prevnar* dose **Caution:** [C, +] w/ ↓ plt **CI:** Sensitivity to components/diphtheria toxoid, febrile illness **Disp:** Inj **SE:** Local Rxns, anorexia, fever, irritability, ↓/↑ sleep, V, D **Interactions:** May ↓ response *W/* immunosuppressant (radiation, chemotherapy, high-dose steroids) **NIPE:** Keep epi (1:1000) available for Rxns; replaces *Prevnar* (has additional spectrum); does not replace *Pneumovax-23* in age > 24 mo w/ immunosuppression

Pneumococcal Vaccine, Polyvalent (Pneumovax-23) [Vaccine/ Inactive Bacteria] Uses: *Immunization against pneumococcal Infxns in pts at high risk (all pts > 65 y, also asplenia, sickle cell Dz, HIV & other immunocompromised & w/ chronic illness)* **Action:** Active immunization **Dose:** 0.5 mL IM or SQ **Caution:** [C, ?] **CI:** Do not vaccinate during immunosuppressive Rx **Disp:** Inj 0.5 mL **SE:** Fever, Inj site Rxn, hemolytic anemia w/ other heme conditions, ↓ plt w/ stable ITP, anaphylaxis, Guillain-Barré synd **Interactions:** ↓ Effects *W/* corticosteroids, immunosuppressants **NIPE:** Keep epi (1:1000) available for Rxns. Revaccinate q3–5y if very high risk (eg, asplenia, nephrotic synd), consider revaccination if > 6 y since initial or if previously vaccinated w/ 14-valent vaccine

Podophyllin (Podocon-25, Condylox Gel 0.5%, Condylox) [Antimitotic Effect] Uses: *Topical Rx of benign growths (genital & perianal warts [condylomata acuminata]*, papillomas, fibromas) **Action:** Direct antimitotic effect; exact mechanism unknown **Dose:** *Condylox Gel & Condylox:* Apply bid for 3 consecutive d/wk then hold for 4 d may repeat 4×0.5 mL/d max *Podocon-25:* Use sparingly on the lesion, leave on for only 30-40 min for 1st application, then 1–4 h on subsequent applications, thoroughly wash off; limit < 5 mL or < 10 cm²/Rx **Caution:** [X, ?] Immunosuppression **CI:** DM, bleeding lesions **Disp:** *Podocon-25* (w/ benzoin) 15-mL bottles; *Condylox Gel* 0.5% 35-g clear gel; *Condylox soln* 0.5% 35-g clear **SE:** Local Rxns, sig absorption; anemias, tachycardia, paresthesias, GI upset, renal/hepatic damage **NIPE:** *Podocon-25* applied by the clinician; do not dispense directly to pt; ⊘ use on warts on mucous membranes; ⊘ use near eyes

Polyethylene Glycol [PEG]-Electrolyte Soln (GoLYTELY, CoLyte) [Laxative] **Uses:** *Bowel prep prior to exam or surgery* **Action:** Osmotic cathartic **Dose:** *Adults.* Following 3–4-h fast, drink 240 mL of soln q10min until 4 L consumed or until BMs are clear *Peds.* 25–40 mL/kg/h for 4–10 h until BM clear; max dose 4L **Caution:** [C, ?] **CI:** GI obst, bowel perforation, megacolon, UC **Disp:** Powder for recons to 4 L **SE:** Cramping or N, bloating **NIPE:** Instruct pt to drink Sol rapidly q10min until finished; 1st BM should occur in approximately 1 h; chilled soln more palatable; clear liquids only after admin

Polyethylene Glycol [PEG] 3350 (MiraLAX [OTC]) [Osmotic Laxative] **Uses:** *Occasional constipation* **Action:** Osmotic laxative **Dose:** 17-g powder (1 heaping tsp) in 8 oz (1 cup) of H_2O & drink; max 14 d **Caution:** [C, ?] Rule out bowel obst before use **CI:** GI obst, allergy to PEG **Disp:** Powder for reconstitution; bottle cap holds 17 g **SE:** Upset stomach, bloating, cramping, gas, severe D, hives **NIPE:** May take qd for no more than 7 d for BM; can add to H_2O, juice, soda, coffee, or tea

Pomalidomide (Pomalyst) **WARNING:** Contraindicated in PRG; a thalidomide analog, a known human teratogen. Exclude PRG before/during Tx; use 2 forms of contraception; available only through a restricted program; DVT/PE w/ multiple myeloma treated w/ pomalidomide **Uses:** *Multiple myeloma previously treated w/ at least 2 regimens including lenalidomide and bortezomib w/ progression w/in 60 d of last therapy* **Action:** Immunomodulatory drug w/ antineoplastic action **Dose:** *Adults.* 4 mg 1 ×/d, d 1–21 in a 28 d cycle, until Dz prog; hold/reduce dose w/ ↓ WBC/plts **Caution:** [X, –] Hematologic toxicity, especially w/ ↓ WBC **CI:** PRG **Disp:** Caps 1, 2, 3, and 4 mg **SE:** Birth defects; ↓ WBC/plts/Hgb; DVT/PE; neuropathy; confusion, dizziness, HA; fever, fatigue, N/V/D, constipation; rash **Notes:** Avoid w/ CYP1A2 Inhib; cannot donate blood/sperm **NIPE:** ⊘ PRG/breast-feeding; r/o + PRG before Tx; use 2 effective contraceptive methods or abstinence during Tx & 1 mo after Tx; male pts use condoms/spermicide; take w/o food 2 h ac or 2 h pc; ⊘ break/crush/dissolve/open capsule; avoid use w/ Cr >3.0 mg/dL; change position slowly; ⊘ ETOH; ⊘ smoking; ✓ & teach S/Sx of DVT

Ponatinib (Iclusig) **WARNING:** Venous/arterial occlusion (27%); DVT/PE, MI, CVA, PVD, often need revascularization; heart failure & hepatotoxicity w/ liver failure and death, (monitor cardiac & hepatic Fxn) **Uses:** *T315I + CML; + Philadelphia chromosome ALL (Ph + ALL); CML or Ph + ALL w/ no other TKI indicated* **Action:** TKI **Dose: Adults.** 45 mg 1 × /d, DC and then ↓ dose for toxicity **Caution:** [D, –] ↓ WBC; vascular occlusion; heart failure; hepatotoxicity; pancreatitis; ↑ BP; neuropathy; ocular toxicity including blindness; arrhythmias, bradycardia, & SVT; edema; tumor lysis; poor wound healing; GI perforation **CI:** None **Disp:** Tabs, 15, 45 mg **SE:** ↑ BP, fever, rash, HA, fatigue, arthralgias, N, abd pain, constipation, pneumonia; sepsis; ↑ QT interval; anemia, ↓ plts, ↓ WBC, ↓ neutrophils, ↓ lymphs; ↑ AST, ↑ ALT, ↑ alk phos, ↑ bilirubin, ↑ lipase, ↑ glucose, ↑/↓ K^+, ↓ Na^+, ↓ HCO_3^-, ↑ creatinine, ↑ Ca^{++}, ↓ phos ↓ albumin **Notes:** CBC q2wk × 3 mo; ✓ following baseline and periodically; eye exam, LFTs, BP; lipase q2wk × 2 mo; monitor BP; w/ CYP3A4 Inhib ↓ dose; avoid w/ CYP3A inducers & meds that ↑ gastric pH **NIPE:** Take w/o regard to food; ⊘ PRG; temporarily hold Tx for major surgery; ensure adequate hydration; ✓ for arrhythmias; comprehensive eye exam at baseline & during Tx; ✓ for peripheral neuropathy

Posaconazole (Noxafil) [Anti-Infective/Antifungal] **Uses:** *Prevent Aspergillus and Candida Infxns in severely immunocompromised; Rx oropharyngeal Candida* **Action:** ↓ Cell membrane ergosterol synth **Dose: Adults.** Invasive fungal prophylaxis: 200 mg PO tid Oropharyngeal candidiasis: 100 mg bid on d 1, then 100 mg daily × 13 d Peds > 13 y. See adult dose **Caution:** [C, ?] Multiple drug interactions; ↑ QT, cardiac Dzs, severe renal/liver impair **CI:** Component hypersensitivity; w/ many drugs including alfuzosin, astemizole, alprazolam, phenothiazine, terfenadine, triazolam, others **Disp:** Soln 40 mg/mL **SE:** ↑ QT, ↑ LFTs, hepatic failure, fever, N/V/D, HA, Abd pain, anemia, ↓ plt, ↓ K^+, rash, dyspnea, cough, anorexia, fatigue **Interactions:** ↑ Effects OF CCB, cyclosporine, midazolam, sirolimus, statins, tacrolimus, vinca alkaloids; ↓ effects W/ cimetidine, phenytoin, rifabutin **Labs:** ↑ LFTs; ↑ K^+, plts; monitor LFTs, lytes, CBC **NIPE:** Monitor for breakthrough fungal Infxns; ⊘ for children < 13 y; ⊘ PRG/breastfeeding; take w/in 20 min of full meal or carbonated drink; ensure adequate oral hygiene

Potassium Citrate (Urocit-K) [Urinary Alkalinizer] **Uses:** *Alkalinize urine, prevention of urinary stones (uric acid, calcium stones if hypocitraturic)* **Action:** Urinary alkalinizer **Dose:** 30–60 mEq/d based on severity of hypocitraturia. Max 100 mEq/d **Caution:** [A, +] **CI:** Severe renal impair, dehydration, ↑ K^+, peptic ulcer; w/ K^+-sparing diuretics, salt substitutes **Disp:** Tabs 5, 10, 15 mEq/d **SE:** GI upset, ↓ Ca^{2+}, ↑ K^+, metabolic alkalosis **Interactions:** ↑ Risk of hyperkalemia W/ ACEIs, K^+-sparing diuretics **Labs:** ↑ K^+, ↓ Ca^{2+} **NIPE:** Take w/in 30 min of meals or hs snack; tabs 540 mg = 5 mEq, 1080 mg = 10 mEq; ✓ ECG for hyperkalemia (peaked T waves)

Potassium Iodide [Lugol Soln] (Iosat, SSKI, Thyro-Block, Thyro-Safe, ThyroShield) [OTC] [Iodine Supplement] **Uses:** *Thyroid storm*, ↓ vascularity before thyroid surgery, block thyroid uptake of radioactive iodine (nuclear scans or nuclear emergency), thin bronchial secretions **Action:** Iodine supl **Dose:** *Adults & Peds > 2 y.* Pre-op thyroidectomy: 50–100 mg PO tid (1–2 gtts or 0.05–0.1 mL SSKI); give 10 d pre-op *Protection:* 130 mg/d **Peds.** *Protection: < 1 y:* 16.25 mg qd *1 mo–3 y.* 32.5 mg qd *3–18y.* 65 mg once daily **Caution:** [D, +] ↑ K⁺, TB, PE, bronchitis, renal impair **CI:** Iodine sensitivity **Disp:** Tabs 65, 130 mg; soln (saturated soln of potassium iodide [SSKI]) 1 g/mL; Lugol soln, strong iodine 100 mg/mL; syrup 325 mg/5 mL **SE:** Fever, HA, urticaria, angioedema, goiter, GI upset, eosinophilia **Interactions:** ↑ Risk of hypothyroidism *W/* antithyroid drugs & Li; ↑ risk of hyperkalemia *W/* ACEIs, K⁺-sparing diuretics, K⁺supls **Labs:** May alter TFTs **NIPE:** Take pc w/ food or milk; w/ nuclear radiation emergency, give until radiation exposure no longer exists; ✓ for hyperkalemia (peaked T waves)

Potassium Supplements (Kaon, Kaochlor, K-Lor, Slow-K, Micro-K, Klorvess, Generic) [Potassium Supplement/Electrolyte] **Uses:** *Prevention or Rx of ↓ K⁺* (eg, diuretic use) **Action:** K⁺ supl **Dose:** *Adults.* 20–100 mEq/d PO ÷ 1–4 ×/d; IV 10–20 mEq/h, max 40 mEq/h & 150 mEq/d (monitor K⁺ levels frequently and in presence of continuous ECG monitoring w/ high-dose IV) **Peds.** Calculate K⁺ deficit; 1–3 mEq/kg/d PO ÷ 1–4 ×/d; IV max dose 0.5–1 mEq/kg × 1–2 h **Caution:** [A, +] Renal Insuff, use w/ NSAIDs & ACE Inhib **CI:** ↑ K⁺ **Disp:** PO forms (Table 6); Inj **SE:** GI irritation; ↓ HR, ↓ K⁺, heart block **Interactions:** ↑ Effects *W/* ACE Inhib, K⁺-sparing diuretics, salt substitutes **Labs:** ↑ K⁺, monitor K⁺, monitor ECG for hyperkalemia (peaked T waves) **NIPE:** Take w/ food; mix powder & Liq w/ beverage (unsalted tomato juice, etc); swallow tabs whole; Cl⁻ salt OK w/ alkalosis; w/ acidosis use acetate, bicarbonate, citrate, or gluconate salt; do not administer IV K⁺ undiluted

Pralatrexate (Folotyn) [Folate Analogue Inhibitor] **Uses:** *Tx refractory T-cell lymphoma* **Action:** Folate analogue metabolic Inhib; ↓ dihydrofolate reductase **Dose:** *Adults.* IV pushover 3–5 min: 30 mg/m² once weekly for 6 wk **Caution:** [D, –] **Disp:** Inj 20 mg/mL (1 mL, 2 mL) **SE:** ↓ Plt anemia, mucositis, N/V/D, edema, fever, fatigue, rash **Interactions:** ↑ Effects *W/* probenecid, NSAIDs, TMP/sulfamethoxazole **Labs:** ↓ Plt, ↓ WBC; monitor CBC weekly; monitor renal & hepatic Fxn < the 1st & 4th dose per cycle **NIPE:** Give folic acid 1–1.25 mg prior to 1st Tx & continue qd. Give vit B₁₂ 1 mg IM approx 10 wk before 1st Tx & q8–10wk ongoing; ⊘ PRG

Pramipexole (Mirapex, Mirapex ER, Generic) [Anti-Parkinson Agent/Dopamine Agonist] **Uses:** *Parkinson Dz (Mirapex, Mirapex ER),* RLS (*Mirapex*)* **Action:** Dopamine agonist **Dose:** *Mirapex* 1.5–4.5 mg/d PO, initial 0.375 mg/d in 3 ÷ doses; titrate slowly; *RLS:* 0.125–0.5 mg PO 2–3 h before bedtime. *Mirapex ER* start 0.375PO daily, ↑ dose q5–7d to 0.75, then by 0.75 mg to max 4.5 mg/d **Caution:** [C, ?/–] Daytime falling asleep, ↓ BP **CI:** None **Disp:** *Mirapex* Tabs 0.125, 0.25, 0.5, 0.75, 1, 1.5 mg; *Mirapex ER* 0.375, 0.75, 1.5, 2.25, 3, 3.75, 4.5 mg **SE:** Somnolence, N, constipation, dizziness, fatigue, hallucinations, dry mouth, muscle spasms, edema **Interactions:** ↑ Drug levels & effects W/ cimetidine, diltiazem, ranitidine, triamterene, verapamil, quinidine, quinine; ↑ effects OF levodopa; ↑ CNS depression W/ CNS depressants, EtOH; ↓ effects W/ antipsychotics, butyrophenones, metoclopramide, phenothiazine, thioxanthenes; ↓ effects W/ DA antagonists (eg, neuroleptics, metoclopramide) **NIPE:** ⊘ Abrupt cessation/withdraw over 1 wk; ↑ risk of hallucinations in elderly; take w/ food w/ nausea; ER tab—swallow whole; report new or ↑ in impulsive behaviors

Pramoxine (Anusol Ointment, ProctoFoam-NS, Others) [Topical Anesthetic] Uses: *Relief of pain & itching from hemorrhoids, anorectal surgery*; topical for burns & dermatosis **Action:** Topical anesthetic **Dose:** Apply freely to anal area 3–5 ×/d **Caution:** [C, ?] **Disp:** [OTC] All 1%; foam (Procto-Foam-NS), cream, oint, lotion, gel, pads, spray **SE:** Contact dermatitis, mucosal thinning w/ chronic use **NIPE:** ⊘ Use on large areas

Pramoxine + Hydrocortisone (ProctoFoam-HC) [Topical Anesthetic/Anti-Inflammatory] Uses: *Relief of pain & itching from hemorrhoids* **Action:** Topical anesthetic, anti-inflammatory **Dose:** Apply freely to anal area tid–qid **Caution:** [C, ?/–] **Disp:** Cream: Pramoxine 1%, acetate 1%/2.5%/2.35% Foam: Pramoxine 1%, hydrocortisone 1%; Lotion: Pramoxine 1%, hydrocortisone 1/2.5%; Ointment: Oramoxine 1%, & hydrocortisone 1/2.5% **SE:** Contact dermatitis, mucosal thinning w/ chronic use **NIPE:** ⊘ Use on large areas

Prasugrel (Effient) [Platelet Inhibitor] WARNING: Can cause significant, sometimes fatal, bleeding; do not use w/ planned CABG w/ active bleeding, Hx TIA or stroke or pts > 75 y Uses: *↓ Thrombotic CV events (eg, stent thrombosis) post-PCI* administer ASAP in ECC setting w/ high-risk ST depression or T-wave inversion w/ planned PCI **Action:** ↓ Plt aggregation **Dose:** 10 mg/d; wgt < 60 kg, consider 5 mg/d; 60 mg PO loading dose in ECC; use at least 12 mo w/ cardiac stent (bare or drug eluting); consider > 15 mo w/ drug eluting stent **Caution:** [B, ?] Active bleeding; ↑ bleed risk; w/ CYP3A4 substrates **CI:** Active bleed, Hx TIA/stroke risk factors ≥ 75 y, propensity to bleed, Wt < 60 kg, CABG, meds that ↑ bleeding **Disp:** Tabs 5, 10 mg **SE:** ↑ Bleeding time, ↑ BP, GI intolerance, HA, dizziness, rash, ↓ WBC **Interactions:** ↑ Risk of bleeding W/ heparin, warfarin, fibrinolytics, chronic NSAIDs use **Labs:** ↓ WBC **NIPE:** Plt aggregation to baseline ~ 7 d after D/C, plt transfusion reverses acutely; ⊘ crush tab; take w/o regard to food

Pravastatin (Pravachol) [Antilipemic/HMG-CoA Reductase Inhibitor] Uses: *↓ Cholesterol* **Action:** HMG-CoA reductase Inhib **Dose:** 10–80 mg PO hs; ↓ in sig renal/hepatic impair **Caution:** [X, –] w/ Gemfibrozil **CI:** Liver Dz or persistent LFTs ↑ **Disp:** Tabs 10, 20, 40, 80 mg **SE:** Use caution w/ concurrent gemfibrozil; HA, GI upset, hep, myopathy, renal failure **Interactions:** ↑ Risk of myopathy & rhabdomyolysis W/ clarithromycin, clofibrate, cyclosporine, danazol, erythromycin, fluoxetine, gemfibrozil, niacin, nefazodone, troleandomycin; ↑ effects W/ azole antifungals, cimetidine, grapefruit juice; ↑ effects

OF warfarin; ↑ CNS effects & liver tox w/ concurrent EtOH use; ↓ effects *W/* cholestyramine, isradipine **Labs:** ↑ LFTs **NIPE:** ⊘ PRG, breast-feeding; take w/o regard to food; full effect may take up to 4 wk; ↑ risk of photosens—use sunblock

Prazosin (Minipress) [Antihypertensive/Alpha-Blocker] Uses: *HTN* **Action:** Peripherally acting α-adrenergic blocker **Dose:** *Adults.* 1 mg PO tid; can ↑ to 20 mg/d max PRN *Peds.* 0.05–0.1 mg/kg/d in 3 ÷ doses; max 0.5 mg/kg/d **Caution:** [C, ?] Use w/ phosphodiesterase-5 (PDE5) Inhib (eg, sildenafil) can cause ↓ BP **CI:** Component allergy, concurrent use of PDE5 Inhib **Disp:** Caps 1, 2, 5 mg; tabs ER 2.5, 5 mg **SE:** Dizziness, edema, palpitations, fatigue, GI upset **Interactions:** ↑ Hypotension *W/* antihypertensives, diuretics, verapamil, nitrates, EtOH; ↓ effects *W/* NSAIDs, butcher's broom **Labs:** ↑ Serum Na levels; alters test for Pheo **NIPE:** ⊘ D/C abruptly; can cause orthostatic ↓ BP, take the 1st dose hs; tolerance develops to this effect; tachyphylaxis may result; concurrent use w/ Viagra-type drugs can cause life-threatening hypotension

Prednisolone (Flo-Pred, Omnipred, Orapred, Pediapred, Generic) [See Steroids Table 2]

Prednisone (Generic) [See Steroids Table 2]

Pregabalin (Lyrica) [Antinociceptive/Antiseizure] Uses: *DM peripheral neuropathy pain; postherpetic neuralgia; fibromyalgia; adjunct w/ adult partial-onset Szs* **Action:** Nerve transmission modulator, antinociceptive, antiseizure effect; mechanism ?; related to gabapentin **Dose:** *Neuropathic pain:* 50 mg PO tid, ↑ to 300 mg/d w/in 1 wk based on response, 300 mg/d max *Postherpetic neuralgia:* 75–150 mg bid, or 50–100 mg tid; start 75 mg bid or 50 mg tid; ↑ to 300 mg/d w/in 1 wk PRN; if pain persists after 2–4 wk, ↑ to 600 mg/d *Partial-onset Sz:* Start 150 mg/d (75 mg bid or 50 mg tid) may ↑ to max 600 mg/d; ↓ w/ CrCl < 60; w/ or w/o food **Caution:** [C, −] w/ Sig renal impair (see PI), w/ elderly & severe CHF avoid abrupt D/C **CI:** Hypersensitivity **Disp:** Caps 25, 50, 75, 100, 150, 200, 225, 300 mg; soln 20 mg/mL **SE:** Dizziness, drowsiness, xerostomia, edema, blurred vision, wgt gain, difficulty concentrating; suicidal ideation **NIPE:** Avoid abrupt D/C—can cause Szs; w/ D/C, taper over at least 1 wk; ⊘ ETOH; ⊘ crush/open capsule

Probenecid (Probalan, Generic) [Uricosuric/Analgesic] Uses: *Prevent gout & hyperuricemia; extends effects of PCNs & cephalosporins* **Action:** Uricosuric, renal tubular blocker of weak organic anions **Dose:** *Adults. Gout:* 250 mg bid × 1 wk, then 500 mg PO bid; can ↑ by 500 mg/mo up to 2–3 g/d *Antibiotic effect:* 1–2 g PO 30 min before dose *Peds > 2 y.* 25 mg/kg, then 40 mg/kg/d PO qid **Caution:** [B, ?] **CI:** Uric acid, kidney stones, initiations during acute gout attack, coadministration of salicylates, age < 2y, MDD, renal impair **Disp:** Tabs 500 mg **SE:** HA, GI upset, rash, pruritus, dizziness, blood dyscrasias **Interactions:** ↑ Effects *OF* acyclovir, allopurinol; ↑ effects *OF* benzodiazepines, cephalosporins, ciprofloxacin, clofibrate, dapsone, dyphylline, MTX, NSAIDs, olanzapine, rifampin, sulfonamides, sulfonylureas zidovudine; ↓ effects

W/ niacin, EtOH; ↑ effects *OF* penicillamine **Labs:** False(+) urine glucose; false ↑ level of theophylline **NIPE:** Take w/ food, ↑ fluids to 2–3 L/d; do not use during acute gout attack; caution when used concurrently w/ benzodiazepines; use low-purine diet

Procainamide (Generic) [Antiarrhythmic]   WARNING: Positive ANA titer or SLE w/ prolonged use; only use in life-threatening arrhythmias; hematologic tox can be severe, follow CBC

Uses: *Supraventricular/ventricular arrhythmias* **Action:** Class Ia antiarrhythmic (Table 9) **Dose:** *Adults. Recurrent VF/VT:* 20–50 mg/min IV (total 17 mg/kg max) *Maint:* 1–4 mg/min *Stable wide-complex tachycardia of unknown origin, AF w/ rapid rate in WPW:* 20 mg/min IV until arrhythmia suppression, ↓ BP, or QRS widens > 50%, then 1–4 mg/min. *Recurrent VF/VT:* 20–50 mg/min IV; max total 17 mg/kg. *ECC 2010: Stable monomorphic VT, refractory reentry SVT, stable wide-complex tachycardia, AFib w/ WPW:* 20 mg/min IV until one of the **SE:** Arrhythmia stopped, hypotension, QRS widens > 50%, total 17 mg/kg; then maintenance Inf of 1–4 mg/min *Peds. ECC 2010: SVT, aflutter, VT (w/ pulses):* 15 mg/kg IV/IO over 30–60 min **Caution:** [C, +] ↓ In renal/hepatic impair **CI:** Complete heart block, 2nd-/3rd-degree heart block w/o pacemaker, torsades de pointes, SLE **Disp:** Inj 100, 500 mg/mL **SE:** ↓ BP, lupus-like synd, GI upset, taste perversion, arrhythmias, tachycardia, heart block, angioneurotic edema, blood dyscrasias **Notes:** *Levels: Trough:* Just before next dose *Therapeutic:* 4–10 mcg/mL; *N*-acetyl procainamide (NAPA) + procaine 5–30 mcg/mL *Toxic:* > 10 mcg/mL; NAPA + procaine > 30 mcg/mL *1/2-life:* Procaine 3–5 h, NAPA 6–10 h **Interactions:** ↑ Effects *W/* acetazolamide, amiodarone, cimetidine, ranitidine, TMP; ↑ effects *OF* anticholinergics, antihypertensives; ↑ effects *W/* procaine, EtOH **Labs:** ↑ LFTs **NIPE:** Take w/ food if GI upset; ⊘ crush SR tab; ✓ BP q5–10min during infusion; ✓ EKG for widening QRS, prolongation of PR & QT intervals

Procarbazine (Matulane) [Antineoplastic/Alkylating Agent]   WARNING: Highly toxic; handle w/ care; should be administered under the supervision of an experienced CA chemotherapy physician

Uses: *Hodgkin Dz*, NHL, brain & lung tumors **Action:** Alkylating agent; ↓ DNA & RNA synth **Dose:** Per protocol **Caution:** [D, ?] w/ EtOH ingestion **CI:** Inadequate BM reserve **Disp:** Caps 50 mg **SE:** ↓ BM, hemolytic Rxns (w/ G6PD deficiency), N/V/D; disulfiram-like Rxn; cutaneous & constitutional Sxs, myalgia, arthralgia, CNS effects, azoospermia, cessation of menses **Interactions:** ↑ CNS depression *W/* antihistamines, barbiturates, CNS depressants, narcotics, phenothiazine; ↑ risk of HTN *W/* guanethidine, levodopa, MAOIs, methyldopa, sympathomimetics, TCAs, caffeine, tyramine-containing foods (aged cheese/meats, red wine, beer, dried fruits); ↓ effects *OF* digoxin **NIPE:** Disulfiram-like Rxn w/ EtOH (tachycardia, N/V, sweating, flushing, HA, blurred vision, confusion); ↑ fluids to 2–3 L/d; ↑ risk of photosens—use sunblock; ⊘ exposure to Infxn; avoid foods w/ high tyramine content (wine, yogurt, ripe cheese, bananas)

Prochlorperazine (Compro, Procomp) [Antiemetic, Antipsychotic/Phenothiazine] **WARNING:** ↑ Mortality in elderly pts w/ dementia-related psychosis **Uses:** *N/V, agitation, & psychotic disorders* **Action:** Phenothiazine; blocks postsynaptic dopaminergic CNS receptors **Dose:** *Adults.* *Antiemetic:* 5–10 mg PO 3–4 ×/d or 25 mg PR bid or 5–10 mg deep IM q4–6h *Antipsychotic:* 10–20 mg IM acutely or 5–10 mg PO 3–4 ×/d for maint; ↑ doses may be required for antipsychotic effect *Peds.* 0.1–0.15 mg/kg/dose IM q4–6h or 0.4 mg/kg/24 h PO PRN ÷ 3–4 ×/d **Caution:** [C, +/–] NAG, severe liver/cardiac Dz **CI:** Phenothiazine sensitivity, BM suppression; age < 2 y or wgt < 9 kg **Disp:** Tabs 5, 10, mg; syrup 5 mg/5 mL; supp 25 mg; Inj 5 mg/mL **Interactions:** Rx w/ diphenhydramine or benztropine **Interactions:** ↑ Effects *W/* chloroquine, indomethacin, narcotics, procarbazine, SSRIs, pyrimethamine; ↑ effect *OF* antidepressants, BBs, EtOH; ↓ effects *W/* antacids, anticholinergics, barbiturates, tobacco; ↓ effects *OF* anticoagulants, guanethidine, levodopa, Li **Labs:** False(+) urine bilirubin, amylase, PKU, ↑ serum prolactin **NIPE:** ⊘ D/C abruptly; risk of photosens—use sunblock; urine may turn pink/red; over sedation w/ anticholinergics, CNS depressants & EtOH; ✓ EPS S/Sx

Promethazine (Promethegan) [Antihistamine, Antiemetic, Sedative/Phenothiazine] **WARNING:** Do not use in pts < 2 y; resp depression risk; tissue damage, including gangrene w/ extravasation **Uses:** *N/V, motion sickness, adjunct to post-op analgesics, sedation, rhinitis* **Action:** Phenothiazine; blocks CNS postsynaptic mesolimbic dopaminergic receptors **Dose:** *Adults.* 12.5–50 mg PO, PR, or IM 2–4 ×/d PRN *Peds > 2 y.* 0.1–0.5 mg/kg/dose PO/ or IM 4–6h PRN **Caution:** [C, +/–] Use w/ agents w/ resp depressant effects **CI:** Component allergy, NAG, age < 2 y **Disp:** Tabs 12.5, 25, 50 mg; syrup 6.25 mg/5 mL; supp 12.5, 25, 50 mg; Inj 25, 50 mg/mL **SE:** Drowsiness, tardive dyskinesia, EPS, lowered Sz threshold, ↓ BP, GI upset, blood dyscrasias, photosens, resp depression in children **Interactions:** ↑ Effects *W/* CNS depressants, MAOIs, EtOH; ↑ effects *OF* antihypertensives; ↓ effects *W/* anticholinergics, barbiturates, tobacco; ↓ effect *OF* levodopa **Labs:** Effects skin allergy tests **NIPE:** Deep IM preferred route; not SQ or intra-arterial; use sunblock for photosens; may lower Sz threshold; ⊘ ETOH/other CNS depressants

Propafenone (Rythmol, Rhythmol SR) [Antiarrhythmic] **WARNING:** Excess mortality or nonfatal cardiac arrest rate possible; avoid use w/a symptomatic & symptomatic non–life-threatening ventricular arrhythmias **Uses:** *Life-threatening ventricular arrhythmias, AF* **Action:** Class Ic antiarrhythmic (Table 9) **Dose:** *Adults.* 150–300 mg PO q8h *Peds.* 8–10 mg/kg/d ÷ in 3–4 doses; may ↑ 2 mg/kg/d, 20 mg/kg/d max **Caution:** [C, ?] w/ Ritonavir, MI w/in 2 y, w/ liver/renal impair, safety in Peds not established **CI:** Uncontrolled CHF, bronchospasm, cardiogenic shock, AV block w/o pacer **Disp:** Tabs 150, 225, 300 mg; ER caps 225, 325, 425 mg **SE:** Dizziness, unusual taste, 1st-degree heart block, arrhythmias, prolongs QRS & QT intervals; fatigue, GI upset, blood dyscrasias

Interactions: ↑ Effects *W/* cimetidine, quinidine; ↑ effects *OF* anticoagulants, BBs, digitalis glycosides, theophylline; ↓ effects *W/* rifampin, phenobarbital, rifabutin **Labs:** ↑ ANA titers; monitor ECG for ↑ QT interval **NIPE:** Take w/o regard to food; associated w/ a high cardiac arrest rate & mortality; take whole capsule

Propantheline (Pro-Banthine) [Antimuscarinic] Uses: *PUD*, symptomatic Rx of small intestine hypermotility, spastic colon, ureteral spasm, bladder spasm, pylorospasm **Action:** Antimuscarinic **Dose:** *Adults.* 15 mg PO ac & 30 mg PO hs; ↓ in elderly *Peds.* 2–3 mg/kg/24 h PO ÷ 3–4 ×/d **Caution:** [C, ?] **CI:** NAG, UC, toxic megacolon, GI atony in elderly, MG, GI/GU obst **Disp:** Tabs 15 mg **SE:** Anticholinergic (eg, xerostomia, blurred vision) **Interactions:** ↑ Anticholinergic effects *W/* antihistamines, antidepressants, atropine, haloperidol, phenothiazines, quinidine, TCAs; ↑ effects *OF* atenolol, digoxin (monitor ECG); ↑ adverse effects when used w/ procainamide; ↓ effects *W/* antacids **NIPE:** May cause heat intolerance—avoid exposure to high temperatures; ↑ risk of photosens—use sunblock

Propofol (Diprivan) [Anesthetic] Uses: *Induction & maint of anesthesia; sedation in intubated pts* **Action:** Sedative–hypnotic; mechanism unknown; acts in 40 s **Dose:** *Adults.* Anesthesia: 2–2.5 mg/kg (also *ECC 2005*), then 100–200 mcg/kg/min Inf *ICU sedation:* 5 mcg/kg/min IV, ↑ PRN 5–10 mcg/kg/min q5–10min, 5–50 mcg/kg/min cont Inf *Peds.* Anesthesia: 2.5–3.5 mg/kg induction; then 125–300 mcg/kg/min; ↓ in elderly, debilitated, ASA II/IV pts **Caution:** [B, –] **CI:** If general anesthesia CI, sensitivity to egg, egg products, soybeans, soybean products **Disp:** Inj 10 mg/mL **SE:** May ↑ triglycerides w/ extended dosing; ↓ BP, pain at site, apnea, anaphylaxis **Interactions:** ↑ Effects *W/* anesthetics, opioids, hypnotics, EtOH **Labs:** ↓ Serum cortisol levels; may ↑ triglycerides w/ extended dosing **NIPE:** 1 mL has 0.1 g fat; N if Hx of allergy to egg/soybean products; monitor BP for hypotension; monitor for resp depression

Propoxyphene (Darvon-N); Propoxyphene & Acetaminophen (Darvocet); Propoxyphene & Aspirin (Darvon Compound-65, Darvon-N w/ Aspirin) [C-IV] [Opioid + Analgesic] In November 2010 the FDA banned all products containing propoxyphene d/t the ↑ risk of abnormal & potentially fatal heart rhythm disturbances. *http://www.fda. gov/Safety/MedWatch/SafetyInformation/SafetyAlertsforHumanMedicalProducts/ ucm234389.htm*

Propranolol (Inderal LA, Innopran XL) [Antihypertensive, Antianginal, Antiarrhythmic/Beta-Blocker] Uses: *HTN, angina, MI, hyperthyroidism, essential tremor, hypertrophic subaortic stenosis, pheochromocytoma; prevents migraines & atrial arrhythmias*, *thyrotoxicosis;* **Action:** β-Adrenergic receptor blocker, β₁, β₂; only β-blocker to block conversion of T_4 to T_3 **Dose:** *Adults.* Angina: 80–320 mg/d PO ÷ 2–4 ×/d or 80–320 mg/d SR. *Arrhythmia:* 10–30 mg/dose PO q6–8h or 1 mg IV slowly, repeat q5min, 5 mg max *HTN:* 40 mg PO bid or 60–80 mg/d SR, weekly to max 640 mg/d *Hypertrophic* *subaortic stenosis:* 20–40 mg PO 3–4 ×/d *MI:* 180–240 mg PO ÷ 3–4 ×/d *Migraine prophylaxis:* 80 mg/d ÷ 3–4 ×/d, ↑ weekly 160–240 mg/d ÷ tid–qid max; wean if no response in 6 wk *Pheochromocytoma:* 30–60 mg/d ÷ 3–4 ×/d *Thyrotoxicosis:* 1–3 mg IV × 1; 10–40 mg PO q6h *Tremor:* 40 mg PO bid, ↑ PRN 320 mg/d max *ECC 2010:* SVT: 0.5–1 mg IV given over 1 min; repeat PRN up to 0.1 mg/kg **Peds.** *Arrhythmia:* 0.5–1.0 mg/kg/d ÷ 3–4 ×/d, ↑ PRN q3–7d to 8 mg/kg max; 0.01–0.1 mg/kg IV over 10 min, 1 mg max infants, 3 mg max children *HTN:* 0.5–1.0 mg/kg/d ÷ 3–4 ×/d, PRN q3–7d to 8 mg/kg/d max; ↓ in renal impair **Caution:** [C (1st tri, D if 2nd or 3rd tri), +] **CI:** Uncompensated CHF, cardiogenic shock, HR, heart block, PE, severe resp Dz **Disp:** Tabs 10, 20, 40, 80 mg; SR caps 60, 80, 120, 160 mg; oral soln 4, 8, mg/mL; Inj 1 mg/mL **SE:** ↓ HR, ↓ BP, fatigue, GI upset, ED **Interactions:** ↑ Effects *W/* antihypertensives, cimetidine, hydralazine, neuroleptics, nitrates, propylthiouracil, theophylline, EtOH; ↑ effects *OF* benzodiazepines, CCB, digitalis, glycosides, hypoglycemics, hydralazine, lidocaine, neuroleptics; ↓ effects *W/* NSAIDs, phenobarbital, phenytoin, rifampin, tobacco **Labs:** ↑ LFTs, BUN; ↑/↓ serum glucose; ↓ plts, thyroxine **NIPE:** ⊘ D/C abruptly—may ↑ angina; concurrent use of epi may cause severe HTN/bradycardia; ↑ cold sensitivity; change position slowly

Propylthiouracil [PTU] [Antithyroid Agent/Thyroid Hormone Antagonist] WARNING: Severe liver failure reported; use only if pt cannot tolerate methimazole; d/t fetal anomalies w/ methimazole, PTU may be DOC in 1st tri Uses: *Hyperthyroidism* Action: ↓ Production of T₃ & T₄ & conversion of T₄ to

Propylthiouracil [PTU] [Antithyroid Agent/Thyroid Hormone Antagonist] **WARNING:** Severe liver failure reported; use only if pt cannot tolerate methimazole; d/t fetal anomalies w/ methimazole, PTU may be DOC in 1st tri **Uses:** *Hyperthyroidism* **Action:** ↓ Production of T_3 & T_4 & conversion of T_4 to T_3 **Dose:** **Adults.** *Initial:* 100 mg PO q8h (may need up to 1200 mg/d); after pt euthyroid (6–8 wk), taper dose by 1/2 q4–6wk to maint, 50–150 mg/24 h; can usually D/C in 2–3 y; ↓ in elderly **Peds.** *Initial:* 5–7 mg/kg/24 h PO ÷ q8h **Maint:** 1/3–2/3 of initial dose **Caution:** [D, –] See Warning **CI:** Allergy **Disp:** Tabs 50 mg **SE:** Fever, rash, leukopenia, dizziness, GI upset, taste perversion, SLE-like synd **Interactions:** ↑ Effects *W/* iodinated glycerol, Li, KI, NaI **Labs:** ↑ LFTs, PT; ↑ effects of anticoagulants; monitor TFT & LFT **NIPE:** Take w/ food for GI upset; omit dietary sources of I; full effects take 6–12 wk; ✓ pulse, wgts qd

Protamine (Generic) [Heparin Antagonist] **Warning:** Severe ↓ BP, CV collapse, noncardiogenic pulmonary edema, pulm vasoconstriction, and pulm HTN can occur; risk factors: high dose/overdose, repeat doses, prior protamine use, current or use of prior protamine-containing product (eg, NPH or protamine zinc insulin, some beta-blockers), fish allergy, prior vasectomy, severe LV dysfunction, abnormal pulm testing; weigh risk/benefit in pts w/ 1 or more risk factors; resuscitation equipment must be available. **Uses:** *Reverse heparin effect* **Action:** Neutralize heparin by forming a stable complex **Dose:** Based on degree of heparin reversal; give IV slowly; 1 mg reverses ~ 100 units of heparin given in the preceding 30 min; 50 mg max **Caution:** [C, ?] **CI:** Allergy **Disp:** Inj 10 mg/mL **SE:** Follow coagulation markers; anticoagulant effect if given w/o heparin; ↓ BP, ↓ HR, dyspnea, hemorrhage **Interactions:** Incompatible *W/* many penicillins &

cephalosporins—⊘ mix **Labs:** ✓ aPTT ~ 15 min after use to assess response **NIPE:** Give by slow IV Inj over 10 min; antidote for heparin tox

Prothrombin Complex Concentrate, Human (Kcentra)
WARNING: Risk vit K antag reversal W/ a thromboembolic event, must be weighed against the risk of NOT reversing vitamin K antag; this risk is higher in those who have had a prior thromboembolic event. Fatal and nonfatal arterial and venous thromboembolic events have occurred. Monitor. May not be effective in pts w/ thromboembolic events in the prior 3 mo **Uses:** *Urgent reversal of acquired coagulation factor deficiencies caused by vit K antagonists; only for acute major bleeding* **Action:** Reverse vit K antag coagulopathy; replaces Factor I,VII, IX, X & Protein C & S **Dose:** Based on INR & wgt: INR 2–4, 25 units/kg, 2500 units max; INR 4–6, 35 units/kg, 3500 units max; INR > 6, 50 unit/kg, 5000 units max; 100 mg/kg max; give w/ vit K **Caution:** [C, ?] Hypersensitivity Rxn; arterial/venous thrombosis; risk of viral Infxn including variant CJD **CI:** Anaphylaxis/reactions to: heparin, albumin, or coag factors (Protein C & S, antithrombin III); known HIT DIC **Disp:** Single vial; to reconstitute, see package; separate IV for Inf **SE:** Thromboembolic events (stroke, DVT/PE); DIC; ↓ BP, HA, N/V, HA, arthralgias **Notes:** INR should be < 1.3 w/in 30 min; risk of transmitting variant CJD, viral Dz (human blood product), and other Infxn (Hep A, B, & C, HIV, etc) **NIPE:** ✓ for S/Sx thromboembolic events; use dedicated IV line for infusion; ✓ for risk of allergic Rxn

Pseudoephedrine (Many OTC Mono and Combination Brands) [OTC] [Decongestant/Sympathomimetic] Uses: *Decongestant*, **Action:** Stimulates α-adrenergic receptors w/ vasoconstriction **Dose:** *Adults. IR:* 60 mg PO q4–6h, PRN ER: 120 mg PO q12h, 240 mg/d max *Peds 2–5 y:* 15 mg q 4–6 h, 60 mg/24 h max *6–12 y:* 30 mg q4–6h, 120 mg/24 h max; ↓ w/ renal Insuff **Caution:** [C, +] Not rec for use in Peds < 2 y **CI:** Poorly controlled HTN or CAD, w/ MAOIs w/in 14 d, urinary retention **Disp:** Tabs 30, 60 mg ER: Caplets 60, 120 mg ER: Tabs 120, 240 mg; Liq 15, 30 mg/5 mL; syrup: 15, 30 mg/5 mL; multiple combo OTC products **SE:** HTN, insomnia, tachycardia, arrhythmias, nervousness, tremor **Interactions:** ↑ Risk of HTN crisis W/ MAOIs; ↑ effects W/ BBs, sympathomimetics; ↓ effects W/ TCAs; ↓ effect OF methyldopa, reserpine **NIPE:** Found in many OTC cough/cold preps; OTC restricted distribution by state (illicit ingredient in methamphetamine production); ⊘ break, crush, divide ER form

Psyllium (Konsyl, Metamucil) [Laxative] Uses: *Constipation & colonic diverticular Dz* **Action:** Bulk laxative **Dose:** 1.25–30 g/d varies w/ specific product **Caution:** [B, ?] *Effer-Syllium* (effervescent psyllium) usually contains K+, caution w/ renal failure; phenylketonuria (in products w/ aspartame) **CI:** Suspected bowel obst **Disp:** Large variety available: granules; powder, caps, wafers **SE:** D, Abd cramps, bowel obst, constipation, bronchospasm **Interactions:** ↓ Effects OF digitalis glycosides, K+-sparing diuretics, nitrofurantoin, salicylates, tetracyclines, warfarin **NIPE:** Psyllium dust Inh may cause wheezing, runny nose, watery eyes. Maintain adequate hydration; take w/ 8–10 oz H_2O

Pyrazinamide (Generic) [Antitubercular] Uses: *Active TB in combo w/ other agents* Action: Bacteriostatic; unknown mechanism Dose: *Adults.* Dose varies based on Tx option chosen daily 1×2 wk–$3 \times$ wk; dosing based on lean body wgt; ↓ dose in renal/hepatic impair Peds. 20–40 mg/kg/d PO ÷ daily–bid; ↓ w/ renal/hepatic impair Caution: [C, +/–] CI: Severe hepatic damage, acute gout Disp: Tabs 500 mg SE: Hepatotox, malaise, GI upset, arthralgia, myalgia, gout, photosens Interactions: ↓ Effects *OF* probenecid Labs: ↑ Uric acid NIPE: ↑ Risk of photosens—use sunblock; ↑ fluids to 2 L/d; take w/ food to ↓ GI distress; use in combo w/ other anti TB drugs; consult *MMWR* for latest TB recommendations; dosage regimen differs for "daily observed" therapy

Pyridoxine [Vitamin B₆] [Vitamin B₆ Supplement] Uses: *Rx & prevention of vit B₆ deficiency* Action: Vit B₆ supl Dose: *Adults. Deficiency:* 10–20 mg/d PO Drug-induced neuritis: 100–200 mg/d; 25–100 mg/d prophylaxis Peds. 5–25 mg/d × 3 wk Caution: [A (C if doses exceed RDA), +] CI: Component allergy Disp: Tabs 25, 50, 100, 250, 500 mg, tab SR 500 mg; liquid 200 mg, 15 mg; Inj 100 mg/mL; caps 50, 250 Interactions: ↓ Effects *OF* levodopa, phenobarbital, phenytoin Labs: ↑ AST; ↓ folic acid NIPE: Antidote for INH poisoning; risk of sensory nerve damage (numbness, tingling, ↓ sensation)—usually reversed when drug D/C; eat diet ↑ in pyridoxine (eg, eggs, tuna, shrimp, legumes, avocados)

Quetiapine (Seroquel, Seroquel XR) [Antipsychotic] WARNING: Closely monitor pts for worsening depression or emergence of suicidality, particularly in Ped pts; not for use in Peds; ↑ mortality in elderly w/ dementia-related psychosis Uses: *Acute exacerbations of schizophrenia, bipolar Dz* Action: Serotonin & dopamine antagonism Dose: 150–750 mg/d; initiate at 25–100 mg bid–tid; slowly ↑ dose; XR: 400–800 mg PO qPM; start ↑ 300 mg/d, 800 mg/d max ↓ dose w/ hepatic & geriatric pts Caution: [C, –] CI: Component allergy Disp: Tabs 25, 50, 100, 200, 300, 400 mg; tabs XR 50, 150, 200, 300, 400 mg SE: Confusion w/ nefazodone; HA, somnolence, ↑ wgt, ↓ BP, dizziness, cataracts, neuroleptic malignant synd, tardive dyskinesia, ↑ QT interval Interactions: ↑ Effects *W/* azole antifungals, cimetidine, macrolides, EtOH; ↑ effects *OF* antihypertensives, lorazepam; ↓ effects *W/* barbiturates, carbamazepine, glucocorticoids, phenytoin, rifampin, thioridazine; ↓ effects *OF* DA antagonists, levodopa Labs: ↑ LFTs, cholesterol, triglycerides, glucose NIPE: ↑ Risk of cataract formation, tardive dyskinesia; take w/o regard to food; ↓ body temperature regulation ability; ↑ risk of depression/suicide tendencies, esp in Peds; risk of ↑ QT internal—monitor ECG; change position slowly; ⊘ EtOH

Quinapril (Accupril) [Antihypertensive/ACEI] WARNING: ACE Inhib used during PRG can cause fetal injury & death Uses: *HTN, CHF, DN, post-MI* Action: ACE Inhib Dose: 10–80 mg PO daily; ↓ in renal impair Caution : [D, +] w/ RAS, vol depletion CI: ACE Inhib sensitivity, angioedema, PRG Disp: Tabs 5, 10, 20, 40 mg SE: Dizziness, HA, ↓ BP, impaired renal Fxn, angioedema, taste perversion, cough Interactions: ↑ Effects *W/* diuretics, antihypertensives; ↑

effects *OF* insulin, Li; ↓ effects *W/* ASA, NSAIDs; ↓ effects *OF* quinolones, tetracyclines **Labs:** ↑ K+, ↓ LFTs, glucose **NIPE:** ↓ Absorption *W/* high-fat foods; ↑ risk of cough; risk of hyperkalemia—monitor ECG (peaked T waves), EtOH ↑ risk of adverse effects; tabs may be crushed; full effect may take 1–2 wk

Quinidine (Generic) [Antiarrhythmic/Antimalarial] WARNING: Mortality rates increased when used to treat non-life-threatening arrhythmias **Uses:** * Prevention of tachydysrhythmias, malaria* **Action:** Class IA antiarrhythmic **Dose:** *Adults. Antiarrhythmic IR:* 200–400 mg/dose q6h; *ER:* 300 mg q8–12h (sulfate) 324 mg q8–12h (gluconate) *Peds.* 15–60 mg/kg/24 h PO in 4–5 ÷ doses; ↓ in renal impair **Caution:** [C, +] **CI:** TTP, thrombocytopenia, medications that prolong QT interval, digitalis tox & AV block; conduction disorders **Disp:** *Sulfate:* Tabs 200, 300 mg; SR tabs 300 mg *Gluconate:* SR tabs 324 mg; Inj 80 mg/mL **SE:** Extreme ↓ BP w/ IV use; syncope, QT prolongation, GI upset, arrhythmias, fatigue, cinchonism (tinnitus, hearing loss, delirium, visual changes), fever, hemolytic anemia, thrombocytopenia, rash **Notes:** *Levels: Trough:* Just before next dose *Therapeutic:* 2–5 mcg/mL *Toxic:* > 10 mcg/mL *1/2-life:* 6–8 h; sulfate salt 83% quinidine; gluconate salt 62% quinidine **Interactions:** ↑ Effects *W/* acetazolamide, antacids, amiodarone, azole antifungals, cimetidine, K+, macrolides, NaHCO₃, thiazide diuretics, lily of the valley, pheasant's eye herb, scopolia root, squill; ↑ effects *OF* anticoagulants, anticholinergics, dextromethorphan, digitalis glycosides, disopyramide, haloperidol, metoprolol, nifedipine, procainamide, propafenone, propranolol, TCAs, verapamil; ↓ effects *W/* barbiturates, disopyramide, nifedipine, phenobarbital, phenytoin, rifampin, sucralfate **NIPE:** Take w/ food; take w/ 8 oz H₂O; ⊘ supine position × 30 min post med ↑ risk of photosens—use sunblock; use w/ drug that slows AV conduction (eg, digoxin, diltiazem, BB), QT prolongation—monitor ECG

Quinupristin–Dalfopristin (Synercid) [Antibiotic/Streptogramin] Uses: *Vancomycin-resistant Infxns d/t *E faecium* & other gram(+)* **Action:** ↓ Ribosomal protein synth *Spectrum:* Vancomycin-resistant *E faecium,* methicillin-susceptible *S aureus, S pyogenes;* not against *E faecalis* **Dose:** *Adults & Peds.* 7.5 mg/kg IV q12h (central line preferred); incompatible w/ NS or heparin; flush IV w/ dextrose; ↓ w/ hepatic failure **Caution:** [B, M] Multiple drug interactions w/ drugs metabolized by CYP3A4 (eg, cyclosporine) **CI:** Component allergy **Disp:** Inj 500 mg (150 mg quinupristin/350 mg dalfopristin) **SE:** Hyperbilirubinemia, Inf site Rxns & pain, arthralgia, myalgia **Interactions:** ↑ Effects *OF* CCBs, carbamazepine, cyclosporine, diazepam, disopyramide, docetaxel, lovastatin, methylprednisolone, midazolam, paclitaxel, protease Inhibs, quinidine, tacrolimus, vinblastine **Labs:** ↑ ALT, AST, bilirubin **NIPE:** Inf site Rxns & pain; if D—✓ for signs of lytes disturbance/ hypovolemia; ✓ Sx superinfection

Rabeprazole (AcipHex) [Antiulcer Agent/Proton Pump Inhibitor] Uses: *PUD, GERD, ZE* *H pylori* **Action:** Proton pump Inhib **Dose:** 20 mg/d; may ↑ to 60 mg/d; *H pylori* 20 mg PO bid × 7 d (w/ amoxicillin & clarithromycin); do not crush/chew tabs; do not use clopidogrel **Caution:** [B, ?/–] Do not use w/ clopidogrel, possible ↓ effect (controversial) **Disp:** Tabs 20 mg ER **SE:** HA, fatigue, GI upset **Interactions:** ↑ Effects *OF* cyclosporine, digoxin; ↓ effects *OF* ketoconazole **Labs:** ↑ LFTs, TSH **NIPE:** Take w/o regard to food; best taken before breakfast; ⊘ crush, break, split tab; ↑ risk of photosens—use sunblock; risk of hypomagnesemia w/ long-term use, monitor; ? ↑ risk of fxs w/ all PPI

Radium-223 Dichloride (Xofigo) **Uses:** *Castration resistant prostate Ca w/ symptomatic bone mets w/o visceral Dz* **Action:** Alpha-emitter, complexes in bone w/ ↑ turnover **Dose:** 50 kBq/kg, IV q4wk × 6 doses slow IV over 1 min **Caution:** [X, –] NOT for women; ✓ CBC before/during each Tx dose, D/C if no CBC recovery 6–8 wk post-Tx **CI:** PRG **Disp:** Single vial, 1000 kBq/mL or 6000 kBq/vial **SE:** ↓ CBC; N/V/D, edema **Notes:** Follow radiation safety/pharma quality control requirements **NIPE:** Use condoms during & 6 mo post-Tx and female partners should use 1 additional BC method; avoid exposure to infection; check w/ physician before having dental work; ✓ bleeding precautions

Raloxifene (Evista) [Selective Estrogen Receptor Modulator] **WARNING:** Increased risk of venous thromboembolism and death from stroke **Uses:** *Prevent osteoporosis, breast CA prevention* **Action:** Partial antagonist of estrogen, behaves like estrogen **Dose:** 60 mg/d **Caution:** [X, –] **CI:** Thromboembolism, PRG **Disp:** Tabs 60 mg **SE:** CP, insomnia, rash, hot flashes, GI upset, hepatic dysfunction, leg cramps **Interactions:** ↓ Effects *W/* ampicillin, cholestyramine **NIPE:** ⊘ PRG, breast-feeding; take w/o regard to food; ↑ risk of venous thromboembolic effects—esp w/ prolonged immobilization; weight-bearing exercises regularly

Raltegravir (Isentress) [HIV-1 Integrase Strand Transfer Inhibitor] **Uses:** *HIV in combo w/ other antiretroviral agents* **Action:** HIV-integrase strand transfer Inhib **Dose:** 400 mg PO bid, 800 mg PO bid w/ rifampin **Caution:** [C, –] **CI:** None **Disp:** Tabs 400 mg **SE:** Development of immune reconstitution synd: ↑ CK, myopathy, and rhabdomyolysis, insomnia, N/D, HA, fever, ↑ cholesterol, paranoia, and anxiety **Interactions:** ↑ Effects *W/* UGT1A1 Inhibs; ↓ effects *W/* rifampin **Labs:** ↑ Cholesterol, monitor lipids **NIPE:** Take w/o regard to food; ⊘ crush, break, divide film-coated tabs; caution w/ drugs that cause myopathy such as statins; ✓ dose before dialysis sessions; initial therapy may cause immune reconstitution synd (inflammatory response to residual opportunistic Infxns, eg, *M avium*, PCP

Ramelteon (Rozerem) [Hypnotic-Melatonin Receptor Agonist] **Uses:** *Insomnia* **Action:** Melatonin receptor agonist **Dose:** 8 mg PO 30 min before bedtime **Caution:** [C, ?/–] w/ CYP1A2 Inhib **CI:** w/ Fluvoxamine; hypersensitivity **Disp:** 8-mg tabs **SE:** Somnolence, dizziness **Interactions:** ↑ Effects *W/* CYP1A2 Inhibs (fluvoxamine), CYP3A4 Inhibs (ketoconazole), & CYP2C9 Inhibs (fluconazole); ↑ risk of CNS depression w/ EtOH & CNS depressants; ↓ effects *W/* CYP450 inducers (rifampin) **Labs:** ↓ Testosterone levels & ↑ prolactin levels noted **NIPE:** High-fat foods delay effect; ⊘ use in pts w/ severe sleep apnea & severe COPD

Ramipril (Altace) [Antihypertensive/ACEI]   WARNING: ACE Inhib used during PRG can cause fetal injury & death **Uses:** *HTN, CHF, DN, post-MI* **Action:** ACE Inhib **Dose:** 1.25–20 mg/d PO ÷ daily–bid; ↓ in renal failure **Caution:** [C-1st tri/D-2nd & 3rd, +] **CI:** ACE-Inhib-induced angioedema **Disp:** Caps 1.25, 2.5, 5, 10 mg **SE:** Cough, HA, dizziness, ↓ BP, renal impair, angioedema **Interactions:** ↑ Effects *W/* α-adrenergic blockers, loop diuretics; ↑ effects *OF* insulin, Li; ↑ risk of hyperkalemia *W/* K⁺, K⁺-sparing diuretics, K⁺ salt substitutes (monitor ECG for peaked T waves), TMP, ↓ effects *W/* ASA, NSAIDs, food **Labs:** ↑ BUN, Cr, K⁺, ↓ HMG, Hct, cholesterol, glucose **NIPE:** ↑ Risk of photosens—use sunscreen; ↑ risk of cough esp w/ capsaicin; take w/o food; OK in combo w/ diuretics; change position slowly

Ranibizumab (Lucentis) [Vascular Endothelial GF Inhibitor]   Uses: *Neovascular "wet" macular degeneration* **Action:** VEGF Inhib **Dose:** 0.5 mg intravitreal Inj qmo **Caution:** [C, ?] Hx thromboembolism **CI:** Periocular Infxn **Disp:** Inj 10 mg/mL **SE:** Endophthalmitis, retinal detachment/hemorrhage, cataract, intraocular inflammation, conjunctival hemorrhage, eye pain, floaters. **NIPE:** Seek immediate care from ophthalmologist if eye develops redness, light sensitivity, pain, change in vision

Ranitidine (Zantac, Zantac EFFER Dose) [Antiulcer Agent/H₂-Receptor Antagonist]   Uses: *Duodenal ulcer, active benign ulcers, hypersecretory conditions, & GERD* **Action:** H₂-receptor antagonist **Dose:** *Adults.* *Ulcer:* 150 mg PO bid, 300 mg PO hs, or 50 mg IV q6–8h; or 400 mg IV/d cont Inf, then maint of 150 mg PO hs. *Hypersecretion:* 150 mg PO bid, up to 600 mg/d *GERD:* 300 mg PO bid; maint 300 mg PO hs *Dyspepsia:* 75 mg PO daily–bid. *Peds.* 1.5–2 mg/kg/dose IV q6–8h or 2 mg/kg/dose PO q12h; ↓ in renal Insuff/failure **Caution:** [B, +] **CI:** Component allergy **Disp:** Tabs 75, 150 mg [OTC], 150, 300 mg; caps 150, 300 mg; effervescent tabs 25 mg (contains phenylalanine); syrup 15 mg/mL; Inj 25 mg/mL **SE:** Dizziness, sedation, rash, GI upset **Interactions:** ↑ Effects *OF* glipizide, glyburide, procainamide, warfarin; ↓ effects *W/* antacids, tobacco; ↓ effects *OF* diazepam **Labs:** ↑ SCr, ALT **NIPE:** ASA, NSAIDs, EtOH, caffeine ↑ stomach acid production; PO & parenteral doses differ; PO best to give at night or w/ meals

Ranolazine (Ranexa) [Antianginal]   Uses: *Chronic angina* **Action:** ↓ Ischemia-related Na⁺ entry into myocardium **Dose:** *Adults.* 500 mg bid–1000 mg PO bid **CI:** w/ Cirrhosis, CYP3A Inhib/inducers (Table 10) **Caution:** [C, ?/–] HTN may develop w/ renal impair, agents that ↑ QT interval; ↓ K⁺ **Disp:** SR tabs 500, 1000 mg **SE:** Dizziness, HA, constipation, arrhythmias **Interactions:** Risk of ↑ QT interval *W/* diltiazem, verapamil, grapefruit juice **Labs:** ↓ K⁺—monitor ECG (flattened T waves) **NIPE:** Not 1st-line; use w/ amlodipine, nitrates, BB; avoid grapefruit products; ⊘ chew, crush, dissolve, or divide ER tabs

Rasagiline Mesylate (Azilect) [Anti-Parkinson Agent/MAO B Inhibitor] Uses: *Early Parkinson Dz monotherapy; levodopa adjunct w/ advanced Dz* Action: MAOB Inhib Dose: *Adults. Early Dz:* 1 mg PO daily, start 0.5 mg PO daily w/ levodopa; ↓ w/ CYP1A2 Inhib hepatic impair CI: MAOIs, sympathomimetic amines, meperidine, methadone, tramadol, propoxyphene, dextromethorphan, mirtazapine, cyclobenzaprine, St. John's wort, sympathomimetic vasoconstrictors, general anesthetics, SSRIs Caution: [C, ?] Avoid tyramine-containing foods; mod–severe hepatic impair Disp: Tabs 0.5, 1 mg SE: Arthralgia, indigestion, dyskinesia, hallucinations, ↓ wgt, postural ↓ BP, N/V, constipation, xerostomia, rash, sedation, CV conduction disturbances Interactions: ↑ Risk of HTN crisis *W/* tyramine-containing foods (beer, red wine, aged cheese/meat, dried fruit); ↑ effects *W/* ciprofloxacin; ↑ CNS tox/death *W/* TCA, SSRIs, MAOIs Labs: Monitor LFTs NIPE: Rare melanoma reported; do periodic skin exams (skin CA risk); D/C 14 d prior to elective surgery; D/C fluoxetine 5 wk before starting rasagiline; initial ↓ levodopa dose OK; allow at least 14 d after discontinuing rasagiline before starting SSRI, tricyclic, or SNRI

Rasburicase (Elitek) [Antigout Agent/Antimetabolite] WARNING: Anaphylaxis possible; do not use in G6PD deficiency & hemolysis; can cause methemoglobinemia; can interfere w/ uric acid assays; collect blood samples and store on ice Uses: *Reduce ↑ uric acid d/t tumor lysis* Action: Catalyzes uric acid Dose: *Adult & Peds.* 0.20 mg/kg IV over 30 min, daily × 5; do not bolus, redosing based uric acid levels Caution:[C, ?/–] Falsely ↓ uric acid values CI: Anaphylaxis, screen for G6PD deficiency to avoid hemolysis, methemoglobinemia Disp: 1.5, 7.5 mg powder Inj SE: Fever, neutropenia, GI upset, HA, rash Labs: Falsely ↓ uric acid values; ↓ neutrophils NIPE: Place blood test tube for uric acid level on ice to D/C enzymatic Rxn; removed by dialysis; use antiemetics for N/V

Regorafenib (Stivarga) WARNING: May cause severe/fatal hepatotox. Monitor LFTs & dose adjust or D/C for ↑ LFTs or hepatocellular necrosis Uses: *Metastatic colorectal CA & GIST (see labeling/institution protocol)* Action: Kinase Inhib Dose: *Adults.* 160 mg PO qAM on d 1–21 of 28-d cycle; see label for toxicity dose adjust Caution: [D, –] Fetal tox; avoid w/ strong CYP3A4 Inhib/ inducers CI: None Disp: Tabs 40 mg SE: Fatigue, asthenia, N/V/D, Abd pain, ↓ appetite, ↓ wgt, HTN, HFSR, mucositis, dysphonia, Infxn, pain, rash, fever, hemorrhage, wound healing complications, RPLS, cardiac ischemia/infarction, derm tox, GI perforation/fistula NIPE: Take same time each day w/ low-fat food; swallow whole; ⊘ PRG; use contraception w/ Tx and × 2 mo after D/C; ⊘ use of herbal products; ✓ educate S/Sx hepatotox; ⊘ grapefruit products

Repaglinide (Prandin) [Hypoglycemic/Meglitinide] Uses: *Type 2 DM* Action: ↑ Pancreatic insulin release Dose: 0.5–4 mg ac, PO start 1–2 mg, ↑ to 16 mg/d max; take pc Caution: [C, ?/–] CI: DKA, type 1 DM Disp: Tabs 0.5, 1, 2 mg SE: HA, hyper-/hypoglycemia, GI upset Interactions: BB use may mask hypoglycemia NIPE: Take 15 min ac; skip drug if meal skipped

Repaglinide/Metformin (PrandiMet) [Hypoglycemic/Meglitinide + Biguanide] **WARNING:** Associated w/ lactic acidosis, risk ↑ w/ sepsis, dehydration, renal/hepatic impair, ↑ alcohol, acute CHF; Sxs include myalgias, malaise, resp distress, Abd pain, somnolence **Labs:** ↓ pH, ↑ anion gap, ↑ blood lactate; D/C immediately & hospitalize if suspected **Uses:** *Type 2 DM* **Action:** Meglitinide & biguanide (see Metformin) **Dose:** *Adults.* 1/500 mg bid w/in 15 min pc (skip dose w/ skipped meal); max 10/2500 mg/d or 4/1000 mg/meal **Caution:** [C,–] suspend use w/ iodinated contrast, do not use w/ NPH insulin, use w/ cationic drugs & CYP2C8 & CYP3A4 Inhib **CI:** SCr > 1.4 mg/dL (females) or > 1.5 mg/dL (males); metabolic acidosis; w/ gemfibrozil **Disp:** Tabs (repaglinide mg/metformin mg) 1/500, 2/500 **SE:** Hypoglycemia, HA, N/V/D, anorexia, weakness, myalgia, rash, ↓ vit B_{12} **Interactions:** Suspend use w/ iodinated contrast, do not use w/ NPH insulin, use w/ cationic drugs & CYP2C8 & CYP3A4 Inhibs; BB use may mask hypoglycemia; ↑ effects *W/* amiloride, cimetidine, digoxin, furosemide, MAOIs, morphine, procainamide, quinidine, quinine, ranitidine, triamterene, TMP, vancomycin; ↓ effects *W/* corticosteroids, CCBs, diuretics, estrogens, INH, OCPs, phenothiazine, phenytoin, sympathomimetics, thyroid drugs, tobacco **Labs:** Monitor LFTs, BUN/Cr, serum vit B_{12} **NIPE:** Take w/ food; avoid dehydration; ⊘ EtOH; educate pt S/Sx & Tx of ↓ glycemia

Retapamulin (Altabax) [Pleuromutilin Antibiotic] **Uses:** *Topical Rx impetigo in pts > 9 mo* **Action:** Pleuromutilin antibiotic, bacteriostatic, ↓ bacteria protein synth *Spectrum: S aureus* (not MRSA), *S pyogenes* **Dose:** Apply bid × 5 d **Caution:** [B, ?] **Disp:** 1% ointment **SE:** Local irritation **NIPE:** Prolonged use may result in super Infxn; apply in thin layer

Reteplase (Retavase) [Tissue Plasminogen Activator] **Uses:** *Post-AMI* **Action:** Thrombolytic **Dose:** 10 units IV over 2 min, 2nd dose in 30 min, 10 units IV over 2 min *ECC 2010:* 10 units IV bolus over 2 min; 30 min later, 10 units IV bolus over 2 min w/ NS flush before and after each dose **Caution:** [C, ?/–] **CI:** Internal bleeding, spinal surgery/trauma, h/o CNS AVM/CVA, bleeding diathesis, severe uncontrolled ↑ BP, sensitivity to thrombolytics **Disp:** IC it: 10.4 units/2 mL **SE:** Bleeding including CNS, allergic Rxns **Interactions:** ↑ Risk of bleeding *W/* ASA, abciximab, dipyridamole, heparin, NSAIDs, anticoagulants, vit K antagonists **Labs:** ↓ Fibrinogen, plasminogen **NIPE:** Use through dedicated IV line; monitor ECG during Rx for ↑ risk of reperfusion arrhythmias; minimize or avoid invasive testing (venipuncture, Inj) d/t ↑ risk of bleeding

Ribavirin (Copegus, Rebetol, Virazole) [Antiviral/Nucleoside Analogue] **WARNING:** Monotherapy for chronic hep C ineffective; hemolytic anemia possible, teratogenic and embryocidal; use 2 forms of birth control for up to 6 mo after D/C drug; ↓ in resp Fxn when used in infants as Inh **Uses:** *RSV Infxn in infants [Virazole]; hep C (in combo w/ peg-interferon α_{2b}* **Action:** Unknown **Dose:** *RSV:* 6 g in 300 mL sterile H_2O, Inh over 12–18 h *Hep C:* See individual product labeling for dosing based on wgt & genotype **Caution:** [X, ?]

May accumulate on soft contact lenses **CI:** PRG, autoimmune hep, CrCl < 50 mL/min **Disp:** Powder for aerosol 6 g; tabs 200, 400, 600 mg, caps 200 mg, soln 40 mg/mL **SE:** Fatigue, HA, GI upset, anemia, myalgia, alopecia, bronchospasm, ↓ HCT **Interactions:** ↓ Effects *W/* Al, Mg, simethicone; ↓ effect *OF* zidovudine **Labs:** ↑ LFTs; ↓ HMG, Hct, plts, WBC; monitor labs; PRG test monthly **NIPE:** ⊘ PRG, breast-feeding; PRG test monthly—2 tabs birth control; male pts must use condoms; ↑ risk of photosens—use sunblock; take w/o regard to food; Virazole aerosolized by a SPAG; monitor resp Fxn closely; hep C viral genotyping may modify dose; take tabs w/ food; ⊘ ETOH

Rifabutin (Mycobutin) [Antibiotic/Antitubercular] Uses: *Prevent MAC Infxnin AIDS pts w/ CD4 count < 100 mc/L* **Action:** ↓ DNA-dependent RNA polymerase activity **Dose:** *Adults.* 150–300 mg/d PO *Peds ≤ 1 y.* 15–25 mg/kg/d PO *Others:* 5 mg/kg/d, max 800 mg/d **Caution:** [B, ?/–] WBC < 1000 cells/mm³ or plts < 50,000 cells/mm³; ritonavir **CI:** Allergy **Disp:** Caps 150 mg **SE:** Discolored urine, rash, neutropenia, leukopenia, myalgia, ↑ LFTs **Interactions:** ↑ Effects *W/* ritonavir; ↓ effects *OF* anticoagulants, anticonvulsants, barbiturates, benzodiazepines, BBs, corticosteroids, methadone, morphine, OCPs, quinidine, theophylline, TCAs **Labs:** ↑ LFTs **NIPE:** Urine & body fluids may turn reddish brown in color, discoloration of soft contact lenses, use barrier contraception, give w/ food if GI upset; SE/interactions similar to rifampin; avoid crowds, those w/ Infxns

Rifampin (Rifadin, Rimactane) [Antibiotic/Antitubercular] Uses: *TB & Rx & prophylaxis of N meningitidis, H influenzae, or S aureus carriers*; adjunct w/ severe *S aureus* **Action:** ↓ DNA-dependent RNA polymerase **Dose:** *Adults. N meningitides & H influenzae carrier:* 600 mg/d PO for 4 d *TB:* 600 mg PO or IV daily or 2 ×/wk w/ combo regimen. *Peds.* 10–20 mg/kg/dose PO or IV daily–bid; ↓ in hepatic failure **Caution:** [C, +] W/ Fosamprenavir, multiple drug interactions **CI:** Allergy, active *N meningitidis* Infxn, w/ saquinavir/ritonavir **Disp:** Caps 150, 300 mg; Inj 600 mg **SE:** Red-orange-colored bodily fluids, ↑ LFTs, flushing, HA **Interactions:** ↓ Effects *W/* aminosalicylic acid; ↓ effects *OF* APAP, aminophylline, amiodarone, anticoagulants, barbiturates, BBs, CCBs, chloramphenicol, clofibrate, delavirdine, digoxin, disopyramide, doxycycline, enalapril, estrogens, haloperidol, hypoglycemics, hydantoins, methadone, morphine, nifedipine, ondansetron, OCPs, phenytoin, protease Inhibs, quinidine, repaglinide, sertraline, sulfapyridine, sulfones, tacrolimus, theophylline, thyroid drugs, tocainide, TCAs, theophylline, verapamil, zidovudine, zolpidem **Labs:** ↑ LFTs, uric acid **NIPE:** Use barrier contraception; take 1 h ac or 2 h pc w/ 8 oz H₂O; ⊘ ETOH; reddish brown color in urine & body fluids; stains soft contact lenses; never use as single agent w/ activeTB

Rifapentine (Priftin) [Antibiotic/Antitubercular] Uses: *Pulm TB* **Action:** ↓ DNA-dependent RNA polymerase *Spectrum: Mycobacterium tuberculosis* **Dose:** *Intensive phase:* 600 mg PO 2 ×/wk for 2 mo; separate doses by > 3 d

Continuation phase: 600 mg/wk for 4 mo; part of 3–4 drug regimen **Caution:** [C, +/– red-orange breast milk] Strong CYP450 inducer, ↓ protease Inhib efficacy, antiepileptics, β-blockers, CCBs **CI:** Rifamycins allergy **Disp:** 150-mg tabs **SE:** Neutropenia, hyperuricemia, HTN, HA, dizziness, rash, GI upset, blood dyscrasias, ↑ LFTs, hematuria, discolored secretions **Interactions:** ↓ Effects *OF* anticoagulants, BBs, CCBs, corticosteroids, cyclosporine, digoxin, fluoroquinolones, methadone, metoprolol, OCPs, phenytoin, propranolol, protease Inhibs, rifampin, sulfonylureas, TCAs, theophylline, verapamil, warfarin **Labs:** ↑ LFTs—monitor; plts, uric acid; ↓ HMG, neutrophil, WBCs **NIPE:** May take w/ food; body fluids, teeth, tongue, feces may become orange-red; may permanently discolor soft contact lenses; use barrier contraception (d/t ↓ effect of OCPs)

Rifaximin (Xifaxan 550) [Antibiotic/Rifamycin Antibacterial] **Uses:** *Traveler's D (noninvasive strains of *E coli*) in pts > 12 y (*Xifaxan*); hepatic encephalopathy (*Xifaxan 550*) > 18 y* **Action:** Not absorbed, derivative of rifamycin *Spectrum:* E coli **Dose:** Diarrhea (*Xifaxan*): 1 tab PO daily × 3 d; encephalopathy (*Xifaxan 550*) > 500 mg PO bid **Caution:** [C, ?/–] Hx allergy to rifamycins; pseudomembranous colitis; w/ severe (Child–Pugh C) hepatic impair **CI:** Allergy to rifamycins **Disp:** Tabs: *Xifaxan* 200 mg; *Xifaxan 550* 550 mg **SE:** *Xifaxan:* Flatulence, HA, Abd pain, rectal tenesmus and urgency, N *Xifaxan 550:* Edema, N, dizziness, fatigue, ascites, flatulence, HA **Interactions:** None sig **Labs:** None noted **NIPE:** May be taken w/o regard to food; ⊘ crush/chew tabs— swallow whole; D/C if D Sx worsen or persist > 24–48 h, or w/ fever or blood in stool

Rilpivirine (Edurant) **Uses:** *HIV in combo w/ other antiretroviral agents* **Action:** NRTI **Dose:** *Adults.* 25 mg daily **Caution:** [B, –] **CI:** None **Disp:** Tab 25 mg **SE:** HA, depression, insomnia, rash, ↑ AST/ALT, ↑ cholesterol, ↑ SCr **Notes:** Metabolized via CYP3A; CYP3A inducers may ↓ virologic response, CYP3A Inhib may ↑ levels; ↑ gastric pH ↓ absorption **NIPE:** Take w/ food to ↑ absorption; ✓ for rash; ✓ renal/hepatic Fxn; report ↑ depression, suicidal ideation

Rimantadine (Flumadine) [Antiviral] **Uses:** *Prophylaxis & Rx of influenza A viral Infxns* **Action:** Antiviral **Dose:** *Adults & Peds > 9 y.* 100 mg PO bid *Peds 1–9 y.* 5 mg/kg/d PO, 150 mg/d max; daily w/ severe renal/hepatic impair & elderly; initiate w/in 48 h of Sx onset **Caution:** [C, –] w/ Cimetidine; avoid w/ PRG, breast-feeding **CI:** Component & amantadine allergy **Disp:** Tabs 100 mg **SE:** Orthostatic ↓ BP, edema, dizziness, GI upset, ↓ Sz threshold **Interactions:** ↑ Effects *W/* cimetidine; ↓ effects *W/* APAP, ASA; concurrent use w/ EtOH may cause confusion, syncope, light-headedness or hypotension **NIPE:** Give w/o regard to food; ⊘ take w/ ASA or acetaminophen; see CDC (*MMWR*) for current influenza A guidelines

Rimexolone (Vexol Ophthalmic) [Steroid] **Uses:** *Post-op inflammation & uveitis* **Action:** Steroid **Dose:** *Adults & Peds > 2 y. Uveitis:* 1–2 gtt/h daytime & q2h at night, taper to 1 gtt q6h *Post-op:* 1–2 gtt qid × 2 wk **Caution:** [C, ?/–]

Ocular Infxns **Disp:** Susp 1% **SE:** Blurred vision, local irritation **NIPE:** Shake well, ⊘ touch eye w/ dropper; taper dose; space eye medication 5 min apart

Riociguat (Adempas) **WARNING:** Do not administer if PRG; R/O PRG before & q mo during Tx & 1 mo after stopping Tx; prevent PRG with appropriate birth control during & 1 mo post-Tx; for females only available through a restricted program **Uses:** *Persistent pulm HTN due to chronic thromboembolic Dz; adults w/ pulm HTN* **Action:** Guanylate cyclase stimulator; guanylate cyclase NO receptor, leads to ↑ cGMP **Dose:** 1 mg PO TID; start 0.5 mg TID if ↓ BP a concern; ↑ 0.5 mg/dose q2wk PRN; 2.5 mg TID max **Caution:** [X, –] ↓ BP, pulm edema w/ pulm veno-occlusive Dz, D/C if confirmed; bleeding **CI:** PRG; use of nitrates or nitric oxide; use of PDE **Disp:** Tabs 0.5, 1, 1.5, 2, 2.5 mg **SE:** N/V/D, GERD, constipation, gastritis; HA, dizziness; anemia **Notes:** Start 0.5 mg w/ CYP and P-gp/BCRP Inhib; do not take w/ antacids, separate by 1 h; not rec w/ severe liver or kidney Dz; may need ↑ dose in smokers; may need to ↓ dose if quit smoking **NIPE:** Use 2 methods of effective contraception; report suspected PRG immediately; ⊘ breast feeding; females must enroll in Adempas REMS Program; educate pt of potential risk of hemoptysis, report to physician asap; change position slowly

Risedronate (Actonel, Actonel w/Calcium) [Biphosphonate/Hormone] **Uses:** *Paget Dz; Rx/prevention glucocorticoid-induced/postmenopausal osteoporosis; ↑ bone mass in osteoporotic men; w/ calcium only FDA approved for female osteoporosis* **Action:** Bisphosphonate; ↓ osteoclast-mediated bone resorption **Dose:** *Paget Dz:* 30 mg/d PO for 2 mo *Osteoporosis Rx/prevention:* 5 mg daily or 35 mg qwk or 150 mg qmo; 30 min before 1st food/drink of the d; stay upright for at least 30 min after dose **Caution:** [C, ?/–] Ca²⁺ supls & antacids ↓ absorption; jaw osteonecrosis, avoid dental work **CI:** Component allergy, ↓ Ca²⁺ esophageal abnormalities, unable to stand/sit for 30 min, CrCl < 30 mL/min **Disp:** Tabs 5, 30, 35, 150 mg; Risedronate 35 mg (4 tabs)/calcium carbonate 1250 mg (24 tabs) **SE:** Back pain, HA, Abd pain,dyspepsia, arthralgia; flu-like Sxs, hypersensitivity (rash, etc), esophagitis, bone pain, eye inflammation **Interactions:** ↓ Effects W/ antacids, ASA, Ca²⁺, food **Labs:** ↓ Ca²⁺, monitor LFTs, Ca²⁺, PO³⁺, K⁺; interference w/ bone-imaging agents **NIPE:** EtOH intake & cigarette smoking promote osteoporosis; ↑ risk of jaw fx; jaw osteonecrosis, avoid dental work; may ↑ atypical subtrochanteric femur fxs; ⊘ lie down for at least 30 min after taking med

Risedronate, Delayed-Release (Atelvia) [Biphosphonate/Hormone] **Uses:** *Postmenopausal osteoporosis* **Action:** See Risedronate **Dose:** One 35 mg tab 1 × wk; in AM following breakfast w/ 4 oz H₂O; do not lie down for 30 min **Caution:** [C, ?/–] Ca²⁺ & Fe²⁺supls/antacids ↓ absorption; do not use w/ Actonel or CrCl < 30 mL/min; jaw osteonecrosis reported, avoid dental work; may ↑ subtrochanteric femur fractures; severe bone/Jt pain **CI:** Component allergy, ↓ Ca²⁺, esophageal abnormalities, unable to stand/sit for 30 min **Disp:** DR tabs 35 mg **SE:** D, influenza, arthralgia, back/Abd pain; rare hypersens, eye inflame

Interactions: ↓ Absorption W/ Ca or Mg-based supls, antacids, laxatives, or Fe prep **Labs:** Correct ↓ Ca²⁺ before use; ✓ Ca²⁺ **NIPE:** Do not use w/ Actonelor CrCl < 30 mL/min; jaw osteonecrosis reported, avoid dental work; may ↑ subtrochanteric femur fxs; severe bone/Jt pain; may interfere W/ bone imaging agents

Risperidone, Oral (Risperdal, Risperdal M-Tab) [Antipsychotic] WARNING: ↑ Mortality in elderly w/ dementia-related psychosis **Uses:*** Psychotic disorders (schizophrenia)*, dementia of the elderly, bipolar disorder, mania, Tourette disorder, autism **Action:** Benzisoxazole antipsychotic **Dose:** *Adults & Peds.* See PI for Dz specific dosing, ↓ dose w/ elderly, renal/hepatic impair **Caution:** [C, −], ↑ BP w/ antihypertensives, clozapine **CI:** Component allergy **Disp:** Tabs 0.25, 0.5, 1, 2, 3, 4 mg; soln 1 mg/mL *M-Tab* (ODT) tabs 0.5, 1, 2, 3, 4 mg **SE:** Orthostatic ↓ BP, EPS w/ high dose, tachycardia, arrhythmias, sedation, dystonias, neuroleptic malignant synd, sexual dysfunction, constipation, xerostomia, ↓ WBC, neutropenia & agranulocytosis, cholestatic jaundice **Interactions:** ↑ Effects W/ clozapine, CNS depressants, EtOH; ↑ effects OF antihypertensives; ↑ effects w/ carbamazepine; ↓ effects OF levodopa **Labs:** ↑ LFTs, serum prolactin, glucose; ↓ WBC **NIPE:** ↑ Risk photosensitivity—use sunblock, extrapyramidal effects; may alter body temperature regulation; several wk to see effect; risk ↑ QT interval—monitor ECG; ⊘ EtOH

Risperidone, Parenteral (Risperdal Consta) [Antipsychotic] WARNING: Not approved for dementia-related psychosis; ↑ mortality risk in elderly dementia pts on atypical antipsychotics; most deaths d/t CV or infectious events **Uses:** Schizophrenia **Action:** Benzisoxazole antipsychotic **Dose:** 25 mg q2wk IM may ↑ to max 50 mg q2wk; w/ renal/hepatic impair start PO Risperdal 0.5 mg PO bid × 1 wk; titrate weekly **Caution:** [C, −], ↑ BP w/ antihypertensives, clozapine **CI:** Component allergy **Disp:** Inj 25, 37.5, 50 mg/vial **SE:** See Risperidone, oral **Interactions:** ↑ Effects W/ clozapine, CNS depressants, EtOH; ↑ effects OF antihypertensives; ↓ effects W/ carbamazepine; ↑ effects OF levodopa **Labs:** ↑ LFTs, serum prolactin **NIPE:** ⊘ ETOH; ↑ risk of photosens—use sunscreen, extrapyramidal effects; may alter body temperature regulation; several wk to see effect; LA Inj

Ritonavir (Norvir) [Antiretroviral/Protease Inhibitor] WARNING: Life-threatening adverse events when used w/ certain nonsedating antihistamines, sedative hypnotics, antiarrhythmics, or ergot alkaloids d/t Inhib drug metabolism **Uses:** *HIV*combo w/ other antiretrovirals **Actions:** Protease Inhib;↓ maturation of immature noninfectious virions to mature infectious virus **Dose:** *Adults.* Initial 300 mg PO bid, titrate over 1 wk to 600 mg PO bid (titration will ↓ GI SE) *Peds > 1 mo.* Initiate at 250 mg/m²; titrate by 50 mg/m² q2–3d, goal 350–400 mg/m², max 600 mg bid; adjust w/ fosamprenavir, indinavir, nelfinavir, & saquinavir; take w/ food **Caution:** [B, +] w/ Ergotamine, amiodarone, bepridil, bosentan, colchicine, PDE Inhib, flecainide, propafenone, quinidine, pimozide, midazolam, triazolam **CI:** Component allergy **Disp:** Caps & tabs 100 mg; soln

80 mg/mL **SE:** ↑ Triglycerides, ↑ LFTs, N/V/D/C, Abd pain, taste perversion, anemia, weakness, HA, fever, malaise, rash, paresthesias **Interactions:** ↑ Effects W/ erythromycin, ILs, grapefruit juice, food; ↑ effects OF amiodarone, astemizole, atorvastatin, barbiturates, bepridil, bupropion, cerivastatin, cisapride, clorazepate, clozapine, clarithromycin, desipramine, diazepam, encainide, ergot alkaloids, estazolam, flecainide, flurazepam, indinavir, ketoconazole, lovastatin, meperidine, midazolam, nelfinavir, phenytoin, pimozide, piroxicam, propafenone, propoxyphene, quinidine, rifabutin, saquinavir, sildenafil, simvastatin, SSRIs, TCAs, terfenadine, triazolam, troleandomycin, zolpidem; ↑ risk of hypotension W/ concurrent use of Viagra-type drugs; ↓ SEs W/ EtOH; ↓ effects W/ barbiturates, carbamazepine, phenytoin, rifabutin, rifampin, St. John's wort, tobacco; ↓ effects OF didanosine, hypnotics, methadone, OCPs, sedatives, theophylline, warfarin **Labs:** ↑ Serum glucose, LFTs, triglycerides, uric acid **NIPE:** Food ↑ absorption; space doses evenly; use barrier contraception; disulfiram-like Rxn w/ disulfiram, metronidazole; refrigerate

Rivaroxaban (Xarelto)
WARNING: May ↑ risk of spinal/epidural hematoma w/ paralysis & increase risk of stroke w/ premature D/C, monitor closely **Uses:** *Prevention of DVT in knee/hip replacement surgery & prevention of stroke and systemic embolism in pts w/ nonvalvular fib* **Action:** Factor Xa Inhib **Dose:** 10 mg PO qd × 35 d (hip) or 12 d (knee), stroke 20 mg daily; w or w/o food **Caution:** [C, –] w/ CYP3A4 Inhib/inducers, other anticoagulants or plt Inhib; avoid w/ CrCl < 30 mL/min or mod/severe hepatic impair **CI:** Active bleeding; component hypersensitivity **Disp:** Tabs 10 mg **SE:** Bleeding **Notes:** See PI for information about timing of stopping or starting dosage in relation to other anticoagulants. **NIPE:** ⊘ D/C abruptly; take qd w/ evening meal w/ Afib Dx; check with prescribing physician *before* taking any OTC, new prescriptions, or herbal products; advise physician immediatly if PRG

Rivastigmine (Exelon) [Cholinesterase Inhibitor/Anti-Alzheimer Agent]
Uses: *Mild–mod dementia in Alzheimer Dz* **Action:** Enhances cholinergic activity **Dose:** 1.5 mg bid; ↑ to 6 mg bid, w/ ↑ at 2-wk intervals (take w/ food) **Caution:** [B, ?] w/ BBs, CCBs, smoking, neuromuscular blockade, digoxin **CI:** Rivastigmine or carbamate allergy **Disp:** Caps 1.5, 3, 4.5, 6 mg; soln 2 mg/mL **SE:** Dose-related GI effects, N/V/D, dizziness, insomnia, fatigue, tremor, diaphoresis, HA, wgt loss (in 18–26%) **Interactions:** ↑ Risk OF GI bleed W/ NSAIDs; ↓ effects W/ nicotine; ↓ effects OF anticholinergics **NIPE:** Take w/ food; swallow caps whole, do not break/chew/crush; ⊘ EtOH; risk of severe emesis w/ stopping & restarting drug

Rivastigmine Transdermal (Exelon Patch) [Cholinesterase Inhibitor/Anti-Alzheimer Agent]
Uses: *Mild–mod Alzheimer & Parkinson Dz dementia* **Action:** Acetylcholinesterase Inhib **Dose:** *Initial:* 4.6-mg patch/d applied to back, chest, upper arm, ↑ 9.5 mg after 4 wk if tolerated **Caution:** [?, ?] Sick sinus synd, conduction defects, asthma, COPD, urinary obst, Szs; death from multiple

patches at same time reported **CI:** Hypersensitivity to rivastigmine, other carbamates **Disp:** Transdermal patch 5 cm² (4.6 mg/24 h), 10 cm² (9.5 mg/24 h) **SE:** N/V/D **Interactions:** ↑ Risk of GI bleed *W/* NSAIDs; ↓ effects *W/* nicotine; ↓ effects *OF* anticholinergics **NIPE:** Risk of severe emesis *w/* stopping & restarting drug; for initial application, may apply the day after the last oral dose

Rizatriptan (Maxalt, Maxalt MLT) [Antimigraine Agent/5-HT₁ Agonist] Uses: *Rx acute migraine* **Action:** Vascular serotonin receptor agonist **Dose:** 5–10 mg PO, repeat in 2 h, PRN, 30 mg/d max **Caution:** [C, M] **CI:** Angina, ischemic heart Dz, ischemic bowel Dz, hemiplegic/basilar migraine, uncontrolled HTN, ergot or serotonin 5-HT₁ agonist use *w/in* 24 h, MAOI use *w/in* 14 d **Disp:** Tab 5, 10 mg *Maxalt MLT:* OD tabs 5, 10 mg **SE:** CP, palpitations, N, V, asthenia, dizziness, somnolence, fatigue **Interactions:** ↑ Vasospastic effects *W/* ergots, 5-HT agonists; ↑ effects *W/* MAOIs, propranolol **NIPE:** Tx for migraines—not for prophylaxis; acute MIs & arrhythmias have occurred after taking 5-HT₁ drugs; remove from blister pack immediately before taking; take as soon as migraine Sx begin

Rocuronium (Zemuron) [Skeletal Muscle Relaxant] Uses: *Skeletal muscle relaxation during rapid-sequence intubation, surgery, or mechanical ventilation* **Action:** Nondepolarizing neuromuscular blocker **Dose:** *Rapid-sequence intubation:* 0.6–1.2 mg/kg IV *Continous Inf:* 8–12 mcg/kg/min IV; adjust/titrate based on *train of four* monitoring; ↓ in hepatic impair **Caution:** [C, ?] Anaphylactoid reactions can occur. Concomitant use of corticosteroids has been associated *w/* myopathy **CI:** Component or other neuromuscular blocker allergy **Disp:** Inj preservative-free 10 mg/mL **SE:** BP changes, tachycardia **Interactions:** ↑ Effects *W/* MAOIs, propranolol; ↑ vasospastic Rxn *W/* ergot-containing drugs; ↑ risk of hyperreflexia, incoordination, weakness *W/* SSRIs **NIPE:** ⊘ Administer *w/o* facilities for intubation, mechanical ventilation, O₂ therapy, antagonist are immediately available

Roflumilast (Daliresp) Uses: *↓ Exacerbations of severe COPD* **Action:** Selective phosphodiesterase-4 Inhib (PDE4), ↑ cAMP *w/* ↓ inflammation **Dose:** *Adults.* 500 mcg daily **Caution:** [C, –] Metabolized by CYP3A4 and 1A2; CYP3A4 and 1A2 Inhib (cimetidine, erythromycin) ↑ levels, inducers (rifampin, carbamazepine) can ↓ blood levels **CI:** Mod–severe liver impair **Disp:** Tabs 500 mcg **SE:** Worsening depression/suicidal behavior/ideation; N/D, ↓ wgt, HA, insomnia, anxiety **Notes:** Not a bronchodilator, not for acute exacerbations **NIPE:** Take *w/o* regard to food; ⊘ PRG, breast-feeding; ✓ S/Sx dehydration, ensure adequate fluid intake; ✓ report changes in mood or behavior; ✓ wgt loss

Romidepsin (Istodax) [Histone Deacetylase Inhibitor] Uses: *Rx cutaneous T-cell lymphoma in pts who have received at least 1 prior systemic therapy* **Action:** Histone deacetylase (HDAC) Inhib **Dose:** 14 mg/m² IV over 4 h d 1, 8, & 15 of a 28-d cycle; repeat cycles q28d if tolerated; Tx D/C or interruption *w/* or *w/o* dose reduction to 10 mg/m² to manage adverse drug Rxns **Caution:** [D, ?]

Risk of ↑ QT, hematologic tox; strong CYP3A4 Inhibs may ↑ conc **Disp:** Inj 10 mg **SE:** N, V, fatigue, Infxn, anorexia, ↓ plt **Interactions:** May ↑ conc *W/* strong CYP3A4 Inhibs (eg, azole antifungals, protease Inhibs, clarithromycin, nefazodone); caution w/ mod CYP3A4 Inhibs; ↓ *W/* strong CYP3A4 inducers (eg, carbamazepine, phenytoin, phenobarbital, rifampin; avoid) **Labs:** ↑ α Plt; monitor PT/INR *W/* warfarin; monitor lytes, CBC w/ differential **NIPE:** Hazardous agent, precautions for handling & disposal; ⊘ St. John's wort; ⊘ immunizations w/o physician approval; avoid contact w/ those who recently received live vaccine; avoid crowds, those w/ Infxns

Romiplostim (Nplate) [Thrombopoietin Receptor Agonist]
WARNING: ↑ Risk for heme malignancies & thromboembolism. D/C may worsen ↓ plt **Uses:** *Rx ↓ plt d/t ITP w/ poor response to other Tx* **Action:** Thrombopoietic, thrombopoietin receptor agonist **Dose:** *Adults.* 1 mcg/kg SQ weekly, adjust 1 mcg/kg/wk to plt count > 50,000/mm³; max 10 mcg/kg/wk **Caution:** [C, /?] **Contra:** None **Disp:** 500 mcg/mL (250-mcg vial) **SE:** HA, fatigue, dizziness, N/V/D, myalgia, epistaxis **Interactions:** ↑ Risk of bleeding *W/* anticoagulants & antiplt drugs **Labs:** Monitor CBC, plts, & peripheral smears before & weekly while adjustment of dose & monthly w/ stable dose & weekly for 2 wk after D/C drug **NIPE:** D/C if no ↑ plt after 4 wk max dose; ↓ dose w/ plt count > 200,000 cells/mm³ risk of hematologic malignancies; risk of renal or hepatic impair; ✓ bleeding precautions

Ropinirole (Requip, Requip XL) [Dopamine Agonist/Anti-Parkinson Agent]
Uses: *Rx of Parkinson Dz, restless leg syndrome (RLS)* **Action:** Dopamine agonist **Dose:** *Parkinson Dz: IR:* Initial 0.25 mg PO tid, weekly ↑ 0.25 mg/dose, to mg PO tid (may continue to titrate weekly to max dose of 24 mg/d) *ER:* 2 mg PO daily, titrate qwk by 2 mg/d to max 24 mg/d *RLS:* Initial 0.25 mg PO 1–3 h before hs **Caution:** [C,?/−] Severe CV/renal/hepatic impair **CI:** Component allergy **Disp:** Tabs IR 0.25, 0.5, 1, 2, 3, 4, 5 mg; tabs ER 2, 4, 6, 8, 12 mg **SE:** Syncope, postural ↓ BP, N/V, HA, somnolence, dose-related hallucinations, dyskinesias, dizziness **Interactions:** ↑ Risk of bleeding *W/* ASA, NSAIDs, feverfew, garlic, ginger, horse chestnut, red clover, EtOH, tobacco; ↑ effects *OF* amitriptyline, Li, MTX, theophylline, warfarin; ↑ risk of photosens *W/* dong quai—use sunscreen, St. John's wort; ↓ effects *W/* antacids, rifampin; ↓ effects *OF* ACEIs, diuretics **Labs:** ↑ ALT, AST **NIPE:** Take *W/* food; D/C w/ 7-d taper; change position slowly (↑ risk orthostatic hypotension)

Rosiglitazone (Avandia) [Hypoglycemic/Thiazolidinedione]
WARNING: May cause or worsen CHF; may ↑ myocardial ischemia **Uses:** *Type 2 DM* **Action:** Thiazolidinedione; ↑ insulin sensitivity **Dose:** 4–8 mg/d PO or in 2 ÷ doses (w/o regard to meals) **Caution:** [C, −] w/ ESRD, CHF, edema **CI:** Severe CHF (NYHA Class III, IV) **Disp:** Tabs 2, 4, 8 mg **SE:** May ↑ CV, CHF & ? CA risk; wgt gain, hyperlipidemia, HA, edema, fluid retention, worsen CHF, hyper-/hypoglycemia, hepatic damage w/ ↑ LFTs **Interactions:** ↑ Risk of

hypoglycemia W/ insulin, ketoconazole, oral hypoglycemics, fenugreek, garlic, ginseng, glucomannan; ↓ effects OF OCPs **Labs:** ↑ LFTs, total cholesterol, LDL, HDL, ↓ HMG, Hct **NIPE:** Use barrier contraception; ⊘ use in pts w/ symptomatic HF; NYHA Class III or IV; caution in pts w/ hepatic impairment, edema, macular edema, diabetic retinopathy, anemia, premenopausal

Rosuvastatin (Crestor) [Antilipemic/HMG-CoA Reductase Inhibitor] **Uses:** *Rx primary hypercholesterolemia & mixed dyslipidemia* **Action:** HMG-CoA reductase Inhib **Dose:** 5–40 mg PO daily; max 5 mg/d w/ cyclosporine, 10 mg/d w/ gemfibrozil CrCl < 30 mL/min (avoid Al-/Mg-based antacids for 2 h after) **Caution:** [X, ?/–] **CI:** Active liver Dz, unexplained ↑ LFTs **Disp:** Tabs 5, 10, 20, 40 mg **SE:** Myalgia, constipation, asthenia, Abd pain, N, myopathy, rarely rhabdomyolysis **Interactions:** ↑ Effects OF warfarin; ↑ risk of myopathy W/ cyclosporine, fibrates, niacin, statins **Labs:** ↑ LFTs; monitor LFTs at baseline, 12 wk, then q6mo; ↑ urine protein, HMG **NIPE:** ⊘ PRG or breast-feeding; use effective contraception ↓ dose in Asian pts; OK w/ grapefruit; ✓ S/Sx of myopathy (muscle tenderness, weakness, pain, fever, malaise)

Rotavirus Vaccine, Live, Oral, Monovalent (Rotarix) [Live Attenuated Human G1P[8] Rotavirus Vaccine] **Uses:** *Prevent rotavirus gastroenteritis in Peds* **Action:** Active immunization w/ live attenuated rotavirus **Dose:** *Peds 6–24 wk.* 1st dose PO at 6 wk of age, wait at least 4 wk, then a 2nd dose by 24 wk of age **Caution:** [C, ?] **CI:** Component sensitivity; uncorrected congenital GI malformation, severe combined immunodeficiency (SCID), intussusception **Disp:** Single-dose vial **SE:** Irritability, cough, runny nose, fever, anaphylactic Rxn, D, ↓ appetite, otitis media **Interactions:** ↓ Response if given W/ immunosuppressants such as irradiation, chemotherapy, high-dose steroids **NIPE:** May give w/ concomitant vaccines such as DTaP, hep B, inactivated poliovirus vaccine combined, Hib conjugated; begin series by age 12 wk, conclude by age 24 wk; can be given to infant in house w/ immunosuppressed family member or mother who is breast-feeding. Safety & effectiveness not studied in immunocompromised infants

Rotavirus Vaccine, Live, Oral, Pentavalent (RotaTeq) [Vaccine] **Uses:** *Prevent rotavirus gastroenteritis* **Action:** Active immunization w/ live attenuated rotavirus **Dose:** *Peds 6–24 wk.* Single dose PO at 2, 4, & 6 mo **Caution:** [?, ?] **CI:** Component sensitivity, uncorrected congenital GI malformation, severe combined immunodeficiency (SCID), intussusception **Disp:** Oral susp 2-mL single-use tubes **SE:** Irritability, cough, runny nose, fever, anaphylactic Rxn, D, ↓ appetite, otitis media, V **Interactions:** ↓ Effects W/ immunosuppressants such as irradiation, chemotherapy or high-dose steroids **NIPE:** Begin series by 12 wk & conclude by 32 wk of age; ⊘ take w/ oral polio vaccine; begin series by age 12 wk & conclude by 32 wk; can be given to infant in house w/ immunosuppressed family member or mother who is breast-feeding. Safety & effectiveness not studied in immunocompromised infants

Rotigotine (Neupro) Uses: *Parkinson Dz, RLS* **Action:** Dopamine agonist **Dose:** *Adults. Parkinson Dz:* 2 mg/24 h (early Dz) or 4 mg/24 h (advanced Dz); ↑ by 2 mg/24 h qwk PRN to max of 6 mg/24 h (early Dz) or 8 mg/24 h (advanced Dz); *RLS:* 1 mg/24 h; ↑ by 1 mg/24 h qwk PRN to max 3 mg/24 h; apply patch 1 ×/d to dry, intact skin; ↓ gradually w/ D/C **Caution:** [C, ?/–] Allergic Rxns w/ sulfite sensitivity **CI:** Hypersensitivity **Disp:** Transdermal sys 1, 2, 3, 4, 6, 8 mg/24 h **SE:** N/V, site Rxn, somnolence, dizziness, anorexia, hyperhidrosis, insomnia, peripheral edema, dyskinesia, HA, postural hypotension, syncope, ↑ HR, ↑ BP, hallucinations, psychotic like/compulsive behavior **Notes:** ⊘ Use same site more than once q14d **NIPE:** Use transdermal patch continuously for 24 h, remove old patch and immediately apply a new one; change position slowly d/t risk of ortostatic changes; remove patch prior to undergoing MRI or cardioversion to prevent skin burns

Rufinamide (Banzel) [Antiepileptic] Uses: *Adjunct Lennox–Gastaut Szs* **Action:** Anticonvulsant **Dose:** *Adults. Initial:* 400–800 mg/d ÷ bid (max 3200 mg/d ÷ bid) *Peds ≥ 4 y. Initial:* 10 mg/kg/d ÷ bid, target 45 mg/kg/d ÷ bid; 3200 mg/d max **Caution:** [C, –/–] **CI:** Familial short QT synd **Disp:** Tab 200, 400 mg; susp 40 mg/mL **SE:** ↓ QT, HA, somnolence, N/V, ataxia, rash **Interactions:** ↑ CNS depression *W/* EtOH & other CNS depressants; ↑ effects *OF* phenobarbital, phenytoin, triazolam; ↑ effects *W/* valproate ↓ effects *OF* carbamazepine, lamotrigine, OC; ↓ effects *W/* carbamazepine, phenobarbital, primidone, phenytoin **NIPE:** Monitor for rash; use w/ OC may lead to contraceptive failure—use barrier contraception; ↑ QT—monitor ECG; take w/ food in 2 equal ÷ doses; monitor for depression or suicidal ideation; ⊘ abrupt withdrawal; ⊘ EtOH

Ruxolitinib (Jakafi) Uses: *Myelofibrosis* **Action:** Inhib Janus-associated kinases, mediators of hematologic & immunologic cytokines & growth factors **Dose:** 20 mg bid if plt > 200,000 × 10^9/L; 15 mg bid if plt 100,000–200,000 × 10^9/L; ↑ based on response, 25 mg bid max; stop Tx if plt < 50,000 × 10^9/L; restart when > 50,000 × 10^9/L; 20 mg bid if plt > 125,000 × 10^9/L; 15 mg bid if plt 100–125,000 × 10^9/L; 10 mg bid if plt 75–100,000 × 10^9/L × 2 wk, if stable ↑ to 15 mg bid; if plt 50–75,000 × 10^9/L, 5 mg bid × 2 wk, if stable ↑ to 10 mg bid if no ↓ in spleen size or Sx D/C after 6 mo **Caution:** [C, –] Do not use if ESRD and not on dialysis; ↓ dose w/ strong CYP3A4 Inhib **CI:** None **Disp:** Tabs 5, 10, 15, 20, 25 mg **SE:** ↓ Plt, ↓ WBC, anemia, bruising, HA, dizziness, serious Infxns including zoster **Notes:** w/ D/C for reason other than ↓ plt, taper 5 mg bid each wk **NIPE:** Take w/o regard to food; ⊘ grapefruit products; ✓ CBC q2–4wk until doses stabilized; ⊘ breast-feeding; if on dialysis, take following dialysis; avoid rectal temps, IM Inj (↑ risk to induce bleeding)

Salmeterol (Serevent Diskus) [Bronchodilator/Sympathomimetic] **WARNING:** LA β_2-agonists, such as salmeterol, may ↑ risk of asthma-related death. Do not use alone, only as additional Rx for pts not controlled on other asthma meds; LA β_2-agonists may ↑ risk of asthma-related hospitalization in pediatric & adolescent pts Uses: *Asthma, exercise-induced asthma, COPD* **Action:** Sympathomimetic bronchodilator, LA β₂-agonist **Dose:** *Adults & Peds > 12 y.* 1 Diskus/dose inhaled bid **Caution:** [C, ?/–] **CI:** Acute asthma; monotherapy concomitant use of inhaled steroid, status astheticus **Disp:** 50 mcg/dose, dry powder discus **SE:** HA, pharyngitis, tachycardia, arrhythmias, nervousness, GI upset, tremors **Interactions:** ↑ CV effects *W/* MAOIs, TCAs; ↓ effects *W/* BBs **Labs:** ↑ Glucose; ↓ serum K⁺—monitor ECG for hypokalemia (flattened T waves) **NIPE:** Shake canister before use, inhale q12h; not for acute attacks; must use w/ steroid or short-acting β-agonist; rinse mouth w/ H₂O immediately after inhalation; wait 1 full min before second inhalation

Saquinavir (Invirase & Fortovase) [Antiretroviral/Protease Inhibitor]
WARNING: Invirase & Fortovase not bioequivalent/interchangeable; must use Invirase in combo w/ ritonavir, which provides saquinavir plasma levels = to those w/ Fortovase **Uses:** *HIV Infxn* **Action:** HIV protease Inhib **Dose:** 1000 mg PO bid w/in 2 h of a full meal (dose w/ ritonavir 100 mg PO bid) w/in 2 h pc (dose adjust w/ delavirdine, lopinavir, & nelfinavir) **Caution:** [B, ?] **CI:** Complete AV block w/o implanted pacemaker; concomitant use antiarrhythmics, ergot derivatives, sedatives/hypnotics, trazodone, sildenafil, statins, rifamins, congenital ↑ QT synd; severe hepatic impair; refractory ↓ K⁺/ ↓ Mg²⁺; anaphylaxis to component **Disp:** Caps 200 mg, tabs 500 mg **SE:** Dyslipidemia, lipodystrophy, rash, hyperglycemia, GI upset, weakness **Interactions:** ↑ Risk of life-threatening arrhythmias *W/* amiodarone, astemizole, bepridil, cisapride, flecainide, propafenone, pimozide, quinidine, terfenadine; ↑ risk of myopathy *W/* HMG-CoA reductase Inhibs; ↑ risk of peripheral vasospasm & ischemia *W/* ergot derivatives; ↑ effects *W/* delavirdine, indinavir, ketoconazole, macrolide antibiotics, nelfinavir, ritonavir, grapefruit juice, garlic, St. John's wort, food; ↑ effects *OF* amitriptyline, benzodiazepines, CCB, lovastatin, macrolide antibiotics, phenytoin, sildenafil, simvastatin, terfenadine, TCAs, verapamil; ↓ effects *W/* barbiturates, carbamazepine, dexamethasone, efavirenz, phenytoin, rifabutin, rifampin, St. John's wort; ↓ effects *OF* OCPs **Labs:** ↑ LFTs, ↓ neutrophils **NIPE:** Take 2 h pc; avoid grapefruit juice; use barrier contraception; ↑ risk of photosensitivity—avoid direct sunlight

Sargramostim [GM-CSF] (Leukine) [Hematopoietic Drug/Colony-Stimulating Factor]
Uses: *Myeloid recovery following BMT or chemotherapy* **Action:** Recombinant GF, activates mature granulocytes & macrophages **Dose:** *Adults & Peds.* 250 mcg/m²/d IV cont until ANC > 1500 cells/m² for 3 consecutive d **Caution:** [C, ?/–] Li, corticosteroids **CI:** > 10% blasts, allergy to yeast, concurrent chemotherapy/RT **Disp:** Inj 250, 500 mcg **SE:** Bone pain, fever, ↑ BP, tachycardia, flushing, GI upset, myalgia **Interactions:** ↑ Effects *W/* corticosteroids, Li **Labs:** ↑ BUN, LFTs **NIPE:** ⊘ Exposure to Infxn; rotate Inj sites; use APAP PRN for pain; ✓ supraventricular arrythmias during administration

Saxagliptin (Onglyza) [Dipeptidyl Peptidase-4 Inhibitor]
Uses: *Monotherapy/combo type 2 DM* **Action:** DDP-4 Inhib, ↑ insulin synth/release

Dose: 2.5 or 5 mg 1 ×/d w/o regard to meals; 2.5 mg 1 ×/d w/ CrCl < 50 mL/min or w/ strong CYP3A4/5 Inhib (eg, atazanavir, clarithromycin, indinavir, itraconazole, ketoconazole, nefazodone, nelfinavir, ritonavir, saquinavir, telithromycin) **Caution:** [B, ?] May cause ↓ glucose when used w/ insulin secretagogues (eg, secretagogues) w/ pancreatitis **CI:** Hypersens Rxn **Disp:** Tabs 2.5, 5 mg **SE:** Peripheral edema, hypoglycemia, UTI, HA, Abd pain **Interactions:** ↑ Effects **W/** strong CYP3A4/5 Inhibs: atazanavir, clarithromycin, indinavir, itraconazole, ketoconazole, nefazodone, nelfinavir, ritonavir, saquinavir, telithromycin; sulfonylurea **Labs:** Monitor BUN/Cr **NIPE:** Take w/o regard to food; grapefruit products ↑ concentration

Saxagliptin/Metformin (Kombiglyze XR) [Dipeptidyl Peptidase-4 Inhibitor + Biguanide] WARNING: Lactic acidosis can occur w/ metformin accumulation; ↑ risk w/ sepsis, vol depletion, CHF, renal/hepatic impair, excess alcohol; if lactic acidosis suspected D/C med & hospitalize **Uses:** *Type 2 DM* **Action:** Dipeptidyl peptidase-4 (DDP-4) Inhib, ↑ insulin synth/release & biguanide; ↓ hepatic glucose production & intestinal absorption of glucose; ↑ insulin sens **Doses:** 5/500 mg–5/2000 mg saxagliptin/metformin HCl XR PO daily w/ evening meal **Caution:** [B, ?/–] w/ 10 diagnosed contrast studies **CI:** SCr > 1.4 mg/dL (females) or > 1.5 mg/dL (males); metacidosis **Disp:** Tabs mg saxagliptin/mg metformin XR 5/500, 5/1000, 2.5/1000 **SE:** Lactic acidosis; ↓ vit B₁₂ levels; ↓ glucose w/ insulin secretagogue; N/V/D, anorexia, HA, URI, UTI, urticaria, myalgia **Interactions:** ↑ Effects **W/** strong CYP3A4/5 Inhibs: atazanavir, clarithromycin, indinavir, itraconazole, ketoconazole, nefazodone, nelfinavir, ritonavir, saquinavir, telithromycin; sulfonylurea **Labs:** Monitor BUN/Cr **NIPE:** Do not exceed 5 mg/2000 mg saxagliptin/metformin HCl XR; do not crush or chew; w/ strong CYP3A4/5 Inhibs do not exceed 2.5 mg saxagliptin/d

Scopolamine Transdermal (Transderm-Scop) [Antiemetic/ Antivertigo/Anticholinergic] Uses: *Prevent N/V associated w/ motion sickness, anesthesia, opiates* **Action:** Anticholinergic, antiemetic **Dose:** 1 mg/72 h, 1 patch behind ear q3d; apply > 4 h before exposure **Caution:** [C, +] w/ APAP, levodopa, ketoconazole, digitalis, KCl **CI:** NAG, GI or GU obst, thyrotoxicosis, paralytic ileus **Disp:** Patch 1.5 mg (releases 1 mg over 72 h) **SE:** Xerostomia, drowsiness, blurred vision, tachycardia, constipation **Interactions:** ↑ Effects **W/** antihistamines, antidepressants, disopyramide, opioids, phenothiazine, quinidine, TCAs, EtOH **NIPE:** Do not blink excessively after dose, wait 5 min before dosing other eye; antiemetic activity w/ patch requires several h; ⊘ D/C abruptly; wear one patch at a time; do not cut patch; wash hands after applying patch; may cause heat intolerance, may cause stroke

Secobarbital (Seconal) [C-II] [Anticonvulsant, Sedative/ Hypnotic/Barbiturate] Uses: *Insomnia, short-term use*, preanesthetic agent **Action:** Rapid-acting barbiturate **Dose:** *Adults.* 100–200 mg hs, 100–300 mg pre-op *Peds.* 2–6 mg/kg/dose, 100 mg/max, ↓ in elderly **Caution:** [D, +] w/ CYP2C9,

3A3/4, 3A5/7 inducer (Table 10); ↑ tox w/ other CNS depressants **CI:** Hypersensitivity to barbiturates, marked hepatic impairment; dyspnea or airway obstruction, porphyria, PRG **Disp:** Caps 100 mg **SE:** Tolerance in 1–2 wk; resp depression, CNS depression, porphyria, photosens **Interactions:** ↑ Effects *W/* MAOIs, valproic acid, EtOH, kava kava, valerian; ↑ effects *OF* meperidine; ↓ effects *OF* anticoagulants, BBs, CCBs, CNS depressants, chloramphenicol, corticosteroids, cyclosporine, digitoxin, disopyramide, doxycycline, estrogen, griseofulvin, methadone, neuroleptics, OCPs, propafenone, quinidine, tacrolimus, theophylline **NIPE:** Tolerance in 1–2 wk; photosens; ⊘ PRG, breast-feeding; use barrier contraception; do not D/C abruptly—may cause withdrawal

Selegiline, Oral (Eldepryl, Zelapar) [Anti-Parkinson Agent/MAOI]

WARNING: Closely monitor for worsening depression or emergence of suicidality, particularly in Ped pts **Uses:** *Parkinson Dz* **Action:** MAOI **Dose:** 5 mg PO bid; 1.25–2.5 once-daily ODT tabs PO qAM (before breakfast w/o Liq) 2.5 mg/d max; ↓ in elderly **Caution:** [C, ?] w/ Drugs that induce CYP3A4 (Table 10) (eg, phenytoin, carbamazepine, nafcillin, phenobarbital, & rifampin); avoid w/ antidepressants **CI:** w/ Meperidine, MAOI, dextromethorphan, tramadol, methadone, general anesthesia w/in 10 d, pheochromocytoma **Disp:** Tabs/caps 5 mg; once-daily tabs 1.25 mg **SE:** N, dizziness, orthostatic ↓ BP, arrhythmias, tachycardia, edema, confusion, xerostomia **Interactions:** ↑ Risk of serotonin synd *W/* dextroamphetamine, dextromethorphan, fenfluramine, meperidine, methylphenidate, sibutramine, venlafaxine; ↑ risk of hypertension *W/* dextroamphetamine, levodopa, methylphenidate, SSRIs, tyramine-containing foods (beer, red wine, aged cheese/meat, dried fruits), EtOH, ephedra, ginseng, ma huang, St. John's wort **Labs:** = + for amphetamine on urine drug screen **NIPE:** ↓ Carbidopa/levodopa if used in combo; see transdermal form; take w/o regard to food

Selegiline, Transdermal (Emsam) [Anti-Parkinson Agent/MAO B Inhibitor]

WARNING: May ↑ risk of suicidal thinking & behavior in children & adolescents w/ MDD **Uses:** *Depression* **Action:** MAOI **Dose:** *Adults.* Apply patch daily to upper torso, upper thigh, or outer upper arm **CI:** Tyramine-containing foods w/ 9- or 12-mg doses; serotonin-sparing agents **Caution:** [C, –] ↑ Carbamazepine & oxcarbazepine levels **Disp:** ER Patches 9, 12 mg **SE:** Local Rxns requiring topical steroids; HA, insomnia, orthostatic, ↓ BP, serotonin synd, suicide risk **Interactions:** ↑ Risk of serotonin synd *W/* dextroamphetamine, dextromethorphan, fenfluramine, meperidine, methylphenidate, sibutramine, venlafaxine; ↑ risk of hypertension *W/* dextroamphetamine, levodopa, methylphenidate, SSRIs, tyramine-containing foods (beer, red wine, aged cheese/ meat, dried fruits), EtOH, ephedra, ginseng, ma huang, St. John's wort **NIPE:** ⊘ EtOH & tyramine-containing foods; rotate site; see oral form

Selenium Sulfide (Exsel Shampoo, Selsun Blue Shampoo, Selsun Shampoo) [Antiseborrheic]

Uses: *Scalp seborrheic dermatitis*, scalp itching & flaking d/t *dandruff*; tinea versicolor **Action:** Antiseborrheic **Dose:**

Dandruff, seborrhea: Massage 5–10 mL into wet scalp, leave on 2–3 min, rinse, repeat; use 2 × wk, then once q1–4wk PRN *Tinea versicolor:* Apply 2.5% daily on area & lather w/ small amounts of H_2O; leave on 10 min, then rinse **Caution:** [C, ?] Avoid contact w/ open wounds or mucous membranes **CI:** Component allergy **Disp:** Shampoo [OTC]; 2.5% lotion **SE:** Dry or oily scalp, lethargy, hair discoloration, local irritation **NIPE:** ⊘ Use on excoriated skin; may cause reversible hair loss; rinse thoroughly after use; do not use more than 2 ×/wk

Sertaconazole (Ertaczo) [Antifungal] **Uses:** *Topical Rx interdigital tinea pedis* **Action:** Imidazole antifungal **Spectrum:** *T rubrum, T mentagrophytes, E floccosum* **Dose:** *Adults & Peds > 12.* Apply between toes & immediate surrounding healthy skin bid × 4 wk **Caution:** [C, ?] Avoid occlusive dressing **CI:** Component allergy **Disp:** 2% Cream **SE:** Contact dermatitis, dry/burning skin, tenderness **NIPE:** Use in immunocompetent pts; not for oral, intravag, ophthal use; avoid occlusive dressings; avoid contact w/ mucous membranes

Sertraline (Zoloft) [Antidepressant/SSRI] **WARNING:** Closely monitor pts for worsening depression or emergence of suicidality, particularly in Ped pts **Uses:** *Depression, panic disorders, PMDD, OCD, PTSD*, social anxiety disorder, eating disorders, premenstrual disorders **Action:** ↓ Neuronal uptake of serotonin **Dose:** *Adults. Depression:* 50–200 mg/d PO *PTSD:* 25 mg PO daily × 1 wk, then 50 mg PO daily, 200 mg/d max *Peds. 6–12 y.* 25 mg PO daily *13–17 y:* 50 mg PO daily **Caution:** [C, ?/–] Serotonin syndrome: ↑ risk w/ concomitant use of serotonin antagonists (haloperidol, etc), hepatic impair **CI:** MAOI use w/in 14 d; concomitant pimozide **Disp:** Tabs 25, 50, 100; 20 mg/mL oral **SE:** Activate manic/hypomanic state, ↑/↓ wgt, insomnia, somnolence, fatigue, tremor, xerostomia, N/D, dyspepsia, ejaculatory dysfunction, ↓ libido, hepatotox **Interactions:** ↑ Effects *W/* cimetidine, tryptophan, St. John's wort; ↑ effects *OF* benzodiazepines, phenytoin, TCAs, warfarin, EtOH; ↑ risk of serotonin synd *W/* MAOIs **Labs:** ↑ LFTs, triglycerides, ↓ uric acid **NIPE:** ⊘ D/C abruptly; give w/ food or milk w/ GI distress; may trigger manic or hypomanic condition in susceptible pts

Sevelamer Carbonate (Renvela) [Phosphate Binder] **Uses:** *Control ↑ PO_4^{3-} in ESRD* **Action:** Intestinal phosphate binder **Dose:** *Initial:* PO_4^{3-} Start 0.8 or 1.6 g PO tid w/ meals; titrate 0.8 g/meal for target PO_4^{3-} 3.5–5.5 mg/dL; switch g/g among sevelamer forms, titrate PRN **Caution:** [C, ?] w/ Swallow disorders, bowel problems, may ↓ absorption of vits D, E, K, ↓ ciprofloxacin & other medicine levels **CI:** Bowel perf **Disp:** Tab 800 mg, powder 0.8/2.4 g **SE:** N/V/D, dyspepsia, Abd pain, flatulence, constipation **Interactions:** ↓ Effects *OF* ciprofloxacin. Monitor narrow therapeutic index drugs esp antiarrhythmics & antiepileptics **Labs:** Monitor serum bicarbonate, chloride levels **NIPE:** Separate other meds (esp narrow therapeutic index drugs) 1 h before or 3 h after sevelamer carbonate; take w/food.

Sevelamer HCl (Renagel) [Phosphate Binder] **Uses:** *↓ PO_4^{3-} in ESRD* **Action:** Binds intestinal PO_4^{3-} **Dose:** *Initial:* PO_4^{3-} > 5.5 & < 7.5 mg/dL:

800 mg PO tid; ≥ 7.5 mg/dL: 1200–1600 mg PO tid *Switching from sevelamer carbonate:* per-g basis; titrate ↑/↓ 1 tab/meal 2-wk intervals PRN; take w/ food 2–4 caps PO tid w/ meals; adjust based on PO_4^{3-}; max 4 g/dose **Caution:** [C, ?] May ↓ absorption of vits D, E, K, ↓ ciprofloxacin & other medicine levels **CI:** ↓ PO_4^{3-}, bowel obst **Disp:** Tab 400, 800 mg **SE:** N/V/D, dyspepsia, ↑ Ca^{2+} **Interactions:** ↓ Effects *OF* antiarrhythmics, anticonvulsants, ciprofloxacin when given *W/* sevelamer **Labs:** ↑ Alk phos **NIPE:** Must be administered w/ meals; take daily multivitamin, may ↓ fat-soluble vit absorption; take 1 h before or 3 h after other meds; do not open or chew caps; 800 mg sevelamer = 667 mg Ca acetate

Short   Ragweed   Pollen   Allergen   Extract   (Ragwitek)
WARNING: Can cause life-threatening allergic Rxn (anaphylaxis, laryngopharyngeal edema); DO NOT use w/ severe unstable/uncontrolled asthma; observe for 30 min after 1st dose; Rx & train to use auto-injectable epi; may not be suitable for pts unresponsive to epi or inhaled bronchodilators (pts on BBs or w/ certain conditions that could ↓ ability to respond to severe allergic Rxn **Uses:** *Immunotherapy of short ragweed pollen-induced allergic rhinitis w/ or w/o conjunctivitis confirmed by + skin test or pollen-specific IgE Ab* **Action:** Allergen immunotherapy **Dose:** *Adults.* 1 tab SL/d; do not swallow for 1 min **Peds.** Not approved **Caution:** [C, ?/–] Discuss severe allergic Rxn; if oral lesions, stop Tx, restart after healed **CI:** Severe uncontrolled/unstable asthma; hx severe systemic/local allergic reaction to SL allergen immunotherapy; eosinophilic esophagitis; component hypersensitivity **Disp:** Tabs, 30/90 day blister packs **SE:** Throat irritation, oral/ear/tongue pruritus, mouth edema, oral paraesthesia **NIPE:** 1st dose in healthcare setting; start 12 wk before expected onset of Sx; give auto-injectable epi; D/C with ↑ local symptoms & seek care; only for adults 18–65 y

Sildenafil   (Viagra,   Revatio)   [Vasodilator/PDE5   Inhibitor]
Uses: *Viagra:* *ED*; *Revatio:* *Pulm artery HTN (adult only)* **Action:** ↓ Phosphodiesterase type 5 (PDE5) (responsible for cGMP breakdown); ↑ cGMP activity to relax smooth muscles & ↑ flow to corpus cavernosum & pulm vasculature; ? antiproliferative on pulm artery smooth muscle **Dose:** *ED:* 25–100 mg PO 1 h before sexual activity, max 1/d; ↓ if > 65 y *Revatio:* Pulm HTN: 20 mg PO tid or 10 mg IV tid **Caution:** [B, ?] w/ CYP3A4 Inhib (Table 10), retinitis pigmentosa; hepatic/severe renal impair; w/ sig hypo-/hypertension **CI:** w/ Nitrates or if sex not advised; w/ protease Inhib **Disp:** Tabs 25, 50, 100 mg, tabs *Revatio:* Tabs 20 mg; Inj 5–10 mg/vial **SE:** HA; flushing; dizziness; blue haze visual change, hearing loss, priapism **Interactions:** ↑ Effects *W/* amlodipine, cimetidine, erythromycin, indinavir, itraconazole, ketoconazole, nelfinavir, protease Inhibs, ritonavir, saquinavir, grapefruit juice; ↑ risk of hypotension *W/* amlodipine, antihypertensives, nitrates; ↓ effects *W/* rifampin **NIPE:** High-fat food delays absorption; ↑ risk of cardiac arrest if used w/ nitrates; cardiac events in absence of nitrates debatable; transient global amnesia reports; do not use nitrogen w/in 24 h of this drug; obtain Tx immediately if erection lasts > 4 h

Silodosin (Rapaflo) [Selective Alpha-1 Adrenergic Receptor Antagonist] Uses: *BPH* Action: α-blockers of prostatic α_{1a} Dose: 8 mg/d; 4 mg/d w/ CrCl 30–50 mL/min; take w/ food Caution: [B, ?] Not for use in females; do not use w/ other α-blockers or w/ glycoprotein Inhib (ie, cyclosporine); R/O PCa before use; IFIS possible w/ cataract surgery CI: Severe hepatic/renal impair (CrCl < 30 mL/min), w/ CYP3A4 Inhib (eg, ketoconazole, clarithromycin, itraconazole, ritonavir) Disp: Caps 4, 8 mg SE: Retrograde ejaculation, dizziness, D, syncope, somnolence, orthostatic ↓ BP, nasopharyngitis, nasal congestion Interactions: ↑ Risk of hepatic/renal impair W/ CYP3A4 Inhibs (eg, ketoconazole, clarithromycin, itraconazole, ritonavir) NIPE: Not for use as antihypertensive; no effect on QT interval; change position slowly (↑ risk orthostatic BP)

Silver Nitrate (Generic) [Antiseptic/Astringent] Uses: *Removal of granulation tissue & warts; prophylaxis in burns* Action: Caustic antiseptic & astringent Dose: *Adults & Peds.* Apply to moist surface 2–3 ×/wk for 2–3 wk or until effect Caution: [C, ?] CI: Do not use on broken skin Disp: Topical impregnated applicator sticks, soln 0.5, 10, 25, 50%; topical ointment 10% SE: May stain tissue black, usually resolves; local irritation, methemoglobinemia NIPE: D/C if redness or irritation develops; no longer used in US for newborn prevention of gonococcus conjunctivitis

Silver Sulfadiazine (Silvadene, Others) [Antibiotic] Uses: *Prevention & Rx of Infxn in 2nd- & 3rd-degree burns* Action: Bactericidal Dose: *Adults & Peds.* Aseptically cover the area w/ 1/16-in coating bid Caution: [B unless near term, ?/–] CI: Infants < 2 mo, PRG near term Disp: Cream 1% SE: Itching, rash, skin discoloration, blood dyscrasias, hep, allergy Interactions: May inactivate topical proteolytic enzymes Labs: ↓ WBCs; monitor LFTs, BUN, Cr NIPE: Photosens—use sunscreen; systemic absorption w/ extensive application; obtain baseline CBC, renal, hepatic labs

Simeprevir (Olysio) Uses: *Hep C w/ genotype 1 & compensated liver Dz in combo w/ ribavirin & peginterferon alpha* Action: NS3/4A protease Inhib Dose: *Adults.* 150 mg Q D w/ food Caution: [C, –] Note: Ribavirin & peginterferon alpha are [X, –] BOTH embryofetal toxic; avoid PRG (patient or in partner) PRG before & 6 mo post CI: PRG or males w/ PRG partner Disp: Caps 150 mg SE: Photosens, rash, pruritus, N, dyspnea Notes: DO NOT use as monotherapy; use w/ ribavirin & peginterferon alpha; monitor w/ P & SE from other meds; screen for NS3 Q80K polymorphism; do not use w/ CYP3A inducers/Inhib; monitor HCV RNA levels NIPE: Take w/ food; swallow whole; use 2 forms of effective contraception & q mo PRG test; ⊘ PRG ⊘ breast-feeding; ⊘ ETOH

Simethicone (Generic) [OTC] [Antiflatulent] Uses: *Flatulence* Action: Defoaming, alters gas bubble surface tension Dose: *Adults & Peds > 12 y.* 40–360 mg PO after meals & at bedtime PRN; 500 mg/d max *Peds < 2 y.* 20 mg PO qid PRN *2–12 y.* 40 mg PO qid PRN Caution: [C, ?] CI: GI perforation or obst Disp: [OTC] Tabs 80, 125 mg; caps 125 mg; caps 125 mg; susp 40 mg/0.6 mL;

chew tabs 80, 125 mg; caps: 125, 180 mg; ODT strip: 40, 62.5 mg SE: N/D Interactions: ↑ Effects *OF* topical proteolytic enzymes NIPE: Available in combo products OTC; ∅ carbonated beverages

Simvastatin (Zocor) [Antilipemic/HMG-CoA Reductase Inhibitor] Uses: ↓ Cholesterol Action: HMG-CoA reductase Inhib Dose: *Adults.* 5–40 mg PO qpm; w/ meals; ↓ in renal Insuff, w/o grapefruit juice *Peds 10–17 y.* 10 mg, 40 mg/d max Caution: [X,–] Max 10 mg daily w/ verapamil, diltiazem; max 20 mg daily w/ amlodipine, ranolazine, amiodarone; 80 mg dose restricted to those taking > 12 mo w/o muscle tox; w/ Chinese pt on lipid-modifying meds CI: PRG, liver Dz, strong CYP3A4 Inhib Disp: Tabs 5, 10, 20, 40, 80 mg SE: HA, GI upset, myalgia, myopathy (pain, tenderness weakness w/ creatine kinase 10 × ULN), & rhabdomyolysis hep Interactions: ↑ Effects *OF* digoxin, warfarin; ↑ risk of myopathy/rhabdomyolysis *W/* amiodarone, cyclosporine, CYP3A4 Inhibs, fibrates, HIV protease Inhibs, macrolides, niacin, verapamil, grapefruit juice; ↓ effects *W/* cholestyramine, colestipol, fluvastatin, isradipine, propranolol Labs: ↑ LFTs, monitor NIPE: Take w/ food & in the evening; ∅ PRG, breast-feeding; combo w/ ezetimibe/simvastatin); pt to report muscle pain; use effective contraception

Sipuleucel-T (Provenge) [Autologous Cellular Immunotherapy] Uses: *Asymptomatic/minimally symptomatic metastatic castrate-resistant PCa* Action: Autologous (pt specific) cellular immunotherapy Dose: 3 doses 1 mo at 2-wk intervals; premed w/ APAP & diphenhydramine Caution: [N/A, N/A] Confirm identity/expir date before Inf; acute transfusion Rxn possible; not tested for transmissible Dz CI: None Disp: 50 MU autologous CD54+ cells activated w/ PAP GM-CSF, in 250 mL LR SE: Chills, fatigue, fever, back pain, N, Jt ache, HA Interactions: ↓ Effects *W/* concomitant chemotherapy or immunosuppressive therapy NIPE: Pt must undergo leukapheresis, w/ shipping & autologous cell processing at manufacturing facility before each Inf

Sirolimus [Rapamycin] (Rapamune) [Immunosuppressant] WARNING: Use only by physicians experienced in immunosuppression; immunosuppression associated w/ lymphoma, ↑ Infxn risk; do not use in lung transplant (fatal bronchial anastomotic dehiscence); do not use in liver transplant: ↑ risk hepatic artery thrombosis, graft failure, & mortality (w/ evidence of Infxn) Uses: *Prevent organ rejection in newTx pts* Action: ↓ T-lymphocyte activation & proliferation Dose: *Adults > 40 kg.* 6 mg PO on d 1, then 2 mg/d PO *Peds < 40 kg & ≥ 13 y.* 3 mg/m² load, then 1 mg/m²/d (in H₂O/orange juice; no grapefruit juice w/ sirolimus); take 4 h after cyclosporine; ↓ in hepatic impair Caution: [C, ?/–] Impaired wound healing & angioedema; grapefruit juice, ketoconazole CI: Component allergy Disp: Soln 1 mg/mL, tabs 0.5, 1, 2 mg SE: HTN, edema, CP, fever, HA, insomnia, acne, rash,↑ cholesterol, ↑/↓ K⁺, Infxns, blood dyscrasias, arthralgia, tachycardia, renal impair, graft loss & death in liver transplant (hepatic artery thrombosis), ascites Notes: Levels: *Trough:* 4–20 ng/mL; can vary based on assay & use of other immunosuppression agents Interactions: ↑ Effects *W/* azole

antifungals, cimetidine, cyclosporine, diltiazem, macrolides, nicardipine, protease Inhibs, verapamil, grapefruit juice; ↓ effects *W/* carbamazepine, phenobarbital, phenytoin, rifabutin, rifapentine, rifampin; ↓ effects *OF* live virus vaccines **Labs:** ↑ LFTs, BUN, Cr, cholesterol, triglycerides; ↑/↓ K⁺ **NIPE:** Take w/o regard to food; if on cyclosporine, take meds 4 h apart; ⊘ PRG while taking drug & for 12 wk after drug D/C; avoid crowds, those w/Infxn; avoid those who have received recent nasal Flu or oral polio vaccines

Sitagliptin (Januvia) [Hypoglycemic/DPP-4 Inhibitor] Uses: *Monotherapy or combo for type 2 DM* **Action:** Dipeptidyl peptidase-4 (DPP-4) Inhib, ↑ insulin synth/release **Dose:** 100 mg PO daily; CrCl 30–50: 50 mg PO daily; CrCl < 30 mL/min: 25 mg PO daily **Caution:** [B, ?] May cause ↓ blood sugar when used w/ insulin secretagogues such as sulfonylureas **CI:** Component hypersens **Disp:** Tabs 25, 50, 100 mg **SE:** URI; peripheral edema, asopharyngitis **Interactions:** ↑ Risk of hypoglycemia *W/* sulfonylureas **Labs:** Monitor LFTs, BUN/Cr **NIPE:** ⊘ Children < 18 y; monitor renal Fxn before starting therapy; start drug at low dose & periodically ↑; monitor for severe pancreatitis; no evidence for ↑ CV risk; take w/o regard to food, swallow whole

Sitagliptin/Metformin (Janumet) [Hypoglycemic/DPP-4 Inhibitor/Biguanide] WARNING: See Metformin **Uses:** *Adjunct to diet & exercise in type 2 DM* **Action:** See individual agents **Dose:** 1 tab PO bid, titrate; 100 mg sitagliptin & 2000 mg metformin/d max; take w/ meals **Caution:** [B, ?/–] **CI:** Type 1 DM, DKA, male Cr > 1.5; female Cr > 1.4 mg/dL **Disp:** Tabs 50/500, 50/1000 mg **SE:** Nasopharyngitis, N/V/D, flatulence, Abd discomfort, dyspepsia, asthenia, HA **Interactions:** ↑ Effects *W/* amiloride, cimetidine, digoxin, furosemide, MAOIs, morphine, procainamide, quinidine, quinine, ranitidine, triamterene, TMP, vancomycin; ↓ effects *W/* corticosteroids, CCBs, diuretics, estrogens, INH, OCPs, phenothiazine, phenytoin, sympathomimetics, thyroid drugs, tobacco; monitor digoxin levels **Labs:** Monitor LFTs, BUN/Cr, CBC **NIPE:** ⊘ Children < 18 y; monitor renal Fxn; start drug at low dose & periodically ↑; hold w/ contrast study; monitor for severe pancreatitis; BB may mask hypoglycemia; take w/ meals; swallow whole

Sitagliptin/Simvastatin (Juvisync) Uses: *DM2 & hyperlipidemia* **Action:** ↑ Insulin synth/release & ↓ cholesterol, ↓ VLDL, ↓ triglycerides, ↑ HDL; dipeptidyl peptidase-4 (DPP-4) Inhib w/HMG-CoA reductase Inhib **Dose:** Start 100 mg/40 or maintain simvastatin dose **Caution:** [X, –] ↑ AST/ALT; myopathy (↑ risk of myopathy w/ age > 65 y, female, renal impair, meds (eg, niacin, amiodarone, CCBs, fibrates, colchicine); renal failure, hypoglycemia w/ sulfonylureas, or insulin; pancreatitis, anaphylaxis **CI:** Hx hypersensitivity Rxn; w/ CYP3A4 Inhib, gemfibrozil, cyclosporine, danazol, ketoconazole, itraconazole, erythromycin, clarithromycin, HIV protease Inhib; liver Dx; PRG or women who may get PRG; nursing **Disp:** Tabs mg sitagliptin/mg simvastatin 100/10, 100/20, 100/40, 50/10, 50/20, 50/40 **SE:** *Simvastatin:* HA, GI upset, myalgia, myopathy (pain, tenderness, weakness w/ creatine kinase 10 × ULN) & rhabdomyolysis, hep; sitagliptin: URI, nasopharyngitis, UTI, HA **Notes:** ↑ Myopathy w/ coadministration of CYP3A4 Inhib; risk of myopathy dose related **NIPE:** ⊘ PRG, breast-feeding; use effective contraception w/ use; avoid grapefruit products; teach S/Sx myopathy; take in evening, swallow tablet whole; ✓ renal/hepatic fxn

Smallpox Vaccine (ACAM2000) [Vaccine] WARNING: Acute myocarditis w/ other infectious complications possible; CI in immunocompromised, eczema or exfoliative skin conditions, infants < 1 y **Uses:** Immunization against smallpox (variolavirus) **Action:** Active immunization (live attenuated cowpox virus) **Dose:** *Adults primary & revaccination:* 15 punctures w/ bifurcated needle dipped in vaccine into deltoid, ✓ site for Rxn in 6–8 d; if major Rxn, site scabs, & heals, leaving scar **Caution:** [D, ?] **CI:** *Nonemergency use:* Febrile illness, immunosuppression, Hx eczema & in household contacts *Emergency:* No absolute CI **Disp:** Vial for reconstitution: 100 mill pock-forming units/mL **SE:** Malaise, fever, regional lymphadenopathy, encephalopathy, rashes, spread of inoculation to other sites, SJS, eczema vaccinatum w/ severe disability **NIPE:** Virus transmission possible until scab separates from skin (14–21 d); avoid infant contact or household contacts w/ PRG for 14 d; avoid PRG w/in 4 wk; intradermal use only; restricted distribution

Sodium Bicarbonate [NaHCO₃] [Antacid/Alkalinizing Agent] Uses: *Alkalinization of urine, RTA, metabolic acidosis, ↑ K⁺, TCA OD* **Action:** Alkalinizing agent **Dose:** *Adults. ECC 2010: Cardiac arrest w/ good ventilation, hyperkalemia, OD of TCAs, ASA, cocaine, diphenhydramine:* 1 mEq/kg IV bolus; repeat ½ dose q10min PRN *Metabolic acidosis:* 2–5 mEq/kg IV over 8 h & PRN based on acid–base status. ↑ K⁺: 50 mEq IV over 5 min *Alkalinize urine:* 4 g (48 mEq) PO, then 12–24 mEq q4h; adjust based on urine pH; 2 amp (100 mEq)/1 L D₅W at 100–250 mL/h IV, monitor urine pH & serum bicarbonate *CRF:* 1–3 mEq/kg/d *Distal RTA:* 0.5–2 mEq/kg/d in 4–5 ÷ doses *Peds. Sodium bicarbonate ECC 2010: Severe metabolic acidosis, hyperkalemia:* 1 mEq/kg IV slow bolus; 4.2% conc in infants < 1 mo *CRF:* See Adult dosage *Distal RTA:* 2–3 mEq/kg/d PO *Proximal RTA:* 5–10 mEq/kg/d; titrate based on serum bicarbonate *Urine alkalinization:* 84–840 mg/kg/d (1–10 mEq/kg/d) in ÷ doses; adjust based on urine pH **Caution:** [C, ?] **CI:** Alkalosis, ↑ Na⁺, severe pulm edema, ↓ Ca²⁺ **Disp:** Powder, tabs; 325 mg = 3.8 mEq; 650 mg = 7.6 mEq; Inj 1 mEq/mL, 4.2% (5 mEq/10 mL), 7.5% (8.92 mEq/mL), 8.4% (10 mEq/10 mL) vial or amp **SE:** Belching, edema, flatulence, ↑ Na⁺, metabolic alkalosis **Interactions:** ↑ Effects *OF* anorexiants, amphetamines, ephedrine, flecainide, mecamylamine, pseudoephedrine, quinidine, sympathomimetics; ↓ effects *OF* Li, MTX, salicylates, tetracyclines **Labs:** ↑ K⁺, Na⁺, lactate **NIPE:** 1 g Neutralizes 12 mEq of acid; 50 mEq bicarbonate = 50 mEq Na; can make 3 amps in 1 L D₅W to = D₅NS w/ 150 mEq bicarbonate; ⊘ take w/in 2 h of other drugs; PO take 1–3 h after meals; ↑ risk of milk-alkali synd w/ long-term use or when taken w/ milk

Sodium Citrate/CitricAcid (Bicitra, Oracit) [Alkalinizing Agent] Uses: *Chronic metabolic acidosis, alkalinize urine; dissolve uric acid & cysteine stones* **Action:** Urinary alkalinizer **Dose: Adults.** 10–30 mL in 1–3 oz H₂O pc & hs **Peds.** 5–15 mL in 1–3 oz H₂O pc & hs; best after meals **Caution:** [?, ?] **CI:** Severe renal impair or Na-restricted diets **Disp:** 15- or 30-mL unit **Dose:** 16 (473 mL) or 4 fl oz **SE:** Tetany, metabolic alkalosis, ↑ K⁺, GI upset; avoid use of multiple 50-mL amps; can cause ↑ Na⁺/hyperosmolality **Interactions:** ↑ Effects *OF* amphetamines, ephedrine, flecainide, pseudoephedrine, quinidine; ↓ effects *OF* barbiturates, chlorpropamide, Li, salicylates **Labs:** ↑ K⁺, monitor ECG for hyperkalemia (peaked T waves) **NIPE:** 1 mL = 1 mEq Na & 1 mEq bicarbonate; dilute w/ H₂O

Sodium Oxybate/Gamma Hydroxybutyrate/GHB (Xyrem) [C-III] [Inhibitory Neurotransmitter] WARNING: Known drug of abuse even at recommended doses; confusion, depression, resp depression may occur Uses: *Narcolepsy-associated cataplexy* **Action:** Inhibitory neurotransmitter **Dose: Adults & Peds > 16 y.** 2.25 g PO qhs, 2nd dose 2.5–4 h later; may ↑ 9 g/d max **Caution:** [C,?/–] **CI:** Succinic semialdehyde dehydrogenase deficiency; potentiates EtOH & other CNS depressants **Disp:** 500-mg/mL (180-mL) PO soln **SE:** Confusion, depression, ↓ diminished level of consciousness, incontinence, sig V, resp depression, psychological Sxs **Interactions:** ↑ Risk of CNS depression *W/* sedatives, hypnotics, EtOH **NIPE:** Dilute w/ 2 oz H₂O, ⊘ eat w/in 2 h of taking this drug; may lead to dependence; synonym for hydroxybutyrate (GHB), abused as a "date rape drug"; controlled distribution (prescriber & pt registration); must be administered when pt in bed; available through restricted program only "Xyrem Success Program"; take 1st dose 2 h pc

Sodium Phosphate (Osmoprep, Visicol) [Laxative] WARNING: Acute phosphate nephropathy reported w/ permanent renal impair risk; w/ ↑ age, hypovolemia, bowel obstr or colitis, baseline kidney Dz, w/ meds that affect renal perf/Fxn (diuretics, ACE Inhib, ARB, NSAIDs) Uses: *Bowel prep prior to colonoscopy*, short-term constipation **Action:** Hyperosmotic laxative **Dose:** 3 tabs PO w/ at least 8 oz clear Liq q15min for 6 doses; then 2 additional tabs in 15 min, 3–5 h prior to colonoscopy; 3 tabs q15 min for 6 doses, then 2 additional tabs in 15 min **Caution:** [C, ?] Renal impair, electrolyte disturbances **CI:** Megacolon, bowel obst **Disp:** Tabs 0.398, 1.102 g (32/bottle) **SE:** ↑ QT, ↑ PO₄³⁻, ↓ calcium, D, flatulence, cramps, Abd bloating/pain **Interactions:** May bind w/ Al- & Mg-containing antacids & sucralfate; ↑ risk of hypoglycemia *W/* bisphosphonates; ↓ absorption *OF* other meds **Labs:** Monitor lytes—↑ PO₄³⁻, ↓ K⁺, Na; ↑ QT—monitor ECG **NIPE:** Drink clear Liq 12 h before start of this med; ⊘ take w/ drugs that prolong QT interval, ⊘ take w/ other laxatives; maintain adeq hydration

Sodium Polystyrene Sulfonate (Kayexalate, Kionex) [Potassium-Removing Resin] Uses: *Rx of ↑ K⁺* **Action:** Na⁺/K⁺ ion-exchange resin **Dose: Adults.** 15–60 g PO or 30–50 g PR q6h based on serum K⁺ **Peds.** 1 g/kg/dose PO or PR q6h based on serum K⁺ **Caution:** [C, ?] **CI:** Obstructive bowel disease; ↑ Na⁺; neonates w/ ↓ gut motility **Disp:** Powder; susp 15 g/60 mL sorbitol **SE:** ↑ Na⁺, ↓ K⁺, GI upset, fecal impaction **Interactions:** ↑ Risk of systemic alkalosis *W/* Ca- or Mg-containing antacids **Labs:** ↑ Na⁺, ↓ K⁺ **NIPE:** Mix w/chilled fluid other than orange juice; enema acts more quickly than PO; PO most effective; onset of action > 2 h; ✓ ECG for hypokalemia (flattened T waves); ✓ serum K⁺ freq under Tx to determine when to D/C; use w/caution in pts w/ severe HF, severe HTN, marked edema

Sofosbuvir (Sovaldi) Uses: *Chronic hepatitis C, genotypes, 1, 2, 3, & 4 & co-infection w/ HIV* **Action:** Nucleotide analog NS5B RNA polymerase Inhibit **Dose:** *Adults.* 400 mg 1 ×/d w/ ribavirin (genotype 2 & 3; for 12 & 24 wk) or ribavirin + pegylated interferon (genotype 1 or 4 for 12 wk) **Caution:** [X, −] embryofetal toxic; avoid PRG (patient or in partner) PRG before & 6 mo post; use at least 2 birth control methods & monthly PRG test **CI:** PRG or may become PRG; men w/ PRG partner **Disp:** Tabs 400 mg **SE:** (SE from combo) HA, fatigue, insomnia, N, anemia, pancytopenia, depression **Notes:** Avoid w/ P-gp inducers; use in post-liver transplant or w/ CrC < 30 mL/min not studied **NIPE:** ◯ PRG; use 2 forms of contraception during & 6 mo after Tx; neg PRG test required before starting; take w/o regard to food; stress importance of adherence w/ regular dosing schedule; may alter taste of food, ↓ appetite

Solifenacin (Vesicare) [Antispasmodic/Muscarinic Receptor Antagonist] Uses: *OAB* **Action:** Antimuscarinic, ↓ detrusor contractions **Dose:** 5 mg PO daily, 10 mg/d max; ↓ w/ renal/hepatic impair **Caution:** [C, ?/−] BOO or GI obst, UC, MyG, renal/hepatic impair, QT prolongation risk **CI:** NAG, urinary/gastric retention **Disp:** Tabs 5, 10 mg **SE:** Constipation, xerostomia, dyspepsia, blurred vision, drowsiness **Interactions:** ↑ Effects *OF* azole antifungals & other CYP3A4 Inhibs; ↑ risk of prolonged QT interval *W/* amiodarone, amitriptyline, bepridil, disopyramide, erythromycin, gatifloxacin, haloperidol, imipramine, moxifloxacin, quinidine, pimozide, procainamide, sparfloxacin, thioridazine; other drugs that prolong QT **Labs:** Monitor BUN, CR, LFTs **NIPE:** Take w/o regard to food; swallow whole w/ H₂O; do not ↑ dose w/ severe renal/mod hepatic impair; recent concern over cognitive effects; monitor ECG for ↑ QT interval; assess for anticholinergic side effects (constipation, urinary retention, blurred vision, heat prostration); avoid exposure to heat

Somatropin (Genotropin, Nutropin AQ, Omnitrope, Saizen, Serostim, Zorbtive) [Growth Hormone] Uses: *HIV-assoc wasting/cachexia* **Action:** Anabolic peptide hormone **Dose:** 0.1 mg/kg SQ hs; max 6 mg/d **Caution:** [B, ?] Lipodystrophy (rotate sites) **CI:** Active neoplasm; acute critical illness post-op; benzyl alcohol sensitivity; hypersensitivity **Disp:** 4, 5, 6 mg powder for Inj **SE:** Arthralgia, edema, ↑ blood glucose **Labs:** ↑ Blood glucose **NIPE:** Use under guidance of healthcare provider trained in AIDs management; provide appropriate training on adminstration, safe handling/disposal of needles

Sorafenib (Nexavar) [Antineoplastic/Kinase Inhibitor]
Uses: *Advanced RCC* metastatic liver CA **Action:** Tyrosine kinase Inhib **Dose:** *Adults.* 400 mg PO bid on empty stomach **Caution:** [D, –] w/ Irinotecan, doxorubicin, warfarin; avoid conception (male/female); avoid inducers **Disp:** Tabs 200 mg **SE:** Hand–foot synd; Tx-emergent hypertension; bleeding, ↑ INR, cardiac infarction/ischemia; ↑ pancreatic enzymes, hypophosphatemia, lymphopenia, anemia, fatigue, alopecia, pruritus, D, GI upset, HA, neuropathy **Interactions:** ↑ Effects *OF* warfarin **NIPE:** ⊘ PRG; monitor BP 1st 6 wk; may require ↓ dose (daily or qod); impaired metabolism in pt of Asian descent; unknown effect on wound healing, D/C before major surgery; ✓ bleeding precautions

Sorbitol (Generic) [Laxative] **Uses:** *Constipation* **Action:** Osmotic laxative **Dose:** 30–150 mL PO of a 20–70% soln PRN **Caution:** [C, ?] **CI:** Anuria **Disp:** Liq 70% **SE:** Edema, lyte loss, lactic acidosis, GI upset, xerostomia **NIPE:** ⊘ Use unless soln clear; may be vehicle for many Liq formulations (eg, zinc, Kayexalate)

Sotalol (Betapace, Sorine) [Antiarrhythmic, Antihypertensive/Beta-Blocker] **WARNING:** To minimize risk of induced arrhythmia, pts initiated/reinitiated on Betapace AF should be placed for a minimum of 3 d (on their maint) in a facility that can provide cardiac resuscitation, cont ECG monitoring, & calculations of CrCl. Betapace should not be substituted for Betapace AF because of labeling; adjust dose base on CrCl. Can cause life-threatening ventricular tachycardia w/ prolonged QT. Do not initiate if QT > 450 ms. If QTc > 500 ms during Tx, ↓ dose **Uses:** *Ventricular arrhythmias, AF* **Action:** β-Adrenergic blocking agent **Dose:** *Adults.* CrCl > 60 mL/min: 80 mg PO bid, may ↑ to 240–320 mg/d *CrCl 30–60 mL/min:* 80 mg q24h *CrCl 10–30 mL/min:* Dose 80 mg q36–48h **ECC 2010:** SVT & ventricular arrhythmias: 1–1.5 mg/kg IV over 5 min **Peds. < 2 y.** Dosing dependent on age, renal Fxn, heart rate, QT interval ≥2 y: 30 mg/m² tid; to max dose of 60 mg/m² tid; ↓ w/ renal impair **Caution:** [B, + (monitor child)] **CI:** Asthma, ↓ HR, prolonged QT interval, 2nd-/3rd-degree heart block w/o pacemaker, cardiogenic shock, uncontrolled CHF **Disp:** Tabs 80, 120, 160, 240 mg **SE:** ↓ HR, CP, palpitations, fatigue, dizziness, weakness, dyspnea **Interactions:** ↑ Effects *W/* ASA, antihypertensives, nitrates, OCPs, fluoxetine, prazosin, sulfinpyrazone, verapamil, EtOH; ↑ risk of prolonged QT interval *W/* amiodarone, amitriptyline, bepridil, disopyramide, erythromycin, gatifloxacin, haloperidol, imipramine, moxifloxacin, quinidine, pimozide, procainamide, sparfloxacin, thioridazine; ↑ effects *OF* lidocaine; ↓ effects *W/* antacids, clonidine, NSAIDs, thyroid drugs; ↓ effects *OF* hypoglycemics, terbutaline, theophylline **Labs:** ↑ BUN, serum glucose, triglycerides, K⁺, uric acid **NIPE:** May ↑ sensitivity to cold; D/C MAOIs 14 d before drug; take w/o food; Betapace should not be substituted for Betapace AF because of differences in labeling; ✓ arrythmias, hypotension, ↓ pulse

Sotalol (Betapace AF) [Antiarrhythmic, Antihypertensive/Beta-Blocker] **WARNING:** See Sotalol (Betapace) **Uses:** *Maintain sinus rhythm for symptomatic AF/A flutter* **Action:** β-Adrenergic blocking agent **Dose:** **Adults.** CrCl > 60 mL/min: 80 mg PO q12h, max 320 mg/d CrCl 40–60 mL/min: 80 mg PO q24h; ↑ to 120 mg during hospitalization; monitor QT interval 2–4 h after each dose, dose reduction or D/C if QT interval ≥ 500 ms **Peds. < 2 y:** Dose adjusted based on logarithmic scale (refer to pkg insert) > **2 y:** 9 mg/m²/d tid, may ↑ to 180 mg/m²/d **Caution:** [B, +] When converting from other antiarrhythmic **CI:** Asthma, ↓ HR, ↑ QT interval, 2nd-/3rd-degree heart block w/o pacemaker, cardiogenic shock, K⁺ < 4, sick sinus synd, baseline QT > 450 ms uncontrolled CHF, CrCl < 40 mL/min **Disp:** Tabs 80, 120, 160 mg **SE:** ↓ HR, CP, palpitations, fatigue, dizziness, weakness, dyspnea **Interactions:** ↑ Risk of prolonged QT interval **W/** amiodarone, amitriptyline, bepridil, disopyramide, erythromycin, gatifloxacin, haloperidol, imipramine, moxifloxacin, quinidine, pimozide, procainamide, sparfloxacin, TCAs, thioridazine; ↑ effects **W/** general anesthesia, phenytoin administered IV, verapamil ↑ effects **OF** insulin, oral hypoglycemics; ↑ risk of hypotension **W/** antihypertensives, ASA, bismuth subsalicylate, Mg salicylate, sulfinpyrazone, nitrates, OCPs, EtOH; ↑ CV Rxns CCB, digoxin; ↑ risk **OF** severe HTN if used w/in 14 d of MAOIs; ↓ effects **W/** antacids; ↑ effects **OF** β-adrenergic bronchodilators, DA, dobutamine, theophylline **Labs:** ↑ ANA titers, BUN, K⁺, serum glucose, LFTs, triglycerides, uric acid; monitor QT interval; follow renal Fxn **NIPE:** ⊘ D/C abruptly after long-term use; take w/o food; administer antacids 2 h < or > sotalol; Betapace should not be substituted for Betapace AF because of differences in labeling; ✓ w/ prescribing provider before using new prescription or OTC meds

Spinosad (Natroba) [Pediculicide]

Uses: *Head lice* **Action:** Neuronal excitation of lice, w/ paralysis & death **Dose:** Cover dry scalp w/ suspension, then apply to dry hair; rinse off in 10 min; may repeat after 7 d; unlabeled to use < 4 y **Caution:** [B; ?/–] **Disp:** 0.9% topical susp **SE:** Scalp/ocular erythema **NIPE:** Shake well before use; use w/overall lice management program; in benzyl alcohol, serious Rxns in neonates, in breast milk, pump, & discard milk for 8 h after use; wash hands after application

Spironolactone (Aldactone) [Potassium-Sparing Diuretic] WARNING:

Tumorogenic in animal studies; avoid unnecessary use **Uses:** *Hyperaldosteronism, HTN, Class III/IV CHF, ascites from cirrhosis* **Action:** Aldosterone antagonist; K⁺-sparing diuretic **Dose: Adults.** CHF (NYHA Class III–IV) 12.5–25 mg/d (w/ ACE & loop diuretic) HTN 25–50 mg/d Ascites:100–400 mg qAM w/ 40–160 mg of furosemide, start w/ 100 mg/40 mg, wait at least 3 d before ↑ dose **Peds.** 1–3.3 mg/kg/24 h PO ÷ q12–24h, take w/ food **Caution:** [C, + (D/C breast-feeding)] **CI:** ↑ K⁺, acute renal failure, anuria **Disp:** Tabs 25, 50, 100 mg **SE:** ↑ K⁺ & gynecomastia, arrhythmia, sexual dysfunction, confusion, dizziness, D/N/V, abnormal menstruation **Interactions:** ↑ Risk of hyperkalemia **W/** ACEIs, K⁺ supls, K⁺-sparing diuretics, ↑ K⁺ diet; ↑ effects **OF** Li; ↓ effects **W/** salicylates; ↓ effects **OF** anticoagulants **Labs:** ↑ K⁺ BUN **NIPE:** Take w/ food; ↑ risk of gynecomastia; max effects of drug may take 2–3 wk; monitor ECG for hyperkalemia (peaked T waves); avoid K+ rich foods; ⊘ ETOH

Starch, Topical, Rectal (Tucks Suppositories [OTC]) [Protectant] Uses: *Temporary relief of anorectal disorders (itching, etc)* **Action:** Topical protectant **Dose: *Adults & Peds ≥ 12 y.*** Cleanse, rinse, & dry, insert 1 supl rectally 6 ×/d × 7 d max. **Caution:** [?, ?] **CI:** None **Disp:** Supp **SE:** D/C w/ or if rectal bleeding occurs or if condition worsens or does not improve w/in 7 d **NIPE:** D/C w/ if rectal bleeding occurs or if condition worsens or does not improve w/ in 7 d

Stavudine (Zerit) [Antiretroviral/Reverse Transcriptase Inhibitor] **WARNING:** Lactic acidosis & severe hepatomegaly w/ steatosis & pancreatitis reported w/ didanosine Uses: *HIV in combo w/ other antiretrovirals* **Action:** RT Inhib **Dose: *Adults > 60 kg.*** 40 mg bid *< 60 kg.* 30 mg bid *Peds Birth–13 d.* 0.5 mg/kg q12h *> 14 d & < 30 kg.* 1 mg/kg q12h *≥ 30 kg.* Adult dose; ↓ w/ renal Insuff **Caution:** [C, –] **CI:** Allergy **Disp:** Caps 15, 20, 30, 40 mg; soln 1 mg/mL **SE:** Peripheral neuropathy, HA, chills, rash, GI upset, anemias, lactic acidosis, ↑ LFTs, pancreatitis **Interactions:** ↑ Risk of pancreatitis *W/* didanosine; ↑ effects *W/* probenecid; ↓ effects *W/* zidovudine **Labs:** ↑ LFTs **NIPE:** Take w/o regard to food; take w/ plenty of H₂O; monitor for S/Sxs of lactic acidosis (tachypnea, altered breathing, lethargy); may cause peripheral neuropathy (numbness, tingling in extremities); ✓ for wgt loss

Steroids, Systemic [Glucocorticoid] (See also Table 2) The following relates only to the commonly used systemic glucocorticoids Uses: *Endocrine disorders* (adrenal Insuff), rheumatoid disorders, collagen-vascular Dzs, derm Dzs, allergic states, cerebral edema*, nephritis, nephrotic synd, immunosuppression for transplantation, ↑ Ca²⁺, malignancies (breast, lymphomas), pre-op (pt who has been on steroids in past year, known hypoadrenalism, pre-op for adrenalectomy); Inj into Jts/tissue **Action:** Glucocorticoid **Dose:** Varies w/ use & institutional protocols:

• *Adrenal Insuff, acute: Adults. Hydrocortisone:* 100 mg IV, then 300 mg/d ÷ q8h for 48 h, then convert to 50 mg PO q8h × 6 doses, taper to 30–50 mg/d ÷ bid *Peds. Hydrocortisone:* 1–2 mg/kg IV, then 150–250 mg/d ÷ q6–8h

• *Adrenal Insuff, chronic (physiologic replacement):* May need mineralocorticoid supl such as Florinef *Adults. Hydrocortisone:* 20 mg PO qᴀᴍ, 10 mg PO qᴘᴍ; *cortisone* 25–35 mg PO daily; *dexamethasone* 0.03–0.15 mg/kg/d or 0.6–0.75 mg/m²/d ÷ q6–12h PO, IM, IV *Peds. Hydrocortisone:* 8–10 mg/m²/d q8h; some may require up to 12 mg/m²/d; *hydrocortisone succinate* 0.25–0.35 mg/kg/d IM

• *Asthma, acute: Adults. Methylprednisolone:* 40–80 mg/d in 1–2 ÷ dose PO/IV or *dexamethasone* 12 mg IV q6h *Peds. Prednisolone* 1–2 mg/kg/d or *prednisone* 1–2 mg/kg/d ÷ daily–bid for up to 5 d; *methylprednisolone* 12 mg/kg/d IV ÷ tid; *dexamethasone* 0.1–0.3 mg/kg/d ÷ q6h

- *Congenital adrenal hyperplasia:* **Peds.** Initial *hydrocortisone* 10–20 mg/m^2/d ÷ 3 ÷ doses
- *Extubation/airway edema:* **Adults.** *Dexamethasone* 0.5–2 mg/kg/d IM/IV ÷ q6h (start 24 h prior to extubation; continue × 4 more doses) **Peds.** *Dexamethasone:* 0.5–2 mg/kg/d ÷ q6h (start 24 h before & cont for 4–6 doses after extubation)
- *Immunosuppressive/anti-inflammatory:* **Adults & Older Peds.** *Hydrocortisone:* 15–240 mg PO, IM, IV q12h; *methylprednisolone* 2–60 mg/d PO in 1-4 ÷ doses, taper to lowest effective dose; *methylprednisolone Na succinate* 10–80 mg/d IM or 10–40 mg/d IV **Adults.** *Prednisone* or *prednisolone* 5–60 mg/d PO ÷ daily–qid **Infants & Younger Children.** *Hydrocortisone* 2.5–10 mg/kg/d PO ÷ q6–8h; 1–5 mg/kg/d IM/IV ÷ bid–daily
- *Nephrotic synd:* **Peds.** *Prednisolone* or *prednisone:* 2 mg/kg/d PO tid–qid until urine is protein-free for 5 d, use up to 28 d; for persistent proteinuria, 4 mg/kg/ dose PO qod max120 mg/d for an additional 28 d; maint 2 mg/kg/dose qod for 28 d; taper over 4–6 wk (max 80 mg/d)
- *Septic shock (controversial):* **Adults.** *Hydrocortisone* 50 mg IV q6h; max 300 mg/d; some suggest 200 mg/d cont Inf **Peds.** *Hydrocortisone:* 1–2 mg/kg/d intermittent or continuous Inf; may titrate up to 50 mg/kg/d
- *Status asthmaticus:* **Adults & Peds.** *Hydrocortisone* 1–2 mg/kg/dose IV q6h for 24 h; then ↓ by 0.5–1 mg/kg qod
- *Rheumatic Dz:* **Adults.** *Intra-articular: Hydrocortisone acetate:* 25–37.5 mg large Jt, 10–25 mg small Jt; *methylprednisolone acetate* 20–80 mg large Jt, 4–10 mg small Jt *Intrabursal: Hydrocortisone acetate* 25–37.5 mg *Intraganglial: Hydrocortisone acetate:* 25–37.5 mg *Tendon sheath: Hydrocortisone acetate:* 5–12.5 mg
- *Perioperative steroid coverage: Hydrocortisone:* 100 mg IV night before surgery, 1 h pre-op, intraoperative, & 4, 8, & 12 h post-op; post-op d 1 100 mg IV q6h; postop day 2 100 mg IV q8h; post-op day 3 100 mg IV q12h; post-op day 4 50 mg IV q12h; postop day 5 25 mg IV q12h; resume prior PO dosing if chronic use or D/C if only perioperative coverage required
- *Cerebral edema: Dexamethasone:* 10 mg IV; then 4 mg IV q4–6h

Caution: [C/ D,?] **CI:** Active varicella Infxn, serious Infxn except TB, fungal Infxns **Disp:** Table 2 **SE:** ↑ Appetite, hyperglycemia, ↓ K$^+$ osteoporosis, nervousness, insomnia, "steroid psychosis," adrenal suppression **Labs:** ↓ K$^+$, ↑ glucose **NIPE:** Hydrocortisone succinate for systemic, acetate for intra-articular; never abruptly D/C steroids, taper dose; also used for bacterial & TB meningitis; can ↑ Infxn risk & fx risk from osteoporosis; risk of GI perforation w/ chronic use; avoid exposure chicken pox/measles when taking immunosuppressant doses

Steroids, Topical [Glucocorticoid] (See Also Table 3) Uses: *Steroid-responsive dermatoses (seborrheic/atopic dermatitis, neurodermatitis, anogenital pruritus, psoriasis)* **Action:** Glucocorticoid; ↓ capillary permeability, stabilizes lysosomes to control inflammation; controls protein synthesis; ↓ migration of leukocytes, fibroblasts **Dose:** Use lowest potency produce for shortest period for effect (See Table 3) **Caution:** [C, +] Do not use occlusive dressings; high potency topical products not for rosacea, perioral dermatitis; not for use on face, groin, axillae; none for use in a diapered area **CI:** Component hypersensitivity **Disp:** See Table 3 **SE:** Skin atrophy w/ chronic use; chronic administration or application over large area may cause adrenal suppression or hyperglycemia

Streptokinase (Generic) [Plasminogen Activator/Thrombolytic Enzyme] **Uses:** *Coronary artery thrombosis, acute massive PE, DVT, & some occluded vascular grafts* **Action:** Activates plasminogen to plasmin that degrades fibrin **Dose:** *Adults. PE:* Load 250,000 units peripheral IV over 30 min, then 100,000 units/h IV for 24–72 h *Coronary artery thrombosis:* 1.5 MU IV over 60 min *DVT or arterial embolism:* Load as w/ PE, then 100,000 units/h for 24 h *ECC 2010:* AMI: 1.5 MU over 1 h *Peds.* 1000–2000 units/kg over 30 min, then 1000 units/kg/h for up to 24 h *Occluded catheter (controversial):* 10,000–25,000 units in NS to final vol of catheter (leave in for 1 h, aspirate & flush w/ NS) **Caution:** [C, +] **CI:** Streptococcal Infxn or streptokinase in last 6 mo, active bleeding, CVA, TIA, spinal surgery/trauma in last mo, vascular anomalies, severe hepatic/renal Dz, severe uncontrolled HTN **Disp:** Powder for Inj 250,000, 750,000, 1,500,000 units **SE:** Bleeding, ↓ BP, fever, bruising, rash, GI upset, hemorrhage, anaphylaxis **Interactions:** ↑ Risk of bleeding *W/* anticoagulants, ASA, heparin, indomethacin, NSAIDs, dong quai, feverfew, garlic, ginger, horse chestnut, red clover **Labs:** ↑ PT, PTT **NIPE:** If Inf inadequate to keep clotting time 2–5 × control, see package insert for adjustments; Abs remain 3–6 mo following dose; reconstitute w/ NS & roll (not shake) to mix; most effective w/ AMI w/in 4 h; most effective for PE/DVT w/in 1 d; ✓ for bleeding/allergic rxn

Streptomycin [Antibiotic/Aminoglycoside] **WARNING:** Neuro-/oto-/renal tox possible; neuromuscular blockage w/ resp paralysis possible **Uses:** *TB combo Rx therapy* streptococcal or enterococcal endocarditis **Action:** Aminoglycoside; ↓ protein synth **Dose:** *Adults. IM route. Endocarditis:* 1 g q12h 1–2 wk, then 500 mg q12h 1–4 wk in combination w/ PCN *TB:* 15 mg/kg/d (up to 1 g), directly observed therapy DOT 2 ×/wk 20–30 mg/kg/dose (max 1.5 g), DOT 2 ×/wk 25–30 mg/kg/dose (max 1.5 g) Peds. 20-40 mg/kg/d 1 g/d max; DOT 2×/wk 20–30 mg/kg/dose (max 1.5 g/d); w/ renal Insuff, either IM (preferred) or IV over 30–60 min **Caution:** [D, −] **CI:** PRG **Disp:** Inj 400 mg/mL (1-g vial) **SE:** ↑ Incidence of vestibular & auditory tox, ↑ neurotox risk in pts w/ impaired renal Fxn **Notes:** Monitor levels: *Peak:* 20–30 mcg/mL *Trough:* < 5 mcg/mL *Toxic peak:* > 50 mcg/mL *Trough:* > 10 mcg/mL IV over 30–60 min **Interactions:** ↑ Risk of nephrotox w/ amphotericin B, cephalosporins, cisplatin, methoxyflurane, polymyxin B, vancomycin; ↑ risk of ototox w/ carboplatin, furosemide, mannitol, urea; ↑ effects *OF* anticoagulants **Labs:** False(+) urine glucose, false ↑ urine protein **NIPE:** ↑ Fluid intake; assess for Sx ototox (hearing loss, tinnitus, vertigo)

Streptozocin (Zanosar) [Alkylating Agent/Nitrosourea]
WARNING: Administer under the supervision of a physician experienced in the use of chemotherapy. Renal tox dose-related/cumulative & may be severe or fatal. Other major tox: N/V, & may be Tx-limiting; liver dysfunction, D, hematologic changes possible. Streptozocin is mutagenic. **Uses:** *Pancreatic islet cell tumors* & carcinoid tumors **Action:** DNA–DNA (interstrand) cross-linking; DNA, RNA, & protein synth Inhib **Dose:** Per protocol; ↓ in renal failure **Caution:** w/ Renal failure [D, −] **CI:** w/ PRG **Disp:** Inj 1 g **SE:** N/V/D, duodenal ulcers, depression, ↓ BM rare (20%) & mild; nephrotox (proteinuria & azotemia dose related), ↑ LFT hypophosphatemia dose limiting; hypoglycemia; Inj site Rxns **Interactions:** ↑ Risk of nephrotox *W/* aminoglycosides, amphotericin B, cisplatin, vancomycin; ↑ effects *OF* doxorubicin; ↓ effects *W/* phenytoin **Labs:** Monitor SCr, ↑ LFTs, hypophosphatemia dose limiting, hypoglycemia **NIPE:** Irritating to tissues, extravasation may cause severe tissue lesions/necrosis; ⊘ PRG, breast-feeding; ↑ fluid intake to 2–3 L/d

Succimer (Chemet) [Chelating Agent] **Uses:** *Lead poisoning (levels > 50 mcg/mL w/ significant symptoms)* **Action:** Heavy-metal chelating agent **Dose:** *Adults & Peds.* 10 mg/kg/dose q8h × 5 d, then 10 mg/kg/dose q12h for 14 d **Caution:** [C, ?] w/ Hepatic/renal Insuff **CI:** Allergy **Disp:** Caps 100 mg **SE:** Rash, fever, GI upset, hemorrhoids, metallic taste, drowsiness, ↑ LFTs **Labs:** ↑ LFTs; monitor lead levels **NIPE:** ⊘ Take w/ other chelating agents; ↑ fluid intake to 2–3 L/d; may open caps; ✓ for S/Sx Infxn

Succinylcholine (Anectine, Quelicin) [Skeletal Muscle Relaxant] **WARNING:** Acute rhabdomyolysis w/ hyperkalemia followed by ventricular dysrhythmias, cardiac arrest, & death. Seen in children w/ skeletal muscle myopathy (Duchenne muscular dystrophy) **Uses:** *Adjunct to general anesthesia, facilitates ET intubation; induce skeletal muscle relaxation during surgery or mechanical ventilation* **Action:** Depolarizing neuromuscular blocker; rapid onset, short duration (3–5 min) **Dose:** *Adults.* Rapid sequence intubation 1–1.5 mg/kg IV over 10–30 s or 3–4 mg/kg IM (up to 150 mg) *(ECC 2010)* *Peds.* 1–2 mg/kg/dose IV, then by 0.3–0.6 mg/kg/dose q5min; ↓ w/ severe renal/hepatic impair **Caution:** See Warning [C, ?] **CI:** w/ Malignant hyperthermia risk, myopathy, recent major burn, multiple trauma, extensive skeletal muscle denervation **Disp:** Inj 20, 100 mg/mL **SE:** Fasciculations, ↑ IOP, ↑ ICP, intragastric pressure, salivation, myoglobinuria, malignant hyperthermia, resp depression, prolonged apnea; multiple drugs potentiate CV effects (arrhythmias, ↓ BP, brady/tachycardia) **Interactions:** ↑ Effects *W/* amikacin, gentamicin, neomycin, streptomycin, Li, MAOIs, opiates; ↓ effect *W/* diazepam **Labs:** ↑ Serum K+ **NIPE:** May be given IV push/Inf/IM deltoid

Sucralfate (Carafate) [Antiulcer Agent/Pepsin Inhibitor] **Uses:** *Duodenal ulcers*, gastric ulcers, stomatitis, GERD, preventing stress ulcers, esophagitis **Action:** Forms ulcer-adherent complex that protects against acid, pepsin, & bile acid **Dose:** *Adults.* 1 g PO qid, 1 h prior to meals & hs *Peds.*

40–80 mg/kg/d ÷ q6h; continue 4–8 wk unless healing demonstrated by x-ray or endoscopy; separate from other drugs by 2 h; take on empty stomach ac **Caution:** [B, ?] **CI:** Component allergy **Disp:** Tabs 1 g; susp 1 g/10 mL **SE:** Constipation, GI, dizziness, xerostomia **Interactions:** ↓ Effects *OF* cimetidine, digoxin, levothyroxine, phenytoin, quinolones, quinidine, ranitidine, tetracyclines, theophylline, warfarin **NIPE:** Take w/o food; Al may accumulate in renal failure

Sucroferricoxyhydroxide (Velphoro) Uses: *↓ Phos in ESRD/CKD*
Action: Binds phosphate **Dose:** *Adults.* Chew 500 mg TID w/ meals; may ↑ dose weekly to target phos < 5.5 mg/dL; max dose studied 3000 mg/d **Caution:** [B, +] ✓ Fe^{+2} w/ peritonitis during peritoneal dialysis, hepatic or GI disorders, post-GI surgery or Dz resulting in Fe^{+2} accumulation **CI:** None **Disp:** Tab 500 mg **SE:** D, discolored feces **Notes:** ⊘ Prescribe with levothyroxine or vit D; take alendronate or doxycycline 1 h before taking this med **NIPE:** Take w/ meals; take other PO meds 1 h before administration; chew tablet, can crush; do not swallow whole; dark-colored feces (due to Fe content) expected, can mask GI bleed—obtain stool guaiac if suspected

Sulfacetamide (Bleph-10, Cetamide, Klaron) [Antibiotic/ Sulfonamide] Uses: *Conjunctival Infxns*, topical acne, seborrheic dermatitis
Action: Sulfonamide antibiotic **Dose:** Ophthal soln: 1–2 gtt q2–3h while awake for 7–10 d; 10% oint apply qid & hs; soln for keratitis apply q2h based on severity **Caution:** [C, M] **CI:** Sulfonamide sensitivity; age < 2 mo **Disp:** Opthal: Oint soln 10%; topical cream 10%; foam, gel, lotion, pad all 10% **SE:** Irritation, burning, blurred vision, brow ache, SJS, photosens **Interactions:** ↓ Effects *W/* tetracyclines **NIPE:** Not compatible w/ Ag-containing preps; purulent exudate inactivates drug; ↑ risk of photosensitivity—use sunblock

Sulfacetamide/Prednisolone (Blephamide, Others) [Antibiotic, Anti-Inflammatory] Uses: *Steroid-responsive inflammatory ocular conditions w/ Infxn or a risk of Infxn* Action: Antibiotic & anti-inflammatory Dose:
Adults & Peds > 2 y. Apply oint lower conjunctival sac daily–qid; soln 1–3 gtt q4h while awake **Caution:** [C, ?/–] Sulfonamide sensitivity; age < 2 mo **Disp:** *Oint:* sulfacetamide 10%/prednisolone 0.2% *Susp:* Sulfacetamide 10%/prednisolone 0.2% **SE:** Irritation, burning, blurred vision, brow ache, SJS, photosens **Interactions:** ↑ Effects *W/* tetracyclines **NIPE:** Not compatible w/ Ag-containing preps; purulent exudate inactivates drug; ↑ risk of sensitivity to light; ⊘ D/C abruptly; OK ophthal susp use as otic agent; instruct on correct administration technique

Sulfasalazine (Azulfidine, Azulfidine EN) [Anti-Inflammatory, Antirheumatic (DMARD)/Sulfonamide] Uses: *UC, RA, juvenile RA*
Action: Sulfonamide; actions unclear **Dose:** *Adults. Ulcerative colitis:* Initial, 1 g PO tid–qid; ↑ to a max of 4–6 g/d in 4 ÷ doses; maint 500 mg PO qid *RA:* (EC tab) 0.5–1 g/d, ↑ weekly to maint 2 g ÷ bid *Peds. Ulcerative colitis:* Initial, 40–60 mg/kg/24 h PO ÷ q4–6h; maint 30 mg/kg/24 h PO ÷ q6h *RA > 6 y:* 30–50 mg/kg/d in 2 doses, start w/ 1/4–1/3 maint dose, ↑ weekly until dose reached at 1 mo, 2 g/d

max **Caution:** [B, M] Not rec w/ renal or hepatic impair **CI:** Sulfonamide or salicylate sensitivity, porphyria, GI or GU obst **Disp:** Tabs 500 mg; EC DR tabs 500 mg **SE:** GI upset; discolors urine; dizziness, HA, photosens, oligospermia, anemias, SJS **Interactions:** ↑ Effects *OF* oral anticoagulants, oral hypoglycemics, MTX, phenytoin, zidovudine; ↓ effects *W/* antibiotics; ↓ effects *OF* digoxin, folic acid, Fe, procaine, proparacaine, sulfonylureas, tetracaine **Labs:** ↑ LFTs, BUN, Cr; ↓ plts, WBCs **NIPE:** Take pc; ↑ fluids to 2–3 L/d; ↑ risk of photosensitivity—use sunblock & avoid sunlight exposure; may cause yellow-orange skin/contact lens discoloration; space doses evenly; take w/food; swallow tab whole

Sulindac (Clinoril) [Analgesic, Anti-Inflammatory, Antipyretic/ NSAID] **WARNING:** May ↑ risk of CV events & GI bleeding; do not use for post-CABG pain control **Uses:** *Arthritis & pain* **Action:** NSAID; ↓ prostaglandins **Dose:** 150–200 mg bid, 400 mg/d max; w/ food **Caution:** [B (D if 3rd tri or nearterm), ?] Not rec w/ severe renal impair **CI:** Allergy to component ASA or any NSAID, post-op pain in CABG surg **Disp:** Tabs 150, 200 mg **SE:** Dizziness, rash, GI upset, pruritus, edema, ↓ renal blood flow, renal failure (? fewer renal effects than other NSAIDs), peptic ulcer, GI bleeding **Interactions:** ↑ Effects *W/* NSAIDs, probenecid; ↑ effects *OF* aminoglycosides, anticoagulants, cyclosporine, digoxin, Li, MTX, K⁺-sparing diuretics; ↑ risk of bleeding *W/* ASA, anticoagulants, NSAIDs, thrombolytics, EtOH, dong quai, feverfew, garlic, ginger, horse chestnut, red clover; ↓ effects *W/* antacids, ASA; ↓ effects *OF* antihypertensives, diuretics, hydralazine **Labs:** ↑ LFTs, BUN, Cr, K⁺ **NIPE:** Take w/ food; ↑ risk of photosens—use sunblock; may take several wk for full drug effect; monitor ECG for hyperkalemia (peaked T waves); ⊘ ETOH, ASA

Sumatriptan (Alsuma, Imitrex Injection, Imitrex, Imitrex Statdose, Imitrex Nasal Spray, Sumavel Dosepro) [Antimigraine Agent/ Selective 5-HT₁ Receptor Agonist] **Uses:** *Rx acute migraine & cluster HA* **Action:** Vascular serotonin receptor agonist **Dose:** *Adults. SQ:* 6 mg SQ as a single-dose PRN; repeat PRN in 1 h to a max of 12 mg/24 h *PO:* 25–100 mg, repeat in 2 h, PRN, 200 mg/d max *Nasal spray:* 1 spray into 1 nostril, repeat in 2 h to 40 mg/24 h max *Peds. Nasal spray: 6–9 y.* 5–20 mg/d *10–17 y.* 5–20 mg, up to 40 mg/d **Caution:** [C, ?] **CI:** IV use, angina, ischemic heart Dz, CV syndromes, PUD, vascular Dz, uncontrolled HTN, severe hepatic impair, ergot use, MAOI use w/in 14 d, hemiplegic or basilar migraine **Disp:** *Imitrex Oral* OD tabs 25, 50, 100 mg; *Imitrex Injection* 4, 6 mg/0.5 mL; ODTs 25, 50, 100 mg; *Imitrex nasal spray* 5, 20 mg/spray *Alsuma Auto-Injector* 6 mg/0.5 mL **SE:** Pain & bruising at Inj site; dizziness, hot flashes, paresthesias, CP, weakness, numbness, coronary vasospasm, HTN **Interactions:** ↑ Effects of weakness, incoordination & hyperreflexia *W/* ergots, MAOIs & SSRIs, horehound, St. John's wort **Labs:** ↑ LFTs **NIPE:** Administer drug as soon as possible after onset of migraine; ⊘ more than 2 inj/24 h; 1 h in between inj

Sumatriptan/Naproxen Sodium (Treximet) [Selective 5-HT$_{1B/1D}$ Receptor Agonist + NSAID] **WARNING:** ↑ Risk of serious CV (MI, stroke) serious GI events (bleeding, ulceration, perforation) of the stomach or intestines **Uses:** *Prevent migraines* **Action:** Anti-inflammatory NSAID w/ 5-HT$_1$ receptor agonist, constricts CNS vessels **Dose:** *Adults.* 1 tab PO; repeat PRN after 2 h; max 2 tabs/24 h, w/ or w/o food **Caution:** [C, −] CI: Sig CV Dz, severe hepatic impair, severe ↑ BP **Disp:** Tab naproxen/sumatriptan 500 mg/85 mg **SE:** Dizziness, somnolence, paresthesia, N, dyspepsia, dry mouth, chest/neck/throat/jaw pain, tightness, pressure **Interactions:** ↑ Risk of serotonin synd *W/* SSRIs (citalopram, escitalopram, fluoxetine, fluvoxamine) & SNRIs (eg, duloxetine, venlafaxine); ↑ effects *OF* methotrexate, Li; ↑ risk of renal tox *W/* ACEIs, diuretics; ↑ risk of GI bleed *W/* oral corticosteroids, anticoagulants, smoking, EtOH; ↓ effects *OF* diuretics, antihypertensives **Labs:** May interfere w/ tests for 17-ketogenic steroids, 5-HIAA **NIPE:** Do not split/crush/chew; ⊘ take w/in 24 h of ergot-type drugs or other 5-HT$_1$ agonists; ⊘ take during or w/in 2 wk after discontinuing MAO type A Inhibs

Sumatriptan Needleless System (Sumavel DosePro) [Antimigraine Agent/Selective 5-HT$_1$ Receptor Agonist] **Uses:** *Rx acute migraine & cluster HA* **Action:** Vascular serotonin receptor agonist **Dose:** *Adults.* *SQ:* 6 mg SQ as a single dose PRN; repeat PRN in 1 h to a max of 12 mg/24 h; administer in abdomen/thigh **Caution:** [C, M] CI: See Sumatriptan **Disp:** Needle free SQ Injector 6 mg/0.5 mL **SE:** Injection site Rxn, tingling, warm/hot/burning sensation, feeling of heaviness/pressure/tightness/numbness, feeling strange, lightheadedness, flushing, tightness in chest, discomfort in nasal cavity/sinuses/jaw, dizziness/vertigo, drowsiness/sedation, HA **Interactions:** ↑ Risk of serotonin synd *W/* SSRIs (eg, citalopram, escitalopram, fluoxetine, fluvoxamine, paroxetine, sertraline) or SNRIs (eg, duloxetine, venlafaxine) **NIPE:** Do not give during or w/ in 2 wk after D/C MAOIs; supervise 1st dose & consider ECG monitoring in pts w/ unrecognized CAD (postmenopausal women, hypercholesterolemia, men > 40 y, HTN, obesity, DM, smokers, strong family Hx); take at onset of Sx

Sunitinib (Sutent) [Kinase Inhibitor] **WARNING:** Hepatotox that may be severe &/or result in fatal liver failure **Uses:** *Advanced GI stromal tumor (GIST) refractory/intolerant of imatinib; advanced RCC; well-differentiated pancreatic neuroendocrine tumors unresectable, locally advanced, metastatic* **Action:** TKI; VEGF Inhib **Dose:** *Adults.* 50 mg PO daily × 4 wk, followed by 2 wk holiday = 1 cycle; ↓ to 37.5 mg w/ CYP3A4 Inhib (Table 10), to ↑ 87.5 mg or 62.5 mg/d w/ CYP3A4 inducers **CI:** None **Caution:** [D, −] Multiple interactions require dose modification (eg, St. John's wort) **Disp:** Caps 12.5, 25, 50 mg **SE:** ↓ WBC & plt, bleeding, ↑ BP, ↓ ejection fraction, ↑ QT interval, pancreatitis, DVT, Szs, adrenal insufficiency, N/V/D, skin discoloration, oral ulcers, taste perversion, hypothyroidism **Labs:** ↓ WBC & plt, monitor CBC, plts, chemistries at cycle onset; baseline cardiac Fxn OK; monitor LVEF, ECG, CBC/plts, chemistries (K$^+$/Mg^{2+}/phosphate);

TFT & LFTs periodically **NIPE:** ↓ Dose in 12.5-mg increments if not tolerated; avoid crowds, those w/ Infxn; ⊘ immunizations w/o physician approval; ⊘ PRG, use effective contraception; ✓ CBC

Tacrolimus (Prograf) [Immunosuppressant/Macrolide]   WARNING: ↑ Risk of Infxn & lymphoma. Only physicians experienced in immunosuppression should prescribe **Uses:** *Prevent organ rejection (kidney/liver/heart)* **Action:** Calcineurin Inhib/immunosuppressant **Dose:** *Adults.* IV: 0.03–0.05 mg/kg/d in kidney & liver, 0.01 mg/kg/d in heart IV *Inf Peds:* IV: 0.03–0.05 mg/kg/d as cont Inf *PO:* 0.15–0.2 mg/kg/d PO ÷ q12h. *Adults & Peds. Eczema:* ↓ w/ hepatic/renal impair **Caution:** [C, –] w/ Cyclosporine; avoid topical if < 2 y; neuro & nephrotox, ↑ risk opportunistic Infxns **CI:** Component allergy, castor oil allergy w/ IV form **Disp:** Caps 0.5, 1, 5 mg; Inj 5 mg/mL **SE:** HTN, edema, HA, insomnia, fever, pruritus, ↑/↓ K⁺, GI upset, anemia, leukocytosis, tremors, paresthesias, pleural effusion, Szs, lymphoma, posterior reversible encephalopathy syndrome (PRES), BK nephropathy, PML **Labs:** ↑/↓ K⁺, hyperglycemia, monitor drug levels *Trough* 5–12 ng/mL based on indication & time since transplant **NIPE:** Reports of ↑ CA risk; ⊘ PRG/breast-feeding; take on empty stomach; avoid grapefruit juice; ↑ photosens, avoid sun exposure/use sunscreen

Tacrolimus, Ointment (Protopic) [Immunosuppressant/Macrolide] WARNING: Long-term safety of topical calcineurin Inhibs not established. Avoid long-term use. ↑ Risk of Infxn & lymphoma. Not for Peds < 2 y **Uses:** *2nd-line mod-severe atopic dermatitis* **Action:** Topical calcineurin Inhib/immunosuppressant **Dose:** *Adult & Peds > 15 y.* Apply thin layer (0.03–0.1%) bid; D/C when S/Sxs clear *Peds 2–15 y.* Apply thin layer (0.03%) bid, D/C when S/Sxs clear **Caution:** [C, –] Reevaluate if no response in 6 wk; not for < 2 y; avoid cont long-term use, ↑ risk opportunistic Infxns **CI:** Component allergy **Disp:** Oint 0.03, 0.1% **SE:** Local irritation **NIPE:** Avoid occlusive dressing; rub gently onto dry, clean skin; only use 0.03% in Peds; topical use for short term & 2nd line

Tadalafil (Adcirca)   Uses: *Pulmonary artery hypertension* **Action:** PDE5 Inhib, ↑ cyclic guanosine monophosphate & NO levels; relaxes pulm artery smooth muscles **Dose:** 40 mg 1 × d w/o regard to meals; ↓ w/ renal/hepatic Insuff **Caution:** [B, –] w/ CV Dz, impaired autonomic control of BP, aortic stenosis α-blockers (except tamsulosin); use w/ CYP3A4 Inhib/inducers (eg, ritonavir, ketoconazole); monitor for sudden ↓loss of hearing or vision (NAION), tinnitus, priapism **CI:** w/ Nitrates, component hypersensitivity **Disp:** Tabs 20 mg **SE:** HA **Notes:** See Tadalafil (*Cialis*) for ED **NIPE:** Give dose at same time daily for PAH

Tadalafil (Cialis) [Anti-Impotence Agent/PDE5]   Uses: *ED, BPH* **Action:** PDE5 Inhib, ↑ cyclic guanosine monophosphate & NO levels; relaxes smooth muscles, dilates cavernosal arteries **Dose:** *Adults. PRN:* 10 mg PO before sexual activity (5–20 mg max based on response) 1 dose/24 h *Daily dosing:* 2.5 mg qd may ↑to 5 mg qd, BPH; 5 mg PO qd; w/o regard to meals; ↓ w/ renal/hepatic

Insuff **Caution:** [B, −] w/ α-blockers (except tamsulosin); use w/ CYP3A4 Inhib (Table 10) (eg, ritonavir, ketoconazole, itraconazole) 2.5 mg/daily dose or 5 mg PRN dose; CrCl < 30 mL/min/hemodialysis/severe hepatic impair; do not use daily dosing **CI:** Nitrates **Disp:** Tabs 2.5, 5, 10, 20 mg **SE:** HA, flushing, dyspepsia, back/limb pain, myalgia, nasal congestion, urticaria, SJS, dermatitis, visual field defect, NIAON, sudden √/loss of hearing, tinnitus **Interactions:** ↑ Effects **W/** ketoconazole, ritonavir, & other cytochrome P450 CYP3A4 Inhibs; ↑ hypotension **W/** antihypertensives, nitrates, EtOH; ↓ effects **W/** P450 CYP3A4 inducers such as rifampin, antacids; daily dosing may ↑ drug interactions **NIPE:** ↑ Risk of priapism; use barrier contraception to prevent STDs; longest acting of class (36 h); daily dosing may ↑ drug interactions; excessive EtOH may ↑ orthostasis; transient global amnesia reports

Tafluprost (Zioptan) **Uses:** *Open-angle glaucoma* **Action:** ↓ IOP by ↑ uveoscleral outflow; prostaglandin analog **Dose:** 1 gtt evening **Caution:** [C, ?/–] **CI:** None **Disp:** Soln 0.0015% **SE:** Periorbital/iris pigmentation, eyelash darkening thickening; ↑ number eye redness **Notes:** Pigmentation maybe permanent **NIPE:** Do not exceed once daily dosing; discard remaining content after admin

Talc (Sterile Talc Powder) [Sclerosing Agent] **Uses:** *√↓ Recurrence of malignant pleural effusions (pleurodesis)* **Action:** Sclerosing agent **Dose:** *Mix slurry:* 50 mL NS w/ 5-g vial, mix, distribute 25 mL into two 60-mL syringes, vol to 50 mL/syringe w/ NS. Inf each into chest tube, flush w/ 25 mL NS. Keep tube clamped; have pt change positions q15min for 2 h, unclamp tube; aerosol 4–8 g intrapleurally **Caution:** [B, ?] **CI:** Planned further surgery on site **Disp:** 5-g powder; (Sclerosol) 400 mg/spray **SE:** Pain, Infxn **NIPE:** May add 10–20 mL 1% lidocaine/syringe; must have chest tube placed, monitor closely while tube clamped (tension pneumothorax), not antineoplastic; monitor for MI, PE, resp distress

Taliglucerase Alfa (Elelyso) **Uses:** *Long-term enzyme replacement for type 1 Gaucher Dz* **Action:** Catalyzes hydrolysis of glucocerebroside to glucose & ceramide **Dose:** *Adults.* 60 units/kg IV every other wk; Inf over 1–2 h **Caution:** [B, ?/–] **CI:** None **Disp:** Inj 200 units/vial **SE:** Inf Rxns (allergic, HA, CP, asthenia, fatigue, urticaria, erythema, ↑ BP, back pain, arthralgia, flushing), anaphylaxis, URI, pharyngitis, influenza, UTI, extremity pain **Notes:** For Rxns: ↓ Inf rate, give antihistamines/antipyretics or D/C **NIPE:** Pre-treatment with antihistamines &/or steriods may be avoid subsequent Rxns

Tamoxifen (Generic) [Antineoplastic/Antiestrogen] **WARNING:** CA of the uterus or endometrium, stroke, & blood clots can occur **Uses:** *Breast CA [postmenopausal, estrogen receptor (+)], ↓ risk of breast CA in high-risk, met male breast CA*, ovulation induction **Action:** Nonsteroidal antiestrogen; mixed agonist–antagonist effect **Dose:** 20–40 mg/d; doses > 20 mg ÷ bid *Prevention:* 20 mg PO/d × 5 y **Caution:** [D, −] w/ ↓ WBC, ↓ plts, hyperlipidemia **CI:** PRG, w/ warfarin,

Hx thromboembolism **Disp:** Tabs 10, 20 mg **SE:** Uterine malignancy & thrombotic events noted in breast CA prevention trials; menopausal Sxs (hotflashes, N/V) in premenopausal pts; Vag bleeding & menstrual irregularities; skin rash, pruritus vulvae, dizziness, HA, peripheral edema; acute flare of bone metastasis pain & ↑ Ca²⁺; retinopathy reported (high dose) **Interactions:** ↑ Effects *W/* bromocriptine, grapefruit juice; ↑ effects *OF* cyclosporine, warfarin; ↓ effects *W/* antacids, aminoglutethimide, estrogens **Labs:** ↑ Ca²⁺, BUN, Cr, LFTs; ↓ WBC, ↓ plts **NIPE:** ⊘ PRG or breast-feeding; use barrier contraception; ↑ risk of photosens—use sunscreen; ↑ risk of PRG in premenopausal women (induces ovulation); brand Nolvadex suspended in US; take w/o regard to food

Tamsulosin (Flomax, Generic) [Smooth Muscle Relaxant/ Anti-adrenergic] Uses: *BPH* Action: Antagonist of prostatic α-receptors **Dose:** 0.4 mg/d, may ↑ to 0.8 mg PO daily **Caution:** [B, ?] Floppy iris syndrome w/ cataract surgery **Disp:** Caps 0.4 mg **SE:** HA, dizziness, syncope, somnolence, ↓ libido, GI upset, retrograde ejaculation, rhinitis, rash, angioedema, IFIS **Interactions:** ↑ Effects *W/* cimetidine; ↑ hypotension *W/* doxazosin, prazosin, terazosin **NIPE:** Not for use as antihypertensive; ⊘ open/crush/chew; approved for use w/ dutasteride for BPH; change position slowly (ortho hypotension risk)

Tapentadol (Nucynta) [Opioid] [C-II] WARNING: Provider should be alert to problems of abuse, misuse, & diversion. Avoid use w/ alcohol. Uses: *Mod–severe acute pain* Action: Mu-opioid agonist & norepinephrine reuptake Inhib **Dose:** 50–100 mg PO q4–6h PRN (max 600 mg/d); w/ mod hepatic impair: 50 mg q8h PRN (max 3 doses/24 h) ER dosing: initial 50 mg PO bid (max daily dose 500 mg) **Caution:** [C, –] Hx of Szs, CNS depression; ↑ ICP, severe renal impair, biliary tract Dz, elderly, serotonin synd w/ concomitant serotonergic agents **CI:** ↓ Pulm Fxn, use w/ or w/in 14 d of MAOI, Ileus **Disp:** Tabs 50, 75, 100 mg, ER: 50, 100, 150, 200, 250 mg **SE:** N/V, dizziness, somnolence, HA, constipation **Interactions:** ↑ CNS depression *W/* general anesthetics, hypnotics, phenothiazines, sedatives, EtOH; ↑ risk of serotonin synd *W/* MAOIs, SNRIs, SSRIs, TCA, triptans **NIPE:** Taper dose w/ D/C; ⊘ during or w/in 14 d of MAOI; up ↑ risk of Szs; do not crush/break/divide ER tabs; take w/o regard to food; ⊘ EtOH

Tasimelteon (Hetlioz) Uses: *Insomnia* Acts: Melatonin agonist at MT₁ & MT₂ receptors **Dose:** *Adults.* 20 mg **Caution:** [C, ?] May cause somnolence & impair performance **CI:** None **Disp:** Caps 20 mg **SE:** Somnolence, ↓ attention to task, HA, unusual dreams or nightmares, URI, UTI **Notes:** avoid use w/ strong CYP3A4 Inhib or inducers; no dose adjustment w/ ESRD or mild to mod hepatic impairment (class sleep aid, insomnia, melatonin-like) **NIPE:** Take w/o food at hs; ⊘ break/crush/chew; may take several wk/mo to work

Tazarotene (Avage, Fabior, Tazorac,) [Keratolytic/Reti-noid] Uses: *Facial acne vulgaris; stable plaque psoriasis up to 20% BSA* Action: Keratolytic **Dose:** *Adults & Peds > 12 y. Acne:* Cleanse face, dry, apply

thin film qhs lesions *Psoriasis:* Apply qhs **Caution:** [X, ?/–] **CI:** Retinoid sensitivity, PRG, use in women of childbearing age unable to comply w/ birth control requirements **Disp:** Gel 0.05, 0.1%; cream 0.05, 0.1%; foam 0.1% **SE:** Burning, erythema, irritation, rash, photosens, desquamation, bleeding, skin discoloration **Interactions:** ↑ Risk of photosensitivity *W/* quinolones, phenothiazine, sulfonamides, tetracyclines, thiazide diuretics **NIPE:** ⊘ PRG or breast-feeding; use contraception; use sunscreen for ↑ photosens risk; D/C w/ excessive pruritus, burning, skin redness, or peeling until Sxs resolve; do not cover with dressing

Teduglutide [rDNA Origin] (Gattex)   **Uses:** *Short bowel synd dependent on parenteral support* **Action:** GLP-2 analog ↑ intestine & portal blood flow & ↓ gastric acid secretion **Dose:** *Adults.* 0.05 mg/kg SQ daily; ↓ 50% w/ mod–severe renal impair; alt Inj site between Abd, thighs, arms **Caution:** [B, ?/–] Acceleration neoplastic growth (colonoscopy baseline, 1 y, & q5y); D/C w/ intestinal obstr; biliary/pancreatic Dz (baseline & q6mo bilirubin, alk phos, lipase, amylase); may ↑ absorption oral meds **CI:** None **Disp:** Inj vial 5 mg **SE:** N/V, Abd pain, Abd distention, Inj site Rxn, HA, URI, fluid overload **NIPE:** Instruct pt on prep & admin/observe for correct technique; report Sx jaundice, N, V, severe Abd pain, wgt loss, change in stool

Telaprevir (Incivek)   **Uses:** *Hep C virus, genotype 1, w/ compensated liver Dz including naive to Tx, nonresponders, partial responders, relapsers; w/ peginterferon & ribavirin* **Action:** Hep C antiviral; NS3/4A protease Inhib **Dose:** *Adults.* 750 mg tid, w/ food, must be used w/ peginterferon & ribavirin × 12 wk, then peginterferon & ribavirin × 12 wk (if Hep C undetectable at 4 & 12 wk) or 36 wk (if Hep C detectable at 4 &/or 12 wk) **Caution:** [X, –] **CI:** All CIs to peginterferon & ribavirin; men if PRG female partner; w/ CYP3A metabolized drugs (eg, alfuzosin, sildenafil, tadalafil, lovastatin, simvastatin, ergotamines, cisapride, midazolam, rifampin, St. John's wort) **Disp:** Tabs 375 mg **SE:** Rash > 50% of pts, include SJS, drug rash w/ eosinophilia (DRESS); pruritus, anemia, N, V, D, fatigue, anorectal pain, dysgeusia, hemorrhoids **Notes:** Must not be used as monotherapy **NIPE:** ⊘ PRG/breast-feeding; females must use 2 methods of birth control (eg, IUD, diaphragm w/ spermacide, barrier methods) during Tx & 6 mo thereafter; hormonal birth control—may reduce effectiveness; give w/ meal w/ at least 20 g of fat; ⊘ EtOH

Telavancin (Vibativ) [Antibacterial/Lipoglycopeptide]   **WARNING:** Fetal risk; must have PRG test prior to use in childbearing age **Uses:** *Complicated skin/skin structure Infxns d/t susceptible gram(–) bacteria* **Action:** Lipoglycopeptide antibacterial *Spectrum:* Good gram(±) aerobic & anaerobic include MRSA, MSSA, some VRE; poor gram(–) **Dose:** 10 mg/kg IV q24h; 7.5 mg/kg q24h w/ CrCl 30–50 mL/min; 10 mg/kg q48h w/ CrCl 10–30 mL/min **Caution:** [C, ?] Nephrotox, *C difficile*–associated diarrhea, insomnia, HA, ↑ QTc, interferes w/ coag tests **CI:** None **Disp:** Inj 250, 750 mg **SE:** Insomnia, psychiatric disorder, taste disturbance, HA, N, V, foamy urine **Interactions:** ↑ Risk of renal tox *W/* NSAIDs, ACE I, loop diuretics **Labs:** May interfere w/ coagulation tests (eg, PT/ INR, aPPT, ACT, coagulation-based factor Xa tests) & some urine protein tests **NIPE:** ↓ Efficacy w/ mod/severe renal impair; use contraception during Tx; obtain C&S prior to 1st dose; avoid rapid infusion to prevent "red-man syndrome"

Telbivudine (Tyzeka) [Antiretroviral, NRTI] **WARNING:** May cause lactic acidosis & severe hepatomegaly w/ steatosis when used alone or w/ antiretrovirals; D/C of the drug may lead to exacerbations of hep B; monitor LFTs **Uses:** *Rx chronic hep B* **Action:** Nucleoside RT Inhib **Dose:** *CrCl > 50 mL/min:* 600 mg PO daily; *CrCl 30–49 mL/min:* 600 mg q48h; *CrCl < 30 mL/min:* 600 mg q72h *ESRD:* 600 mg q96h; dose after hemodialysis **Caution:** [B, ?/–] May cause myopathy; follow closely w/ other myopathy-causing drugs **Disp:** Tabs 600 mg **SE:** Fatigue, Abd pain, N/V/D, HA, URI, nasopharyngitis, ↑ LFTs/CPK, myalgia/ myopathy, flu-like Sxs, dizziness, insomnia, dyspepsia **Interactions:** Use w/ PEG-interferon may ↑ peripheral neuropathy risk; ↑ risk of myopathy *W/* azole antifungals, chloroquine, corticosteroids, cyclosporine, erythromycin, fibrates, hydroxychloroquine, niacin, penicillamine, statins, zidovudine; ↑ risk of renal impair *W/* cyclosporine, tacrolimus **Labs:** ↑ LFTs, CPK **NIPE:** Not a cure for HBV, does not reduce transmission of HBV by sexual contact or blood contamination; monitor for liver tox/hep (jaundice, rash, hepatomegaly, fatigue)

Telithromycin (Ketek) [Antibiotic/Macrolide Derivative] **WARNING:** CI in MyG **Uses:** *Mild–mod CAP* **Action:** Unique macrolide, blocks ↓ protein synth; bactericidal **Spectrum:** *S aureus, S pneumoniae, H influenzae, M catarrhalis, C pneumoniae, M pneumoniae* **Dose:** *CAP:* 800 mg (2 tabs) PO daily × 7–10 d **Caution:** [C, ?] Pseudomembranous colitis, ↑ QTc interval, visual disturbances, hepatic dysfunction; dosing in renal impair unknown **CI:** Macrolide allergy, w/ pimozide or cisapride; Hx of hep or jaundice, w/ macrolide abx, w/ MyG **Disp:** Tabs 300, 400 mg **SE:** N/V/D, dizziness, blurred vision **Interactions:** ACYP450 Inhib = multiple drug interactions; hold statins d/t ↑ risk of myopathy; avoid rifampin, ergots, simvastatin, lovastatin, atorvastatin (suspend during therapy). Do not use w/ Class Ia (eg, quinidine, procainamide) or Class III (eg, dofetilide) antiarrhythmics; ↑ QTc interval & arrhythmias *W/* antiarrhythmics, mesoridazine, quinolone antibiotics, thioridazine; ↑ effects *OF* alprazolam, atorvastatin, benzodiazepines, CCBs, carbamazepine, cisapride, colchicine, cyclosporine, digoxin, ergot alkaloids, felodipine, lovastatin, mirtazapine, midazolam, nateglinide, nefazodone, pimozide, sildenafil, simvastatin, sirolimus, tacrolimus, tadalafil, triazolam, vardenafil, venlafaxine, verapamil, warfarin; ↓ effects *W/* azole antifungals, ciprofloxin, clarithromycin, diclofenac, doxycycline, erythromycin, imatinib, INH, nefazodone, nicardipine, propofol, protease Inhibs, quinidine; ↑ effect *W/* aminoglutethimide, carbamazepine, nafcillin, nevirapine, phenobarbital, phenytoin, rifampin, rifamycins **Labs:** ↑ LFTs, plts **NIPE:** Take w/o regard to food; ⊘ chew/crush tabs, monitor

ECG; hold statins d/t ↑ risk of myopathy; take same time qd; may cause fainting in pts w/ severe N/V, lightheadedness

Telmisartan (Micardis) [Antihypertensive/ARB] **WARNING:** Use of renin-angiotensin agents in PRG can cause fetal injury & death, D/C immediately when PRG detected **Uses:** *HTN, CHF* **Action:** Angiotensin II receptor antagonist **Dose:** 40–80 mg qd **Caution:** [C (1st tri; D 2nd & 3rd tri), ?/–] ↑ K⁺ CI: Angiotensin II receptor antagonist sensitivity **Disp:** Tabs 20, 40, 80 mg **SE:** Edema, GI upset, HA, angioedema, renal impair, orthostatic ↓ BP **Interactions:** ↑ Risk of hyperkalemia W/ K⁺ supls, K⁺-sparing diuretics, K⁺- containing salt substitutes; ↑ effects W/ EtOH; ↑ effects OF digoxin; ↓ effects OF warfarin **Labs:** ↑ Cr, ↓ HMG **NIPE:** Take w/o regard to food; ⊘ PRG; use barrier contraception; maintain hydration; ✓ BP/Sx hypotension

Telmisartan/Amlodipine (Twynsta) [Angiotensin II Receptor Blocker + Calcium Channel Blocker] **WARNING:** Use of renin-angiotensin agents in PRG can cause fetal injury & death, D/C immediately when PRG detected **Uses:** *Hypertension* **Action:** CCB: relaxes coronary vascular smooth muscle & angiotensin II receptor antagonist **Dose:** Start 40/5 mg telmisartan/amlodipine; max 80/10 mg PO/d; ↑ dose after 2wk **Caution:** [C (1st tri; D 2nd/3rd), ?/–] ↑ K⁺ CI: PRG **Disp:** Tabs mg telmisartan/mg amlodipine 40/5; 40/10; 80/5; 80/10 **SE:** HA, edema, dizziness, N, ↓ BP **Interactions:** ↑ Effects OF digoxin, Li; CCB w/ CAD may cause ACS **NIPE:** Slow titrate w/ hepatic/renal impair; avoid w/ ACE/other ARBs; correct hypovolemia before; w/ CHF monitor; ⊘ PRG

Temazepam (Restoril) [C-IV] [Sedative/Hypnotic/Benzodiazepine] **Uses:** *Insomnia*, anxiety, depression, panic attacks **Action:** Benzodiazepine **Dose:** 15–30 mg PO hs PRN; ↓ in elderly **Caution:** [X, ?/–] Potentiates CNS depressive effects of opioids, barbs, EtOH, antihistamines, MAOIs, TCAs **CI:** NAG, PRG **Disp:** Caps 7.5, 15, 22.5, 30 mg **SE:** Confusion, dizziness, drowsiness, hangover **Interactions:** ↑ Effects W/ cimetidine, disulfiram, kava kava, valerian; ↑ CNS depression W/ anticonvulsants, CNS depressants, EtOH; ↑ effects OF haloperidol, phenytoin; ↓ effects W/ aminophylline, dyphylline, OCPs, oxtriphylline, rifampin, theophylline, tobacco; ↓ effects OF levodopa **NIPE:** Abrupt D/C after > 10 d use may cause withdrawal; ⊘ use in PRG or breast-feeding; assess for paradoxical effect in elderly; ⊘ ETOH; take 30 min before hs

Temozolomide (Temodar) [Alkylating Agent] **Uses:** *Glioblastoma multiforme (GBM), refractory anaplastic astrocytoma* **Action:** Alkylating agent **Dose:** *GBM, new*: 75 mg/m² PO/IV/d × 42 d w/ RT, maint 150 mg/m²/d days 1–5 of 28-d cycle × 6 cycles; may ↑ to 200 mg/m²/d × 5 d q28d in cycle 2 *Refractory astrocytoma*: 150 mg/m² PO/IV/d × 5 d/28-d cycle; adjust dose based on ANC & plt count (see PI & local protocols) **Caution:** [D, ?/–] w/ Severe renal/hepatic impair, myelosuppression (monitor ANC & plt), myelodysplastic synd, secondary malignancies, PCP pneumonia (PCP prophylaxis required) **CI:** Hypersensitivity to components or dacarbazine **Disp:** Caps 5, 20, 100, 140, 180, & 250 mg; powder for Inj 100 mg **SE:** N/V/D, fatigue, HA, asthenia, Sz, hemiparesis, fever, dizziness, coordination abnormality, alopecia, rash, constipation, anorexia, amnesia, insomnia, viral Infxn, ↓ WBC, plt **Interactions:** ↑ Effects W/ valproic acid **Labs:** ↓ WBC, plt; monitor CBC—do CBC on 22nd d of each cycle & weekly until recovery if ANC or plts below nl limits **NIPE:** Inf over 90 min; swallow caps whole w/ H₂O; if caps open avoid Inh & contact w/ skin/mucous membranes; to reduce N—take on empty stomach at hs, take antiemetics before dosing; avoid immunizations w/o physician approval; ⊘ PRG

Temsirolimus (Torisel) [mTOR Kinase Inhibitor] Uses: *Advanced RCC* **Action:** Multikinase Inhib, ↓ mTOR (mammalian target of rapamycin), ↓ hypoxic-induced factors, ↓ VEGF **Dose:** 25 mg IV 30–60 min 1 ×/wk. Hold w/ ANC < 1000 cells/mcL, plt < 75,000 cells/mcL, or NCI grade 3 tox. Resume when tox grade 2 or less, restart w/ dose ↓ 5 mg/wk; not < 15 mg/wk *w/ CYP3A4 Inhib:* ↓ 12.5 mg/wk *w/ CYP3A4 inducers:* ↑ 50 mg/wk **Caution:** [D, –] Avoid live vaccines, ↓ wound healing, avoid periop **CI:** Bilirubin > 1.5 × ULN **Disp:** Inj 25 mg/mL w/ 250 mL diluent **SE:** Rash, asthenia, mucositis, N, bowel perforation, angioedema, impaired wound healing; interstitial lung Dz anorexia, edema, ↑ lipids, ↑ glucose, ↑ triglycerides, ↑ LFTs, ↑ Cr, ↓ WBC, ↓ HCT, ↓ plt, ↓ PO₄ **Interactions:** ↑ Effects W/ strong CYP3A4 Inhibs such as ketoconazole, itraconazole, clarithromycin, atazanavir, indinavir, nefazodone, nelfinavir, ritonavir, saquinavir, telithromycin, voriconazole, grapefruit juice; ↓ effects W/ strong CYP3A4 inducers such as dexamethasone, phenytoin, carbamazepine, rifampin, rifabutin, rifampicin, phenobarbital, St. John's wort **Labs:** ↑ Lipids, ↑ glucose, ↑ triglycerides, ↑ LFTs, ↑ Cr, ↓ WBC, ↓ HCT, ↓ plt, ↓ PO₄; monitor Cr, CBC, plts, lipids, glucose **NIPE:** Combine only w/ provided diluent for IV administration; premedicate w/ antihistamine; w/ sunitinib & anticoagulants dose-limiting tox likely; females use w/ contraception; ⊘ live vaccines or people recently immunized w/ live vaccines; ✓ Sx of Infxn/bruising/bleeding

Tenecteplase (TNKase) [Thrombolytic/Recombinant Tissue Plasminogen Activator] Uses: *Restore perfusion & ↓ mortality w/ AMI* **Action:** Thrombolytic; TPA **Dose:** 30–50 mg; see table on next page **Caution:** [C, ?], Bleeding w/ NSAIDs, ticlopidine, clopidogrel, GP IIb/IIIa antagonists **CI:** Bleeding, ANA aneurysm, CVA, CNS neoplasm, uncontrolled ↑ BP, major surgery (intracranial, intraspinal) or trauma w/in 2 mo **Disp:** Inj 50 mg, reconstitute w/ 10 mL sterile H₂O only **SE:** Bleeding, allergy **Interactions:** ↑ Risk of bleeding W/ heparin, ASA, clopidogrel, dipyridamole, indomethacin, vit K antagonists, GP IIb/IIIa Inhibs; ↓ effects W/ aminocaproic acid **Labs:** ↑ PT, PTT, INR **NIPE:** Eval for S/Sxs bleeding; do not shake w/ reconstitution; start ASA ASAP, IV heparin ASAP w/ aPTT 50–70; ✓ EKG for arrythmias

Tenecteplase Dosing (From one vial of reconstituted TNKase)

Weight (kg)	TNKase (mg)	TNKase Volume (mL)
<60	30	6
60–69	35	7
70–79	40	8
80–89	45	9
≥90	50	10

Tenofovir (Viread) [Antiretroviral/NRTI]   **WARNING:** Lactic acidosis/hepatomegaly w/ steatosis (some fatal) reported w/ the use of NRTI. Exacerbations of hepatitis reported w/ HBV patients who D/C hep B Rx, including VIREAD. ✓ LFT in these patients & may need to resume hep B Rx **Uses:** *HIV & chronic hep B Infxn* **Action:** NRTI **Dose:** 300 mg PO daily w/ or w/o meal; CrCl 30–49 mL/min q48h, CrCl 10–29 mL/min 2 ×/wk **Caution:** [B, –] Didanosine, lopinavir, ritonavir w/ known risk factors for liver Dz **CI:** Hypersensitivity **Disp:** Tabs 300 mg **SE:** GI upset, metabolic synd, hepatotoxicity; insomnia, rash, ↑ CK, Fanconi synd **Interactions:** ↑ Effects *W/* acyclovir, cidofovir, ganciclovir, indinavir, lopinavir, ritonavir, valacyclovir, food **Labs:** ↑ LFTs, triglycerides **NIPE:** Take w/o regard to food; take 2 h before or 1 h after didanosine, lopinavir/ritonavir; combo product w/ emtricitabine is Truvada

Tenofovir/Emtricitabine (Truvada) [Antiretroviral, Dual NRTI] **WARNING:** Lactic acidosis/severe hepatomegaly w/ steatosis, (some fatal) reported w/ the use of NRTI. Not approved for chronic hep B. Exacerbations of hepatitis reported w/ HBV pts who D/C *Truvada*. May need to resume hep B Rx. If used for pre-exposure prophylaxis (PrEP), confirm (–) HIV before & q3mo. Drug-resistant HIV-1 variants have been identified **Uses:** *HIV Infxn PrEP for HIV-1* **Action:** Dual nucleotide RT Inhib **Dose:** 1 tab PO daily w/ or w/o a meal; adjust w/ renal impair **Caution:** [B, ?/–] Known risk factors for liver Dz **CI:** None **Disp:** Tabs 200 mg emtricitabine/300 mg tenofovir **SE:** GI upset, rash, metabolic synd, hepatotoxicity, Fanconi synd; OK Peds > 12 y **Interactions:** ↑ Effects *W/* acyclovir, cidofovir, ganciclovir, indinavir, lopinavir, ritonavir, valacyclovir, food; ↓ effects *OF* didanosine, lamivudine, ritonavir **Labs:** ↑ LFTs, triglycerides **NIPE:** Take w/ food, take 2 h before or 1 h after didanosine, lopinavir/ritonavir; causes redistribution & accumulation of body fat; take w/ other antiretrovirals; not a cure for HIV or prevention of opportunistic Infxns; DC with Sx of lactic acidosis or hepatoxicity

Terazosin (Hytrin) [Antihypertensive/Peripherally Acting Anti-adrenergic]   **Uses:** *BPH & HTN* **Action:** α_1-Blocker (blood vessel & bladder neck/prostate) **Dose:** Initial, 1 mg PO hs; ↑ 20 mg/d max; may ↓ w/ diuretic or other BP medicine **Caution:** [C, ?] w/ BBs, CCB, ACE Inhib; use w/ phosphodiesterase-5 (PDE5) Inhib (eg, sildenafil) can cause ↓ BP, intra op floppy iris synd w/ cataract surgery **CI:** α-Antagonist sensitivity **Disp:** Tabs 1, 2, 5, 10 mg; caps 1, 2, 5, 10 mg angina **SE:** Angina, ↓ BP, & syncope following 1st dose or w/ PDE5 Inhib; dizziness, weakness, nasal congestion, peripheral edema, palpitations, GI upset **Interactions:** ↑ Effects *W/* antihypertensives, diuretics; ↑ effects *OF* finasteride; ↓ effects *W/* NSAIDs, α-blockers, ephedra, garlic, ginseng, saw palmetto, yohimbe; ↓ effects *OF* clonidine; use w/ PDE5 Inhib (eg, sildenafil) can cause ↓ BP **Labs:** ↓ Albumin, HMG, Hct, WBCs **NIPE:** Take w/o regard to food, ⊘ D/C abruptly; caution w/ 1st dose syncope; if for HTN, combine w/ thiazide diuretic; ⊘ EtOH; change position slowly

Terbinafine (Lamisil, Lamisil AT, Generic [OTC]) [Antifungal] **Uses:** *Onychomycosis, athlete's foot, jock itch, ringworm*, cutaneous candidiasis, pityriasis versicolor **Action:** ↓ Squalene epoxidase resulting in fungal death **Dose:** *PO:* 250 mg/d PO for 6–12 wk *Topical:* Apply to area tinea pedis bid, tinea cruris, & corporus daily–bid, tinea versicolor soln bid; ↓ PO in renal/hepatic impair **Caution:** [B, –] PO ↑ effects of drug metabolism by CYP2D6, w/ liver/renal impair **CI:** CrCl < 50 mL/min, WBC < 1000 cells/mm³, severe liver Dz **Disp:** Tabs 250 mg; oral granules 125 mg/pkt, 187.5 mg/pkt Lamisil AT [OTC] cream, gel, soln 1% **SE:** HA, N dizziness, rash, pruritus, alopecia, GI upset, taste perversion, neutropenia, retinal damage, SJS, ↑ LFTs **Interactions:** ↑ Effects *W/* cimetidine; ↑ effects *OF* dextromethorphan, theophylline, caffeine; ↓ effects *W/* rifampin; ↓ effects *OF* cyclosporine **Labs:** ↑ LFTs; follow CBC/LFTs w/ oral med **NIPE:** Effect may take mo d/t need for new nail growth; do not use occlusive dressings; topical not for nails; rare reports of liver failure

Terbutaline   (Generic)   [Bronchodilator/Sympathomimetic] **WARNING:** Not approved & should not be used > 48–72 h for tocolysis. Serious adverse Rxns possible, including death. **Uses:** *Reversible bronchospasm (asthma, COPD); inhibit labor* **Action:** Sympathomimetic; tocolytic **Dose:** *Adults. Bronchodilator:* 2.5–5 mg PO qid or 0.25 mg SQ; repeat in 15 min PRN; max 0.5 mg in 4 h. Max 15 mg/24 h PO *Metered-dose inhaler:* 1 puff PRN, repeat after 5 min PRN; 6 inhal/24 h max *Premature labor:* 0.25 mg SQ every 1–4 h × 24 h, 5 mg max/24 h; 2.5–5 mcg/min IV, ↑ 5 mcg/min q10min as tolerated, 25 mcg/min max. When controlled ↓ to lowest effective dose; SQ pump: basal 0.05–0.10 mg/h, bolus over 25 mg PRN *Peds. PO:* 0.05–0.15 mg/kg/dose PO tid; max 5 mg/24 h; ↓ in renal failure **Caution:** [C, +] ↑ Tox w/ MAOIs, TCAs; DM, HTN, hyperthyroidism, CV Dz, convulsive disorders, K⁺ **CI:** Component allergy, prolonged tocolysis **Disp:** Tabs 2.5, 5 mg; Inj 1 mg/mL; metered-dose inhaler **SE:** HTN, hyperthyroidism, β₁-adrenergic effects w/ high dose, nervousness, trembling, tachycardia, arrhythmia, HTN, dizziness, ↑ glucose **Interactions:** ↑ Toxicity *W/* MAOIs, TCAs; ↓ effects *W/* BBs **Labs:** ↑ LFTs; serum glucose; ↓ K⁺—monitor labs **NIPE:** Take oral dose w/ food; tablets can be crushed; monitor ECG for hypokalemia (flattened T waves), tocolysis requires close monitoring of mother & fetus; avoid excessive caffine

Terconazole (Terazol 3, Terazol 7) [Antifungal] Uses: *Vag fungal Infxns* **Action:** Topical triazole antifungal **Dose:** 1 applicator-full or 1 supp intravag hs × 3–7 d **Caution:** [C, ?] **CI:** Component allergy **Disp:** Vag cream (Tersznol 7) 0.4, (Terzsol 3) 0.8%, (Terszol 3) Vag sup 80 mg **SE:** Vulvar/Vag burning **NIPE:** Insert cream or supp high into Vag, complete full course of Rx, ⊘ intercourse during drug Rx, ↑ risk of breakdown of latex condoms & diaphragms w/ drug

Teriflunomide (Aubagio) **WARNING:** Hepatotx; ✓ LFT baseline & ALT qmo × 6 mo. D/C w/ liver injury & begin accelerated elimination procedure; CI in PRG & women of childbearing potential w/o reliable contraception Uses: *Relapsing MS* **Acts:** Pyrimidine synth Inhib **Dose:** *Adults.* 7 or 14 mg PO daily **Caution:** [X, –] w/ CYP2C8, CYP1A2 metab drugs, warfarin, ethinylestradiol, levonorgestrel; ↑ elimin w/ cholestyramine or activated charcoal × 11 d; **CI:** PRG; severe hepatic impair; w/ leflunomide **Disp:** Tabs 7, 14 mg **SE:** ↑ ALT, alopecia, N/D, influenza, paresthesia, ↓ WBC, neuropathy, ↑ BP, SJS, TEN, ARF, ↑ K+ **NIPE:** ⊘ PRG; ✓ CBC & TB screen prior to Rx; ✓ BP, S/Sxs of Infxn; do not give w/ live vaccines; give w/o regard to food

Teriparatide (Forteo) [Antiosteoporotic/Parathyroid Hormone] **WARNING:** ↑ Osteosarcoma risk in animals, use only where potential benefits outweigh risks Uses: *Severe/refractory osteoporosis* **Action:** PTH (recombinant) **Dose:** 20 mcg SQ daily in thigh or Abd **Caution:** [C,–] Caution in urolithiasis **Disp:** 250 mcg/mL in 2.4-mL prefilled syringe **SE:** Orthostatic ↓ BP on administration, N/D, Ca2+; leg cramps, ↑ uric acid **Labs:** ↑ Serum Ca2+, uric acid, urine Ca2+ **NIPE:** ⊘ Take if h/o Paget Dz, bone mets or malignancy, or h/o radiation therapy; take w/o regard to food; not used to prevent osteoporosis; 2 y max use; refrigerate; change position slowly; monitor ECG for cardiac conduction changes related to ↑ Ca2+

Tesamorelin (Egrifta) [Growth Hormone–Releasing Factor Analog] Uses: *↓ Excess body fat in HIV-infected patients w/ lipodystrophy* **Action:** Binds/stimulates growth hormone–releasing factor receptors **Dose:** 2 mg SQ/d **Caution:** [X; HIV-infected mothers should not breast-feed] **CI:** Hypothalamic-pituitary axis disorders; hypersensitivity to tesamorelin, mannitol, or any component, head radiation/trauma; malignancy; PRG; child w/ open epiphyses **Disp:** Vial 1 mg **SE:** Arthralgias, Inj site Rxn, edema, myalgia, ↑ glucose, N, V **Labs:** ↑ Glucose, ✓ glucose **NIPE:** ? ↑ Mortality w/ acute critical illness; ↑ IGF; ⊘ PRG/breast-feeding; rotate Inj sites

Testosterone (AndroGel, 1%, AndroGel 1.62% Androderm, Axiron, Fortesta, Striant, Testim, Testopel) [C-III] [Androgen Replacement] **WARNING:** Virilization reported in children exposed to topical testosterone products. Children to avoid contact w/ unwashed or unclothed application sites Uses: *Male hypogonadism (congenital/acquired)

Action: Testosterone placement; ↑ lean body mass, libido **Dose:** All daily applications *AndroGel 1%*: 50 mg (4 pumps); *AndroGel 1.62%*: 40.5 mg (2 pumps); apply to clean skin on upper body only *Androderm:* Two 2.5-mg or one 5-mg patch daily *Axiron* 60 mg (1 pump = 30 mg each axilla) qAM *Fortesta:* 40 mg (4 pumps) on clean dry thighs; adjust from 1–7 pumps based on blood test 2 h after (days 14 & 35) *Striant:* 30-mg buccal tabs bid *Testim:* One 5-g gel tube *Testopel:* 150–150 mg (2–6 pellets) SQ implant q3–6mo (implant two 75-mg pellets for each 25-mg testosterone required weekly; eg: for 75 mg/wk, implant 450 mg (6 pellets) **Caution:** [X, −] May cause polycythemia, worsening of BPH Sx **CI:** PCa, male breast CA, women **Disp:** *AndroGel 1% 12.5 mg/pump; AndroGel 1.62%: 20.25 mg/ pump; Androderm:* 2.5-, 5-mg patches *Axiron* metered-dose pump 30 mg/pump *Fortesta:* Metered-dose gel pump 10 mg/pump *Striant:* 30-mg buccal tab *Testopel:* 75 mg/implant **SE:** Site Rxns, acne, edema, wgt gain, gynecomastia, HTN, ↑ sleep apnea, prostate enlargement, ↑ PSA **Interactions:** ↑ Effects *OF* anticoagulants, cyclosporine, insulin, hypoglycemics, oxyphenbutazone; ↑ effects *W/* grapefruit juice; ↓ effects *W/* St. John's wort **Labs:** ↑ AST, Cr, Hgb, Hct, LDL, serum alk phos, bilirubin, Ca, K⁺, & Na; ↓ thyroid hormones **NIPE:** IM testosterone enanthate (*Delatestryl; Testro-L.A.*) & cypionate (*Depo-Testosterone*) dose q14–28d w/ variable serum levels; PO agents (methyltestosterone & oxandrolone) associated w/ hepatic tumors; transdermal/mucosal forms preferred; wash hands stat after topical applications; *Andro Gel* formulations not equivalent; ✓ levels & adjust PRN (300–1000 ng/dL nl testosterone range); ✓ daily wgts

Testosterone, Nasal Gel (Natesto) [C-III] **WARNING:** Virilization reported in children exposed to topical testosterone products. Children to avoid contact w/ unwashed or unclothed application sites **Uses:** *Adult male hypogonadism (congenital/acquired)* **Action:** Testosterone replacement **Dose:** 2 pumps each nostril (11 mg testosterone/actuation) one in each nostril TID (total 33 mg/d) **Caution:** [X, −] Avoid w/ nasal pathology; monitor BPH Sx & for DVT; may cause azoospermia, edema, sleep apnea; not rec if < 18 y **CI:** Prostate CA, male breast CA, women **Disp:** Metered-dose pump; 1 pump = 5.5 mg of testosterone **SE:** ↑ PSA, headache, rhinorrhea, epistaxis, nasal discomfort, nasopharyngitis, bronchitis, URI, sinusitis, nasal scab. 1 pump actuation delivers 5.5 mg of testosterone **Notes:** Previously known as Compleo TRT; may minimize exposure of testosterone to women or children; monitor testosterone, PSA, Hgb, LFTs, & lipids periodically **NIPE:** Blow nose prior to use; completely depress pump 1 × in each nostril; ⊘ blow nose/sniff I h after admin; ⊘ males w/breast CA; ⊘ females/children

Testosterone Undecanoate, Injectable (Aveed) **WARNING:** POME (pulmonary oil microembolism) reactions (urge to cough, dyspnea, throat tightening, chest pain, dizziness, syncope) & episodes of anaphylaxis, including life-threatening reactions, have been reported after the administration; observe patients for 30 min after dosing **Uses:** *Male hypogonadism (congenital/ acquired)* **Action:** Testosterone replacement; ↑ lean body mass, libido **Dose:** 3 mL (750 mg)

IM (gluteal) initially, at 4 wk, every 10 wk thereafter; observe for 30 min for POME or aphylaxis **Caution:** [X, –] May worsen BPH Sx, azoospermia possible, edema with pre-existing cardiac/renal/hepatic Dz, sleep apnea with other risk factors, monitor PSA, hgb/Hct, lipids periodically; may reduce insulin requirements, monitor INR if on warfarin; w/ steroids may cause fluid retention **CI:** PCa, male breast CA, women, component sensitivity **Disp:** 3-mL (750 mg) in castor oil & benzyl benzoate **SE:** Acne, injection site pain, PSA & estradiol, hypogonadism, fatigue, irritability, ↑ hemoglobin, insomnia, mood swings **Notes:** Available only through a restricted program (Aveed REMS); other IM forms not commonly used: testosterone enanthate (*Delatestryl; Testro-L.A.*) & cypionate (*Depo-Testosterone*) dose q14–28d w/ variable serum levels **NIPE:** Risk of POME/anaphylaxis—observe × 30 min after admin; ⊘ females/Ped pts

Tetanus Immune Globulin [Tetanus Prophylaxis/Immune Serum] **Uses:** Prophylaxis *passive tetanus immunization* (suspected contaminated wound w/ unknown immunization status, see Table 7), or Tx of tetanus **Action:** Passive immunization **Dose:** *Adults & Peds.* Prophylaxis: 250 mg units IM × 1 Tx: 500–6000 (30–300 units/kg) units IM **Caution:** [C, ?] Anaphylaxis Rxn **CI:** Thimerosal sensitivity **Disp:** Inj 250-unit vial/syringe **SE:** Pain, tenderness, erythema at site; fever, angioedema **Interactions:** ↓ Immune response when administration w/ Td **NIPE:** Give Td booster q10y; may begin active immunization series at different Inj site if required; slight soreness/warmth at Inj site may occur

Tetanus Toxoid (TT) [Tetanus Prophylaxis/Vaccine] **Uses:** *Tetanus prophylaxis* **Action:** Active immunization **Dose:** Based on previous immunization, Table 7 **Caution:** [C, ?/–] **CI:** Thimersal hypersensitivity, neurologic Sxs w/ previous use, active Infxn w/ routine primary immunization **Disp:** Inj tetanus toxoid fluid, 5 Lf units/0.5 mL; tetanus toxoid, adsorbed, 5 units/0.5 mL **SE:** Inj site erythema, induration, sterile abscess, arthralgias, fever, malaise, neurologic disturbances **Interactions:** Delay of active immunity if given **W/** tetanus immune globulin; ↓ immune response if given to pts taking corticosteroids or immunosuppressive drugs **NIPE:** Stress the need of timely completion of immunization series; DTaP rather than TT or Td all adults 19–64 y who have not previously received 1 dose of DTaP (protection adult pertussis); also use DT or Td instead of TT to maintain diphtheria immunity; if IM, use only preservative-free Inj; do not confuse Td (for adults) w/ DT (for children)

Tetrabenazine (Xenazine) [Monoamine Depletory] **WARNING:** ↑ Risk of depression, suicide w/ Huntington Dz **Uses:** *Rx chorea in Huntington Dz* **Action:** Monoamine depleter **Dose:** 25–100 mg/d ÷ doses; 12.5 mg PO/d × 1 wk, ↑ to 12.5 mg bid, may ↑ to 12.5 mg TID if > 37.5 mg/d after 1 wk; if > 50 mg needed, ✓ for CYP2D6 gene; if poor metabolizer, 25 mg max; 50 mg/d max; extensive/indeterminate metabolizer 37.5 mg dose max, 100 mg/d max **Caution:** [C; ?/–] ½ dose w/ strong CYP2D6 Inhib 50 mg/d max (paroxetine, fluoxetine) **CI:** Wait 20 d after reserpine D/C before use, suicidality, untreated, or inadequately treated depression; hepatic impair; w/ MOAI or reserpine **Disp:** Tabs 12.5, 25 mg **SE:** Sedation, insomnia, depression, anxiety, irritability, akathisia, Parkinsonism, balance difficulties, neuroleptic malignant synd, fatigue, N, V, dysphagia, ↑ QT, EPS Szs, falls **Interactions:** ↑ Risk of QT prolongation *W/* chlorpromazine, thioridazine, ziprasidone, moxifloxacin, quinidine, procainamide, amiodarone, sotalol; ↑ effects *W/* CYP2D6 Inhibs (eg, paroxetine, fluoxetine); ↑ risks of neuroleptic malignant synd & extrapyramidal synd *W/* neuroleptics, DA antagonists; ↑ CNS depression *W/* EtOH & other CNS depressants **NIPE:** Give w/o regard to meals; can DC w/o tapering; report increased depression/suicidality; ⊘ EtOH

Tetracycline (Generic) [Antibiotic/Tetracycline] Uses: *Broad-spectrum antibiotic* **Action:** Bacteriostatic; ↓ protein synth *Spectrum:* Gram(+): Staphylococcus, Streptococcus Gram(−): H pylori Atypicals: Chlamydia, Rickettsia, & Mycoplasma **Dose:** *Adults.* 250–500 mg PO bid–qid *Peds > 8 y.* 25–50 mg/kg/24 h PO q6–12h; ↓ w/ renal/hepatic impair, w/o food preferred **Caution:** [D, −] **CI:** PRG, children < 8 y **Disp:** Cap 100, 250, 500 mg; tabs 250, 500 mg; PO susp 250 mg/5 mL **SE:** Photosens, GI upset, renal failure, pseudotumor cerebri, hepatic impair **Interactions:** ↑ Effects *OF* anticoagulants, digoxin; ↓ effects *W/* antacids, cimetidine, laxatives, penicillin, Fe supl, dairy products; ↓ effects *OF* OCPs **Labs:** False(−) of urinary glucose, serum folate; false ↑ serum glucose **NIPE:** ⊘ Take w/ dairy products; take w/o food; use barrier contraception; can stain tooth enamel & depress bone formation in children; use sunblock

Thalidomide (Thalomid) [Immunomodulatory Agent] WARNING: Restricted use; use associated w/ severe birth defects & ↑ risk of venous thromboembolism Uses: *Erythema nodosum leprosum (ENL)*, GVHD, aphthous ulceration in HIV(+) **Action:** ↓ Neutrophil chemotaxis, ↓ monocyte phagocytosis **Dose:** *GVHD:* 50–100 tid, max 600–1200 mg/d *Stomatitis:* 200 mg bid for 5 d, then 200 mg daily up to 8 wk *Erythema nodosum leprosum:* 100–300 mg PO qhs **Caution:** [X, −] May ↑ HIV viral load; Hx Szs **CI:** PRG or females not using 2 forms of contraception **Disp:** Caps 50, 100, 150, 200 mg caps **SE:** Dizziness, drowsiness, rash, fever, orthostasis, SJS, peripheral neuropathy, Szs **Interactions:** ↑ Effects *OF* barbiturates, CNS depressants, chlorpromazine, reserpine, EtOH; ↑ peripheral neuropathy *W/* INH, Li, metronidazole, phenytoin **Labs:** Monitor LFTs, WBC, differential, PRG test before start of Tx & monthly during Tx **NIPE:** If also taking drugs that ↓ hormonal contraceptives (carbamazepine, griseofulvin, phenytoin, rifabutin, rifampin) use 2 other contraceptive methods; male pts use latex condoms; take 1 h pc with H_2O; take in evening/hs (causes drowsiness)—food will affect absorption; photosens—use sunblock; ⊘ PRG & breast-feeding; healthcare provider must register w/ STEPS risk management program; informed consent necessary; stat D/C if rash develops

Theophylline (Theo24, Theochron, Theolair) [Bronchodilator/Xanthine Derivative] Uses: *Asthma, bronchospasm* **Action:** Relaxes smooth muscle of the bronchi & pulm blood vessels **Dose: *Adults.*** 900 mg PO ÷ q6h; SR products may be ÷ q8–12h (maint) ***Peds.*** 16–22 mg/kg/24 h PO ÷ q6h; SR products may be ÷ q8–12h (maint); ↓ in hepatic failure **Caution:** [C, +] Multiple interactions (eg, caffeine, smoking, carbamazepine, barbiturates, BBs, ciprofloxacin, E-mycin, INH, loop diuretics, arrhythmia, hyperthyroidism, uncontrolled Szs **CI:** Corn allergy **Disp:** Elixir 80 mg/15 mL; soln 80 mg/15 mL; ER 1 h caps: 300 mg; ER 12 h tabs: 200, 100, 300, 480 mg; ER 24 h caps: 100, 200, 300, 400 mg; ER 24 h tabs: 400, 600 mg **SE:** N/V, tachycardia, Szs, nervousness, arrhythmias **Notes:** *Levels IV:* Sample 12–24 h after Inf started *Therapeutic:* 5–15 mcg/mL *Toxic:* > 20 mcg/mL *Levels PO:* Trough just before next dose *Therapeutic:* 5–15 mcg/mL **Interactions:** ↑ Effects *W/* allopurinol, BBs, CCBs, cimetidine, corticosteroids, macrolide antibiotics, OCPs, quinolones, rifampin, tacrine, tetracyclines, verapamil, zileuton; ↑ effects *OF* digitalis; ↓ effects *W/* barbiturates, loop diuretics, thyroid hormones, tobacco, St. John's wort; ↓ effects *OF* benzodiazepines, Li, phenytoin **Labs:** ↑ Glucose **NIPE:** Use barrier contraception; take w/ food if GI upset; ⊘ crush/break ER tabs; caffeine foods ↑ drug effects; smoking ↓ drug effects; adeq hydration

Thiamine [Vitamin B₁] [Vitamin] **Uses:** *Thiamine deficiency (beriberi), alcoholic neuritis, Wernicke encephalopathy* **Action:** Dietary supl **Dose: *Adults.*** *Deficiency:* 5–30 mg IM or IV TID then 5–30 mg/d for 1 mo *Wernicke encephalopathy:* 100 mg IV single dose, then 100 mg/d IM for 2 wk **Peds.** 10–25 mg/d IM for 2 wk, then 5–10 mg/24 h PO for 1 mo **Caution:** [A, +] **CI:** Component allergy **Disp:** Tabs 50, 100, 250, 500 mg; Inj 100 mg/mL **SE:** Angioedema, paresthesias, rash, anaphylaxis w/rapid IV **Interactions:** ↑ Effects *OF* neuromuscular blocking drugs **Labs:** Interference w/ theophylline levels **NIPE:** IV use associated w/ anaphylactic Rxn; give IV slowly; PO take w/o regard to food

Thioguanine [6-TG] (Tabloid) [Purine Antimetabolite] **Uses:** *AML, ALL, CML* **Action:** Purine-based antimetabolite (substitutes for natural purines interfering w/ nucleotide synth) **Dose: Adult:** 2–3 mg/kg/d **Peds:** 60 mg/m²/d for 14 d no renal adjustment in peds; D/C if pt develops jaundice, VOD, portal hypertension; ↓ in severe renal/hepatic Impair **Caution:** [D,–] **CI:** Resistance to mercaptopurine **Disp:** Tabs 40 mg **SE:** ↓ BM (leukopenia/thrombocytopenia), N/V/D, anorexia, stomatitis, rash, hyperuricemia, rare hepatotox **Interactions:** ↑ Bleeding *W/* anticoagulants, NSAIDs, salicylates, thrombolytics **Labs:** ↑ Serum & urine uric acid **NIPE:** Take w/o food; ↑ fluids to 2–3 L/d; ⊘ exposure to Infxn; lower doses w/ hepatic/renal impairment; ⊘ PRG

Thioridazine (Mellaril) [Antipsychotic/Phenothiazine] **WARNING:** Dose-related QT prolongationelderly pts w/ dementia-related psychosis **Uses:** *Schizophrenia*, psychosis **Action:** Phenothiazine antipsychotic **Dose: *Adults.*** Initial: 50–100 mg PO tid; maint 200–800 mg/24 h PO in 2–4 ÷ doses **Peds > 2 y.** 0.5–3 mg/kg/24 h PO in 2–3 ÷ doses **Caution:** [C, ?] Phenothiazines, QTc-prolonging agents, Al **CI:** Phenothiazine sensitivity, severe CNS depression, severe ↑ BP, heart DZ, coma, combo w/ drugs that prolong QTc or CYPZD6 Inhib; pt w/ congenital prolonged QTc or Hx cardiac arrhythmia **Disp:** Tabs 10, 15, 25, 50, 100 mg **SE:** Low incidence of EPS; ventricular arrhythmias; ↓ BP, dizziness, drowsiness, neuroleptic malignant synd, Szs, skin discoloration, photosens, constipation, sexual dysfunction, blood dyscrasias, pigmentary retinopathy, hepatic impair **Interactions:** ↑ Effects *OF* anticholinergics, antihistamines, antihypertensives, antihistamines, CNS depressants, nitrates, EtOH; ↓ effects *W/* barbiturates, Li, tobacco; ↓ effects *OF* levodopa **Labs:** ↑ Serum LFTs; ↓ HMG, Hct, plts, WBC **NIPE:** ↑ Risk of photosens—use sunblock, take w/ food; ⊘ D/C abruptly; ↓ temperature regulation; urine color change to reddish brown; avoid EtOH, dilute PO conc in 2–4 oz Liq; monitor ECG for ↑ QT interval

Thiothixene (Generic) [Antipsychotic/Thioxanthene] WARNING: Not for dementia-related psychosis; ↑ mortality risk in elderly on antipsychotics Uses:
Psychosis **Action:** ? May antagonize dopamine receptors **Dose:** *Adults & Peds > 12 y.* Mild–mod psychosis: 2 mg PO tid, up to 20–30 mg/d. Rapid tranquilization for agitated pts: 5–10 mg q30–60min; avg: 15–30 mg total *Severe psychosis:* 5 mg PO bid; ↑ to max of 60 mg/24 h PRN *IM use:* 16–20 mg/24 h ÷ bid–qid; max 30 mg/d *Peds < 12 y.* 0.25 mg/kg/24 h PO ÷ q6–12h **Caution:** [C, ?] Avoid w/ ↑ QT interval or meds that can ↑ QT **CI:** Severe CNS depression; circulatory collapse; blood dyscrasias, phenothiazine sensitivity **Disp:** Caps 1, 2, 5, 10 mg **SE:** Drowsiness, EPS most common; ↓ BP, dizziness, drowsiness, neuroleptic malignant synd, Szs, skin discoloration, photosens, constipation, sexual dysfunction, leukopenia, neutropenia & agranulocytosis, pigmentary retinopathy, hepatic impair **Interactions:** ↑ Effects *W/* BBs; ↑ effects *OF* anticholinergics, antihistamines, antihypertensives, CNS depressants, nitrates, EtOH; ↓ effects *W/* barbiturates, Li, tobacco, caffeine; ↓ effects *OF* levodopa **Labs:** ↑ LFTs **NIPE:** ↑ Risk of photosens—use sunblock; take w/ food or H₂O; ✓ BP/peripheral edema; ⊘ D/C abruptly; ↓ temperature regulation; darkens urine color to reddish brown; dilute PO conc stat before use

Tiagabine (Gabitril) [Anticonvulsant] Uses: *Adjunct in partial Szs*,
bipolar disorder **Action:** Antiepileptic, enhances activity of GABA **Dose:** *Adults & Peds ≥ 12 y.* (*Dose if already on enzyme-inducing AED; use lower dose if not on AED*) Initial 4 mg/d PO, ↑ by 4 mg during 2nd wk; ↑ PRN by 4–8 mg/d based on response, 56 mg/d max; take w/ food **Caution:** [C,–] May ↑ suicidal risk **CI:** Component allergy **Disp:** Tabs 2, 4, 12, 16 mg **SE:** Dizziness, HA, somnolence, memory impair, tremors, N **Interactions:** ↑ Effects *W/* valproate; ↓ effects *OF* CNS depressants, EtOH; ↓ effects *W/* barbiturates, carbamazepine, phenobarbital, phenytoin, primidone, rifampin, ginkgo **NIPE:** Take w/ food; ⊘ D/C abruptly— use gradual withdrawal; used in combo w/ other anticonvulsants; change position slowly

Ticagrelor (Brilinta) WARNING: ↑ Bleeding risk; can be fatal; daily aspirin
> 100 mg may ↓ effectiveness; do not start w/ active bleeding, Hx intracranial bleed, planned CABG; if hypotensive & recent procedure, suspect bleeding;

manage any bleed w/o D/C of ticagrelor **Uses:** *↓ CV death & heart attack in ACS* **Acts:** Oral antiplatelet; reversibly binding ADP receptor antagonist Inhib **Dose:** Initial 180 mg PO w/ ASA 325 mg, then 90 mg bid w/ ASA 75–100 mg/d **Caution:** [C, –] w/ Mod hepatic impair; w/ strong CYP3A Inhib or CYP3A inducers **CI:** Hx intracranial bleed, active pathologic bleeding, severe hepatic impair **Disp:** Tabs 90 mg **SE:** Bleeding, SOB **Notes:** REMS; D/C 5 days pre-op **NIPE:** Give w/o regard to meals; bleeding precautions; notify physician of planned dental or surgical procedures

Ticarcillin/Potassium Clavulanate (Timentin) [Antibiotic/Penicillin, Beta-Lactamase Inhibitor]

Uses: *Infxns of the skin, bone, resp, & urinary tract, Abd, sepsis* **Action:** Carboxy-PCN; bactericidal; ↓ cell wall synth; clavulanic acid blocks β-lactamase *Spectrum:* Good gram(+), not MRSA; good gram(−) & anaerobes **Dose:** *Adults.* 3.1 g IV q4–6h max 24 g ticarcillin component/d *Peds.* ≤ *60 kg* (if ≥ 60 kg, adult dose). 200–300 mg/kg/d IV ÷ q4–6h; ↓ in renal failure **Caution:** [B, +/–] PCN sensitivity **Disp:** Inj ticarcillin/clavulanate acid 3.1-g/0.1-g vial **SE:** Hemolytic anemia, false(+) proteinuria **Interactions:** ↑ Effects *W/* probenecid; ↑ effects *OF* anticoagulants, MTX; ↓ effects *W/* tetracyclines, ↓ effects *OF* aminoglycosides, OCPs **Labs:** False ↑ urine glucose, false(+) urine proteins **NIPE:** Monitor for S/Sxs super Infxn; frequent loose stools may be d/t pseudomembranous colitis; use barrier contraception; often used in combo w/ aminoglycosides; penetrates CNS w/ meningeal irritation; use extra form of birth control if on OCP (eg, condoms)

Ticlopidine (Ticlid) [Antiplatelet/Platelet Aggregation Inhibitor]

WARNING: Neutropenia/agranulocytosis, TTP, aplastic anemia reported **Uses:** *↓ Risk of thrombotic stroke*, protect grafts status post-CABG, diabetic microangiopathy, ischemic heart Dz **Action:** Plt aggregation Inhib **Dose:** 250 mg PO bid w/ food **Caution:** [B, ?/–], ↑ Tox of ASA, anticoagulation, NSAIDs, theophylline; do not use w/ clopidogrel (↑ effect) **CI:** Bleeding, hepatic impair, neutropenia, ↓ plt **Disp:** Tabs 250 mg **SE:** Bleeding, GI upset, rash **Interactions:** ↑ Effects *W/* anticoagulants, cimetidine, dong quai, evening primrose oil, feverfew, garlic, ginkgo, ginseng, red clover; ↑ effects *OF* ASA, phenytoin, theophylline; ↓ effects *W/* antacids; ↓ effects *OF* cyclosporine, digoxin **Labs:** ↑ LFTs; ↓ plts, RBCs, WBCs; monitor CBC for 1st 3 mo **NIPE:** Take w/ food; minimize or avoid invasive procedures (IV insertion, IM Inj, etc), compress venipuncture sites up to 30 min

Tigecycline (Tygacil) [Antibiotic/Related to Tetracycline]

Uses: *Rx complicated skin & soft-tissue Infxns, & comp intra-Abd Infxns* **Action:** A glycycycline; binds 30 S ribosomal subunits, ↓ protein synthesis *Spectrum:* Broad gram(+), gram(−), anaerobic, some mycobacterial; *E coli, E faecalis* (vancomycin-susceptible isolates), *S aureus* (methicillin-susceptible/resistant), *Streptococcus* (*agalactiae, anginosus* grp, *pyogenes*), *Citrobacter freundii, Enterobacter cloacae, B fragilis* group, *C perfringens, Peptostreptococcus* **Dose:** 100 mg, then 50 mg q12h IV over 30–60 min **Caution:** [D, ?] Hepatic impair, monotherapy w/ intestinal perforation, not OK in peds, w/ tetracycline allergy **CI:** Component sensitivity **Disp:** Inj 50-mg vial **SE:** N/V, Inj site Rxn, anaphylaxis **Interactions:** ↑ Risk of bleeding *W/* warfarin; ↓ effectiveness *OF* hormonal contraceptives **Labs:** ↑ LFTs, BUN, Cr, PT, PTT, INR; ↓ K⁺, HMG, Hct, WBCs **NIPE:** ⊘ w/ Children; ↑ risk of photosens; monitor ECG for hypokalemia (flattened T waves); ✓ super Infxn

Timolol (Generic) [Antihypertensive/Beta-Blocker] WARNING: Exacerbation of ischemic heart Dz w/ abrupt D/C **Uses:** *HTN & MI* **Action:** β-Adrenergic receptor blocker, β₁,β₂ **Dose:** *HTN:* 10–20 mg bid or up to 60 mg/d *MI:* 10 mg bid **Caution:** [C (1st tri; Dif 2nd or 3rd tri), +] **CI:** CHF, cardiogenic shock, ↓ HR, heart block, COPD, asthma **Disp:** Tabs 5, 10, 20 mg **SE:** Sexual dysfunction, arrhythmia, dizziness, fatigue, CHF **Interactions:** ↑ Effects *W/* antihypertensives, ciprofloxacin, fentanyl, nitrates, quinidine, reserpine; ↑ bradycardia & myocardial depression *W/* cardiac glycosides, diltiazem, reserpine, tacrine, verapamil; ↑ effects *OF* epinephrine, ergots, flecainide, lidocaine, nifedipine, phenothiazine, prazosin, verapamil; ↓ effects *W/* barbiturates, cholestyramine, colestipol, NSAIDs, penicillin, rifampin, salicylates, sulfinpyrazone, theophylline; ↓ effect *OF* hypoglycemics, sulfonylureas, theophylline **Labs:** ↑ BUN, K⁺, LFTs, uric acid **NIPE:** ⊘ D/C abruptly; ↑ cold sensitivity; monitor ECG for hyperkalemia (peaked T waves)

Timolol, Ophthalmic (Betimol, Timoptic, Timoptic XE) [Antiglaucoma Agent/Beta-Blocker] Uses: *Glaucoma* **Action:** β-Blocker **Dose:** 0.25% 1 gtt bid; ↓ to daily when controlled; use 0.5% if needed; 1 gtt/d gel **Caution:** [C, ?/+] **Disp:** Soln 0.25/0.5%; Timoptic XE (0.25) gel-forming soln **SE:** Local irritation **NIPE:** Depress lacrimal sac 1 min after administration to lessen systemic absorption; administer other drops 10 min apart; ✓ BP/pulse

Timothy Grass Pollen Allergen Extract (Grastek) WARNING: Can cause life-threatening allergic Rxn (anaphylaxis, laryngopharyngeal edema); DO NOT use w/ severe unstable/uncontrolled asthma; observe for 30 min after 1st dose; Rx & train to use auto-injectable epi; may not be suitable for pts unresponsive to epi or inhaled bronchodilators (pts on BBs) or w/ certain conditions that could ↓ ability to respond to severe allergic Rxn **Uses:** *Immunotherapy of grass pollen-induced allergic rhinitis w/ or w/o conjunctivitis confirmed by + skin test or pollen-specific IgE Ab* **Action:** Allergen immunotherapy **Dose:** *Adults* & *Peds. 5–17 y:* 1 tab SL/d; do not swallow for 1 min; for sustained effect 1 pollen season after D/C may take qd × 3 consecutive y **Caution:** [B, ?/–] discuss severe allergic Rxn; if oral lesions, stop Rx, restart after healed **CI:** Severe uncontrolled/unstable asthma; hx severe systemic/local allergic reaction to SL allergen immunotherapy; component hypersensitivity **Disp:** Tabs, 30-day blister pack **SE:** Ear/oral/tongue pruritus, mouth edema, throat irritation **Notes:** 1st dose in healthcare setting; start 12 wk before expected onset of Sx; give auto-injectable epi; Peds give only w/ adult supervision; D/C with ↑ local Sx & seek care **NIPE:** Remove tab from blister immediately before taking; ⊘ touch w/dry hands; ⊘ eating/drinking 5 min after med is dissolved; wash hands after taking med; ⊘ severe asthma

Tinidazole (Tindamax) **WARNING:** Carcinogenicity has been seen in mice & rats treated chronically with metronidazole, another nitroimidazole agent **Uses:** *Trichomoniasis, giardiasis, & amebiasis: in pts age 3 & older; bacterial vaginosis: in non-PRG, adult women* **Action:** Nitroimidazole antimicrobial **Dose:** *Adults. Trichomoniasis, giardiasis:* 2 g PO w/ food × 1. For trichomoniasis, treat sexual partners *Bacterial vaginosis:* Non-PRG adult women: 2 g daily for 2 d w/ food, or 1 g once daily for 5 d w/ food *Peds > 3 y.* *Giardiasis:* 50 mg/kg (up to 2 g) × 1 w/ food *Amebiasis:* 50 mg/kg/d (up to 2 g/d) × 3 d w/ food *Amebic liver abscess:* Same up to 5 d **Caution:** [C, ?] Seizures/nephropathy reported; Vag candidiasis **CI:** Component allergy; 1st tri pregnancy, breast-feeding **Disp:** Tabs 250, 500 mg **SE:** Metallic/bitter taste, N, anorexia dyspepsia, weakness/fatigue, HA, dizziness **NIPE:** Take w/ food; ⊘ EtOH; use extra form of contraception (eg, condoms) w/ OCP use; notify physician/DDS of use before any medical or dental procedures/surgery

Tioconazole (Generic) [Antifungal] **Uses:** *Vag fungal Infxns* **Action:** Topical antifungal **Dose:** 1 applicator-full intravag hs (single dose) **Caution:** [C, ?] **CI:** Component allergy **Disp:** Vag oint 6.5% **SE:** Local burning, itching, soreness, polyuria **Interactions:** Risk *OF* inactivation of nonoxynol-9 spermicidal **NIPE:** Insert high into Vag canal; may cause staining of clothing; refrain from intercourse during drug Tx; risk of latex breakdown of condoms & diaphragm; ⊘ concurrent use w/ tampons; douches; spermicides; other Vag products

Tiotropium (Spiriva) [Bronchodilator/Anticholinergic] **Uses:** Bronchospasm w/ COPD, bronchitis, emphysema **Action:** Synthetic anticholinergic-like atropine **Dose:** 1 caps/d inhaled using HandiHaler, **do not** use w/ spacer **Caution:** [C, ?/−] BPH, NAG, MyG, renal impair **CI:** Acute bronchospasm **Disp:** Inh caps 18 mcg **SE:** URI, xerostomia **Interactions:** ↑ Effects *W/* other anticholinergic drugs **Labs:** Monitor FEV_1 or peak flow **NIPE:** ⊘ For acute resp episode; take daily at same time; rinse mouth w/ H_2O after inhalation; avoid excessive caffine products

Tirofiban (Aggrastat) [Antiplatelet Agent] **Uses:** *Acute coronary synd* **Action:** Glycoprotein IIB/IIIa Inhib **Dose:** Initial 0.4 mcg/kg/min for 30 min, followed by 0.1 mcg/kg/min 12–24 h; use in combo w/ heparin; *ECC 2010:* ACS or P **CI:** 0.4 mcg/kg/min IV for 30 min, then 0.1 mcg/kg/min for 18–24 h post PCI ↓ in renal Insuff **Caution:** [B, ?/−] **CI:** Bleeding, intracranial neoplasm, vascular malformation, stroke/surgery/trauma w/ in last 30 d, severe HTN, acute pericarditis **Disp:** Inj 50, 250 mcg/mL **SE:** Bleeding, bradycardia, coronary dissection, pelvic pain, rash **Interactions:** ↑ Bleeding risks *W/* anticoagulants, antiplts, NSAIDs, salicylates, dong quai, feverfew, garlic, ginger, ginkgo, horse chestnut; ↓

effects W/ levothyroxine, omeprazole **Labs:** ↓ HMG, Hct, plts **NIPE:** ⊘ Breast-feeding; bleeding precautions; ✓APTT prior to Tx

Tizanidine (Zanaflex) [Alpha-2-Adrenergic Agonist] Uses: *Rx spasticity* **Action:** α₂-Adrenergic agonist **Dose:** *Adults.* 4 mg q6–8h, ↑ 2–4 mg PRN max 12 mg/dose or 36 mg/d; ↓ w/ CrCl < 25 mL/min **Peds:** Not rec **Caution:** [C, ?/–] Do not use w/ potent CYP1A2 Inhib or other α₂-adrenergic agonists **CI:** w/ Fluvoxamine, ciprofloxacin; hypersensitivity **Disp:** Caps 2, 4, 6 mg; tabs 2, 4 mg **SE:** ↓ BP, ↓ HR, somnolence, hepatotox **Interactions:** ↑ Hypotension W/ other antihypertensives; ↑ CNS depression W/ baclofen, benzodiazepines, other CNS depressants; EtOH; ↑ effects W/ CYP1A2 Inhibs (amiodarone, mexiletine, propafenone, verapamil, cimetidine, famotidine, other fluoroquinolones, acyclovir, ticlopidine, zileuton, OCP) **Labs:** ↑ AST, ALT, ✓ LFT **NIPE:** ⊘ D/C abruptly; taper dose; tabs ≠ caps; ↓ BP (hypotension); change position slowly; ⊘ EtOH

Tobramycin (Nebcin) [Antibiotic/Aminoglycoside] Uses: *Serious gram(−) Infxns* **Action:** Aminoglycoside; ↓ protein synth **Spectrum:** Gram(−) bacteria (including *Pseudomonas*) **Dose:** *Adults.* Conventional dosing: 1–2.5 mg/kg/dose IV q8–12h *Once-daily dosing:* 5–7 mg/kg/dose q24h *Peds.* 2.5 mg/kg/dose IV q8h; ↓ w/ renal Insuff **Caution:** [D, –] **CI:** PRG lt; aminoglycoside sensitivity **Disp:** Inj 10, 40 mg/mL **SE:** Nephro/ototox **Notes:** Levels: *Peak:* 30 min after Inf *Trough:* < 0.5 before next dose *Therapeutic conventional: Peak:* 5–10 mcg/mL *Trough:* < 2 mcg/mL **Interactions:** ↑ Effects W/ indomethacin; ↑nephro-, neuro-, &/or ototox effects W/ aminoglycosides, amphotericin B, cephalosporins, cisplatin, IV loop diuretics, methoxyflurane, vancomycin **Labs:** ↑ BUN, Cr; ↓ serum K⁺, Na⁺, Ca²⁺, Mg²⁺, plt, WBC; follow CrCl & levels **NIPE:** ✓ Fluids to 2–3 L/d; monitor for super Infxn; monitor ECG for hypokalemia (flattened T waves); ✓ hrg; visual; balance; GU disturbance; ✓ Sx super Infxn

Tobramycin, Inhalation (TOBI, TOBI Podhaler) Uses: *CF pts w/ P aeruginosa* **Acts:** Aminoglycoside; ↓ protein synth **Spectrum:** Gram (–) bacteria **Dose:** *Adults/Peds > 6 y.* 300 mg inhal q12h by nebulizer, cycle 28 d on 28 d off **Caution:** [D, –] w/ Renal/auditory/vestibular/neuromuscular dysfunction; avoid w/ other neuro/nephro/ototoxic drugs **CI:** Aminoglycoside sensitivity **Disp:** 300 mg vials for nebulizer *TOBI Podhaler:* 4-wk supply (56 blister caps w/ inhaler device plus reserve) **SE:** Cough, productive cough, lung disorders, dyspnea, pyrexia, oropharyngeal pain, dysphonia, hemoptysis, ↓ hearing **Notes:** Do not mix w/ dornase alfa in nebulizer; safety not established in Peds < 6 y, or w/ FEV₁ < 25% or > 80%, or if colonized w/ *Burkholderia cepacia* **NIPE:** Store soln in refrigerator at 36–46°F; use last if taking other inhaled medications (eg, bronchodilator)

Tobramycin Ophthalmic (AKTob, Tobrex) [Antibiotic/Aminogly-coside] Uses: *Ocular bacterial Infxns* **Action:** Aminoglycoside **Dose:** 1–2 gtt q2–4h; oint bid–tid; if severe, use oint q3–4h, or 2 gtt q60 min, then less frequently **Caution:** [B, –] **CI:** Aminoglycoside sensitivity **Disp:** Oint & soln tobramycin 0.3% **SE:** Ocular irritation **NIPE:** Depress lacrimal sac for 1 min to prevent systemic absorption; ↑ risk of blurred vision & burning; ✓ for redness; swelling; itching; tearing

Tobramycin & Dexamethasone Ophthalmic (TobraDex) [Antibiotic/Anti-Inflammatory] Uses: *Ocular bacterial Infxns associated w/ sig inflammation* Action: Antibiotic w/ anti-inflammatory Dose: 0.3% oint apply q6–8h or soln 0.3% apply 1–2 gtt q4–6h (↑ to q2h for first 24–48 h) Caution: [C, M] CI: Aminoglycoside sensitivity, viral, fungal, or mycobacterium Infxn of eye Disp: Oint & susp 2.5, 5, & 10 mL tobramycin 0.3% & dexamethasone 0.1% SE: Local irritation/edema NIPE: Eval IOP & lens if prolonged use; use under ophthalmologist's direction

Tocilizumab (Actemra) [Interleukin-6 Receptor Inhibitor] WARNING: May cause serious Infxn (TB, bacterial, invasive fungal, viral, opportunistic); w/ serious Infxn stop tocilizumab until Infxn controlled Uses: *Mod–severe RA, SJIA* Action: IL-6 receptor Inhib Dose: RA 4–8 mg/kg q4wk; SJIA if < 30 kg 12 mg/kg q2wk; if > 30 kg 8 mg/kg q2wk Caution: [C; ?/–] ANC < 2000/mm³, plt count < 100,000, AST/ALT > 1.5 ULN; serious Infxn; high-risk bowel perforation CI: Hypersensitivity Disp: Inj 20 mg/mL SE: URI, nasopharyngitis, HA, HTN, ↑ ALT, ↑ AST, rash, D, ↑ LDL ↓ ANC Interactions: ↑ Risk of Infxn *W/* concomitant immunosuppressants (eg, TNF antagonists IL-1R antagonists, anti-CD20 MoAb, selective costimulation modulators) Labs: ↑ ALT, ↑ AST, ↑ LDL ↓ ANC; ✓ CBC/plt counts, LFTs, lipids; monitor lipids 4–8 wk after initiation, then every 6 mo NIPE: Do not give live vaccines; PPD, if + treat before starting, w/ prior Hx retreat unless adequate Tx confirmed, monitor for TB, even if –PPD; ↓ mRNA expression of several CYP450 isoenzymes (CYP3A4); D/C w/ acute Infxn; OI; sepsis

Tofacitinib (Xeljanz) WARNING: Serious Infxns (bacterial, viral, fungal, TB, opportunistic) possible. D/C w/ severe Infxn until controlled; test for TB w/ Tx; lymphoma/other CA possible; possible EBV-associated renal transplant lymphoproliferative disorder Uses: *Mod–severe RA w/ inadequate response/ intolerance to MTX* Action: Janus kinase Inhib Dose: *Adults.* 5 mg PO bid; ↓ 5 mg once daily w/ mod–severe renal & mod hepatic impair, w/ potent Inhib CYP3A4, w/ meds w/ both mod Inhib CYP3A4 & potent Inhib CYP2C19 Caution: [C, –] Do not use w/ active Infxn, w/ severe hepatic impair, w/ biologic DMARDs, immunosuppressants, live vaccines, w/ risk of GI perforation CI: None Disp: Tabs 5 mg SE: D, HA, URI, nasopharyngitis, ↑ LFTs, HTN, anemia Notes: OK w/ MTX or other nonbiologic DMARDs; ✓ CBC, LFTs, lipids NIPE: Take w/o regard to food; consider D/C w/ acute Infxn; OI; sepsis; ⊘ breast feeding; ⊘ live virus vaccines

Tolazamide (Generic) [Hypoglycemic/Sulfonylurea] Uses: *Type 2 DM* Action: Sulfonylurea; ↑ pancreatic insulin release; ↑ peripheral insulin sensitivity; ↓ hepatic glucose output Dose: 100–500 mg/d (no benefit > 1 g/d) Caution: [C, ?/–] Elderly, hepatic or renal impair; G6PD deficiency = ↑ risk for hemolytic anemia CI: Component hypersensitivity, DM type 1, DKA Disp: Tabs

250, 500 mg **SE:** HA, dizziness, GI upset, rash, hyperglycemia, photosens, blood dyscrasias **Interactions:** BB may mask hypoglycemia; ↑ effects *W/* chloramphenicol, cimetidine, clofibrate, insulin, MAOIs, phenylbutazone, probenecid, salicylates, sulfonamides, garlic, ginseng; ↓ effects *W/* diuretics **NIPE:** Risk of disulfiram-type Rxn w/ EtOH; take with 1st meal of the day; use sunblock

Tolbutamide (Generic) [Hypoglycemic/Sulfonylurea] **Uses:** *Type 2 DM* **Action:** Sulfonylurea; ↑ pancreatic insulin release; ↑ peripheral insulin sensitivity; ↓ hepatic glucose output **Dose:** 500–1000 mg bid; 3 g/d max; ↓ in hepatic failure **Caution:** [C, −] G6PD deficiency = ↑ risk hemolytic anemia **CI:** Sulfonylurea sensitivity **Disp:** Tabs 500 mg **SE:** HA, dizziness, GI upset, rash, photosens, blood dyscrasias, hypoglycemia, heartburn **Interactions:** ↑ Effects *W/* anticoagulants, azole antifungals, chloramphenicol, insulin, H₂-antagonists, MAOIs, metformin, phenylbutazone, probenecid, salicylates, sulfonamides, TCAs; ↓ effects *W/* BBs (can mask hypoglycemia), CCBs, cholestyramine, corticosteroids, hydantoins, INH, OCPs, phenothiazine, phenytoin, rifampin, sympathomimetics, thiazides, thyroid drugs **NIPE:** Risk of disulfiram-type Rxn w/ EtOH; take w/ food; use barrier contraception; ↑ risk of photosensitivity—use sunblock.

Tolcapone (Tasmar) [Anti-Parkinson Agent/COMT Inhibitor]
WARNING: Cases of fulminant liver failure resulting in death have occurred **Uses:** *Adjunct to carbidopa/levodopa in Parkinson Dz* **Action:** Catechol-*O*-methyltransferase Inhib slows levodopa metabolism **Dose:** 100 mg PO tid w/ 1st daily levodopa/carbidopa dose, then dose 6 &12 h later; ↓ w/ renal Insuff **Caution:** [C, ?] **CI:** Hepatic impair; w/ nonselective MAOI; nontraumatic rhabdomyolysis or hyperpyrexia **Disp:** Tabs 100 mg **SE:** Constipation, xerostomia, vivid dreams, hallucinations, anorexia, N/D, orthostasis, liver failure, rhabdomyolysis **Interactions:** ↑ Effects *OF* CNS depressants, SSRIs, TCAs, warfarin, EtOH; ↑ risk of hypertension crisis *W/* nonselective MAOIs (phenelzine, tranylcypromine) **Labs:** Monitor LFTs **NIPE:** May give w/o regard to food; bioavailability of drug; may experience hallucinations; ⊘ abruptly D/C or ↓ dose; change position slowly; ✓ S/Sx hepatotoxicity

Tolmetin (Generic) [Analgesic, Anti-Inflammatory, Antipyretic/ NSAID] **WARNING:** May ↑ risk of CV events & GI bleeding **Uses:** *Arthritis & pain* **Action:** NSAID; ↓ prostaglandins **Dose:** 400 mg PO tid titrate up max 1.8 g/d max **Caution:** [C, −] **CI:** NSAID or ASA sensitivity; use for pain CABG **Disp:** Tabs 200, 600 mg; caps 400 mg **SE:** Dizziness, rash, GI upset, edema, GI bleeding, renal failure **Interactions:** ↑ Effect *OF* aminoglycosides, anticoagulants, cyclosporine, digoxin, insulin, Li, MRX, K⁺-sparing diuretics, sulfonylureas; ↓ effect *W/* ASA, food; ↓ effect *OF* furosemide, thiazides **Labs:** ↑ ALT, AST, serum K⁺, BUN, ↓ HMG, Hct **NIPE:** Take w/ food if GI upset; ↑ risk of photosensitivity— use sunblock; monitor ECG for hyperkalemia (peaked T waves)

Tolnaftate (Tinactin) [OTC] [Antifungal] **Uses:** *Tinea pedis, cruris, corporis, manus, versicolor* **Action:** Topical antifungal **Dose:** Apply to area bid for 2–4 wk **Caution:** [C, ?] **CI:** Nail & scalp Infxns **Disp:** OTC 1% liq; gel; powder; topical cream; ointment, powder, spray skin **SE:** Local irritation **NIPE:** Avoid ocular contact; Infxn should improve in 7–10 d; ⊘ w/ children < 2 y

Tolterodine (Detrol, Detrol LA) [Anticholinergic/Muscarinic Antagonist] Uses: *OAB (frequency, urgency, incontinence)* **Action:** Anticholinergic **Dose:** *Detrol:* 1–2 mg PO bid; *Detrol LA:* 2–4 mg/d **Caution:** [C,–] w/ CYP2D6 & 3A3/4 Inhib (Table 10) w/ QT prolongation **CI:** Urinary retention, gastric retention, or uncontrolled NAG **Disp:** Tabs 1, 2 mg; *Detrol LA* tabs 2, 4 mg **SE:** Xerostomia, blurred vision, HA, constipation **Interactions:** ↑ Effects **W/** azole antifungals, macrolides, grapefruit juice, food; ↑ anticholinergic effects **W/** amantadine, amoxapine, bupropion, clozapine, cyclobenzaprine, disopyramide, olanzapine, phenothiazine, TCAs **NIPE:** May cause blurred vision/dizziness; LA form may see "intact" pill in stool

Tolvaptan (Samsca) [Vasopressin V$_2$-Receptor Antagonist] **WARNING:** Hospital use only w/ close monitoring of Na$^+$; too rapid Na$^+$ correction can cause severe neurologic Sx. Correct slowly w/ ↑ risk (malnutrition, alcoholism, liver Dz) Uses: *Hypervolemic or euvolemic ↓ Na$^+$* **Action:** Vasopressin V$_2$-receptor antagonist **Dose:** *Adults.* 15 mg PO daily; after ≥ 24 h, may ↑ to 30 mg × 1 daily; max 60 mg × d; titrate at 24-h intervals to Na$^+$ goal **Caution:** [C, –] Monitor Na$^+$, volume, neurologic status; GI bleed risk **W/** cirrhosis, avoid w/ CYP3A inducers & moderate Inhib, ↓ dose **W/** P-gp Inhib, ↑ K$^+$ **CI:** Hypovolemic hyponatremia; urgent need to raise Na$^+$; in pts incapable of sensing/reacting to thirst; anuria; **W/** strong CYP3A Inhib **Disp:** Tabs 15, 30 mg **SE:** N, xerostomia, pollakiuria, polyuria, thirst, weakness, constipation, hyperglycemia **Interactions:** Do not use **W/** strong Inhibs of CYP3A (amiodarone, amprenavir, atazanavir, ciprofloxacin, cisapride, clarithromycin, diltiazem, erythromycin, fluconazole, fluvoxamine, indinavir, itraconazole, ketoconazole, nefazodone, verapamil, grapefruit juice); avoid concomitant use **W/** CYP3A inducers (carbamazepine, efavirenz, glucocorticoids, macrolides, nevirapine, phenytoin, phenobarbital, rifabutin, rifapentine, rifampin, St. John's wort) (see Table 10) **NIPE:** Pts can't drink in response to thirst; too rapid correction of serum Na (> 12 mEq/L/24 h) can cause serious neurologic sequelae (osmotic demyelination resulting in dysarthria, mutism, dysphagia, lethargy, effective changes, spastic quadriparesis, Szs, coma & death)

Topiramate (Topamax, Trokendi XR, Generic) Uses: *Initial monotherapy or adjunctive for complex partial Szs & tonic–clonic Szs; adjunct for Lennox-Gastaut synd*, bipolar disorder, neuropathic pain, migraine prophylaxis **Action:** Anticonvulsant **Dose:** *Adults. Seizures:* Total dose 400 mg/d; see PI for 8-wk schedule. *Migraine Px:* Titrate 100 m/d total. *Peds 2–9.* See label; ↓ w/ renal impair **Caution:** [D, ?/–] visual field defects unrelated to ↑ ocular pressure, nystagmus, acute glaucoma requires D/C; memory impair, psychomotor slowing, suicidal ideation/behavior, metabolic acidosis, kidney stones, hyperthermia,

↓ sweating, embryofetal toxicity, ↑ ammonia w/ encephalopathy **CI:** Component allergy; for ER recent EtOH use or w/ metabolic acidosis **Disp:** Tabs 25, 50, 100, 200 mg; caps sprinkles 15, 25 mg; ER Caps 25, 50, 100, 200 mg **SE:** Somnolence, fatigue, paresthesias, wgt loss, GI upset, tremor, ↓ serum HCO_3^- **Notes:** If metabolic acidosis, ↓ dose or D/C or give alkali Tx; ✓ bicarbonate; when D/C must taper; ✓ efficacy of OCPs; use w/ phenytoin or carbamazepine ↓ topiramate levels; monitor HCO_3^- if on carbonic anhydrase Inhib; Li levels ↑, ✓ if taking both; avoid other CNS depressants **NIPE:** Take w/o regard to food; ○ break/crush tabs; ○ D/C abruptly; ○ EtOH; use alternative contraception method w/OCP (eg, condoms)

Topotecan (Hycamtin) [Antineoplastic] WARNING: Chemotherapy precautions, for use by physicians familiar w/ chemotherapeutic agents, BM suppression possible **Uses:** *Ovarian CA (cisplatin-refractory), cervical CA, NSCLC*, sarcoma, ped NSCLC **Action:** Topoisomerase I Inhib; ↓ DNA synth **Dose:** 1.5 mg/m²/d as a 1-h IV Inf × 5 d, repeat q3wk; ↓ w/ renal impair **Caution:** [D, –] **CI:** PRG, breast-feeding, severe bone marrow suppression **Disp:** Inj 4-mg vials; caps 0.25, 1.0 mg **SE:** ↑ BM, N/V/D, drug fever, skin rash, interstitial lung disease **Interactions:** ↑ Myelosuppression **W/** cisplatin, other neoplastic drugs, radiation therapy; ↑ in duration of neutropenia **W/** filgrastim **Labs:** ↑ AST, ALT, bilirubin; ↓ HMG, Hct, plt, WBCs **NIPE:** Monitor CBC; ○ PRG, breast-feeding, immunizations; ○ exposure to Infxn; barrier contraception; rash loss is reversible

Torsemide (Demadex) [Antihypertensive/Loop Diuretic] **Uses:** *Edema, HTN, CHF, & hepatic cirrhosis* **Action:** Loop diuretic; ↓ reabsorption of Na^+ & Cl^- in ascending loop of Henle & distal tubule **Dose:** 5–20 mg/d PO or IV; 200 mg/d max **Caution:** [B, ?] **CI:** Sulfonylurea sensitivity, anuria **Disp:** Tabs 5, 10, 20, 100 mg; Inj 10 mg/mL **SE:** Orthostatic ↓ BP, HA, dizziness, photosens, electrolyte imbalance, blurred vision, renal impair **Interactions:** ↑ Risk of ototox **W/** aminoglycosides, cisplatin; ↑ effects **W/** thiazides; ↓ effects **OF** anticoagulants, antihypertensives, Li, salicylates; ↓ effects **W/** barbiturates, carbamazepine, cholestyramine, NSAIDs, phenytoin, phenobarbital, probenecid, dandelion **Labs:** Monitor lytes, BUN, Cr, glucose, uric acid **NIPE:** Take w/o regard to food; take in AM; monitor for S/Sxs tinnitus; 10–20 mg torsemide = 40 mg furosemide = 1 mg bumetanide; monitor ECG for hypokalemia (flattened T waves)

Tramadol (Rybix ODT, Ryzolt ER, Ultram, Ultram ER) [Centrally Acting Analgesic/Nonnarcotic] **Uses:** *Mod–severe pain* **Action:** Centrally acting synthetic opiod analgesic **Dose:** *Adults.* 50–100 mg PO q4–6h PRN, start 25 mg PO qAM, ↑ q3d to 25 mg PO qid; ↑ 50 mg q3d, 400 mg/d max (300 mg if > 75 y); ER 100–300 mg PO daily; Rybix ODT individualize ↑ 50 mg/d q3d to 200 mg/d or 50 mg qid; after titration 50–100 mg q4–6 PRN, 400 mg/d max **Peds.** (ER form not rec) 1–2 mg/kg q4–6h PRN (max dose 100 mg); ↓ w/ renal Insuff **Caution:** [C, –] Suicide risk in addiction prone, w/ tranquilizers or antidepressants; ↑ Szs risk w/ MAOI; seratonin syndrome **CI:** Opioid dependency; w/ MAOIs; sensitivity to opioids, acute alcohol intoxication, hypnotics, centrally acting analgesics, or w/ psychotropic drugs **Disp:** Tabs 50 mg; ER 100, 200, 300 mg; Rybix ODT 50 mg **SE:** Dizziness, HA, somnolence, GI upset, resp depression, anaphylaxis **Interactions:** ↑ Effects *W/* antihistamines, CNS depressants, phenothiazine, quinidine, TCAs, EtOH; ↑ risk of serotonin synd *W/* MAOIs, St. John's wort; ↑ effects *OF* digoxin,warfarin; ↓ effects *W/* carbamazepine **Labs:** ↑ Cr, LFTs, ↓ HMG **NIPE:** Take w/ regard to food; ⊘ cut, chew ODT tabs; ↓ Sz threshold; tolerance/dependence may develop; has mu-opioid agonist activity; monitor for abuse; ⊘ EtOH

Tramadol/Acetaminophen (Ultracet) [Centrally Acting Analgesic/Nonnarcotic] Uses: *Short-term Rx acute pain (< 5 d)* Action: Centrally acting opioid analgesic w/ APAP **Dose:** 2 tabs PO q4–6h PRN; 8 tabs/d max *Elderly/renal impair:* Lowest possible dose; 2 tabs q12h max if CrCl < 30 mL/min **Caution:** [C, −] Szs, hepatic/renal impair, suicide risk in addiction prone, w/ tranquilizers or antidepressants **CI:** Acute intoxication, w/ ethanol, hypnotics, central acting analgesics or psychotropic drugs, hepatic dysfunction **Disp:** Tab 37.5 mg tramadol/325 mg APAP **SE:** SSRIs, TCAs, opioids, MAOIs ↑ risk of Szs; dizziness, somnolence, tremor, HA, N/V/D, constipation, xerostomia, liver tox, rash, pruritus, ↑ sweating, physical dependence **Interactions:** ↑ Effects *W/* CNS depressants, MAOIs, phenothiazines, quinidine, TCAs, EtOH; ↑ risk of serotonin synd *W/* MAOIs, St. John's wort; ↑ effects *OF* digoxin, warfarin; ↓ effects *W/* carbamazepine **Labs:** ↑ Cr, LFTs **NIPE:** Take w/o regard to food; ⊘ take other APAP-containing drugs; ⊘ EtOH; has mu-opioid agonist activity; monitor for abuse

Trametinib (Mekinist) Uses: *Metastatic melanoma w/ BRAF V600E or V600K mutations; single drug or combo w/ dabrafenib* **Action:** TKI **Dose:** *Adults.* 2 mg 1 ×/d; may need to reduce dose or hold or discontinue for SEs or toxicity **Caution:** [D, −] w/ dabrafenib new cutaneous & noncutaneous Ca can occur, bleeding, DVT/PE, cardiomyopathy; ocular toxicity, retinal vein thrombosis; cardiomyopathy; ocular toxicity, ILD, serious skin reactions; ↑ glu; embryofetal toxicity **CI:** None **Disp:** Tabs 0.5, 1, 2 mg **SE:** Fever, chills, night sweats, N/V/D, constipation, abd pain, anorexia, fatigue, HA, arthralgias/myalgias, cough; rash; lymphedema; hemolytic anemia w/ G6PD def; ↑glucose; ↑AST, ↑ALT, ↑alk phos, ↓ albumin, ↓ WBC, plt **Notes:** Not a single agent if prior BRAF-Inhib Tx; ✓ LV function before, 1 mo after start & q2–3mo; hold w/ pulm Sx; ✓ glu & monitor w/ DM or ↑glu; D/C w/ retinal vein thrombosis, ILD, pneumonitis or rash, grade 2, 3, or 4 not improved after off 3 wk; w/ dabrafenib avoid Inhib or inducers CYP3A4/CYP2C8; use contraception during & 4 mo post-Tx; w/ dabrafenib, must use nonhormonal contraception (class kinase Inhib) **NIPE:** Take 1 h ac/2 h pc; ✓ skin for new lesions

Trandolapril (Mavik) [Antihypertensive/ACEI] WARNING: Use in PRG in 2nd/3rd tri can result in fetal death **Uses:** *HTN*, heart failure, LVD, post-AMI **Action:** ACE Inhib **Dose:** *HTN:* 1–4 mg/d *Heart failure/LVD:* Start 1 mg/d, titrate to 4 mg/d; ↓ w/ severe renal/hepatic impair **Caution:** [C first, D in 2nd + 3rd, −] ACE Inhib sensitivity, angioedema w/ ACE Inhib **Disp:** Tabs 1, 2, 4 mg

SE: ↓ BP, ↓ HR, dizziness, ↑ K⁺; GI upset, renal impair, cough, angioedema **Interactions:** ↑ Effects *W/* diuretics; ↑ effects *OF* insulin, Li; ↓ effects *W/* ASA, NSAIDs **Labs:** ↑ K⁺ **NIPE:** ⊘ PRG or breast-feeding; ⊘ K⁺-containing salt substitutes; minimum dose is 2 mg in African Americans vs 1 mg in whites; monitor ECG for hyperkalemia (peaked T waves)

Tranexamic Acid (Lysteda) [Antifibrinolytic]
Uses: *↓ Cyclic heavy menstrual bleeding* **Action:** ↓ Dissolution of hemostatic fibrin by plasmin **Dose:** 2 Tabs tid (3900 mg/d) 5 d max during monthly menstruation; ↓ w/ renal impair (see label) **Caution:** [B, +/−] ↑ thrombosis risk **CI:** Component sensitivity; active or ↑ thrombosis risk **Disp:** Tabs 650 mg; Inj 100 mg/mL **SE:** HA, sinus & nasal symptoms, Abd pain, back/musculoskeletal/Jt pain, cramps, migraine, anemia, fatigue, retinal/ocular occlusion; allergic Rxns **Interactions:** ↑ Risk of MI/ CVA *W/* hormonal contraceptives, Factor IX products, anti-Inhib coagulant concentrates, oral tretinoin **NIPE:** Take w/o regard to food w/ 8 oz H₂O; ⊘ crush/break/ chew tab

Tranylcypromine (Parnate) [MAOI]
WARNING: Antidepressants ↑ risk of suicidal thinking & behavior in children & adolescents w/ MDD & other psychiatric disorders **Uses:** *Depression* **Action:** MAOI **Dose:** 30 mg/d PO ÷ doses, may ↑ 10 mg/d over 1–3 wk to max 60 mg/d **Caution:** [C; +/−] Minimize foods w/ tyramine **CI:** CV Dz, cerebrovascular defects, Pheo, w/ MAOIs, TCAs, SSRIs, SNRIs, sympathomimetics, bupropion, meperidine, dextromethorphan, buspirone **Disp:** Tabs 10 mg **SE:** Orthostatic hypotension, ↑ HR, sexual dysfunction, xerostomia **Interactions:** ↑ Risk of hypertensive crisis *W/* sympathomimetics (eg, amphetamines, pseudoephedrine), levodopa, high-tyramine foods (eg, cheese, salami, chocolate, wine, beer, yogurt, broadbeans, yeast); ↑ CNS depression *W/* other CNS depressants (eg, MAOIs, TCAs, SSRI, SNRIs, EtOH, opiates, buspirone); ↑ risk of psychosis *W/* dextromethorphan; ↑ risk of circulatory collapse, coma/death *W/* meperidine **Labs:** False(+) amphetamine drug test **NIPE:** Minimize foods w/ tyramine; ⊘ abruptly D/C; may mask angina pain; may potentiate anxiety or agitation

Trastuzumab (Herceptin) [Antineoplastic/Monoclonal Antibody]
WARNING: Can cause cardiomyopathy & ventricular dysfunction; Inf Rxns & pulm tox reported; use during PRG can lead to pulm hypoplasia, skeletal malformations, & neonatal death **Uses:** *Met breast CA that overexpress the HER2/neu protein*, breast CA adjuvant, w/ doxorubicin, cyclophosphamide, & paclitaxel if pt HER2/neu(+) **Action:** MoAb; binds human EGFR 2 protein (HER2); mediates cellular cytotoxicity **Dose:** Per protocol, typical 2 mg/kg/IV/wk **Caution:** [D, −/−] CV dysfunction, allergy/Inf Rxns **CI:** None **Disp:** Inj 440 mg **SE:** Anemia, cardiomyopathy, nephrotic synd, pneumonitis, N/V/D, rash, pain, fever, HA, insomnia **Interactions:** ↑ Risk of cardiac dysfunction *W/* anthracyclines, cyclophosphamide, doxorubicin, epirubicin **Labs:** Monitor cardiac Fxn cardiomyopathy, ventricular dysfunction, & pulm tox have been reported; ↓ HMG, Hct,

WBCs **NIPE:** ⊘ Use dextrose Inf soln; ⊘ breast-feed; ⊘ immunizations w/o physician approval; ✓ cardiac function decline for 6 mo following drug therapy; Inf-related Rxns minimized w/ APAP, diphenhydramine, & meperidine

Trazodone (Oleptro) [Antidepressant] **WARNING:** Closely monitor for worsening depression or emergence of suicidality, particularly in pts < 24 y; Oleptro not approved in peds **Uses:** *Depression*, hypnotic, augment other antidepressants **Action:** Antidepressant; ↓ reuptake of serotonin & norepinephrine **Dose: *Adults & Adolescents. Desyrel:*** 50–150 mg PO daily–tid; max 600 mg/d *Sleep:* 25–50 mg PO, qhs, PRN *Adults. Oleptro:* Start 150 mg PO qd, may ↑ by 75 mg q3d; take qhs on empty stomach **Caution:** [C, ?/–] Serotonin/neuroleptic malignant syndromes reported; ↑ QTc; may activate manic states; syncope reported; may ↑ bleeding risk; avoid w/in 14 d of MAOI **CI:** Component allergy **Disp:** *Desyrel:* Tabs 50, 100, 150, 300 mg; *Oleptro:* Scored tabs 150, 300 mg **SE:** Dizziness, HA, sedation, N, xerostomia, syncope, confusion, libido, ejaculation dysfunction, tremor, hep, EPS **Interactions:** ↑ Effects W/ fluoxetine, phenothiazines; ↑ risk of serotonin synd W/ MAOIs, SSRIs, venlafaxine, St. John's wort; ↑ CNS depression W/ barbiturates, CNS depressants, opioids, sedatives, EtOH; ↑ hypotension W/ antihypertensive, neuroleptics; nitrates, EtOH; ↑ effects *OF* clonidine, digoxin, phenytoin; ↓ effects W/ potent CYP3A4 inducers (carbamazepine) (Table 10); CYP3A4 Inhibs to ↑ trazodone conc (nefazodone, ritonavir, indinavir, ketoconazole, itraconazole) (see Table 10) **NIPE:** ↑ Fluids to 2–3 L/d; ⊘ D/C abruptly; takes 1–2 wk for Sx improvement

Treprostinil (Remodulin, Tyvaso) [Antihypertensive/Vasodilator] **Uses:** *NYHA Class II–IV pulm arterial HTN* **Action:** Vasodilation, ↓ plt aggregation **Dose:** *Remodulin.* 0.625–1.25 ng/kg/min cont Inf/SQ (preferred), titrate to effect *Tyvaso:* Initial: 18 mcg (3 Inh) q4h 4 ✍/d; if not tolerated, ↓ to 1–2 inhals, then ↑ to 3 inhal *Maint:* ↑ additional 3 inhal 1–2 wk intervals; 54 mcg (or 9 inhal) 4 ✕/d max **Caution:** [B, ?/–] Component allergy **Disp:** *Remodulin* Inj 1, 2.5, 5, 10 mg/mL *Tyvaso:* 0.6 mg/mL (2.9 mL) ~ 6 mg/Inhal **SE:** Additive effects w/ anticoagulants, antihypertensives; Inf site Rxns; D, N, HA, ↓ BP **Interactions:** ↑ Effects W/ CYP2C8 Inhibs (eg, gemfibrozil); ↑ risk of hypotension W/ antihypertensives, diuretics, other vasodilators; ↑ risk of bleeding W/ anticoagulants; ↓ effects W/ CYP2C8 inducers (eg, rifampin) **NIPE:** Teach care of Inf site & pump; use barrier contraception; once med vial used discard after 14 d; initiate in monitored setting; ⊘ D/C use or ↓ dose abruptly (risk of rebound HTN)

Treprostinil, Extended Release (Orenitram) **Uses:** *Pulm arterial ↑ BP to improve exercise capacity* **Action:** Vasodilator **Dose: *Adults.*** Start 0.25 mg bid; ↑ by 0.25 or 0.5 mg bid or 0.125 mg tid q3–4d; max dose based on tolerance **Caution:** [C, ?/–] ↑ risk of bleeding; ⊘ take with EtOH; ⊘ abruptly DC; tabs may lode in colonic diverticulum **CI:** Severe hepatic Dz **Disp:** ER Tabs 0.125, 0.25, 1, 2.5 mg **SE:** HA, N, D, Abd pain, flushing, pain in jaw or extrem, ↓ K+ **Notes:** Risk of ↓ BP w/ antihypertensive drugs; if co-admin w/ strong CYP2C8 Inhib starting dose 0.125 mg bid; Inhib plt aggregation

Tretinoin, Topical [Retinoic Acid] (Avita, Retin-A, Renova, Retin-A Micro) [Retinoid/Antineoplastic] Uses: *Acne vulgaris, sun-damaged skin, wrinkles* (photo aging), some skin CAs Action: Exfoliant retinoic acid derivative Dose: *Adults & Peds > 12 y.* Apply daily hs (w/ irritation, ↓ frequency) *Photoaging:* Start w/ 0.025%, ↑ to 0.1% over several mo (apply only q3d if on neck area; dark skin may require bid use) Caution: [C, ?] CI: Retinoid sensitivity Disp: Cream 0.02, 0.025, 0.05, 0.0375, 0.1%; gel 0.01, 0.025, 0.05%; microformulation gel 0.1, 0.04% SE: Avoid sunlight; edema; skin dryness, erythema, scaling, changes in pigmentation, stinging, photosens Interactions: ↑ Photosens W/ quinolones, phenothiazines, sulfonamides, tetracyclines, thiazides, dong quai. St. John's wort; ↑ skin irritation W/ topical sulfur, resorcinol, benzoylperoxide, salicylic acid; ↑ effects W/ vit A supl & foods W/ excess vit A such as fish oils NIPE: ⊘ Apply to mucous membranes, wash skin & apply med after 30 min, wash hands after application; ⊘ breastfeeding, PRG use contraception; use sunblock; ⊘ use on sunburned skin

Triamcinolone/Nystatin (Mycolog-II) [Anti-Inflammatory, Antifungal/Corticosteroid] Uses: *Cutaneous candidiasis* Action: Antifungal & anti-inflammatory Dose: Apply lightly to area bid; max 25 mg/d Caution: [C, ?] CI: Varicella; systemic fungal Infxns Disp: Cream & oint; triamcinolone 1 mg/g & 100,000 units nystatin/g SE: Local irritation, hypertrichosis, pigmentation changes Interactions: ↓ Effects W/ barbiturates, phenytoin, rifampin; ↓ effects OF salicylates, vaccines NIPE: ⊘ Eyes; ⊘ apply to open skin/wounds, mucous membranes; for short-term use (< 7 d); apply sparingly.

Triamterene (Dyrenium) [Diuretic/Potassium-Sparing Agent] WARNING: Hyperkalemia can occur Uses: *Edema associated w/ CHF, cirrhosis* Action: K+-sparing diuretic Dose: *Adults.* 100–300 mg/24 h PO ÷ daily–bid *Peds. HTN:* 2–4 mg/kg/d in 1–2 ÷ doses; ↓ w/ renal/hepatic impair Caution: [C (Expert opinion), ?] CI: ↑ K+, renal impair; caution w/ other K+-sparing diuretics Disp: Caps 50, 100 mg SE: ↓ K+, ↓ BP, bradycardia, cough, HA Interactions: ↑ Risk of hyperkalemia W/ ACEIs, K+ supls, K+-sparing drugs, K+-containing drugs, K+ salt substitutes; ↑ effects W/ cimetidine, indomethacin; ↑ effects OF amantadine, antihypertensives, Li; ↓ effects OF digitalis Labs: ↑ LFTs, BUN, Cr, glucose, uric acid; ↓ HMG, Hct, plt, K+ NIPE: Take w/ food in AM; blue discoloration of urine, ↑ risk of photosens—use sunblock; avoid foods high in K+, salt substitutes

Triazolam (Halcion) [C-IV] [Sedative/Hypnotic/Benzodiazepine] Uses: *Short-term management of insomnia* Action: Benzodiazepine Dose: 0.125–0.25 mg/d PO hs PRN; ↓ in elderly Caution: [X, ?/–] CI: Concurrent fosamprenavir, ritonavir, indinavir, itraconazole, ketoconazole, nefazodone, or other moderate/strong CYP3A4 Inhib; PRG Disp: Tabs 0.125, 0.25 mg SE: Tachycardia, CP, drowsiness, fatigue, memory impair, GI upset Interactions: ↑ Effects W/ azole antifungals, cimetidine, clarithromycin, ciprofloxin, CNS depressants, disulfiram, digoxin, erythromycin, fluvoxamine, INH, protease Inhibs, troleandomycin, verapamil, EtOH, grapefruit juice, kava kava, valerian; additive CNS depression **W/** EtOH & other CNS depressants; ↓ effects **OF** levodopa; ↓ effects **W/** carbamazepine, phenytoin, rifampin, theophylline **NIPE:** ⊘ PRG or breast-feeding; ⊘ D/C abruptly after long-term use; do not prescribe > 1 mo supply; ⊘ grapefruit juice

Triethylenethiophosphoramide (Thiotepa, Thioplex, Tespa, TSPA) [Alkylating Agent]
Uses: *Breast, ovarian CAs, lymphomas (infrequently used) preparative regimens for allogeneic & ABMT w/ high doses, intravesical for bladder CA, intracavitary effusion control* **Action:** Polyfunctional alkylating agent **Dose:** Per protocol typical 0.3–0.4 mg/kg IV q1–4wk *Effusions:* Intracavitary 0.6–0.8 mg/kg; 60 mg into the bladder & retained 2 h q1–4wk; 900–125 mg/m² in ABMT regimens (highest dose w/o ABMT is 180 mg/m²); ↓ in renal failure **Caution:** [D, –] w/ BM suppression, renal & hepatic impair **CI:** Component allergy **Disp:** Inj 15 mg/vial **SE:** ↓ BM, N/V, dizziness, HA, allergy, paresthesias, alopecia **Interactions:** ↑ Tox **W/** concomitant or sequential alkylating agents (nitrogen mustards, cyclophosphamide), radiation, myelosuppressants **Labs:** Monitor LFT, BUN, SCr; Monitor HMG & plts weekly during Tx & 3 wk > therapy; D/C if WBC ≤ 3000/mm³ or plt ≤ 150,000/mm³ **NIPE:** Caution w/ handling/preparing med (cytotoxic); use effective contraception; notify physician of S/Sx blding (bruising, epitaxis, black stool)

Trifluoperazine (Generic) [Antipsychotic/Phenothiazine]
WARNING: ↑ Mortality in elderly patients **W/** dementia-related psychosis **Uses:** *Psychotic disorders* **Action:** Phenothiazine; blocks postsynaptic CNS dopaminergic receptors **Dose:** *Adults. Schizophrenia/psychosis:* Initial 1–2 mg PO bid (out pt) or 2–5 mg PO bid (in pt). Typical 15–20 mg/d, max 40 mg/d *Non-psychotic anxiety:* 1–2 mg PO/d, 6 mg/d max *Peds 6–12 y.* 1 mg PO daily–bid initial, gradually ↑ to 15 mg/d; ↓ in elderly/debilitated pts **Caution:** [C, ?/–] [±] w/ BM dyscrasias; phenothiazinesens; severe hepatic Dz **Disp:** Tabs 1, 2, 5, 10 mg **SE:** Orthostatic ↓ BP, EPS, dizziness, neuroleptic malignant synd, skin discoloration, lowered Sz threshold, photosens, blood dyscrasias **Interactions:** ↑ CNS depression **W/** barbiturates, benzodiazepines, TCAs, EtOH; ↑ effects **OF** antihypertensives, propranolol, ↓ effects **OF** anticoagulants ↓ effects **W/** antacids **Labs:** ↑ LFTs; ↓ WBCs **NIPE:** ↑ Risk of photosens—use sunblock; urine color may change to pink to reddish-brown; PO conc must be diluted to 60 mL or more prior to administration; requires several wk for onset of effects; ⊘ EtOH

Trifluridine Ophthalmic (Viroptic) [Antiviral]
Uses: *Herpes simplex keratitis & conjunctivitis* **Action:** Antiviral **Dose:** 1 gtt q2h, max 9 gtt/d; ↑ to 1 gtt q4h × 7 d after healing begins; Rx up to 21 d **Caution:** [C, ?] **CI:** Component allergy **Disp:** Soln 1% **SE:** Local burning, stinging **NIPE:** ⊘ < 6 y of age; reeval if no improvement in 7 d

Trihexyphenidyl (Generic) [Anti-Parkinson Agent/Anticholinergic]
Uses: *Parkinson Dz, drug-induced EPS* **Action:** Blocks excess acetylcholine

at cerebral synapses **Dose:** *Parkinson:* 1 mg PO daily, ↑ by 2 mg q3–5d to usual dose 6–10 mg/d in 3–4 ÷ doses. *EPS:* 1 mg PO daily ↑ to 5–15 mg/d 3–4 ÷ doses **Caution:** [C, –] **CI:** NAG, GI obst, MyG, BOO Dzgn **Disp:** Tabs 2, 5 mg; elixir 2 mg/5 mL **SE:** Dry mouth, constipation, xerostomia, photosens, tachycardia, arrhythmias **Interactions:** ↑ Effects *W/* MAOIs, phenothiazine, quinidine, TCAs; ↑ effects *OF* amantadine, anticholinergics, digoxin; ↓ effects *OF* antacids, tacrine; ↓ effects *OF* chlorpromazine, haloperidol, tacrine **NIPE:** Take w/ food; monitor for urinary hesitancy or retention; ⊘ D/C abruptly; ↑ risk of heat stroke; ↑ risk of CNS depression w/ concurrent EtOH use; ✓ elderly for paradoxical effect

Trimethobenzamide (Tigan) **[Antiemetic/Anticholinergic]**
Uses: *N/V* **Action:** ↓ Medullary chemoreceptor trigger zone **Dose:** *Adults.* 300 mg PO or 200 mg IM tid–qid PRN **Caution:** [C, ?] **CI:** Benzocaine sensitivity; children < 40 kg **Disp:** Caps 300 mg; Inj 100 mg/mL **SE:** Drowsiness, ↓ BP, dizziness; hepatic impair, blood dyscrasias, Szs, parkinsonian-like synd **Interactions:** ↑ CNS depression *W/* antidepressants, antihistamines, opioids, sedatives, EtOH; ↑ risk *OF* extrapyramidal effects **NIPE:** In the presence of viral Infxns, may mask emesis or mimic CNS effects of Reye synd

Trimethoprim (Primsol) [Antibiotic/Folate Antagonist] **Uses:** *UTI d/t susceptible gram(+) & gram(−) organisms; Rx PCP w/ dapsone* suppression of UTI **Action:** ↓ Dihydrofolate reductase *Spectrum:* Many gram(+) & (−) except *Bacteroides, Branhamella, Brucella, Chlamydia, Clostridium, Mycobacterium, Mycoplasma, Nocardia, Neisseria, Pseudomonas,* & *Treponema* **Dose:** *Adults.* 100 mg PO bid or 200 mg PO daily; PCP 5 mg/kg ÷ in 3 d w/ dapsone *Peds.* ≥ 2 *mo:* 4–6 mg/kg/d in 2 ÷ doses; otitis media (> or equal to 6 mo): 10 mg/kg/d in 2 ÷ doses × 10 d; ↓ w/ renal failure **Caution:** [C, +] **CI:** Megaloblastic anemia d/t folate deficiency **Disp:** Tabs 100 mg; (Primsol) PO soln 50 mg/5 mL **SE:** Rash, pruritus, megaloblastic anemia, hepatic impair, blood dyscrasias **Interactions:** ↑ Effects *W/* dapsone; ↑ effects *OF* dapsone, phenytoin, procainamide; ↓ efficacy *W/* rifampin **Labs:** ↑ BUN, Cr, bilirubin **NIPE:** ↑ Fluids to 2–3 L/d; ↑ risk of hematologic toxicity (fatigue, fever, pale skin, sore throat, bleeding/bruising), use sunblock

Trimethoprim (TMP)–Sulfamethoxazole (SMX) [Co-Trimoxazole] (Bactrim, Bactrim DS, Septra DS) [Antibiotic/Folate Antagonist] **Uses:** *UTI Rx & prophylaxis, otitis media, sinusitis, bronchitis, prevent PCP pneumonia (w/ CD4 count < 200 cells/mm³)* **Action:** SMX ↓ synth of dihydrofolic acid; TMP ↓ dihydrofolate reductase to impair protein synth *Spectrum:* Includes *Shigella,* PCP, & *Nocardia* Infxns, *Mycoplasma, Enterobacter* sp, *Staphylococcus, Streptococcus,* & more **Dose:** All doses based on TMP *Adults.* 1 DS tab PO bid or 8–20 mg/kg/24 h IV in 1–2 ÷ doses *PCP:* 15–20 mg/kg/d IV or PO (TMP) in 4 ÷ doses *Nocardia:* 10–15 mg/kg/d IV or PO (TMP) in 4 ÷ doses *PCP prophylaxis:* 1 reg tab daily or DS tab 3 × wk *UTI prophylaxis:* 1 PO daily *Peds.* 8–10 mg/kg/24 h PO ÷ in 2 doses or 3–4 doses IV; do not use in < 2 mo; ↓ in renal failure; maintain hydration **Caution:** [C (D if near term), –] **CI:** Sulfonamide sensitivity, porphyria, megaloblastic anemia w/ folate deficiency, PRF, breast-feeding Inf < 2 mo, sig hepatic impair **Disp:** Regular tabs 80 mg TMP/400 mg SMX; DS tabs 160 mg TMP/400 mg SMX PO susp 40 mg TMP/200 mg SMX/5 mL; Inj 80 mg TMP/400 mg SMX/5 mL **SE:** Allergic skin Rxns, photosens, GI upset, SJS, blood dyscrasias, hep **Interactions:** ↑ Effect *OF* dapsone, MTX, phenytoin, sulfonylureas, warfarin, zidovudine; ↓ effects *W/* rifampin; ↓ effect *OF* cyclosporine **Labs:** ↑ Serum bilirubin, alk phos, BUN, Cr **NIPE:** ↑ Risk of photosens—use sunscreen; ↑ fluids to 2–3 L/d; synergistic combo; reinforce need to complete full course of therapy

Triptorelin (Trelstar 3.75, Trelstar 11.25, Trelstar 22.5) [Antineoplastic/Gonadotropin-Releasing Hormone]

Uses: *Palliation of advanced PCa* **Action:** LHRH analogue; ↓ GnRH w/ cont dosing; transient ↑ in LH, FSH, testosterone, & estradiol 7–10 d after 1st dose; w/ chronic use (usually 2–4 wk), sustained ↓ LH & FSH w/ ↓ testicular & ovarian steroidogenesis similar to surgical castration **Dose:** 3.75 mg IM q4wk; or 11.25 mg IM q12wk or 22.5 mg **Caution:** [X, N/A] **CI:** Not indicated in females **Disp:** Inj Depot 3.75 mg; 11.25 mg; 22.5 mg **SE:** Dizziness, emotional lability, fatigue, HA, insomnia, HTN, D/V, ED, retention, UTI, pruritus, anemia, Inj site pain, musculoskeletal pain, osteoporosis, allergic Rxns **Interactions:** ↑ Risk of severe hyperprolactinemia *W/* antipsychotics, metoclopramide **Labs:** ✓ Periodic testosterone levels; suppression of pituitary-gonadal Fxn; monitor for ↑ glucose **NIPE:** May cause hot flashes; initial ↑ bone pain & may cause spinal cord compression leading to paralysis & death; only 6 mo formulation; ✓ worsening S/Sx prostate CA in 1st wk of Tx

Trospium (Sanctura, Sanctura XR) [Antispasmodic/Anticholinergic]

Uses: *OAB w/ Sx of urge incontinence, urgency, frequency* **Action:** Muscarinic antagonist, ↓ bladder smooth muscle tone **Dose:** 20 mg tabs PO bid; 60 mg ER caps PO daily AM, 1 h ac or on empty stomach. ↓ w/ CrCl < 30 mL/min & elderly **Caution:** [C, +/–] w/ EtOH use, in hot environments, UC, MyG, renal/hepatic impair **CI:** Urinary/gastric retention, NAG **Disp:** Tab 20 mg; caps ER 60 mg **SE:** Dry mouth, constipation, HA, rash **Interactions:** ↑ Effects *W/* amiloride, digoxin, morphine, metformin, procainamide, tenofovir, vancomycin; ↑ effects *OF* anticholinergics, amiloride, digoxin, morphine, metformin, procainamide, tenofovir, vancomycin **NIPE:** Take w/o food 1 h ac; ⊘ crush/break tab; ER caps swallow whole; ↑ risk of heat exhaustion/stroke, ↑ drowsiness w/ EtOH

Ulipristal Acetate (Ella) [Progesterone Agonist/Antagonist]

Uses: *Emergency contraceptive for PRG prevention (unprotected sex/contraceptive failure)* **Action:** Progesterone agonist/antagonist, delays ovulation **Dose:** 1 Tab PO (30 mg) PO ASAP w/in 5 d of unprotected sex or contraceptive failure **Caution:** [X, –] CYP3A4 inducers ↓ effect **CI:** PRG **Disp:** Tab 30 mg **SE:** HA, N, Abd, dysmenorrhea **Interactions:** ↑ Effects w/ CYP3A4 Inhibs (eg, ketoconazole, itraconazole); ↓ effectiveness *W/* CYP3A4 inducers (barbiturates, bosentan, carbamazepine, felbamate, griseofulvin, oxcarbazepine, phenytoin, rifampin, topiramate, St. John's wort) **NIPE:** Not for routine contraception; fertility after use unchanged, maintain routine contraception; use any ⍉ of menstrual cycle; ⊘ PRG; ⊘ menopause

Umeclidinium/Vilanterol (Anoro Ellipta) WARNING: LABA, such as vilanterol, ↑ risk of asthma-related death; the safety & efficacy in asthma has not been established **Uses:** *Maintenance COPD* **Action:** Combo antimuscarinic (anticholinergic) & LABA (B₂) **Dose:** 1 inhal/D **Caution:** [C, ?/–] May cause asthma-related death; not for acute exacerbations or deteriorations; do not use w/ other LABA; paradoxical bronchospasm; caution w/ CV Dz, seizure hx, thyrotoxicosis, DM, ketoacidosis, NAG, & Hx of urinary retention or BPH **CI:** hypersensitivity to milk proteins **Disp:** Inhaler w/ double-foil blister strips of powder, 62.5 mcg umeclidinium & 25 mg vilanterol **SE:** Sinusitis, pharyngitis, resp Infxn, D, constipation, pain (chest, neck, extremities); ↓ K⁺, á glucose **Notes:** DO NOT use to Tx asthma; caution w/ MAOIs, TCA, BBs (may block bronchodilator effect); diuretics (may potentiate ↓ K⁺); other anticholinergic meds; strong P450 3A4 Inhib **NIPE:** Do not use for acute Sx; do not stop w/o physician guidance; ⊘ use of additional LABA

Ustekinumab (Stelara) [Interleukin-12 & Interleukin-23 Antagonist] Uses: *Mod–severe plaque psoriasis* **Action:** Human IL-12 & IL-23 antagonist **Dose:** Wt < 100 kg, 45 mg SQ initially & 4 wk later, then 90 mg q12wk. Wgt > 100 kg, 90 mg SQ initially & 4 wk later, then 90 mg q12wk **Caution:** [B/ ?] **Disp:** Prefilled syringe & single-dose vial 45 mg/0.5 mL, 90 mg/1 mL **SE:** Nasopharyngitis, URI, HA, fatigue **Interactions:** W/ Concomitant live vaccines, other immunosuppressants, phototherapy **NIPE:** Do not use w/ live vaccines; do not give BCG vaccines during or w/in 1 y of starting or stopping ustekinumab; do not start w/ active Infxns; D/C if serious Infxn develops; instruct on Inj techniques; 1st self-Inj under supervision

Valacyclovir (Valtrex, Generic) [Antiviral/Synthetic Purine Nucleoside] Uses: *Herpes zoster; genital herpes; herpes labialis* **Action:** Prodrug of acyclovir; ↓ viral DNA replication **Spectrum:** Herpes simplex I & II **Dose:** Zoster: 1 g PO tid × 7 d Genital herpes (initial episode): 1 g bid × 7–10 d, (recurrent) 500 mg PO bid × 3 d. Herpes prophylaxis: 500–1000 mg/d Herpes labialis: 2g PO q12h × 1 d ↓ w/ renal failure **Caution:** [B, +] ↑ CNS effects in elderly **Disp:** Caplets 500, 1000 mg; tab 500, 1000 mg **SE:** HA, GI upset, ↑ LFTs, dizziness, pruritus, photophobia **Interactions:** ↑ Effects W/ cimetidine, probenecid **Labs:** ↑ LFTs, Cr ↓ HMG, Hct, plt, WBCs **NIPE:** Take w/o regard to food; ↑ fluids to 2–3 L/d; begin drug at 1st sign of S/Sxs; dose evenly; complete full Tx course

Valganciclovir (Valcyte) [Antiviral/Synthetic Nucleoside] WARNING: Granulocytopenia, anemia, & thrombocytopenia reported. Carcinogenic, teratogenic, & may cause aspermatogenesis **Uses:** *CMV retinitis & CMV prophylaxis in solid-organ transplantation* **Action:** Ganciclovir prodrug; ↓ viral DNA synth **Dose:** *CMV Retinitis induction:* 900 mg PO bid w/ food × 21 d, then 900 mg PO daily *CMV prevention:* 900 mg PO daily × 100 d post transplant, ↓ w/ renal dysfunction **Caution:** [C, ?/–] Use w/ imipenem/cilastatin, nephrotoxic drugs; ANC < 500 cells/mL; plt < 25,000 cells/mcL; Hgb < 8 g/dL **CI:** Allergy to acyclovir, ganciclovir, valganciclovir **Disp:** Tabs 450 mg; oral solution: 50 mg/mL **SE:** BM suppression, HA, GI upset **Interactions:** ↑ Effects *W/* cytotoxic drugs, immunosuppressive drugs, probenecid; ↑ risks of nephrotox *W/* amphotericin B, cyclosporine; ↑ effects *W/* didanosine **Labs:** ↑ Cr; monitor CBC & Cr, monitor glucose for hypoglycemia **NIPE:** Take w/ food; ⊘ PRG, breast-feeding, EtOH, NSAIDs; use contraception for at least 3 mo after drug Rx; ✓ CBC; ✓ vision

Valproic Acid (Depakene, Depakote, Stavzor, Generic) [Anticonvulsant/Carboxylic Acid Derivative]   WARNING: Fatal hepatic failure (usually during first 6 mo of Tx, peds < 2 y high risk, monitor LFTs at baseline & frequent intervals), teratogenic effects, & life-threatening pancreatitis reported

Uses: *Rx epilepsy, mania; prophylaxis of migraines*, Alzheimer behavior disorder **Action:** Anticonvulsant; ↑ availability of GABA **Dose:** *Adults & Peds. Szs:* 10–15 mg/kg/24 h PO ÷ tid (after initiation by 5–10 mg/kg/d weekly basis until therapeutic levels) *Mania:* 750 mg in 3 ÷ doses, ↑ 60 mg/kg/d max *Migraines:* 250 mg bid, ↑ 1000 mg/d max; ↓ w/ hepatic impair **Caution:** [D, –] Multiple drug interactions **CI:** Severe hepatic impair, urea cycle disorder **Disp:** Caps 250 mg; caps w/ coated particles 125 mg; tabs DR 125, 250, 500 mg; tabs ER 250, 500 mg; caps DR (Stavzor) 125, 250, 500 mg; syrup 250 mg/5 mL; Inj 100 mg/mL **SE:** Somnolence, dizziness, GI upset, diplopia, ataxia, rash, thrombocytopenia, ↓ plt hep, pancreatitis, ↑ bleeding times, alopecia, ↑ wgt, ↑ hyperammonemic encephalopathy in pts w/ urea cycle disorders; if taken during PRG may cause lower IQ tests in children **Notes:** *Trough:* Just before next dose *Therapeutic: Peak:* 50–100 mcg/mL *Toxic trough:* > 100 mcg/mL *1/2-life:* 5–20 h; phenobarbital & phenytoin may alter levels **Interactions:** ↑ Effects *W/* clarithromycin, erythromycin, felbamate, INH, phenytoin, salicylates, troleandomycin; ↑ effects *OF* anticoagulants, lamotrigine, nimodipine, phenobarbital, phenytoin, primidone, zidovudine; ↑ CNS depression *W/* CNS depressants, haloperidol, loxapine, maprotiline, MAOIs, phenothiazine, thioxanthenes, TCAs, EtOH; ↓ effects *W/* cholestyramine, colestipol; ↓ effects *OF* clozapine, rifampin **Labs:** ↑ LFTs; altered TFTs; monitor LFTs & serum levels **NIPE:** Take w/ food for GI upset; ⊘ PRG, breast-feeding; ⊘ D/C abruptly—↑ risk of Szs; reinforce strict adherence; report suicidal ideation

Valsartan (Diovan) [Antihypertensive/ARB]   WARNING: Use during 2nd/3rd tri of PRG can cause fetal harm

Uses: HTN, CHF, DN **Action:** Angiotensin II receptor antagonist **Dose:** 80–160 mg/d, max 320 mg/d **Caution:** [D, ?/–] w/ K⁺-sparing diuretics or K⁺ supls **CI:** Severe hepatic impair, biliary cirrhosis/obst, primary hyperaldosteronism, bilateral RAS **Disp:** Tabs 40, 80, 160, 320 mg **SE:** ↓ BP, dizziness, HA, viral Infxn, fatigue, Abd pain, D, arthralgia, fatigue, back pain, hyperkalemia, cough, ↑ Cr **Interactions:** ↑ Effects

W/ diuretics, Li; ↑ risk of hyperkalemia *W/* K⁺-sparing diuretics, K⁺ supls, TMP **Labs:** ↑ K⁺, ↑ Cr **NIPE:** Take w/o regard to food; ⊘ PRG, breast-feeding; use contraception; monitor ECG for hyperkalemia (peaked T waves); do not use K⁺ supplements/salt substitutes

Vancomycin (Vancocin, Generic) [Antibiotic/Glycopeptide]
Uses: *Serious MRSA Infxns; enterococcal Infxns; PO Rx of S aureus & C difficile pseudomembranous colitis* **Action:** ↓ Cell wall synth **Spectrum:** Gram(+) bacteria & some anaerobes (includes MRSA, *Staphylococcus*, *Enterococcus*, *Streptococcus* sp, *C difficile*) **Dose:** *Adults.*15–20 mg/kg IV q8–48h based on CrCl, 15–20 mg/kg/ dose *C difficile:* 125–500 mg PO q 6h × 7 d *Peds.* 40–60 mg/kg/d IV in ÷ doses q6–12h *C difficile:* 40 mg/kg/d PO in ÷ 3–4 doses × 7–10 d **Caution:** [B oral + C Inj, −] **CI:** Component allergy; avoid in Hx hearing loss **Disp:** Caps 125, 250 mg; powder for Inj **SE:** Oto-/nephrotox, GI upset (PO) **Labs:** Levels: *Peak:* 1 h after Inf *Trough:* < 0.5 h before next dose *Therapeutic: Peak:* 20–40 mcg/mL *Trough:* 10–20 mcg/mL *Toxic peak:* > 50 mcg/mL *Trough:* > 20 mcg/mL *1/2-life:* 6–8 h **Interactions:** ↑ Ototox & nephrotox *W/* ASA, aminoglycosides, cyclosporine, cisplatin, loop diuretics; ↓ effects *OF* MRX **Labs:** ↑ BUN, Cr; ↓ WBC **NIPE:** Take w/ food, ↑ fluid to 2–3 L/d; not absorbed PO, local effect in gut only; give IV dose slowly (over 1–3 h) to prevent "red-man synd" (flushing of head/neck/upper torso); IV product used PO for colitis; ✓ rash; hearing; dose evenly; complete full Tx course

Vandetanib (Caprelsa) WARNING: Can ↑ QT interval, torsades de pointes, sudden death; do not use in pts w/ ↑ K⁺, ↓ Ca²⁺, ↓ Mg²⁺, prolonged QT, avoid drugs that prolong QT, monitor QT baseline, 2-4 wk, 8–12 wk, then q3mo **Uses:** *Advanced medullary thyroid CA* **Action:** Multi-TKI Inhib **Dose:** *Adults.* 300 mg/d; ↓ dose w/ ↓ renal Fxn **Caution:** [D, –] Can ↑ QT; avoid w/ CYP3A inducers or drugs that ↑ QT (eg, amiodarone, sotalol, clarithromycin); avoid w/ mod–severe liver impair **CI:** Prolonged QT synd **Disp:** Tabs 100, 300 mg **SE:** Anorexia, Abd pain, N/V, HA, ↑ BP, reversible posterior leukoencephalopathy synd (PRES), fatigue, rash (eg, acne), ↑ QT interval, ILD **Notes:** Half-life 19 d; restricted distribution, providers and pharmacies must be certified; may need ↑ thyroid replacement **NIPE:** ✓ EKG wk 2–4, 8–12 then q3mo; ✓ lytes; ✓ visual acuity; ⊘ PRG, breast-feeding

Vardenafil (Levitra, Staxyn, Generic) [Anti-Impotence Agent/ PDE5] Uses: *ED* **Action:** PDE5 Inhib, increases cyclic guanosine monophosphate (cGMP) & NO levels; relaxes smooth muscles, dilates cavernosal arteries **Dose:** *Levitra* 10 mg PO 60 min before sexual activity; titrate; max × 1 = 20 mg; 2.5 mg w/ CYP3A4 Inhib (Table 10) *Staxyn* 1 (10 mg ODT) 60 min before sex, max 1 ×/d **Caution:** [B, –] w/ CV, hepatic, or renal Dz or if sex activity not advisable; potentiate the hypotensive effects of nitrates, alpha-blockers, and antihypertensives **CI:** w/ Nitrates **Disp:** *Levitra* Tabs 2.5, 5, 10, 20 mg tabs; *Staxyn* 10 mg ODT (contains phenylalanine) **SE:** ↑ QT interval, ↓ BP, HA, dyspepsia, priapism, flushing, rhinitis, sinusitis, flu synd, sudden ↓/loss of hearing, tinnitus,

NIAON **Interactions:** ↑ Effects W/ erythromycin, ketoconazole indinavir, ritonavir; ↑ risk of hypotension W/ α-blockers, nitrates **NIPE:** Take w/o regard to food; ↑ risk of priapism; transient global amnesia reported; place Staxyn on tongue to disintegrate w/o Liqs; ODT not equal to oral pill; gets higher levels; do not take with nitrates/grapefruit juice

Varenicline (Chantix) [Nicotinic Acetylcholine Receptor Partial Agonist] **WARNING:** Serious neuropsychiatric events (depression, suicidal ideation/attempt) reported **Uses:** *Smoking cessation* **Action:** Nicotine receptor partial agonist **Dose:** *Adults.* 0.5 mg PO daily × 3 d, 0.5 mg bid × 4 d, then 1 mg PO bid for 12 wk total; after meal w/ glass of H_2O **Caution:** [C, ?/–] ↓ Dose w/ renal impair, may increase risk of CV events in pts w/ CV Dz **Disp:** Tabs 0.5, 1 mg **SE:** Serious psychological disturbances, N, V, insomnia, flatulence, constipation, unusual dreams **Interactions:** May affect metabolism of warfarin, theophylline, insulin; ↑ effects W/ nicotine-replacement drugs **NIPE:** Slowly ↑ dose to ↓ N; initiate 1 wk before desired smoking cessation date; monitor for changes in behavior; use of additional smoking cessation OTC nicotine-replacement drugs may ↑ adverse effects; take w/ food & 8 oz H_2O; ⊘ crush, break, or dissolve

Varicella Immune Globulin (VariZIG) [Investigational, call (800) 843-7477] **WARNING:** Prepared from pools of human plasma, which may contain causative agents of hep & other viral Dz; may cause rare hypersensitivity w/ shock (investigational, call (800) 843-7477) **Uses:** Postexposure prophylaxis for persons w/o immunity, exposure likely to result in Infxn (household contact > 5 min) & ↑ risk for severe Dz (immunosuppression, PRG) **Action:** Passive immunization **Dose:** 125 units/10 kg up to 625 units IV (over 3–5 min) or IM (deltoid or proximal thigh); give w/in 4–5 d (best < 72 h) of exposure **Caution:** [?, –] Indicated for PRG women exposed to varicella zoster **CI:** IgA deficiency, Hx, anaphylaxis to immunoglobulins; known immunity to varicella zoster **Disp:** Inj 125-mg unit vials **SE:** Inj site Rxn, dizziness, fever, HA, N; ARF, thrombosis rare **NIPE:** Wait 5 mo before varicella vaccination after varicella immune globulin; may ↓ vaccine effectiveness; observe for varicella for 28 d; if VariZIG administration not possible w/in 96 h of exposure, consider administration of IGIV (400 mg/kg); ⊘ use with h/o anaphylactic reactions to other human immune globulin preparations

Varicella Virus Vaccine (Varivax) [Vaccine] **Uses:** *Prevent varicella (chickenpox)* **Action:** Active immunization w/ live attenuated virus **Dose:** *Adults & Peds > 12 mo.* 0.5 mL SQ, repeat 4–8 wk **Caution:** [C, M] **CI:** Immunosuppression; PRG, fever, untreated TB, neomycin-anaphylactoid Rxn; **Disp:** Powder for Inj, acute febrile Infxn **SE:** Varicella rash, generalized or at Inj site, arthralgias/myalgias, fatigue, fever, HA, irritability, GI upset **Interactions:** ↓ Effects W/ acyclovir, immunosuppressant drugs **NIPE:** OK for all children & adults who have not had chickenpox; ⊘ salicylates for 6 wk after immunization; ⊘ PRG for 3 mo after immunization; do not give w/in 3 mo of immunoglobulin

(IgG) & no IgG w/in 2 mo of vaccination; avoid high-risk people for 6 wk after vaccination

Vasopressin [Antidiuretic Hormone, ADH] (Pitressin, Generic) [Antidiuretic Hormone/Posterior Pituitary Hormone] Uses: *DI; Rx post-op Abd distention*; adjunct Rx of GI bleeding & esophageal varices; asystole, PEA, pulseless VT & VF, adjunct systemic vasopressor (IV drip) **Action:** Posterior pituitary hormone, potent GI & peripheral vasoconstrictor **Dose:** ***Adults & Peds. DI:*** 5–10 units SQ or IM bid–tid *GI hemorrhage:* 0.2–0.4 units/min; ↓ in cirrhosis; caution in vascular Dz *VT/VF:* 40 units IV push × 1 *Vasopressor:* 0.01–0.03 units/min *Peds. (ECC 2010). Cardiac arrest:* 0.4–1 unit/kg IV/IO bolus; max dose 40 units *Hypotension:* 0.2–2 MU/kg/min cont Inf **Caution:** [C, +] w/ Vascular Dz **CI:** Allergy **Disp:** Inj 20 units/mL **SE:** HTN, arrhythmias, fever, vertigo, GI upset, tremor **Interactions:** ↑ Vasopressor effects *W/* guanethidine, neostigmine; ↑ antidiuretic effects *W/* carbamazepine, chlorpropamide, clofibrate, phenformin urea, TCAs; ↓ antidiuretic effects *W/* demeclocycline, epi, heparin, Li, phenytoin, EtOH **Labs:** ↑ Cortisol level **NIPE:** ✓ I&O; ✓ wgts at baseline & daily; ✓ VS; ✓ Sx of GI bleeding

Vecuronium (Generic) [Skeletal Muscle Relaxant/Nondepolarizing Neuromuscular Blocker] WARNING: To be administered only by appropriately trained individuals **Uses:** *Skeletal muscle relaxation* **Action:** Nondepolarizing neuromuscular blocker; onset 2–3 min **Dose:** *Adults & Peds.* 0.1–0.2 mg/kg IV bolus (also rapid intubation *ECC 2010*); maint 0.010–0.015 mg/kg after 25–40 min; additional doses q12–15min PRN; ↓ w/ severe renal/hepatic impair **Caution:** [C, ?] Drug interactions cause ↑ effect (eg, aminoglycosides, tetracycline, succinylcholine) **CI:** Component hypersensitivity **Disp:** Powder for Inj 10, 20 mg **SE:** ↓ HR, ↓ BP, itching, rash, tachycardia, CV collapse, muscle weakness **Interactions:** ↑ Neuromuscular blockade *W/* amikacin, clindamycin, gentamicin, neomycin, streptomycin, tobramycin, general anesthetics, quinidine, tetracyclines; ↑ resp depression *W/* opioids; ↓ effects *W/* phenytoin **NIPE:** Will not provide pain relief or sedation; fewer cardiac effects than succinylcholine; synergistic effects with opioids, anesthetics or sedatives

Vemurafenib (Zelboraf) **Uses:** *Unresectable metastatic melanoma w/ BRAF mutation* **Action:** BRAF serine-threonine kinase Inhib **Dose:** *Adults.* 960 mg bid **Caution:** [D, –] If on warfarin, monitor closely **CI:** None **Disp:** Tab 240 mg **SE:** Rash including SJS; anaphylaxis, pruritus, alopecia, photosens, arthralgias, skin SCC (> 20%), ↑ QT **Notes:** ✓ Derm exams q2mo for SCC; monitor ECG 15 days and qmo × 3; if QTc > 500 ms, D/C temporarily; mod CYP1A2 Inhib, weak CYP2D6 Inhib and CYP3A4 inducer **NIPE:** Give w/o regard to food; do not crush, break or dissolve; ⊘ PRG; ✓ skin changes; use contraception during Tx

Venlafaxine (Effexor, Effexor XR, Generic) [Antidepressant/Serotonin, Norepinephrine, & Dopamine Reuptake Inhibitor] WARNING: Monitor for worsening depression or emergence of suicidality, particularly in ped pts **Uses:** *Depression, generalized anxiety, social anxiety disorder; panic disorder*, OCD, chronic fatigue synd, ADHD, autism **Action:** Potentiation of CNS neurotransmitter activity **Dose:** 75–225 mg/d ÷ in 2–3 equal doses (IR) or daily (ER); 375 mg IR or 225 mg ER max/d ↓ w/ renal/hepatic impair **Caution:** [C, ?/–] **CI:** MAOIs **Disp:** Tabs IR 25, 37.5, 50, 75, 100 mg; ER caps 37.5, 75, 150 mg **SE:** HTN, ↑ HR, HA, somnolence, xerostomia, insomnia, GI upset, sexual dysfunction; actuates mania or Szs **Interactions:** ↑ Effects *W/* cimetidine, desipramine, haloperidol, MAOIs; ↑ risk of serotonin synd *W/* sumatriptan, trazodone, St. John's wort **NIPE:** XR caps swallow whole—⊘ chew; take w/ food; ⊘ use EtOH; ⊘ D/C abruptly; D/C MAOI 14 d before start of this drug; ↑ fluids to 2–3L/d; may take 2–3 wk for full; report suicidal ideation/increase in depression effects; frequent edema & wgt gain; may ↑ risk of mania & hypomania

Vernal, Orchard, Perennial Rye, Timothy and Kentucky Blue Grass Mixed Pollens Allergenic Extract (Oralair)
WARNING: Can cause life-threatening allergic Rxn (anaphylaxis, laryngopharyngeal edema); ⊘ use w/ severe unstable/uncontrolled asthma; observe for 30 min after 1st dose; Rx and train to use auto-injectable epi; may not be suitable for pts unresponsive to epi or inhaled bronchodilators (pts on BBs) or w/ certain conditions that could ↓ ability to respond to severe allergic Rxn **Uses:** *Immunotherapy of grass pollen-induced allergic rhinitis w/ or w/o conjunctivitis confirmed by + skin test or pollen-specific IgE Ab* **Action:** Allergen immunotherapy **Dose:** *Adults.* 300 IR SL × 1/d *Peds.* 100 IR SL d 1, 2 × 100 IR SL d 2, and then 300 IR SL qd starting d 3 (not approved age < 10 y) **Caution:** [B, ?/–] Discuss severe allergic Rxn; if oral lesions, stop Tx, restart after healed **CI:** Severe uncontrolled/unstable asthma; h/o severe systemic allergic reaction or severe local reaction to SL allergen immunotherapy; hypersensitivity **Disp:** Tabs 100, 300 IR **SE:** Pruritus of mouth, tongue, or ear; mouth/lip edema, throat irritation, oropharyngeal pain, cough **Notes:** 1st dose in healthcare setting; ⊘ eat w/in 5 min of admin; start Tx 4 mo before expected onset of Sx; have auto-injectable epi available **NIPE:** ✓ For 30 min after initial dose; wash hands before/after taking tablet; leave under tongue × 5 min before swallowing

Verapamil (Calan, Covera HS, Isoptin, Verelan, Generic) [Antihypertensive, Antianginal, Antiarrhythmic/CCB] **Uses:** *Angina, HTN, PSVT, AF, atrial flutter*, migraine prophylaxis, hypertrophic cardiomyopathy, bipolar Dz **Action:** CCB **Dose:** *Adults.* **Arrhythmias:** 2nd line for PSVT w/ narrow QRS complex & adequate BP 2.5–5 mg IV over 1–2 min; repeat 5–10 mg in 15–30 min PRN (30 mg max) *Angina:* 80–120 mg PO tid, ↑ 480 mg/24 h max *HTN:* 80–180 mg PO tid or SR tabs 120–240 mg PO daily to 240 mg bid *ECC 2010:* Reentry SVT w/ narrow QRS: 2.5–5 mg IV over 2 min (slower in older pts); repeat 5–10 mg, in 15–30 min PRN max of 20 mg; or 5-mg bolus q15min (max 30 mg) *Peds <1 y.* 0.1–0.2 mg/kg IV over 2 min (may repeat in 30 min) *1–16 y.* 0.1–0.3 mg/kg IV over 2 min (may repeat in 30 min); 5 mg max *PO:* 3–4 mg/kg/d PO ÷ in 3 doses, max 8 mg/kg/d up to 480 mg/d *> 5 y.* 80 mg q6–8h; ↓ in renal/hepatic impair

Caution: [C, +] Amiodarone/β-blockers/flecainide can cause ↓ HR; statins, midazolam, tacrolimus, theophylline levels may be ↑; use w/ clonidine may cause severe ↓ HR w/ elderly pts CI: EF < 30%, severe LV dysfunction, BP < 90 mm HG, SSS, 2nd-, 3rd-AV block AF/atrial flutter w/ bypass tract Disp: *Calan SR:* Caps 120, 180, 240 mg *Verelan SR:* Caps 120, 180, 240, 360 mg *Verelan PM:* Caps (ER) 100, 200, 300 mg *Calan:* Tabs 80, 120 mg *Isoptin* SR 24-h 120, 180, 240 mg; Inj 2.5 mg/mL SE: Gingival hyperplasia, constipation, ↓ BP, bronchospasm, HR or conduction disturbances, edema; ↓ BP and bradyarrhythmias taken w/ telithromycin Interactions: ↑ Effects *W/* antihypertensives, nitrates, quinidine, EtOH, grapefruit juice; ↑ effects *OF* buspirone, carbamazepine, cyclosporine, digoxin, prazosin, quinidine, theophylline; ↓ effects *W/* antineoplastics, barbiturates, NSAIDs; ↓ effects *OF* Li, rifampin; ↓ BP & bradyarrhythmias taken *W/* telithromycin Labs: ↑ ALT, AST, alk phos NIPE: Take w/ food; ↑ fluids & bulk foods to prevent constipation; ⊘ grapefruit juice; ⊘ abrupt D/C

Vigabatrin (Sabril) [Antiepileptic]   WARNING: Vision loss reported; D/C w/in 2–4 wk if no effects seen Uses: *Refractory complex partial Sz disorder, infantile spasms* **Action:** ↓ GABA transaminase (GABA-T) to ↑ levels of brain GABA **Dose:** *Adults.* Initially 500 mg 2 ×/d, then ↑ daily dose by 500 mg at weekly intervals based on response and tolerability; 1500 mg/d max *Peds. Seizures:* 10–15 kg: 0.5–1 g/d ÷ 2 ×/d; 16–30 kg: 1–1.5 g/d ÷ 2 ×/d; 31–50 kg: 1.5–3 g/d ÷ 2 ×/d; > 50 kg: 2–3g/d ÷ 2 ×/d *Infantile spasms:* Initially 50 mg/kg/d ÷ bid, ↑ 25–50 mg/kg/d q3d to 150 mg/kg/d max **Caution:** [C, +/–] ↓ Dose by 25% w/ CrCl 50–80 mL/min, ↓ dose 50% w/ CrCl 30–50 mL/min, ↓ dose 75% w/ CrCl 10–30 mL/min; MRI signal changes reported in some infants **Disp:** Tabs 500 mg, powder/oral soln 500 mg/packet **SE:** Vision loss/blurring, anemia, peripheral neuropathy, fatigue, somnolence, nystagmus, tremor, memory impairment, ↑ wgt, arthralgia, abnormal coordination, confusion **Interactions:** May ↓ phenytoin levels **Labs:** Monitor LFTs **NIPE:** Taper slowly to avoid withdrawal Szs; restricted distribution, to register call (888) 233-2334; take w/ food if GI upset

Vilazodone HCL (Viibryd) [Selective Serotonin Reuptake Inhibitor + 5-HT$_{1A}$ Receptor Partial Agonist]   WARNING: ↑ Suicide risk in children/adolescents/young adults on antidepressants for major depressive disorder (MDD) and other psychological disorders Uses: *MDD* **Action:** SSRI & 5-HT$_{1A}$ receptor partial agonist **Dose:** 40 mg/d; start 10 mg PO/d × 7 d, then 20 mg/d × 7 d, then 40 mg/d; ↓ to 20 mg/d w/ CYP3A4 Inhib **Caution:** [C; ?/–] **CI:** MOAI, < 14 d between D/C MAOI and start **Disp:** Tabs 10, 20, 40 mg **SE:** Serotonin syndrome, neuroleptic malignant syndrome, N/V/D, dry mouth, dizziness, insomnia, restlessness, abnormal dreams, sexual dysfunction **Interactions:** ↑ Risk of serotonin synd *W/* concomitant triptans, MAOIs, SSRIs, SNRIs, buspirone, tramadol, antidopaminergic drugs; ↑ risk of bleeding *W/* ASA, NSAIDs, warfarin, other anticoagulants, ↑ effects *W/* CYP3A4 Inhibs; ↓ effects *W/* CYP3A4 inducers **NIPE:** Not approved for peds; w/ D/C, ↓ dose gradually, do not take w/in 14 d of MAOI; report suicidal ideation, worsening depression; take w/ food

Vinblastine (Generic) [Antineoplastic/Vinca Alkaloid]
WARNING: Chemotherapeutic agent; handle w/ caution; only individuals experienced in use of vinblastine should administer **Uses:** *Hodgkin Dz & NHLs, mycosis fungoides, CAs (testis, renal cell, breast, NSCLC), AIDS-related Kaposi sarcoma*, choriocarcinoma, histiocytosis **Action:** ↓ Microtubule assembly **Dose:** 0.1–0.5 mg/kg/wk (4–20 mg/m²) (based on specific protocol); ↓ in hepatic failure **Caution:** [D, ?] **CI:** Granulocytopenia, bacterial **Disp:** Inj 1 mg/mL in 10-mg vial **SE:** ↓ BM (especially leukopenia), N/V, constipation, neurotox, alopecia, rash, myalgia, tumor pain **Interactions:** ↑ Effects *W/* erythromycin, itraconazole; ↓ effects *W/* glutamic acid, tryptophan; ↓ effects *OF* phenytoin **Labs:** ↑ Uric acid **NIPE:** ↑ Fluids to 2–3L/d; ⊘ PRG or breast-feeding; use contraception for at least 2 mo after drug; photosens—use sunblock; ⊘ administer immunizations; takes several wk for therapeutic effect; ↑ risk of Infxns; ✓ wkly CBC

Vincristine (Marqibo, Vincasar, Generic) [Antineoplastic/Vinca Alkaloid] **WARNING:** Chemotherapeutic agent; handle w/ caution; fatal if administered IT; IV only; administration by individuals experienced in use of vincristine only; sever w/ extrav **Uses:** *ALL, breast & small-cell lung CA, sarcoma (eg, Ewing tumor, rhabdomyosarcoma), Wilms tumor, Hodgkin Dz & NHLs, neuroblastoma, multiple myeloma* **Action:** Promotes disassembly of mitotic spindle, causing metaphase arrest, vinca alkaloid **Dose:** 0.4–1.4 mg/m² (single doses 2 mg/max); ↓ in hepatic failure **Caution:** [D, –] **CI:** Charcot-Marie-Tooth synd **Disp:** Inj 1 mg/mL **SE:** Neurotox commonly dose limiting, jaw pain (trigeminal neuralgia), fever, fatigue, anorexia, constipation & paralytic ileus, bladder atony; no sig ↓ BM w/ standard doses; tissue necrosis w/ extrav; myelosupression **Interactions:** ↑ Effects *W/* CCBs, azole antifungals; ↑ risk of bronchospasm *W/* mitomycin; ↓ effects *OF* digoxin, phenytoin, quinolone antibiotics **Labs:** ↑ Uric acid; ↓ HMG, Hct, plt, WBC **NIPE:** ↑ Fluids to 2–3 L/d; reversible hair loss; ⊘ exposure to Infxns; ⊘ administer immunizations; ↑ risk of Infxns; ✓ vision changes

Vinorelbine (Navelbine, Generic) [Antineoplastic/Vinca Alkaloid] **WARNING:** Chemotherapeutic agent; administration by physician experienced in CA chemotherapy only; severe granulocytopenia possible; extravas may cause tissue irritation and necrosis **Uses:** *Breast CA & NSCLC* (alone or w/ cisplatin) **Action:** ↓ Polymerization of microtubules, impairing mitotic spindle formation; semisynthetic vinca alkaloid **Dose:** 30 mg/m²/wk; ↓ in hepatic failure **Caution:** [D, ?] **CI:** IT use, granulocytopenia (<1000 cells/mm³) **Disp:** Inj 10 mg **SE:** ↓ BM (leukopenia), mild GI, neurotox (6–29%); constipation/paresthesias (rare); tissue damage from extrav **Interactions:** ↑ Risk of granulocytopenia *W/* cisplatin, ↑ pulm effects *W/* mitomycin, paclitaxel **Labs:** ↑ LFTs **NIPE:** ⊘ PRG or breast-feeding; use contraception; avoid infectious environment; ↑ fluids to 2–3 L/d; use bulk in diet

Vismodegib (Erivedge) WARNING: Embryo-fetal death and severe birth defects; verify PRG status before start; advise female and male pts of these risks;

advise females on the need for contraception and males of potential risk of exposure through semen **Uses:** *Metastatic basal cell carcinoma, postsurgery local recurrence, not surgical candidate* **Acts:** Binds/Inhibs transmembrane protein—involved in hedgehog signal transduction **Dose:** 150 mg PO daily **Caution:** [D, –] **CI:** None **Disp:** Caps 150 mg **SE:** N/V/D/C, ↓ wgt, anorexia, dysgeusia, ageusia, arthralgias, muscle spasms, fatigue, alopecia, ↓ Na⁺, ↓ K⁺, azotemia; ↑ SE if coadministered w/ P-gp Inhib **Notes:** w/ Missed dose ⊘ make up missed dose, resume w/ next scheduled dose; ⊘ donate blood while on Tx until 7 mo after last Tx; immediately report exposure if PRG **NIPE:** Take w/o regard to food; ⊘ crush/open capsule; ⊘ PRG/breast-feeding; use contraception

Vitamin B₁ (See Thiamine)
Vitamin B₆ (See Pyridoxine)
Vitamin B₁₂ (See Cyanocobalamin)
Vitamin K (See Phytonadione)
Vitamin, Multi See Multivitamins (Table 12)
Vorapaxar (Zontivity) **WARNING:** ↑ Risk of suicidal behavior/thinking in children, adolescents, & young adults; monitor for ↑ suicidal behaviors or thought; has not been evaluated in peds **Uses:** *Major depressive disorder* **Action:** Inhib serotonin reuptake **Dose:** *Adults.* 10 mg 1 ×/d, ↑ to 20 mg as tolerated; consider 5 mg/d if intolerant to higher doses **Caution:** [C, –] Serotonin syndrome risk ↑ w/ other serotonergic drugs (TCA, tramadol, lithium, triptans, buspirone, St. John's wort); ↑ bleed risk; may induce mania or hypomania; SIADH w/ ↓ Na⁺ **CI:** w/ MAOIs, linezolid or methylene blue (IV); stop MAOIs for 14 d before; stop 21 d before starting MAOIs **Disp:** Tabs 5, 10, 15, 20 mg **SE:** N, V, constipation, sexual dysfunction **Notes:** w/ Strong CYP2D6 Inhib, ↓ dose by ½; w/ strong CYP2D6 inducers for > 2 wk, consider ↑ dose, NOT to exceed 3× original dose **NIPE:** Take w/o regard to food; ✓ bleeding precautions; ⊘ PRG/breast-feeding; do not use w/ h/o of stroke/TIAs; inform MD/DDS of use prior to any procedures

Voriconazole (VFEND, Generic) [Antifungal/Triazole] **Uses:** *Invasive aspergillosis, candidemia, serious fungal Infxns* **Action:** ↓ Ergosterol synth *Spectrum: Candida, Aspergillus, Scedosporium, Fusarium* sp **Dose:** *Adults & Peds > 12 y.* *IV:* 6 mg/kg q2h × 2, then 4 mg/kg bid PO < 40 kg: 100 mg q12h, up to 150 mg > 40 kg: 200 mg q12h, up to 300 mg; w/ mild–mod hepatic impair; IV not rec d/t accumulation of IV diluent; w/ CYP3A4 substrates (Table 10); do not use w/ clopidogrel (↓ effect); **Caution:** [D, ?/–] SJS, electrolyte disturbances **CI:** w/ Terfenadine, astemizole, cisaride, pimozide, quinidine, sirolimus, rifampin, carbamazepine, long-acting barbituates, ritonavir, rifabutin, ergot alkaloids, St. John's wort; in pt w/ galactose intolerance; skeletal events w/ long-term use; w/ proarrhythmic cond **Disp:** Tabs 50, 200 mg; susp 200 mg/5 mL; Inj 200 mg **SE:** Visual changes, fever, rash, GI upset, ↑ LFTs, edema **Interactions:** ↑ Effects *W/* delavirdine, efavirenz; ↑ effects *OF* benzodiazepines, buspirone,

CCBs, cisapride, cyclosporine, ergots, pimozide, quinidine, sirolimus, sulfonyl-ureas, tacrolimus; ↓ effects **W/** carbamazepine, clopidogrel, mephobarbital, phenobarbital, rifampin, rifabutin **Labs:** ↑ LFTs—✓ LFT before and during administration; **NIPE:** ✓ For multiple drug interactions; ✓ vision w/ use q28d; take 1 h ac or pc; ⊘ grapefruit products; ↑ risk of photosens—use sunblock; ⊘ PRG or breast-feeding:

Vorinostat (Zolinza) [Histone Deacetylase Inhibitor] Uses: *Rx cutaneous manifestations in cutaneous T-cell lymphoma* **Action:** Histone deacetylase Inhib **Dose:** 400 mg PO daily w/ food; if intolerant. 300 mg PO d × 5 consecutive days each week **Caution:** [D, ?/−] w/ Warfarin (↑ INR); **CI:** Severe hepatic impair **Disp:** Caps 100 mg **SE:** N/V/D, dehydration, fatigue, anorexia, dysgeusia, DVT, PE, ↓ plt, anemia, ↑ SCr, hyperglycemia, ↑ QTc, edema, muscle spasm **Labs:** ↓ heme, Hct, plt; ↑ serum glucose, SCr; monitor CBC, lytes (K⁺, Mg²⁺, Ca²⁺), glucose, and SCr q2wk × 2 mo then monthly **Interactions:** ↑ Risk of thrombocytopenia & GI bleed **W/** HDAC Inhibs (valproic acid) **Labs:** Monitor CBC, lytes (K⁺, Mg, Ca), glucose, & SCr q2wk × 2 mo, then monthly; baseline, periodic ECGs **NIPE:** Drink 2 L fluid/d; take w/ food; ⊘ PRG/breast-feeding & < 18 y of age; may ↑ QT interval—monitor ECG; ↑ risk of DVT reported

Vortioxetine (Brintellix)   WARNING: ↑ Risk of suicidal behavior/thinking in children, adolescents, and young adults; monitor for ↑ suicidal behaviors or thought; has not been evaluated in peds **Uses:** *Major depressive disorder* **Action:** Inhib serotonin reuptake **Dose:** *Adults.* 10 mg 1 ×/d, ↑ to 20 mg as tolerated; consider 5 mg/d if intolerant to higher doses **Caution:** [C, −] Serotonin syndrome risk ↑ w/ other serotonergic drugs (TCA, tramadol, Li, triptans, buspirone, St. John's wort); ↑ bleed risk; may induce mania or hypomania; SIADH w/ ↓ Na⁺ **CI:** w/ MAOIs, linezolid or methylene blue (IV); stop MAOIs for 14 d before; stop 21 d before starting MAOIs **Disp:** Tabs 5, 10, 15, 20 mg **SE:** N, V, constipation, sexual dysfunction **Notes:** w/ Strong CYP2D6 Inhib, ↓ dose by ½; w/ strong CYP2D6 inducers for > 2 wk, consider ↑ dose, NOT to exceed 3 × original dose **NIPE:** Take w/ food w/ GI upset; ✓ serum Na⁺; ⊘ EtOH; report suicidal ideation/violent behavior

Warfarin (Coumadin, Jantoven, Generic) [Anticoagulant/Coumarin Derivative]   WARNING: Can cause major/fatal bleeding. Monitor INR. Drugs, dietary changes, other factors affect INR. Instruct pts about bleeding risk **Uses:** *Prophylaxis & Rx of PE & DVT, AF w/ embolization*, other post-op indications **Action:** ↓ Vit K–dependent clotting factors in this order: VII-IX-X-II **Dose:** *Adults.* Titrate, INR 2.0–3.0 for most; mechanical valves INR is 2.5–3.5 *American College of Chest Physicians guidelines:* 5 mg initial, may use 7.5–10 mg; ↓ if pt elderly or w/ other bleeding risk factors; maint 2–10 mg/d PO, follow daily INR initial to adjust dosage (Table 8). *Peds.* 0.05–0.34 mg/kg/24 h PO or IV; follow PT/INR to adjust dosage; monitor vit K intake; ↓ w/ hepatic impair/elderly

Caution: [X, +] **CI:** Bleeding, peptic ulcer, PRG **Disp:** Tabs 1, 2, 2.5, 3, 4, 5, 6, 7.5, 10 mg; Inj **SE:** Bleeding d/t overanticoagulation or injury & therapeutic INR; bleeding, alopecia, skin necrosis, purple toe synd **Interactions:** Caution pt on taking **W/** other meds, esp ASA *Common warfarin* **Interactions:** ↑ Action **W/** APAP, EtOH (w/ liver Dz), amiodarone, cimetidine, ciprofloxacin, cotrimoxazole, erythromycin, fluconazole, flu vaccine, INH, itraconazole, metronidazole, omeprazole, phenytoin, propranolol, quinidine, tetracycline. ↓ Action **W/** barbiturates, carbamazepine, chlordiazepoxide, cholestyramine, dicloxacillin, nafcillin, rifampin, sucralfate, high-vit K foods **Labs:** ↑ PTT; false ↓ serum theophylline levels **NIPE:** Monitor/maintain consistent intake of vit K (↓ effect); INR preferred test; ✓ when new meds added; to rapidly correct overanticoagulation: vit K, fresh-frozen plasma, or both; highly teratogenic. Elderly & Asian patients w/ ↑ sensitivity may require ↓ doses; ⊘ OTC meds w/o physician approval; bleeding precautions

Witch Hazel (Tucks Pads, Others [OTC]) Uses: After bowel movement, cleansing to decrease local irritation or relieve hemorrhoids; after anorectal surgery, episiotomy, Vag hygiene **Acts:** Astringent; shrinks blood vessels locally **Dose:** Apply PRN **Caution:** [?, ?] External use only **CI:** None **Disp:** Pre-soaked pads **SE:** Mild itching or burning **NIPE:** Do not insert into rectum

Zafirlukast (Accolate, Generic) [Bronchodilator/Leukotriene Receptor Antagonist] Uses: *Adjunctive Rx of asthma* **Action:** Selective & competitive Inhib of leukotrienes **Dose:** *Adults & Peds > 12 y.* 20 mg bid *Peds 5–11 y.* 10 mg PO bid (empty stomach) **Caution:** [B, −] Interacts w/ warfarin, ↑ INR **CI:** Component allergy, hepatic impair **Disp:** Tabs 10, 20 mg **SE:** Hepatic dysfunction, usually reversible on D/C; HA, dizziness, GI upset; Churg–Strauss synd, neuropsych events (agitation, restlessness, suicidal ideation) **Interactions:** ↑ Effects **W/** ASA; ↑ effects *OF* CCBs, cyclosporine; ↑ risk of bleeding **W/** warfarin; ↓ effects **W/** erythromycin, theophylline, food **Labs:** ↑ ALT **NIPE:** Take 1 h at or 2 h pc; ⊘ breast-feeding; ⊘ use for acute asthma attack; report neuropsych Sx (depression/insomnia) asap

Zaleplon (Sonata, Generic) [C-IV] [Sedative/Hypnotic] Uses: *Insomnia* **Action:** A nonbenzodiazepine sedative/hypnotic, a pyrazolopyrimidine **Dose:** 5–20 mg hs PRN; not w/ high-fat meal; ↓ w/ renal/hepatic Insuff, elderly **Caution:** [C, ?/−] Angioedema, anaphylaxis; w/ mental/psychological conditions **CI:** Component allergy **Disp:** Caps 5, 10 mg **SE:** HA, edema, amnesia, somnolence, photosens **Interactions:** ↑ CNS depression **W/** CNS depressants, imipramine, thoridazine, EtOH; ↓ effects **W/** carbamazepine, phenobarbital, phenytoin, rifampin **NIPE:** Rapid effects of drug, take stat before desired onset; take w/o food; ⊘ D/C abruptly; ⊘ ETOH; ⊘ other CNS depressants

Zanamivir (Relenza) [Antiviral/Neuraminidase Inhibitor] Uses: *Influenza A & B w/ Sxs < 2 d; prophylaxis for influenza* **Action:** ↓ Viral neuraminidase **Dose:** *Adults & Peds > 7 y.* 2 Inh (10 mg) bid × 5 d, initiate w/in 48 h of Sxs *Prophylaxis household:* 10 mg daily × 10 d *Adults & Peds > 12 y. Prophylaxis community:* 10 mg daily × 28 d **Caution:** [C, ?] Not OK for pt w/ airway

Dz, reports of severe bronchospasms **CI:** Component or milk allergy **Disp:** Powder for Inh 5 mg **SE:** Bronchospasm, HA, GI upset, allergic Rxn, abnormal behavior, ear, nose, throat Sx **Labs:** ↑ ALT, AST, CPK **NIPE:** ⊘ use in airway disease (COPD; asthma); does not reduce risk of transmitting virus; use as a Diskhaler for administering dose same time each d; ⊘ use w/ milk protein allergies; ⊘ use w/ nebulizer/mechanical ventilation

Ziconotide   (Prialt)   [Pain   Control   Agent/Nonnarcotic]
WARNING: Psychological, cognitive, neurologic impair may develop over several wk; monitor frequently; may necessitate D/C **Uses:** *IT Rx of severe, refractory, chronic pain* **Action:** N-type CCB in spinal cord **Dose:** Max initial dose 2.4 mcg/d IT at 0.1 mcg/h; may ↑ 2.4 mcg/d 2–3 ×/wk to max 19.2 mcg/d (0.8 mcg/h) by d 21 **Caution:** [C, ?/–] w/ Neuro-/psychological impair **CI:** Psychosis, bleeding, diathesis, spinal canal obst **Disp:** Inj mcg/mL: 100/1, 500/5, 500/20 **SE:** Dizziness, N/V, confusion, psych disturbances, abnormal vision, edema, ↑ SCF, amnesia, ataxia, meningitis; may require dosage adjustment **NIPE:** May D/C abruptly; uses specific pumps; dilute *W/* preservative-free 0.9% NaCl; assess/educate pt to report cognitve impair/neuropsych Sxs asap; do not ↑ more frequently than 2–3 ×/wk

Zidovudine   (Retrovir,   Generic)   [Antiretroviral/NRTI]
WARNING: Neutropenia, anemia, lactic acidosis, myopathy, & hepatomegaly w/ steatosis **Uses:** *HIV Infxn, prevent maternal HIV transmission* **Action:** NRTI **Dose:** *Adults.* 200 mg PO tid or 300 mg PO bid or 1 mg/kg/dose IV q4h *PRG:* 100 mg PO 5 ×/d until labor; during labor 2 mg/kg IV over 1 h then 1 mg/kg/h until cord clamped *Peds 4 wk–18 y.* 160 mg/m²/dose tid or see table on next page; ↓ in renal failure **Caution:** [C, ?/–] w/ Ganciclovir, interferon alfa, ribavirin; may alter many other meds (see PI) **CI:** Allergy **Disp:** Caps 100 mg; tab 300 mg; syrup 50 mg/5 mL; Inj 10 mg/mL **SE:** Hematologic tox, HA, fever, rash, GI upset, malaise, myopathy, fat redistribution **Interactions:** ↑ Effects *W/* fluconazole, phenytoin, probenecid, valproic acid; ↑ hematologic tox *W/* adriamycin, dapsone, ganciclovir, interferon-α; ↓ effects *W/* rifampin, ribavirin, stavudine **NIPE:** Take w/o food; monitor for S/Sxs opportunistic Infxn; monitor for anemia & liver tox/hep; w/severe anemia/neutropenia dosage interruption may be needed; ⊘ other zidovudine containing combo products

Recommended Pediatric Dosage of Retrovir

Dosage Regimen & Dose

Body Weight (kg) Total Daily Dose bid–tid

4–< 9,24 mg/kg/d,12 mg/kg, 8 mg/kg

≥ 9–< 30, 18 mg/kg/d, 9 mg/kg, 6 mg/kg

≥ 30, 600 mg/d, 300 mg, 200 mg

Zidovudine/Lamivudine (Combivir, Generic) [Antiretroviral/NRTI] **WARNING:** Neutropenia, anemia, lactic acidosis, myopathy & hepatomegaly w/ steatosis **Uses:** *HIV Infxn* **Action:** Combo of RT inhib **Dose:** *Adults & peds > 12 y.* 1 tab PO bid; ↓ in renal failure **Caution:** [C, ?/–] **CI:** Component allergy **Disp:** Tab zidovudine 300 mg/lamivudine 150 mg **SE:** Hematologic tox, HA, fever, rash, GI upset, malaise, pancreatitis **Interactions:** ↑ Effects *W/* fluconazole, phenytoin, probenecid, valproic acid; ↑ hematologic tox *W/* adriamycin, dapsone, ganciclovir, interferon-α; ↓ *W/* rifampin, ribavirin, stavudine **NIPE:** Take w/o food; monitor for S/Sxs opportunistic Infxn; monitor for anemia; combo product ↓ daily pill burden; ⊘ pediatric pts < 30 kg; evenly space doses; ⊘ ETOH

Zileuton (Zyflo, Zyflo CR) [Leukotriene Receptor Antagonist] **Uses:** *Chronic Rx asthma* **Action:** Leukotriene Inhib (↓ 5-lipoxygenase) **Dose:** *Adults & peds > 12 y.* 600 mg PO qid; CR 1200 mg bid 1 h after AM/PM meal **Caution:** [C, ?/–] **CI:** Hepatic impair **Disp:** Tabs 600 mg; CR tabs 600 mg **SE:** Hepatic damage, HA, D/N, upper Abd pain, leukopenia, neuropsych events (agitation, restlessness, suicidal ideation) **Interactions:** ↑ Effects *OF* propranolol, terfenadine, theophylline, warfarin **Labs:** ↓ WBCs; ↑ LFTs; monitor LFTs qmo × 3, then q2–3mo **NIPE:** Take w/o regard to food; take on a regular basis; not for acute asthma; ⊘ chew/crush CR; not for acute asthma episodes

Ziprasidone (Geodon, Generic) [Antipsychotic/Piperazine Derivative] **WARNING:** ↑ Mortality in elderly w/ dementia-related psychosis **Uses:** *Schizophrenia, acute agitation bipolar disorder* **Action:** Atypical antipsychotic **Dose:** 20 mg PO bid, may ↑ in 2-d intervals up to 80 mg bid; agitation 10–20 mg IM PRN up to 40 mg/d; separate 10 mg doses by 2 h & 20 mg doses by 4 h (w/ food) **Caution:** [C, –] w/ ↓ Mg²⁺, ↓ K⁺ **CI:** QT prolongation, recent MI, uncompensated HF, meds that ↑ QT interval **Disp:** Caps 20, 40, 60, 80 mg; susp 10 mg/mL; Inj 20 mg/mL **SE:** ↑ HR; rash, somnolence, resp disorder, EPS, wgt gain, orthostatic ↓ BP **Interactions:** ↑ Effects *W/* ketoconazole; ↑ effects *OF* antihypertensives; ↑ CNS depression *W/* anxiolytics, sedatives, opioids, EtOH; TCAs, thioridazine; risk of prolonged QT *W/* cisapride, chlorpromazine, clarithromycin, diltiazem, erythromycin, levofloxacin, mefloquine, pentamidine, TCAs, thioridazine; ↓ effects *W/* amphetamines, carbamazepine; ↓ effects *OF* levodopa **Labs:** ↑ Glucose; monitor lytes **NIPE:** May take wk before full effects, take w/ food, ↑; monitor ECG; may ↑ QT interval; ↑ risk of tardive dyskinesia; ✓ Sx ↑ glycemia; ✓ wgt; ⊘ breast-feeding; ✓ CBC; ↓ Sz threshold

Ziv-Aflibercept (Zaltrap) **WARNING:** Severe/fatal hemorrhage possible including GI hemorrhage; D/C w/ GI perf; D/C w/ compromised wound healing, suspend T × 4 wk prior & after surgery & until surgical wound is fully healed **Uses:** *Metastatic colorectal CA (label/institution protocol)* **Acts:** Binds VEGF-A & PIGF w/ ↓ neovascularization & ↓ vascular permeability **Dose:** 4 mg/kg IV Inf over 1 h q2wk **Caution:** [C, –] Severe D w/ dehydration; D/C w/ fistula, ATE, hypertensive crisis, RPLS; ✓ urine protein, suspend Tx if proteinuria > 2 g/24 h,

D/C w/ nephrotic synd or thrombotic microangiopathy; ✓ neutrophils, delay until > 1.5 ⊘ 10⁹/ L CI: None **Disp:** Inj vial 25 mg/mL (100 mg/4 mL, 200 mg/8 mL) **SE:** D, ↓ WBC, ↓ plts, stomatitis, proteinuria, ↑ ALT/AST, fatigue, epistaxis, Abd pain, ↓ appetite, ↓ wgt, dysphonia, ↑ SCr, HA **Notes:** Males/females: use contraception during Tx & for 3 mo after last dose **NIPE:** Monitor BP ↑ risk HTN; use highly effective contraception during Tx and 3 mo following last dose; ↑ risk of thromboembolic events

Zoledronic Acid (Reclast, Zometa, Generic) [Antihypercalcemic/ Biphosphonate] Uses: *↑ Ca^{2+} of malignancy (HCM), ↓ skeletal-related events in CAP, multiple myeloma, & metastatic bone lesions (*Zometa*)*; *prevent/ Rx of postmenopausal osteoporosis, Paget Dz, ↑ bone mass in men w/ osteoporosis, steroid-induced osteoporosis (*Reclast*)* **Action:** Bisphosphonate; ↓ osteoclastic bone resorption **Dose:** *Zometa HCM:* 4 mg IV over ≥ 15 min; may retrain in 7 d w/ adequate renal Fxn *Zometa bone lesions/myeloma:* 4 mg IV over > 15 min, repeat q3–4wk PRN; extend w/ ↑ Cr *Reclast Rx osteoporosis:* 5 mg IV annually; *Reclast* Prevent postmenopausal osteoporosis 5 mg IV q2y *Paget:* 5 mg IV × 1 **Caution:** [D, ?/–] w/ Diuretics, aminoglycosides; ASA-sensitive asthmatics; avoid invasive dental procedures **CI:** Bisphosphonate allergy; hypocalcemia, angioedema, CrCl < 35 **Disp:** Vial 4 mg, 5 mg **SE:** Fever, flu-like synd, GI upset, insomnia, anemia; electrolyte abnormalities, bone, Jt, muscle pain, AF, osteonecrosis of jaw, atypical femur fx **Interactions:** ↑ Risk of hypocalcemia *W/* diuretics; ↑ risk of nephrotox *W/* aminoglycosides, thalidomide **Labs:** Follow Cr; effect prolonged w/ Cr ↑ **NIPE:** ↑ Fluids to 2–3 L/d; requires vigorous prehydration; do not exceed recommended doses/Inf duration to ↓ renal dysfunction; avoid oral surgery; dental exam recommended prior to therapy; ↓ dose w/renal dysfunction; give Ca^{2+} & vit D supls; may ↑ atypical subtrochanteric femur fxs; ⊘ PRG; breast-feeding; promote good dental hygiene; correct ↓ calcemia prior to Tx

Zolmitriptan (Zomig, Zomig ZMT, Zomig Nasal) [Analgesic Migraine Agent/5-HT₁ Receptor Agonist] Uses: *Acute Rx migraine* **Action:** Selective serotonin agonist; causes vasoconstriction **Dose:** Initial 2.5 mg PO, may repeat after 2 h, 10 mg max in 24 h; nasal 5 mg; if HA returns, repeat after 2 h, 10 mg max 24 h **Caution:** [C, ?/–] **CI:** Ischemic heart Dz, Prinzmetal angina, uncontrolled HTN, accessory conduction pathway disorders, ergots, MAOIs **Disp:** Tabs 2.5, 5 mg; rapid tabs (ZMT) 2.5, 5 mg; nasal 5 mg **SE:** Dizziness, hot flashes, paresthesias, chest tightness, myalgia, diaphoresis, unusual taste, coronary artery spasm **Interactions:** ↑ Effects *W/* cimetidine, MAOIs, OCPs, propranolol; ↑ risk of prolonged vasospasms *W/* ergots; ↑ risk of serotonin synd *W/* sibutramine, SSRIs **NIPE:** Administer to relieve migraines; not for prophylaxis; ⊘ use w/in 2 wk of MAOI use; ⊘ PRG; do not exceed > 10 mg/24 h; follow package insert for admin instructions

Zolpidem (Ambien IR, Ambien CR, Edluar, ZolpiMist, Generic) [C-IV] [Sedative/Hypnotic] Uses: *Short-term Tx of insomnia; *Ambien &*

Edluar w/ difficulty of sleep onset; *Ambien CR* w/ difficulty of sleep onset and/or sleep maint* **Action:** Hypnotic agent **Dose:** *Adults. Ambien:* 5–10 mg or 12.5 mg CR PO qhs *Edluar:* 10 mg SL qhs *Zolpimist:* 10 mg spray qhs; ↓ dose in elderly, debilitated, & hepatic impair (5 mg or 6.25 mg CR) **Caution:** [C, M] May cause anaphylaxis, angioedema, abnormal thinking, CNS depression, withdrawal; evaluate for other comorbid conditions; next-day psychomotor impairment/impaired driving when Ambien is taken w/ less than a full night of sleep remaining (7–8 h) **CI:** None **Disp:** *Ambien IR:* Tabs 5, 10 mg; *Ambien CR* 6.25, 12.5 mg *Edluar:* SL tabs 5, 10 mg *Zolpimist:* Oral soln 5 mg/spray (60 actuations/unit) **SE:** Drowsiness, dizziness, D, drugged feeling, HA, dry mouth, depression **Interactions:** ↑ CNS depresssion **W/** CNS depressants, sertraline, EtOH; ↑ effects **OF** ketoconazole; ↓ effects **OF** rifampin **NIPE:** Take w/o food; be able to sleep 7–8 h *Zolpimist:* Prime w/ 5 sprays initially, & w/ 1 spray if not used in 14 d; store upright; ⊘ D/C abruptly if long-term use; may develop tolerance to drug; may be habit-forming; ⊘ EtOH; ↓ dose in elderly/hepatic impairment

Zonisamide (Zonegran, Generic) [Anticonvulsant/Sulfonamide]

Uses: *Adjunct Rx complex partial Szs* **Action:** Anticonvulsant **Dose:** Initial 100 mg/d PO; may ↑ to 100 mg/d q2wk to 400 mg/d **Caution:** [C, –] ↑ q2wk w/ CYP3A4 Inhib; ↓ levels w/ carbamazepine, phenytoin, phenobarbital, valproic acid **CI:** Allergy to sulfonamides **Disp:** Caps 25, 50, 100 mg **SE:** Metabolic acidosis, dizziness, drowsiness, confusion, ataxia, memory impair, paresthesias, psychosis, nystagmus, diplopia, tremor, anemia, leukopenia; GI upset, nephrolithiasis (? d/t metabolic acidosis), SJS; monitor for ↓ sweating & ↑ body temperature **Interactions:** ↑ Tox **W/** CYP3A4 Inhib; ↓ effects **W/** carbamazepine, phenobarbital, phenytoin, valproic acid **Labs:** ↑ Serum alk phos, ALT, AST, Cr, BUN, ↓ glucose, Na **NIPE:** ⊘ D/C abruptly; swallow caps whole; monitor for ↓ sweating & ↑ body temperature; report rash immediately; ↑ drowsiness—caution w/ driving/operating complex machinery

Zoster Vaccine, Live (Zostavax) [Vaccine]

Uses: *Prevent varicella zoster in adults > 60 y* **Action:** Active immunization (live attenuated varicella) virus **Dose:** *Adults.* 0.65 mL SQ × 1 **CI:** Gelatin, neomycin anaphylaxis; fever, untreated TB, immunosuppression, PRG **Caution:** [C, ?/–] **Disp:** Single-dose vial **SE:** Inj site Rxn, HA **Interactions:** Risk of extensive rash **W/** corticosteroids **NIPE:** ⊘ PRG for at least 3 mo > vaccination; once reconstituted use stat; may be used if previous h/o zoster; do not use in place of varicella virus vaccine in children; contact precautions not necessary; defer administration during acute illness

COMMONLY USED NATURAL AND HERBAL AGENTS

The following is a guide to some common herbal products. These may be sold separately or in combination with other products. According to the FDA, "Manufacturers of dietary supplements can make claims about how their products affect the structure or function of the body, but they may not claim to prevent, treat, cure, mitigate, or diagnose a disease without prior FDA approval." These agents can have significant side effects that RNs & APNs should be aware of. The table below provides a listing of unsafe herbs with known toxicities

Unsafe Herbs with Known Toxicity

Agent	Toxicities
Aconite	Salivation, N/V, blurred vision, cardiac arrhythmias
Aristolochic acid	Nephrotox
Calamus	Possible carcinogenicity
Chaparral	Hepatotox, possible carcinogenicity, nephrotox
"Chinese herbal mixtures"	May contain ma huang or other dangerous herbs
Coltsfoot	Hepatotox, possibly carcinogenic
Comfrey	Hepatotox, carcinogenic
Ephedra/ma huang	Adverse cardiac events, stroke, Sz
Juniper	High allergy potential, D, Sz, nephrotox
Kava kava	Hepatotox
Licorice	Chronic daily amounts (> 30 g/mo) can result in ↓ K+, Na/fluid retention w/ HTN, myoglobinuria, hyporeflexia
Liferoot	Hepatotox, liver CA
Ma huang/ephedra	Adverse cardiac events, stroke, Sz
Pokeweed	GI cramping, N/D/V, labored breathing, ↓ BP, Sz
Sassafras	V, stupor, hallucinations, dermatitis, abortion, hypothermia, liver CA
Usnic acid	Hepatotox
Yohimbine	Hypotension, Abd distress, CNS stimulation (mania & psychosis in predisposed individuals)

Aloe Vera (*Aloe barbadensis*)   **Uses:** Topically for burns, skin irritation, sunburn, wounds; internally used for constipation, amenorrhea, asthma, colds **Action:** Multiple chemical components; aloinosides inhibit H_2O & lytes reabsorption & irritate colon which ↑ peristalsis & propulsion; wound healing d/t ↓ production of thromboxane A2, inhibiting bradykinin & histamine **Available forms:** Apply gel topically 3–5/d PRN; caps 100–200 mg PO hs **CI:** ⊘ Internally if PRG, lactating, or in children < 12 y **Notes/SE:** Abd cramping, D, edema, hematuria, hypokalemia, muscle weakness, dermatitis **Interactions w/ internal use:** ↑ K^+ loss **W/** BB, corticosteroids, diuretics, licorice; ↑ effects **OF** antiarrhythmics, corticosteroids, digoxin, diuretics, hyperglycemias, jimson weed **Labs:** ↓ K^+, BS **NIPE:** Assess for dehydration, lytes imbalance, Abd distress w/ internal use; stimulates uterine contractions & may cause spontaneous abortion; ✓ BG—can ↓ BG levels/ potentiate glucose-lowering medications

Arnica (*Arnica montana*)   **Uses:** ↓ Swelling & inflammation from acne, blunt injury, bruises, rashes, sprains **Action:** Sesquiterpenoids have shown antibacterial, anti-inflammatory, & analgesic properties **Available forms:** Topical cream, spray, oint, tinc; for poultice dilute tinc 3–10 × w/ H_2O & apply PRN **CI:** Poisonous, ⊘ take internally; avoid if pt allergic to arnica, chrysanthemums, marigold, sunflowers **Notes/SE:** Arrhythmias, Abd pain, cardiac arrest, contact dermatitis, coma, death, hepatic failure, HTN, nervousness, restlessness **Interactions:** ↑ Risk of bleeding **W/** ASA, heparin, warfarin, angelica, anise, asafetida, bogbean, boldo, capsicum, celery, chamomile, clove, danshen, fenugreek, feverfew, garlic, ginger, ginkgo, ginseng, horse chestnut, horseradish, licorice, meadowsweet, onion, papain, passion flower, poplar bark, prickly ash, quassia wood, red clover, turmeric, wild carrot, wild lettuce, willow; ↓ effects **OF** antihypertensives **Labs:** None **NIPE:** ⊘ Apply to broken skin, ⊘ use in PRG & lactation, serious liver & kidney damage w/ internal use, ingestion of flowers & root can cause death, prolonged topical use ↑ risk of allergic Rxn

Astragalus (*Astragalus membranaceus*)   **Uses:** Rx of resp Infxns, enhancement of immune system, & HF **Action:** Root saponins ↑ diuresis, ↓ BP; anti-inflammatory action related to the stimulation of macrophages, ↑ Ab formation & ↑ T-lymphocyte proliferation **Available forms:** Caps/tabs 1–4 g tid, PO; Liq extract 4–8 mL/d (1:2 ratio) ÷ doses; dry extract 250 mg (1:8 ratio) tid, PO **Notes/SE:** Immunosuppression w/ doses > 28 g **Interactions:** ↑ Effect **OF** acyclovir, anticoagulants, antihypertensives, antithrombotics, antiplts, IL-2, interferon; ↓ effect **OF** cyclophosphamide **Labs:** ↑ PT, INR **NIPE:** Use cautiously in immunosuppressed pts or those w/ autoimmune Dz; diuretic effect can cause dehydration

Bilberry (*Vaccinium myrtillus*)   **Uses:** Prevent/Tx visual problems such as cataract, retinopathy, myopia, glaucoma, macular degeneration; treat vascular problems such as hemorrhoids, & varicose veins **Action:** Contain anthocyanidins that ↓ vascular permeability, inhibit plt aggregation & thrombus formation, ↑ antioxidant effects on LDLs & liver, ↑ regeneration of rhodopsin in retina

Available forms: Products should have 25% anthocyanoside content; caps, extracts, dried, or fresh fruit, leaves; eye/vascular problems 240–480 mg PO bid/tid; night vision 60–120 mg of extract PO once/day **CI:** ⊘ PRG or lactation; caution in pts w/ DM & bleeding disorders **Notes/SE:** Constipation **Interactions:** ↑ Effects *OF* anticoagulants, antiplts, insulin, NSAIDs, oral hypoglycemics, ↓ effects *OF* Fe **Labs:** ↑ PT; ↓ glucose, plt aggregation **NIPE:** Large dose of leaves for long periods of time may be poisonous/fatal; take w/o regard to food

Black Cohosh (*Cimicifuga racemosa*) **Uses:** Sx of menopause (eg, hot flashes), PMS, hypercholesterolemia, peripheral arterial Dz; has anti-inflammatory & sedative effects **Efficacy:** May have short-term benefit on menopausal Sx **Dose:** 20–40 mg bid **Caution:** May further ↓ lipids &/or BP w/ prescription meds **CI:** PRG (miscarriage, prematurity reports); lactation **SE:** w/ OD, N/V, dizziness, nervous system & visual changes, ↓ HR, & (possibly) Szs, liver damage/failure **Action:** Estrogenic activity w/ some studies showing ↓ in LH; vasodilation activity causing ↑ blood flow & hypotensive effects; antimicrobial activity **Available forms:** Dried root/rhizome caps 40–200 mg once/d; fluid extract (1:1) 2–4 mL or 1 tsp once/d; tinc (1:5) 3–6 mL or 1–2 tsp once/d; powdered extract (4:1) 250–500 mg once/d; Remifemin menopause (standardized extract brand name) 20 mg bid **Notes/SE:** ↓ Hypotension, bradycardia, N/V, anorexia, HA, miscarriage, nervous system & visual disturbances; liver damage/failure **Interactions:** ↑ Effects *OF* antihypertensives, estrogen HRT, OCPs, hypnotics, sedatives; tinc may cause a Rxn *W/* disulfiram & metronidazole; ↑ antiproliferative effect *W/* tamoxifen; ↓ effects *OF* ferrous fumarate, ferrous gluconate, ferrous sulfate **Labs:** May ↓ LH levels & plt counts **NIPE:** Tinc contains large % of EtOH, ⊘ use in PRG or breast-feeding; ⊘ use in children; ⊘ use w/ liver Dz

Bogbean (*Menyanthes trifoliate*) **Uses:** ↑ Appetite; treat GI distress; anti-inflammatory for arthritis **Action:** Several chemical constituents include alkaloids (choline, gentianin, gentianidine), flavonoids (hyperin, kaempferol, quercetin, rutin, trifolioside) that act as an anti-inflammatory, & acids (caffeic, chlorogenic, ferulic, folic, palmitic, salicylic, vanillic) that act as bile stimulants & other elements such as carotene, ceryl alcohol, coumarin, iridoid, scopoletin; 2 compounds produce considerable inhibition of prostaglandin synth **Available forms:** Extract (1:1 dilution) 1–2 mL PO tid w/ fluid; dried leaf as tea 1–3 g PO tid **CI:** ⊘ PRG or lactating **Notes/SE:** N/V, bleeding **Interactions:** ↑ Risk of bleeding *W/* anticoagulants, antiplts, ANA, NSAIDs; ↑ effects *OF* stimulant laxatives; ↓ effects *OF* antacids, H₂-antagonists, PPIs, sucralfate **Labs:** None **NIPE:** May ↑ uterine contractions; extracts contain EtOH; monitor for S/Sxs bleeding or ↑ bruising; N if h/o colitis, anemia; ⊘ use w/ anticoagulants or antiplt drugs

Borage (*Borage officinalis*) **Uses:** Oil used for eczema & dermatitis & as a GLA supl; treat colds, coughs, & bronchitis; anti-inflammatory action used to treat arthritis **Action:** Oil contains GLA & its metabolites produce anti-inflammatory action; topical oil absorbed in skin ↑ fluid retention in stratum corneum; mucilage

& malic acid components have expectorant & diuretic actions; contains alkaloids that are hepatotox **Available forms:** Caps w/ 10–25% GLA; 1.1–1.4 g GLA PO once/day for Jt inflammation; for topical application bid for dermatitis & eczema **CI:** ⊘ PRG, lactation, & pts w/ h/o liver Dz or Sz disorder **Notes/SE:** ↑ Constipation, flatulence, liver dysfunction, Sz **Interactions:** ↑ Risk of bleeding **W/** anticoagulants, antiplts; ↑ effects **OF** antihypertensives; ↓ effects **OF** anticonvulsants, phenothiazine, TCAs; ↓ effects **OF** herb **W/** NSAIDs **Labs:** Monitor LFTs; may ↑ LFTs, PT, & INR **NIPE:** Only use herb w/o UPA alkaloids; ⊘ use in seizure disorders; can ↓ blood glucose; ⊘ PRG or breast-feeding

Bugleweed (*Lycopus virginicus*) **Uses:** ↓ Hyperthyroid Sxs, analgesic, astringent **Action:** Inhibits gonadotropin, prolactin, TSH & IgG Ab activity **Available forms:** Teas, extracts, dried herb **CI:** ⊘ PRG or lactation, pts w/ hypothyroidism, pituitary or thyroid tumors, hypogonadism, & CHF **Notes/SE:** Thyroid gland enlargement **Interactions:** ↑ Effects **OF** insulin, oral hypoglycemics, ↑ thyroid suppressing effects **W/** balm leaf & wild thyme plant; ↓ effect **OF** thyroid hormone **Labs:** ↓ FSH, LH, HCG, TSH; monitor BS **NIPE:** ⊘ N Substitute for antithyroid drugs; avoid if undergoing Tx or diagnostic procedures w/ radioisotopes; ⊘ D/C abruptly

Butcher's Broom (*Ruscus aculeatus*) **Uses:** Rx of circulatory disorders such as PVD, varicose veins, & leg edema; hemorrhoids; diuretic; laxative; inflammation; arthritis **Action:** Vasoconstriction d/t direct activation of the α-receptors of the smooth-muscle cells in vascular walls **Available forms:** Raw extract 7–11 mg once/d, PO; tea 1 tsp in 1 cup H_2O; topical oint apply PRN **Notes/SE:** GI upset, N/V **Interactions:** ↑ Effects **OF** anticoagulants, MAOIs; ↓ effects **OF** antihypertensives **Labs:** None **NIPE:** Hypertensive crisis may occur if administer w/ MAOIs; ⊘ use in PRG & lactation

Capsicum (*Capsicum frutescens*) **Uses:** Topical use includes pain relief from arthritis, diabetic neuropathy, postherpetic neuralgia, postsurgical pain; internal uses include circulatory disorders, GI distress, HTN **Action:** Stimulates skin pain receptors causing burning sensations; desensitization of pain receptors results in pain relief; ↓ lymphocyte production, Ab production, & plt aggregation **Available forms:** Topical creams 0.025–0.25% up to qid; caps 400–500 mg PO tid **CI:** ⊘ On open sores, in PRG, children < 2 y **Notes/SE:** GI irritation, sweating, bronchospasm, resp irritation, topical burning, stinging, erythema **Interactions:** ↑ Effects **OF** anticoagulants, antiplts, theophylline; ↑ risk of cough **W/** ACEIs; ↑ risk of anticoagulant effects **W/** feverfew, garlic, ginger, ginkgo, ginseng; ↑ risk of hypertensive crisis **W/** MAOIs; ↓ effects **OF** clonidine, methyldopa **Labs:** None **NIPE:** Pain relief may take several wk; ⊘ apply heat on areas w/ topical capsicum cream; avoid contact w/ eyes or mucous membranes; ⊘ use w/antiplt drugs

Cascara (*Rhamnus purshiana*) **Uses:** Laxative **Action:** Stimulates large intestine, ↑ bowel motility & propulsion **Available forms:** Liq extract 1–5 mL PO once/day **CI:** NPRG, lactation, & IBD **Notes/SE:** N/V, Abd cramps, urine discoloration, osteomalacia **Interactions:** ↑ Effects *OF* antiarrhythmics, cardiac glycosides; ↑ K$^+$ loss *W/* diuretics, corticosteroids, cardiac glycosides; ↓ effects W/ antacids, milk **Labs:** ↓ Serum K$^+$ **NIPE:** Short-term use; monitor lytes; caution w/ diuretics; ∅ use w/ digoxin d/t ↑ effect

Chamomile (*Matricaria recutita*) Uses: Antispasmodic, sedative, anti-inflammatory, astringent, antibacterial **Dose:** 10–15 g PO daily (3 g dried flower heads tid–qid between meals; can steep in 250 mL hot H$_2$O) **W/P:** w/ Allergy to chrysanthemums, ragweed, asters (family Compositae) **SE:** Contact dermatitis; allergy, anaphylaxis **Interactions:** w/ Anticoagulants, additive w/ sedatives (benzodiazepines); delayed ↑ gastric absorption of meds if taken together (↓ GI motility) **Action:** Ingredients include α-bisabolol oil, which ↓ inflammation, antispasmodic activity, ↑ healing times for burns & ulcers, & inhibits ulcer formation; apigenin contributes to the anti-inflammatory effect, antispasmodic & sedative effect; azulene inhibits histamine release; chamazulene reduces inflammation & has antioxidant & antimicrobial effects **Available forms:** Teas 3–5 g (1 tbsp) flower heads steeped in 250 mL hot H$_2$O tid–qid between meals, also use as a gargle or compress; fluid extract 1:1—45% EtOH 1–3 mL tid **Notes/SE:** Allergic Rxns if pt allergic to Compositae family (chrysanthemums, ragweed, sunflowers, asters) eg, angioedema, eczema, contact dermatitis, & anaphylaxis **Interactions:** ↑ Effects *OF* CNS depressants, EtOH, anticoagulants, antiplts; ↑ risk of miscarriage; ↓ effects *OF* drugs metabolized by CY4503A4, eg, alprazolam, atorvastatin, diazepam, ketoconazole, verapamil **Labs:** Monitor anticoagulant levels **NIPE:** ∅ PRG, lactation, children < 2 y, pt w/ asthma or hay fever; delayed ↓ gastric absorption of meds if taken together (↓ GI motility); ↑ amts can cause diarrhea

Chondroitin Sulfate Uses: Combine w/ glucosamine to Rx arthritis; use as an anticoagulant; draws fluids/nutrients into Jt, "shock absorption" **Action:** Biological polymer, flexible matrix between protein filaments in cartilage; attracts fluid & nutrients into the Jts; inhibits thrombin **Available forms:** 1200 mg once/d, PO, & usually given w/ glucosamine 1500 mg once/d, PO for nl wgt adults **Notes/SE:** D, dyspepsia, HA, N/V, restlessness **Interactions:** ↑ Effects *OF* anticoagulants, ASA, NSAIDs **Labs:** None **NIPE:** ∅ PRG & breast-feeding

Comfrey (*Symphytum officinale*) Uses: Topical Tx of wounds, bruises, sprains, inflammation **Action:** Multiple chemical components, allantoin promotes cell division, rosmarinic acid has anti-inflammatory effects, tannin possesses astringent effects, mucilage is a demulcent w/ anti-inflammatory properties, UPA cause hepatotox **Available forms:** Topical application w/ 5–20% of herb applied on intact skin for up to 10 d **CI:** ∅ Internally d/t hepatotox, ∅ PRG or lactation **Notes/SE:** N/V, exfoliative dermatitis w/ topical use **Interactions:** ↑ Risk of hepatotox *W/* ingestion of borage, golden ragwort, hemp, petasties **Labs:** ↑ LFTs, total bilirubin, urine bilirubin **NIPE:** ∅ Use for more than 6 wk/1 y; ∅ use on broken skin; consult MD and D/C if Sx persist for > 3 d or worsen

Coriander (*Coriandrum sativum*) **Uses:** ↑ Appetite, treat D, dyspepsia, flatulence **Action:** Stimulates gastric secretions, spasmolytic effects **Available forms:** Tinc 10–30 gtts PO once/day **CI:** ⊘ PRG or lactation **Notes/SE:** N/V, fatty liver tumors, allergic skin Rxns **Interactions:** ↑ Effects *OF* oral hypoglycemic **Labs:** Monitor BS **NIPE:** ↑ Risk of photosens—use sunscreen

Cranberry (*Vaccinium macrocarpon*) **Uses:** Prevention & Rx UTI; urinary deodorizer in urinary incontinence **Dose:** 300–400 mg bid in 6-oz juice qid; tincture 1/2–1 tsp up to 3 ×/d, tea 2–3 tsps of dried flowers/cup; creams apply topically 2–3 ×/d PO **Caution:** May ↑ kidney stones in some susceptible individuals, V **SE:** None known **Action:** Interferes w/ bacterial adherence to epithelial cells of the bladder **Available forms:** Caps 300–500 mg PO bid–qid; unsweetened juice 8–16 oz daily; tinc 3–5 mL *or tinc* 1/2–1 tsp up to 3 ×/d, *tea* 2–3 tsps of dried flowers/cup; *creams* apply topically 2–3 ×/d PO **SE:** D, irritation, nephrolithiasis if ↑ urinary Ca oxalate **Interactions:** ↑ Effects *OF* warfarin; ↑ excretion *OF* alkaline drugs such as antidepressants & methotrexate will cause ↓ effectiveness *OF* drug, ↓ effectiveness *OF* Uva-ursi **Labs:** ↑ Urine pH **NIPE:** Possibly effective in treating UTI; tinc contains up to 45% EtOH; only unsweetened form effective; regular use may ↓ frequency of bacteriuria w/ pyria; ↑ amts can cause GI distress/diarrhea

Dong Quai (*Angelica polymorpha, sinensis*) **Uses:** Uterine stimulant; anemia, menstrual cramps, irregular menses, & menopausal Sx; anti-inflammatory, vasodilator, CNS stimulant, immunosuppressant, analgesic, antipyretic, antiasthmatic **Action:** Root extracts contain at least 6 coumarin derivatives that have anticoagulant, vasodilating, antispasmodic, & CNS-stimulating activity. Studies demonstrate weak estrogen-agonist actions of the extract **Efficacy:** Possibly effective for menopausal Sx **Dose:** 3–15 g daily, 9–12 g PO tab bid **Caution:** Avoid in PRG & lactation **Available forms:** Caps 500 mg, 1–2 caps PO, tid; Liq extract 1–2 gtt, tid; tea 1–2 g, tid **Notes/SE:** D, photosens, skin CA **Interactions:** ↑ Effects *OF* anticoagulants, antiplts, estrogens, warfarin; ↑ anticoagulant activity *W/* chamomile, dandelion, horse chestnut, red clover; ↑ risk of disulfiram-like Rxn *W/* disulfiram, metronidazole **Labs:** ↑ INR w/ warfarin **NIPE:** Photosensitivity—use sunscreen, ⊘ breast-feeding or PRG; tincs & extracts contain EtOH up to 60%; D/C herb 14 d prior to dental or surgical procedures

Echinacea (*Echinacea purpurea*) **Uses:** Immune system stimulant; prevention/Rx of colds, flu; supportive care in chronic Infxns of the resp/lower urinary tract **Action:** Stimulates phagocytosis & cytokine production & ↑ resp cellular activity; topically exerts anesthetic, antimicrobial, & anti-inflammatory effects **Efficacy:** Not established; may ↓ severity & duration of URI **Available forms:** Caps w/ powdered herb equivalent to 300–500 mg, PO, tid; pressed juice 6–9 mL, PO, once/d; tinc 2–4 mL, PO, tid (1:5 dilution); tea 2 tsp (4 g) of powdered herb in 1 cup of boiling H_2O **Dose:** Caps 500 mg, 6–9 mL expressed juice or 2–5 g dried root PO **W/P:** Do not use w/ progressive systemic or immune Dzs (eg, TB, collagen–vascular disorders, MS); may interfere w/ immunosuppressive Rx, not OK w/ PRG; do not use > 8 consecutive wk; possible immunosuppression; 3 different commercial forms **SE:** N; rash, Fever, taste perversion, urticaria, angioedema **CI:** ⊘ In pts w/ autoimmune Dz, collagen Dz, progressive systemic Dz (TB, MS, collagen-vascular disorders), HIV, leukemia, may interfere w/ immunosuppressive therapy **Interactions:** ↑ Risk of disulfiram-like Rxn **W/** disulfiram, metronidazole; ↑ risk of exacerbation of HIV or AIDS **W/** Echinacea & amprenavir, other protease Inhibs; ↓ effects **OF** azathioprine, basiliximab, corticosteroids, cyclosporine, daclizumab, econazole Vag cream, muromonab-CD3, mycophenolate, prednisone, tacrolimus **Labs:** ↑ ALT, AST, lymphocytes, ESR **NIPE:** Large doses of herb interferes w/ sperm activity; ⊘ breast-feeding or PRG; ⊘ continuously for longer than 8 wk w/o a 3-wk break in Rx-possible immunosuppression; 3 different commercial forms

Ephedra/Ma Huang
Uses: Stimulant, aid in wgt loss, bronchial dilation **Dose:** Not OK d/t reported deaths (> 100 mg/d can be life-threatening). US sales banned by FDA in 2004; bitter orange w/ similar properties has replaced this compound in most wgt loss supls **Caution:** Adverse cardiac events, strokes, death **SE:** Nervousness, HA, insomnia, palpitations, V, hyperglycemia **Interactions:** Digoxin, antihypertensives, antidepressants, diabetic medications **Labs:** ↑ ALT, AST, total bilirubin, urine bilirubin, serum glucose **NIPE:** Tincs & extracts contain EtOH; linked to several deaths; monitor for behavioral mood changes; ⊘ avoid use in PRG, breast-feeding; ⊘ use in CV Dz, DM, renal Dz

Evening Primrose Oil (*Oenothera biennis*)
Uses: PMS, diabetic neuropathy, ADHD **Action:** Anti-inflammatory, antispasmodic, diuretic, sedative effects related to a high conc of essential fatty acids esp GLA & CLA & their conversion into prostaglandins **Efficacy:** Possibly for PMS, not for menopausal Sx **Available forms:** Caps, gel-caps, Liq dose depends on GLA content *DM neuropathy:* 4000–6000 mg PO once/day *Eczema:* 4000 mg PO once/day *Mastalgia:* 3000–4000 mg PO ÷ doses *PMS:* 2000–4000 mg PO once/day *RA:* Up to 5000 mg PO once/day **Dose:** 2–4 g/d PO **SE:** Indigestion, N, soft stools, flatulence, HA, anorexia, rash **CI:** ⊘ PRG or lactation; ⊘ persons w/ Sz disorders **Interactions:** ↑ Phenobarbital metabolism, ↓ Sz threshold, ↑ effects **OF** diuretics, sedatives **Labs:** None **NIPE:** May take up to 4 mo for max effectiveness, take w/ food; can cause bruising/bleeding w/ concurrent use of antiplatelet/anticoagulant drugs

Feverfew (*Tanacetum parthenium*)
Uses: Prevent/Rx migraine; fever; menstrual disorders; arthritis, toothache; insect bites **Action:** Active ingredient, parthenolide, inhibits serotonin release, prostaglandin synth, plt aggregation, & histamine release from mast cells; several ingredients inhibit activation of polymorphonuclear leukocytes & leukotriene synth **Efficacy:** Weak for migraine prevention **Available forms:** Freeze-dried leaf extract 25 mg once/d; caps 300–400 mg tid PO; tinc 15–30 gtt once/d to 0.2–0.7 mg of parthenolide **Dose:** 125 mg PO

of dried leaf (standardized to 0.2% of parthenolide) PO **Caution:** Do not use in PRG **SE:** Oral ulcers, gastric disturbance, swollen lips, Abd pain; long-term SE unknown **Notes/SE:** Mouth ulcers, muscle stiffness, Jt pain, GI upset, rash **CI:** ⊘ PRG & lactation or w/ ragweed allergy **Interactions:** ↑ Effects *OF* anticoagulants, antiplts, ↓ absorption *OF* Fe **Labs:** ↑ PT, INR, PTT **NIPE:** ⊘ D/C herb abruptly or may experience Jt stiffness & pain, HA, insomnia; ↑ risk of bleeding w/ antiplatelet drugs

Fish Oil Supplements (Omega-3 Polyunsaturated Fatty Acid)

Uses: CAD, hypercholesterolemia, hypertriglyceridemia, type 2 DM, arthritis **Efficacy:** No definitive data on ↓ cardiac risk in general population; may ↑ lipids & help w/ secondary MI prevention **Dose:** One FDA approved (see Lovaza); OTC 1500–3000 mg/d; AHA rec 1 g/d **Caution:** Mercury contamination possible, some studies suggest ↑ cardiac events **SE:** ↑ Bleed risk, dyspepsia, belching, aftertaste **Interactions:** Anticoagulants **NIPE:** Fishy aftertaste; ↑ doses can ↑ immune system activity

Garlic (*Allium sativum*)

Uses: Antioxidant; hyperlipidemia, HTN; anti-infective (antibacterial, antifungal); tick repellant (oral) **Action:** Inhibits gram(+) & (−) organisms, exerts cholesterol lowering by preventing gastric lipase fat digestion & fecal excretion of sterols & bile acids & it inhibits free radicals **Efficacy:** ↓ Cholesterol by 4–6%; soln ↓ BP; possible ↓ GI/CAP risk **Available forms:** Teas, tabs, caps, extract, oil, dried powder, syrup, fresh bulb **Dose:** 2–5 g, fresh garlic; 0.4–1.2 g of dried powder; 2–5 mg oil; 300–1000 mg extract or other formulations = to 2–5 mg of allicin daily, 400–1200 mg powder (2–5 mg allicin) PO **Notes/SE:** ↑ Insulin/lipid/cholesterol levels, anemia, oral burning sensation, dizziness, diaphoresis, HA, N/V/D, hypothyroidism, contact dermatitis, allergic Rxns, systemic garlic odor, ↓ Hgb production, lysis of RBCs **Interactions:** ↑ Effects *OF* anticoagulants, antiplts, insulin, oral hypoglycemics; CYP450 3A4 inducer (may ↑ cyclosporine, HIV antivirals, OCPs; ↓ effects *W/* acidophilus) **Labs:** ↓ Total cholesterol, LDL, triglycerides, plt aggregation, iodine uptake; ↑ PT, serum IgE; monitor CBC, PT **NIPE:** ⊘ PRG—abortifacient, lactation, prior to surgery—D/C 7 d pre-op (bleeding risk), GI disorders; report bleeding, bruising, petechiae, tarry stools

Gentian (*Gentian alutea*)

Uses: ↑ Appetite, treat digestive disorders such as colitis, IBS, flatulence **Action:** Chemical components stimulate digestive juices **Available forms:** Liq extract 2–4 g PO once/day, tinc 1–3 g PO once/day, dried root 2–4 g PO once/day **CI:** ⊘ PRG, lactation, & HTN **Notes/SE:** N/V, HA **Interactions:** ↑ CNS sedation *W/* barbiturates, benzodiazepines, EtOH if extract/tinc contains alcohol; ↓ absorption *OF* Fe salts **Labs:** None **NIPE:** Caution—many herb preps contain up to 60% EtOH; ↑ risk of low BP

Ginger (*Zingiber officinale*)

Uses: Prevent motion sickness; N/V d/t anesthesia; **Action:** Anti-inflammatory effect inhibits prostaglandin, thromboxane, & leukotriene biosynthesis; antiemetic effects d/t action on the GI tract; antiplt effect d/t the inhibition of thromboxane formation; + inotropic effect on CV system **Efficacy:** Benefit in ↓ N/V w/ motion or PRG; weak for post-op or chemotherapy **Available forms:** Dosage form & strength depends on Dz process **Dose:** 1–4 g rhizome or 0.5–2 g powder PO daily *General use:* Dried ginger caps 1 g once/d, PO; fluid extract 0.7–2 mL once/d, PO (2:1 ratio); tabs 500 mg bid–qid, PO; tinc 1.7–5 mL once/d, PO (1:5 ratio) **Caution:** Pt w/ gallstones; excessive dose (↑ depression, & may interfere w/ cardiac Fxn or anticoagulants) **SE:** Heartburn **Interactions:** ↑ Risk of bleeding **W/** anticoagulants, antiplts; ↑ risk of disulfiram-like Rxn **W/** disulfiram, metronidazole **Labs:** ↑ PT **NIPE:** Store herb in cool, dry area; ⊘ PRG, lactation; lack of standardization for herb dosing; can ↑ bleeding risk

Ginkgo (*Ginkgo biloba*)
Uses: Memory deficits, dementia, anxiety, improvement, Sx peripheral vascular Dz, vertigo, tinnitus, asthma/bronchospasm, antioxidant, premenstrual Sx (esp breast tenderness), impotence, SSRI-induced sexual dysfunction **Action:** Extract flavonoids, release neurotransmitters, & inhibit MAO, which enhances cognitive Fxn; vascular protective action results from relaxation of blood vessels, ↑ tissue perfusion, inhibition of plt aggregation; eradicates free radicals & ↓ polymorphonuclear neutrophils **Efficacy:** Small cognition benefit w/ dementia; no other demonstrated benefit in healthy adults **Available forms:** Dosage depends on diagnosis *General use:* Tabs & caps 40–80 mg tid, PO; tinc 0.5 mL tid, PO; extract 40–80 mg tid, PO **Dose:** 1–4 g rhizome or 0.5–2 g powder PO daily **Caution:** ↑ Bleeding risk (antagonism of plt-activating factor), concerning w/ antiplatelet agents (D/C 3 d pre-op); reports of ↑ Sz risk **Notes/SE:** GI upset, HA, dizziness, heart palpitations, rash **Interactions:** ↑ Effect *OF* MAOIs; ↑ risk of bleeding **W/** anisindione, dalteparin, dicumarol garlic, heparin, salicylates, warfarin; ↑ risk of coma **W/** trazodone; ↑ effect *OF* carbamazepine, gabapentin, insulin, oral hypoglycemics, phenobarbital, phenytoin; ↓ Sz threshold **W/** bupropion, TCAs **Labs:** ↑ PT **NIPE:** ⊘ PRG & lactation; tincs contain up to 60% EtOH; ⊘ 2 wk prior to surgery

Ginseng (*Panax quinquefolius*)
Uses: "Energy booster" general; also for pt undergoing chemotherapy, stress reduction, enhance brain activity, & physical endurance (adaptogenic), antioxidant, aid to control type 2 DM; panax ginseng being studied for ED **Action:** Dried root contains ginsenosides, which ↑ natural killer cell activity, & nuclear RNA synth, & motor activity **Efficacy:** Not established **Available forms:** No standard dosage *General use:* Caps 200–500 mg once/d, PO; tea 3 g steeped in boiling H_2O tid PO, tinc 1–2 mg once/d, PO (1:1 dilution); dose: 1–2 g of root or 100–300 mg of extract (7% ginsenosides) PO tid **Caution:** w/ Cardiac Dz, DM, ↓ BP, HTN, mania, schizophrenia, w/ corticosteroids; avoid in PRG; D/C 7 d pre-op (bleeding risk) **SE:** Controversial "ginseng abuse synd" w/ high dose (nervousness, excitation, HA, insomnia); palpitations, Vag bleeding, breast nodules, hypoglycemia **Notes/SE:** Anxiety, anorexia, CP, D, HTN, N/V, palpitations **Interactions:** ↑ Effects *OF* estrogen, hypoglycemics, CNS stimulants, caffeine, ephedra; ↑ risk of bleeding **W/** ibuprofen; ↑ risk of HA,

irritability & visual hallucinations **W/** MAOIs; ↓ effects **OF** anisindione, dicumarol, furosemide, heparin, warfarin **Labs:** ↑ Digoxin level falsely; ↓ glucose, PT, INR **NIPE:** ⊘ Use continuously for > 3 mo; ⊘ PRG or lactation; eval for ginseng abuse synd w/ Sxs of D, depression, edema, HTN, insomnia, rash, & restlessness

Glucosamine Sulfate (Chitosamine) and Chondroitin Sulfate

Uses: Osteoarthritis (glucosamine: rate-limiting step in glycosaminoglycan synth, ↑ cartilage rebuilding; *Chondroitin:* biological polymer, flexible matrix between protein filaments in cartilage; draws fluids/nutrients into joint, "shock absorption") **Efficacy:** Controversial **Action:** Stimulate the production of cartilage components **Available forms:** Caps/tabs 1500 mg once/d, PO & chondroitin sulfate 1200 mg once/d, PO for adults of nl wgt **Dose:** Glucosamine 500 mg PO tid, chondroitin 400 mg PO tid **Caution:** Many forms come from shellfish, so avoid if have shellfish allergy **SE:** ↑ Insulin resistance in DM; concentrated in cartilage, theoretically unlikely to cause toxic/teratogenic effects **Notes/SE:** Abd pain, anorexia, constipation or D, drowsiness, HA, heartburn, N/V, rash **Interactions:** ↑ Effects **OF** hypoglycemic **Labs:** Monitor serum glucose levels in DM **NIPE:** Take w/ food to reduce GI effects; no uniform standardization of herb; ✓ BG w/ DM more freq

Green Tea (*Camellia sinensis*)
Uses: Antioxidant, antibacterial, diuretic; prevention of CA, hyperlipidemia, atherosclerosis, dental caries **Action:** Chemical components include anti-inflammatory, anti-CA, polyphenol, epigallocatechin, & epigallocatechin-3-gallate, which inhibit tumor growth; fluoride & tannins demonstrate antimicrobial action against oral bacteria; antioxidant activity delays lipid peroxidation; antimicrobial action d/t inhibition of growth of various bacteria including *S aureus* **Available forms:** Recommend 300–400 mg polyphenol PO once/day (3 cups tea = 240–320 mg polyphenol) **CI:** Caution ↑ intake may cause tannin-induced asthma **Notes/SE:** Tachycardia, insomnia, anxiety, N/V, ↑ BP **Interactions:** ↑ Effects **OF** doxorubicin, ephedrine, stimulant drugs, theophylline; ↑ risk of hypertensive crisis **W/** MAOIs; ↑ bleeding risk **W/** anticoagulants, antiplts; ↓ effects **W/** antacids, dairy products **Labs:** ↑ PT, PTT **NIPE:** Contains caffeine, can ↑ effects of amphetamines, other caffeine-containing products—caution in PRG, infants, & small children & pts w/ CAD, hyperthyroidism & anxiety disorders; GI distress d/t tannins ↓ w/ the addition of milk; ↑ tannin content d/t ↑ brewing times

Guarana (*Paullinia cupana*)
Uses: Appetite suppressant, CNS stimulant, ↑ sexual performance, ↓ fatigue **Action:** ↑ Caffeine content stimulates cardiac, CNS, & smooth muscle; ↑ diuresis; ↓ plt aggregation **Available forms:** Daily ÷ doses w/ max 3 g PO daily **CI:** Avoid in PRG & lactation, CAD, hyperthyroidism, anxiety disorders d/t high caffeine content **Notes/SE:** Insomnia, tachycardia, anxiety, N/V, HA, HTN, Sz **Interactions:** ↑ Effects **OF** anticoagulants, antiplts, BBs, bronchodilators; ↑ risk of hypertensive crisis **W/** MAOIs; ↑ effects **W/** cimetidine, ciprofloxacin, ephedrine, hormonal contraceptives, theophylline, cola, coffee; ↓ effects **OF** adenosine, antihypertensives, benzodiazepines, Fe, ↓ effects **W/**

smoking **Labs:** ↑ PT, PTT **NIPE:** Tincs contain EtOH; may exacerbate GI disorders & HTN; ∅ use w/ MVP

Hawthorn (*Crataegus laevigata*)

Uses: Rx of HTN, arrhythmias, HF, stable angina pectoris, insomnia **Action:** ↑ Myocardial contraction by ↓ oxygen consumption, ↓ peripheral resistance, dilating coronary blood vessels, ACE inhibition **Available forms:** Tinc 1–2 mL (1:5 ratio) tid, PO; Liq extract 0.5–1 mL (1:1 ratio) tid, PO **Notes/SE:** Arrhythmias, fatigue, hypotension, N/V, sedation **Interactions:** ↑ Effects *OF* antihypertensives, cardiac glycosides, CNS depressants, & herbs such as adonis, lily of the valley, squill; ↓ effects *OF* Fe **Labs:** False ↑ of digoxin **NIPE:** ∅ PRG & lactation; many tincs contain EtOH; ✓ BP, pulse

Horsetail (*Equisetum arvense*)

Uses: ↑ Strength of bones, hair, nails, & teeth; diuretic, treat dyspepsia, gout; topically used to treat wounds **Action:** Multiple chemical components; flavonoids ↑ diuretic activity; contains silica which strengthens bones, hair, & nails **Available forms:** Extract 20–40 gtts in H₂O PO tid–qid; topically 10 g herb/L H₂O as compress PRN **CI:** ∅ PRG, lactation, w/ children, CAD; contains nicotine & large amounts may cause nicotine tox **Notes/SE:** Nicotine tox (N/V, weakness, fever, dizziness, abnormal HR, wgt loss) **Interactions:** ↑ Effects *OF* digoxin, diuretics, Li, adonis, lily of the valley; ↑ CNS stimulation *W/* CNS stimulants, theophylline, coffee, tea, cola, nicotine; ↑ K⁺ depletion *W/* corticosteroids, diuretics, stimulant laxatives, licorice; ↑ risk of thiamine deficiency *W/* EtOH use **Labs:** Monitor digoxin, lytes, thiamine levels **NIPE:** Tinc contains EtOH which may cause disulfiram-like Rxn if taken w/ benzodiazepines or metronidazole; short-term use only; apply directly to skin—active components of herb absorbed through skin

Kava Kava (Kava Kava Root Extract, *Piper methysticum*)

Uses: Anxiety, stress, restlessness, insomnia **Action:** Appears to act directly on the limbic system **Available forms:** Standardized extract (70% kavalactones) 100 mg bid–tid, PO **Efficacy:** Possible mild anxiolytic **Dose:** Standardized extract (70% kavalactones) 100 mg PO bid–tid **Caution:** Hepatotox risk, banned in Europe/Canada. Not OK in PRG, lactation. D/C 24 h pre-op (may ↑ sedative effect of anesthetics) **SE:** Mild GI disturbances; rare allergic skin/rash Rxns, may ↑ cholesterol; ↑ LFTs/jaundice; vision changes, red eyes, puffy face, muscle weakness **Notes/SE:** ↑ Reflexes, HA, dizziness, visual changes, red eyes, puffy face, muscle weakness, hematuria, SOB, mild GI disturbances; rare allergic skin/rash Rxns **Interactions:** ↑ Effects *OF* antiplts, benzodiazepines, CNS depressants, MAOIs, phenobarbital; ↑ absorption when taken *W/* food; ↑ in parkinsonian Sxs *W/* kava kava & antiparkinsonian drugs **Labs:** ↑ ALT, AST, urinary RBCs; ↓ albumin, total protein, bilirubin, urea, plts, lymphocytes **NIPE:** ∅ Take for > 3 mo; ∅ during PRG & lactation; ✓ ↑ depression; D/C 2 wk before surgery

Licorice (*Glycyrrhiza glabra*)

Uses: Expectorant, shampoo, GI complaints **Action:** ↑ Mucus secretions, ↓ peptic activity, ↓ scalp sebum secretion

Available forms: Liq extract, bulk dried root, tea; 15 g once/d PO of licorice root; intake > 50 g once/d may cause tox **Notes/SE:** HTN, arrhythmias, edema, hypokalemia, HA, lethargy, rhabdomyolysis **Interactions:** ↑ Drug effects *OF* diuretics, corticosteroids, may prolong QT interval *W/* loratadine, procainamide, quinidine, terfenadine **Labs:** None **NIPE:** ✓ for lytes & ECG changes, HTN, mineralocorticoid-like effects; tox more likely w/ prolonged intake of small doses than 1 large dose; D/C 2 wk before surgery

Melatonin (MEL) **Uses:** Insomnia, jet lag, antioxidant, immunostimulant **Action:** Hormone produced by the pineal gland in response to darkness; declines w/ age **Available forms:** XR caps 1–3 mg once/d 2 h before hs PO **Efficacy:** Sedation most pronounced w/ elderly pts w/ ↓ endogenous melatonin levels; some evidence for jet lag **Dose:** 1–3 mg 20 min before hs (w/ CR 2 h before hs) **Caution:** Use synthetic rather than animal pineal gland, "heavy head," HA, depression, daytime sedation, dizziness **Notes/SE:** HA, confusion, sedation, HTN, tachycardia, hyperglycemia **Interactions:** ↑ Anxiolytic effects *OF* benzodiazepines; ↑ risk of insomnia *W/* cerebral stimulants, methamphetamine, succinylcholine **Labs:** None **NIPE:** ⊘ PRG & breast feeding; additive sedation w/ use of CNS depressants

Milk Thistle (*Silybum marianum*) **Uses:** Prevent/Rx liver damage (eg, from alcohol, toxins, cirrhosis, chronic hep); preventive w/ chronic toxin exposure (painters, chemical workers, etc), dyspepsia **Action:** Stimulates protein synth, which leads to liver cell regeneration **Available forms:** 80–200 mg PO tid; tinc 70–120 mg (70% silymarin) tid, PO **Efficacy:** Use before exposure more effective than use after damage has occurred **Notes/SE:** D, menstrual stimulation, N/V, GI intolerance **Interactions:** ↑ Effects *OF* drugs metabolized by the cytochrome P-450, CYP3A4, CYP2C9 enzymes **Labs:** ↑ PT; ↓ LFTs, serum glucose **NIPE:** ⊘ PRG & lactation; ⊘ pts allergic to ragweed, chrysanthemums, marigolds, daisies

Nettle (*Urtica dioica*) **Uses:** Allergic rhinitis, asthma, cough, TB, BPH, bladder inflammation, diuretic, antispasmodic, expectorant, astringent, & topically for oily skin, dandruff, & hair stimulant **Action:** Multiple chemical components have different actions; scopoletin has anti-inflammatory action, root extract ↓ BPH, lectins display immunostimulant action **Available forms:** Caps 150–300 mg PO once/day; Liq extract 2–8 mL PO tid **CI:** ⊘ PRG or lactating or in children < 2 y **Notes/SE:** N/V, edema, Abd distress, D, oliguria, edema, local skin irritation **Interactions:** ↑ Effects *OF* diclofenac, diuretics, barbiturates, antipsychotics, opiates, EtOH; ↓ effects *OF* anticoagulants **Labs:** Monitor lytes **NIPE:** Skin contact w/ plant will result in stinging & burning; caution w/ use w/ elderly can cause low BP; ↑ intake of foods high in K⁺

Red Yeast Rice (*Monascus purpureus*) **Uses:** Hyperlipidemia **Efficacy:** HMG-CoA reductase activity, naturally occurring lovastatin; ↓ LDL, ↓ triglycerides, ↑ HDL; ↓ secondary CAD events **Dose:** 1200–1800 mg bid **Caution:** CI w/ PRG, lactation; do not use w/ liver Dz, recent surgery, serious infection; may contain a mycotoxin, citrinin, can cause renal failure **Disp:** Caps 600–1200 mg **SE:** N, V, Abd pain, hepatitis, myopathy, rhabdomyolysis **Interactions:** Possible interactions w/ many drugs, avoid w/ CYP3A4 Inhibs or EtOH **NIPE:** Use only in adults; generic lovastatin cheaper; ↑ risk of liver damage w/ EtOH use

Resveratrol Uses: Cardioprotective, prevent aging ? antioxidant **Efficacy:** Limited human research **Caution:** Avoid w/ Hx of estrogen-responsive CA or w/ CYP3A4 metabolized drugs **Disp:** Caps, tabs 20–500 mg, skins of red grapes, plums, blueberries, cranberries, red wine **SE:** D/N, anorexia, insomnia, anxiety, Jt pain, antiplt aggregation **Interactions:** Avoid w/ other antiplt drugs or anticoagulants; CYP3A4 Inhib **NIPE:** ↑ bleeding risk w/ use of anticoagulants, antiplt and NSAID drugs

Rue (*Ruta graveolens*) Uses: Sedative, spasmolytic for muscle cramps, GI & menstrual disorders, promote lactation, promote abortion via uterine stimulation, anti-inflammatory effect for sports injuries, bruising, arthritis, Jt pain **Action:** Contains essential oils, flavonoids, & alkaloids; shown mutagenic & cytotoxic action on cells; produced CV effects d/t + chronotropic & inotropic effects on atria; vasodilatory effects reduce BP; shown strengthening effect on capillaries; alkaloids produce antispasmodic & abortifacient activity **Available forms:** Caps, extracts, teas, topical creams, topical oils; topical oil for earache; topical creams to affected areas PRN; teas use 1 tsp/1/4 L H₂O; extract 1/4–1 tsp PO tid w/ food; caps 1 PO tid w/ food **Notes/SE:** Dizziness, tremors, hypotension, bradycardia, allergic skin Rxns, spontaneous abortion **CI:** ⊘ During PRG or lactation or give to children; caution in pts w/ CHF, arrhythmias, or receiving antihypertensive medication **Interactions:** ↑ Inotropic effects *OF* cardiac glycosides; ↑ effects *OF* antihypertensives & warfarin; ↓ effects *OF* fertility drugs **Labs:** ↑ BUN, Cr, LFT **NIPE:** Large doses can be toxic or fatal; research does not establish a safe dose; tincs & extracts contain EtOH; no data w/ use in children; avoid if h/o EtOH abuse or liver Dz

Saw Palmetto (*Serenoa repens*) Uses: Rx BPH, hair tonic, PCa prevention (weak 5-α-reductase Inhib like finasteride, dutasteride) **Action:** Theorized that sitosterols Inhib conversion of testosterone to dihydrotestosterone (DHT), which reduces the prostate gland, also competes w/ DHT on receptor sites resulting in antiestrogenic effects **Available forms:** Caps/tabs 160 mg bid PO; tinc 20–30 gtt qid (1:2 ratio); fluid extract, standardized 160 mg bid PO or 320 mg once/d PO **Efficacy:** Small, no sig benefit for prostatic Sx **Caution:** Possible hormonal effects, avoid in PRG, w/ women of childbearing years **SE:** Mild GI upset, mild HA, D w/ large amounts **Notes/SE:** Abd pain, back pain, D, dysuria, HA, HTN, N/V, impotence **CI:** ⊘ PRG, lactation **Interactions:** ↑ Effects *OF* adrenergics, anticoagulants, antiplts, hormones, Fe **Labs:** May affect semen analysis, may cause false(−) PSA **NIPE:** Take w/ meals to ↓ GI upset, do baseline PSA prior to taking herb, no standardization of herb content

Spirulina (*Spirulina sp*) Uses: Rx of obesity & as a nutritional supl **Action:** Contains 65% protein, all amino acids, carotenoids, B-complex vits, essential fatty acids & Fe; has been shown to inhibit replicating viral cells

Available forms: Caps/tabs or powder administer 3–5 g ac PO **Notes/SE:** Anorexia, N/V **Interactions:** ↑ Effects *OF* anticoagulants; ↓ effects *OF* thyroid hormones p/t high iodine content; ↓ absorption *OF* vit B$_{12}$ **Labs:** ↑ Serum Ca, alk phos; monitor PT, INR **NIPE:** May contain ↑ levels of Hg & radioactive ion content; ⊘ autoimmune diseases (eg, MS, RA, SLE)

St. John's Wort (*Hypericum perforatum*) **Uses:** Mild–mod depression, anxiety, gastritis, insomnia, vitiligo, anti-inflammatory; immune stimulant/ anti-HIV/antiviral; **Action:** MAOI in vitro, not in vivo; bacteriostatic & bactericidal, ↑ capillary blood flow, uterotonic activity in animals **Efficacy:** Variable; benefit w/ mild–mod depression in several trials, but not always seen in clinical practice **Available forms:** Teas, tabs, caps, tinc, oil extract for topical use **Dose:** 2–4 g of herb or 0.2–1 mg of total hypericin (standardized extract) daily *Also* 300 mg PO tid (0.3% hypericin) **Caution:** Excess doses may potentiate MAOI, cause allergic Rxn, not OK in PRG **SE:** Photosens, xerostomia, dizziness, constipation, confusion, fluctuating mood w/ chronic use **Notes/SE:** Photosens (use sunscreen) rash, dizziness, dry mouth, GI distress **Interactions:** Enhance MAOI activity, EtOH, narcotics, sympathomimetics **Labs:** ↑ GH; ↓ digoxin, serum Fe, serum prolactin, theophylline **NIPE:** ⊘ PRG, breast-feeding, in children, ⊘ w/ SSRIs, MAOIs, EtOH, ⊘ sun exposure

Stevia (*Stevia rebaudiana*) **Uses:** Natural sweetener, hypoglycemic & hypotensive properties **Actions:** Multiple chemical components; sweetness d/t glycoside stevioside; hypotensive effect may be d/t diuretic action or vasodilation action **Available forms:** Liq extract, powder, caps **Notes/SE:** HA, dizziness, bloating **Interactions:** ↑ Hypotensive effects *W/* antihypertensives esp CCB, diuretics **Labs:** Monitor BS **NIPE:** Monitor BP; does not encourage dental caries

Tea Tree (*Melaleuca alternifolia*) **Uses:** Rx of superficial wounds (bacterial, viral, & fungal), insect bites, minor burns, cold sores, acne **Action:** Broad-spectrum antibiotic activity against *E coli, S aureus, C albicans* **Available forms:** Topical creams, lotions, oint, oil apply topically PRN **Notes/SE:** Ataxia, contact dermatitis, D, drowsiness, GI mucosal irritation **Interactions:** ↓ Effects *OF* drugs that affect histamine release **Labs:** ↑ Neutrophil count **NIPE:** Caution pt to use externally only; ⊘ apply to broken skin; assess for contact dermatitis

Valerian (*Valeriana officinalis*) **Uses:** Anxiolytic, sedative, restlessness, dysmenorrheal **Action:** Inhibits uptake & stimulates release of GABA, which ↑ GABA conc extracellularly & causes sedation **Available forms:** Extract 400–900 mg PO 30 min < hs, tea 2–3 g (1 tsp of crude herb) qid, PRN, tinc 3–5 mL (1/2–1 tsp) (1:5 ratio) PO qid, PRN **Efficacy:** Probably effective sedative (reduces sleep latency) **Dose:** 2–3 g in extract PO daily held added to 2/3 cup boiling H$_2$O, tinc 15–20 drops in H$_2$O, oral 400–900 mg hs (combined w/ OTC sleep product Alluna) **Caution:** Hepatotoxicity w/ long-term use **SE:** Sedation, hangover effect, HA, cardiac disturbances, GI upset **Notes/SE:** GI upset, HA, insomnia, N/V, palpitations, restlessness, vision changes **Interactions:** ↑ Effects *OF* barbiturates, benzodiazepines, opiates, EtOH, catnip, hops, kava kava, passion flower, skullcap); ↓ effects *OF* MAOIs, phenytoin, warfarin **Labs:** ↑ ALT, AST, total bilirubin, urine bilirubin **NIPE:** Periodic check of LFTs, unknown effects in PRG & lactation, full effect may take 2–4 wk, taper herb to avoid withdrawal Sxs after long-term use; additive effects (sedation) when used w/ CNS depressants (eg, EtOH, benzodiazepines)

Yohimbine (*Pausinystalia yohimbe*) **Uses:** Improve sexual vigor, Rx ED **Action:** Peripherally affects autonomic nervous system by ↓ adrenergic activity & ↑ cholinergic activity; ↑ blood flow **Efficacy:** Variable **Available forms:** Tabs 5.4 mg tid PO; doses at 20–30 mg/d may ↑ BP & HR **Dose:** 1 tab = 5.4 mg PO tid (use w/ physician supervision) **Caution:** Do not use w/ renal/hepatic Dz; may exacerbate schizophrenia/mania (if pt predisposed); α_2-adrenergic antagonist (↓ BP, Abd distress, weakness w/ high doses), OD can be fatal; salivation, dilated pupils, arrhythmias **SE:** Anxiety, tremors, dizziness, ↑ BP, ↑ HR **Notes/SE:** Anxiety, dizziness, dysuria, genital pain, HTN, tachycardia, tremors **Interactions:** ↑ Effects *OF* CNS stimulants, MAOIs, SSRIs, caffeine, EtOH; ↑ risk of tox *W/* α-adrenergic blockers, phenothiazines; ↑ yohimbe tox *W/* sympathomimetics; ↑ BP *W/* foods containing tyramine **Labs:** ↑ BUN, Cr **NIPE:** ⊘ w/ caffeine-containing foods w/ herb, may exacerbate mania in pts w/ psychiatric disorders; additive effects w/ MAOIs

Tables

TABLE 1
Local Anesthetic Comparison Chart for Commonly Used Injectable Agents

Agent	Proprietary Names	Onset	Duration	Maximum Dose mg/kg	Maximum Dose Volume in 70-kg Adult[a]
Bupivacaine	Marcaine	7–30 min	5–7 h	3	70 mL of 0.25% solution
Lidocaine	Xylocaine, Anestacon	5–30 min	2 h	4	28 mL of 1% solution
Lidocaine with epinephrine (1:200,000)		5–30 min	2–3 h	7	50 mL of 1% solution
Mepivacaine	Carbocaine	5–30 min	2–3 h	7	50 mL of 1% solution
Procaine	Novocaine	Rapid	30 min–1 h	10–15	70–105 mL of 1% solution

[a] To calculate the maximum dose if not a 70-kg adult, use the fact that a 1% solution has 10 mg/mL drug.

TABLE 2
Comparison of Systemic Steroids (See also pp. 365–366)

Drug	Relative Equivalent Dose (mg)	Relative Mineralo-corticoid Activity	Duration (h)	Route
Betamethasone	0.75	0	36–72	PO, IM
Cortisone	25	2	8–12	PO, IM
Dexamethasone	0.75	0	36–72	PO, IV
Hydrocortisone (Solu-Cortef, Hydrocortone)	20	2	8–12	PO, IM, IV
Methylprednisolone acetate (Depo-Medrol)	4	0	36–72	PO, IM, IV
Methylprednisolone succinate (Solu-Medrol)	4	0	8–12	PO, IM, IV
Prednisone	5	1	12–36	PO
Prednisolone	5	1	12–36	PO, IM, IV

TABLE 3
Topical Steroid Preparations (See also p. 367)

Agent	Common Trade Names Dosage/Strength	Potency	Apply
Alclometasone dipropionate	Aclovate, cream, oint 0.05%	Low	bid/tid
Amcinonide	Cream, lotion, oint 0.1%	High	bid/tid
Betamethasone			
Betamethasone valerate	Cream, lotion, oint 0.1%	Low	q day/bid
Betamethasone valerate	Luxiq foam 0.12%	Intermediate	q day/bid
Betamethasone dipropionate	Cream, lotion, oint 0.05%; aerosol 0.1%	High	q day/bid
Betamethasone dipropionate, augmented	Diprolene oint, lotion, gel 0.05%	Ultrahigh	q day/bid
Clobetasol propionate	Diprolene AF cream 0.05%	Ultrahigh	bid (2 wk max)
	Temovate, Clobex, Cormax cream, gel, oint, lotion, foam, aerosol, shampoo, soln, 0.05%, 00.05%, 0.5%		
Clocortolone pivalate	Cloderm cream 0.1%	Intermediate	q day–qid
Desonide	DesOwen, cream, oint, lotion 0.05%	Low	bid–qid
Desoximetasone			
Desoximetasone 0.05%	Topicort cream, gel 0.05%	Intermediate	q day–qid
Desoximetasone 0.25%	Topicort cream, gel 0.025%	High	q day–bid
Dexamethasone base	Aerosol 0.01%, cream 0.1%	Low	bid–qid
Diflorasone diacetate	ApexiCon cream, oint 0.05%	Ultrahigh	bid/qid
Fluocinolone			
Fluocinolone acetonide 0.01%	Synalar cream, soln 0.01%	Low	bid/tid
	Capex shampoo 0.01%		

436

Drug	Formulation	Potency	Frequency
Fluocinolone acetonide 0.025%	Synalar oint, cream 0.025%	Intermediate	bid/tid
Fluocinonide 0.1%	Vanos cream 0.1%	High	q day/bid
Flurandrenolide	Cordran cream, oint 0.25%	Intermediate	q day
Fluticasone propionate	Cutivate cream, lotion 0.05%, oint 0.005%	Intermediate	bid
Halobetasol	Ultravate cream, oint 0.05%	Very high	bid
Halcinonide	Halog cream oint 0.1%	High	q day–bid
Hydrocortisone	Cortizone, Caldecort, Hycort, Hytone, etc.–aerosol 1%, cream 0.5, 1, 2.5%, gel 0.5%, oint 0.5, 1, 2.5%, lotion 0.5, 1, 2.5%, paste 0.5%, soln 1%	Low	tid/qid
Hydrocortisone acetate	Cream, oint 0.5, 1%	Low	tid/qid
Hydrocortisone butyrate	Locoid oint, cream, lotion soln 0.1%	Intermediate	bid/tid
Hydrocortisone valerate	Cream, oint 0.2%	Intermediate	bid/tid
Mometasone furoate	Elocon cream, oint, lotion, soln 0.1%	Intermediate	q day
Prednicarbate	Dermatop cream, oint 0.1%	Intermediate	bid
Triamcinolone			
Triamcinolone acetonide 0.025%	Cream, oint, lotion 0.025%	Low	tid/qid
Triamcinolone acetonide 0.1%	Cream, oint, lotion 0.1%, Kenalog aerosol 0.147 mg/g	Intermediate	tid/qid
Triamcinolone acetonide 0.5%	Cream, oint 0.5%	High	tid/qid

Table 4
Comparison of Insulins (See also p. 221)

Products are classified based on onset and duration of action. Insulin is 100 units per mL unless otherwise noted. Cartridge volume of insulin pens is 3 mL. Approximate performance characteristics of the different insulins are listed. See individual package inserts for specifics.

Type of Insulin			
Ultra Rapid	Onset < 0.25 h	Peak 0.5–1.5 h	Duration 3–4 h
glulisine [rDNA origin] • Apidra, Apidra SoloSTAR pen			
lispro [rDNA origin] • HumaLOG, HumaLOG KwikPen • HumaPen Luxura HD pen			
aspart [rDNA origin] • NovoLOG, NovoLOG FlexPen • NovoPen Echo			
Rapid (regular insulin)	Onset 0.5–1 h	Peak 2–3h	Duration 4–6 h
regular • HumuLIN R, NovoLIN R			

438

| Intermediate | Onset 1–4 h | Peak 6–10 h | Duration 10–16 h |

NPH
- HumulIN N, HumulIN N Pen
- NovolIN N

| Prolonged | Onset 1–4 h | Peak No peak/ max effect 5 h | Duration 24 h |

glargine [rDNA origin]
- Lantus, Lantus SoloSTAR pen

detemir [rDNA origin]
- Levemir, Levemir FlexPen

| Combination Insulins | Onset < 0.25 h | Peak Dual based on agent | Duration Up to 10 h |

lispro protamine suspension/insulin lispro
- HumaLOG Mix 75/25
- HumaLOG Mix 75/25 KwikPen
- HumaLOG Mix 50/50
- HumaLOG Mix 50/50 KwikPen

(Continued)

Table 4 (continued)
Comparison of Insulins (See also p. 221)

Combination Insulins	Onset < 0.25 h	Peak Dual based on agent	Duration Up to 10 h

aspart protamine suspension/insulin aspart
- NovoLOG Mix 70/30
- NovoLOG Mix 70/30 FlexPen

	Onset 0.5–1 h	Peak Dual based on agent	Duration Up to 10–16 h

NPH/insulin regular
- HumuLIN 70/30
- HumuLIN 70/30 Pen
- NovoLIN 70/30

About insulin pens:

Insulin pens can increase patient acceptance and adherence. Depending on the pen, the insulin cartridges may be prefilled disposable single use OR refillable/reusable. Dosage ranges vary but are typically 1 to 60–80 units, in increments of 1 unit, with *HumaPen Luxura HD* and *NovoPen Echo* offering 0.5-unit increments. Features that are helpful for patients with reduced vision are: a large or magnified dosing window and audible dosing (end of dose click). Many pens allow for adjusting the dose without wasting insulin and prevent dialing a dose that is larger than the number of units remaining in the pen. *NovoPen Echo* is the first pen to record the dose and time of last injection and can accommodate different types of insulin in the cartridges.

Do not confuse *HumaLOG, NovoLOG, HumaLOG Mix,* and *NovoLOG Mix* with each other or with other agents, as serious medication errors can occur. Use "TALL MAN LETTERS" for the 'LOGs and the 'LINs per FDA recommendations to avoid prescribing errors.

440

TABLE 5
Oral Contraceptives (See also pp. 301–302)

(Note: 21 = 21 Active pills; 24 = 24 Active pills; Standard for most products is 28 [unless specified] = 21 Active pills + 7 Placebo[a])

Drug	Note	Progestin (mg)	Estrogen (mcg)	Extra
Monophasics				
Altavera		Levonorgestrel (0.15)	Ethinyl estradiol (30)	
Alyacen 1/35		Norethindrone (1)	Ethinyl estradiol (35)	
Apri		Desogestrel (0.15)	Ethinyl estradiol (30)	
Aviane		Levonorgestrel (0.1)	Ethinyl estradiol (20)	
Balziva		Norethindrone (0.4)	Ethinyl estradiol (35)	
Beyaz	b, c, e	Drospirenone (3)	Ethinyl estradiol (20)	0.451 mg levomefolate in all including 7 placebo
Brevicon		Norethindrone (0.5)	Ethinyl estradiol (35)	
Briellyn		Norethindrone (0.4)	Ethinyl estradiol (35)	
Cryselle		Norgestrel (0.3)	Ethinyl estradiol (30)	
Cyclafem 1/35		Norethindrone (1)	Ethinyl estradiol (35)	
Elinest		Norgestrel (0.3)	Ethinyl estradiol (30)	
Emoquette		Desogestrel (0.15)	Ethinyl estradiol (30)	
Enskyce		Desogestrel (0.15)	Ethinyl estradiol (30)	
Estarylla		Norgestimate (0.25)	Ethinyl estradiol (35)	

(Continued)

TABLE 5 (continued)
Oral Contraceptives (See also pp. 301–302)

(Note: 21 = 21 Active pills; 24 = 24 Active pills; Standard for most products is 28 [unless specified] = 21 Active pills + 7 Placebo[a])

Drug	Note	Progestin (mg)	Estrogen (mcg)	Extra
Monophasics				
Gianvi	c, e	Drospirenone (3)	Ethinyl estradiol (20)	
Gildagia		Norethindrone (0.4)	Ethinyl estradiol (35)	
Falmina		Levonorgestrel (0.1)	Ethinyl estradiol (20)	
Femcon Fe		Norethindrone (0.4)	Ethinyl estradiol (35)	75 mg Fe x 7 d in 28 d
Junel Fe 1/20		Norethindrone acetate (1)	Ethinyl estradiol (20)	75 mg Fe x 7 d in 28 d
Junel Fe 1.5/30		Norethindrone acetate (1.5)	Ethinyl estradiol (30)	75 mg Fe x 7 d in 28 d
Kelnor		Ethynodiol diacetate (1)	Ethinyl estradiol (35)	
Kurvelo		Levonorgestrel (0.15)	Ethinyl estradiol (30)	
Lessina		Levonorgestrel (0.1)	Ethinyl estradiol (20)	
Levlen		Levonorgestrel (0.15)	Ethinyl estradiol (30)	
Levora		Levonorgestrel (0.15)	Ethinyl estradiol (30)	
Lo Minastrin Fe		Norethindrone (1)	Ethinyl estradiol (10)	2 10 mcg est/2 Fe
Loestrin 24 Fe		Norethindrone (1)	Ethinyl estradiol (20)	75 mg Fe x 4 d
Loestrin Fe 1.5/30		Norethindrone acetate (1.5)	Ethinyl estradiol (30)	75 mg Fe x 7 d in 28 d
Loestrin Fe 1/20		Norethindrone acetate (1)	Ethinyl estradiol (20)	75 mg Fe x 7 d in 28 d
Loestrin 1/20		Norethindrone acetate (1)	Ethinyl estradiol (20)	75 mg Fe x 7 d in 28 d

442

Loestrin 1.5/20		Norethindrone acetate (1.5)	Ethinyl estradiol (20)
Lo/Ovral		Norgestrel (0.3)	Ethinyl estradiol (30)
Loryna	c, e	Drospirenone (3)	Ethinyl estradiol (20)
Low-Ogestrel	c	Drospirenone (3)	Ethinyl estradiol (20)
Lutera		Levonorgestrel (0.1)	Ethinyl estradiol (20)
Marlissa		Levonorgestrel (0.15)	Ethinyl estradiol (30)
Microgestin 1/20		Norethindrone acetate (1)	Ethinyl estradiol (20)
Microgestin 1.5/30		Norethindrone acetate (1.5)	Ethinyl estradiol (30)
Microgestin Fe 1/20		Norethindrone acetate (1)	Ethinyl estradiol (20) 75mg Fe x 7 d in 28 d
Microgestin Fe 1.5/30		Norethindrone acetate (1.5)	Ethinyl estradiol (30) 75mg Fe x 7 d in 28 d
Minastrin 24 Fe (chew)		Norethindrone 1 mg	Ethinyl estradiol (20) 75mg Fe x 4 d
Mircette		Desogestrel (0.15)	Ethinyl estradiol (20, 0, 10) 2 inert, 2 ethinyl estradiol 10 mcg
Modicon		Norethindrone (0.5)	Ethinyl estradiol (35)
Mono-Linyah		Norgestimate (0.25)	Ethinyl estradiol (35)
MonoNessa		Norgestimate (0.25)	Ethinyl estradiol (35)
Necon 0.5/35		Norethindrone (0.5)	Mestranol (35)
Necon 1/50		Norethindrone (1)	Mestranol (50)
Necon 1/35		Norethindrone (1)	Ethinyl estradiol (35)
Nordette		Levonorgestrel (0.15)	Ethinyl estradiol (30)
Norethin 1/35E		Norethindrone (1)	Ethinyl estradiol (35)
Norinyl 1/35		Norethindrone (1)	Ethinyl estradiol (35)
Norinyl 1/50		Norethindrone (1)	Mestranol (50)

(Continued)

TABLE 5 (continued)
Oral Contraceptives (See also pp. 301–302)

(Note: 21 = 21 Active pills; 24 = 24 Active pills; Standard for most products is 28 [unless specified] = 21 Active pills + 7 Placebo[a])

Drug	Note	Progestin (mg)	Estrogen (mcg)	Extra
Monophasics				
Nortrel 0.5/35		Norethindrone (0.5)	Ethinyl estradiol (35)	
Nortrel 1/35		Norethindrone (1)	Ethinyl estradiol (35)	
Ocella	c	Drospirenone (3)	Ethinyl estradiol (30)	
Ogestrel 0.5/50		Norgestrel (0.5)	Ethinyl estradiol (50)	
Orsythia		Levonorgestrel (0.1)	Ethinyl estradiol (20)	
Ortho-Cept		Desogestrel (0.15)	Ethinyl estradiol (30)	
Ortho-Cyclen		Norgestimate (0.25)	Ethinyl estradiol (35)	
Ortho-Novum		Norethindrone (1)	Ethinyl estradiol (35)	
Ovcon 35		Norethindrone (0.4)	Ethinyl estradiol (35)	
Ovcon 35 Fe		Norethindrone (0.4)	Ethinyl estradiol (35)	75 mg Fe x 7 d in 28 d
Philith		Norethindrone (0.4)	Ethinyl estradiol (35)	
Pirmella 1/35		Norethindrone (1)	Ethinyl estradiol (35)	
Previfem		Norgestimate (0.25)	Ethinyl estradiol (35)	
Portia		Levonorgestrel (0.15)	Ethinyl estradiol (30)	
Reclipsen		Desogestrel (0.15)	Ethinyl estradiol (30)	
Safyral	b, c	Drospirenone (3)	Ethinyl estradiol (30)	0.451 mg levomefolate in all including 7 placebo

Solia	Desogestrel (0.15)		Ethinyl estradiol (30)	
Sprintec	Norgestimate (0.25)		Ethinyl estradiol (35)	
Sronyx	Levonorgestrel (0.1)		Ethinyl estradiol (20)	
Syeda	Drospirenone (3)	c	Ethinyl estradiol (30)	
Vestura	Drospirenone (3)	c, e	Ethinyl estradiol (20)	
Vyfemla	Norethindrone (0.4)		Ethinyl estradiol (35)	
Wera	Norethindrone (0.5)		Ethinyl estradiol (35)	
Wymza Fe	Norethindrone (0.4)		Ethinyl estradiol (35)	75 mg Fe x 7 in 28 d
Yasmin	Drospirenone (3)	c, d	Ethinyl estradiol (30)	
Yaz	Drospirenone (3)	d, e, f	Ethinyl estradiol (20)	4 inert in 28 d
Zarah	Drospirenone (3)	c	Ethinyl estradiol (30)	
Zenchent	Ethynodiol diacetate (0.4)		Ethinyl estradiol (35)	
Zeosa	Norgestimate (0.25)		Ethinyl estradiol (35)	
Zovia 1/35	Ethynodiol diacetate (1)		Ethinyl estradiol (35)	
Zovia 1/50	Ethynodiol diacetate (1)		Ethinyl estradiol (50)	
Multiphasics				
Alyacen 7/7/7	Norethindrone (0.5, 0.75, 1)		Ethinyl estradiol (35, 35, 35)	
Aranelle	Norethindrone (0.5, 1, 0.5)		Ethinyl estradiol (35, 35, 35)	
Azurette	Desogestrel (0.15, 0, 0)		Ethinyl estradiol (20, 0, 10)	
Caziant	Desogestrel (0.1, 0.125, 0.15)		Ethinyl estradiol (25, 25, 25)	

445

(Continued)

TABLE 5 (continued)
Oral Contraceptives (See also pp. 301–302)
(Note: 21 = 21 Active pills; 24 = 24 Active pills; Standard for most products is 28 [unless specified] = 21 Active pills + 7 Placebo[a])

Drug	Note	Progestin (mg)	Estrogen (mcg)	Extra
Multiphasics				
Cesia		Desogestrel (0.1, 0.125, 0.15)	Ethinyl estradiol (25, 25, 25)	
Cyclafem 7/7/7		Norethindrone (0.5, 0.75, 1)	Ethinyl estradiol (35, 35, 35)	
Cyclessa		Desogestrel (0.1, 0.125, 0.15)	Ethinyl estradiol (25, 25, 25)	
Dasetta 7/7/7		Norethindrone (0.5, 0.75, 1)	Ethinyl estradiol (35, 35, 35)	
Enpresse		Levonorgestrel (0.05, 0.075, 0.125)	Ethinyl estradiol (30, 40, 30)	
Estrostep Fe	e	Norethindrone acetate (1, 1, 1)	Ethinyl estradiol (20, 30, 35)	75 mg Fe × 7 d in 28 d
Generess Fe	e	Norethindrone acetate (0.8)	Ethinyl estradiol (25)	75 mg Fe × 4 d
Kariva		Desogestrel (0.15, 0, 0)	Ethinyl estradiol (20, 0, 10)	
Leena		Norethindrone (0.5, 1,0.5)	Ethinyl estradiol (35, 35, 35)	
Lessina		Levonorgestrel (0.1)	Ethinyl estradiol (20)	

446

Levonest	Levonorgestrel (0.05, 0.075, 0.125)	Ethinyl estradiol (30, 40, 30)
Lo Loestrin Fe	Norethindrone acetate (1.0)	Ethinyl estradiol (10, 10)
Lutera	Levonorgestrel (0.1)	Ethinyl estradiol (20)
Mircette	Desogestrel (0.15, 0, 0)	Ethinyl estradiol (20, 0, 10)
Myzilra	Levonorgestrel (0.05, 0.075, 0.125)	Ethinyl estradiol (30, 40, 30)
Natazia g	Dienogest (0, 2, 3, 0)	Estradiol valerat (3, 2, 2, 1)
Necon 10/11	Norethindrone (0.5, 1)	Ethinyl estradiol (35)
Necon 7/7/7	Norethindrone (0.5, 0.75, 1)	Ethinyl estradiol (35, 35, 35)
Nortrel 7/7/7	Norethindrone (0.5, 0.75, 1)	Ethinyl estradiol (35, 35, 35)
Orsythia	Levonorgestrel (0.1)	Ethinyl estradiol (20)
Ortho-Novum 10/11	Norethindrone (0.5, 1)	Ethinyl estradiol (35)
Ortho-Novum 7/7/7	Norethindrone (0.5, 0.75, 1)	Ethinyl estradiol (35, 35, 35)
Ortho Tri-Cyclen e	Norgestimate (0.18, 0.215, 0.25)	Ethinyl estradiol (25, 25, 25)
Ortho Tri-Cyclen Lo	Norgestimate (0.18, 0.215, 0.25)	Ethinyl estradiol (35, 35, 35)
Pirmella 7/7/7	Norethindrone (0.5, 0.75, 1)	Ethinyl estradiol (35, 35, 35)
Previfem	Norgestimate (0.25)	Ethinyl estradiol (35)

[Continued]

TABLE 5 (continued)
Oral Contraceptives (See also pp. 301–302)

(Note: 21 = 21 Active pills; 24 = 24 Active pills; Standard for most products is 28 [unless specified] = 21 Active pills + 7 Placebo[a])

Drug	Note	Progestin (mg)	Estrogen (mcg)	Extra
Multiphasics				
Tilia Fe		Norethindrone acetate (1, 1, 1)	Ethinyl estradiol (20, 30, 35)	75 mg Fe × 7 d in 28 d
Tri-Estarylla		Norgestimate (0.18, 0.215, 0.25)	Ethinyl estradiol (25, 25, 25)	
Tri-Legest		Norethindrone acetate (1, 1, 1)	Ethinyl estradiol (20, 30, 35)	
Tri-Legest Fe		Norethindrone acetate (1, 1, 1)	Ethinyl estradiol (20, 30, 35)	75 mg Fe × 7 d in 28 d
Tri-Levlen		Levonorgestrel (0.05, 0.075, 0.125)	Ethinyl estradiol (30, 40, 30)	
Tri-Linyah		Norgestimate (0.18, 0.215, 0.25)	Ethinyl estradiol (25, 25, 25)	
Tri-Nessa		Desogestrel (0.1, 0.125, 0.15)	Ethinyl estradiol (25, 25, 25)	
Tri-Norinyl		Norethindrone (0.5, 1, 0.5)	Ethinyl estradiol (35, 35, 35)	
Tri-Previfem		Desogestrel (0.1, 0.125, 0.15)	Ethinyl estradiol (25, 25, 25)	

Tri-Sprintec	Desogestrel (0.1, 0.125, 0.15)	Ethinyl estradiol (25, 25, 25)	
Trivora	Levonorgestrel (0.05, 0.075, 0.125)	Ethinyl estradiol (30, 40, 30)	
Velivet	Desogestrel (0.1, 0.125, 0.15)	Ethinyl estradiol (25, 25, 25)	
Viorele	Desogestrel (0.15, 0, 0)	Ethinyl estradiol (20, 0, 10)	

Progestin Only (aka "mini-pills")

Camila	Norethindrone (0.35)	None
Errin	Norethindrone (0.35)	None
Heather	Norethindrone (0.35)	None
Jencycla	Norethindrone (0.35)	None
Jolivette	Norethindrone (0.35)	None
Micronor	Norethindrone (0.35)	None
Nor-QD	Norethindrone (0.35)	None
Nora-BE	Norethindrone (0.35)	None

Extended-Cycle Combination (aka COCP [combined oral contraceptive pills]) 91 d

Daysee	Levonorgestrel (0.15)	Ethinyl estradiol (30)	7 (0 mg/10 mcg)
Introvale	Levonorgestrel (0.15)	Ethinyl estradiol (30)	7 inert
Jolessa	Levonorgestrel (0.15)	Ethinyl estradiol (30)	7 inert
LoSeasonique	Levonorgestrel (0.1)	Ethinyl estradiol (20, 10)	7 (0 mg/10 mcg)

[Continued]

449

TABLE 5 (continued)
Oral Contraceptives (See also pp. 301–302)

(Note: 21 = 21 Active pills; 24 = 24 Active pills; Standard for most products is 28 [unless specified] = 21 Active pills + 7 Placebo[a])

Drug	Note	Progestin (mg)	Estrogen (mcg)	Extra
Extended-Cycle Combination (aka COCP [combined oral contraceptive pills]) 91 d				
Quasense		Levonorgestrel (0.15)	Ethinyl estradiol (30)	7 inert
Seasonale		Levonorgestrel (0.15)	Ethinyl estradiol (30)	7 inert
Seasonique		Levonorgestrel (0.15)	Ethinyl estradiol (30)	7 (0 mg/10 mcg)
Extended-Cycle Combination, ascending dose				
Quartette 91 d		Ethinyl estradiol	Levonorgestrel	
		0.02 mg (42 d)	0.15 mg (42 d)	
		0.025 mg (21 d)	0.15 mg (21 d)	
		0.03 mg (21 d)	0.15 mg (21 d)	
		0.01 mg (7 d)		

[a] The designations 21 and 28 refer to number of days in regimen available; if not listed, then assume 28.

[b] Raises folate levels to help decrease neural tube defect risk with eventual pregnancy.

[c] Drospirenone-containing pills have increased risk for blood clots compared to other progestins.

[d] Avoid in patients with hyperkalemia risk.

[e] Also approved for acne.

[f] Approved for premenstrual dysphoric disorder (PMDD) in women who use contraception for birth control.

[g] First "four phasic" OCP.

TABLE 6
Oral Potassium Supplements (See also p. 329)

Brand Name	Salt	Form	mEq Potassium/ Dosing Unit
Glu-K	Gluconate	Tablet	2 mEq/tablet
Kaon elixir	Gluconate	Liquid	20 mEq/15 mL
Kaon-Cl 10	KCl	Tablet, SR	10 mEq/tablet
Kaon-Cl 20%	KCl	Liquid	40 mEq/15 mL
K-Dur 20	KCl	Tablet, SR	20 mEq/tablet
KayCiel	KCl	Liquid	20 mEq/15 mL
K-Lor	KCl	Powder	20 mEq/packet
K-lyte/Cl	KCl/bicarbonate	Effervescent tablet	25 mEq/tablet
Klorvess	KCl/bicarbonate	Effervescent tablet	20 mEq/tablet
Klotrix	KCl	Tablet, SR	10 mEq/tablet
K-Lyte	Bicarbonate/ citrate	Effervescent tablet	25 mEq/tablet
Klor-Con/EF	Bicarbonate/ citrate	Effervescent tablet	25 mEq/tablet
K-Tab	KCl	Tablet, SR	10 mEq/tablet
Micro-K	KCl	Capsule, SR	8 mEq/capsule
Potassium Chloride 10%	KCl	Liquid	20 mEq/15 mL
Potassium Chloride 20%	KCl	Liquid	40 mEq/15 mL
Slow-K	KCl	Tablet, SR	8 mEq/tablet
Tri-K	Acetate/ bicarbonate and citrate	Liquid	45 mEq/15 mL
Twin-K	Citrate/gluconate	Liquid	20 mEq/5 mL

SR = sustained release.

Note: Alcohol and sugar content vary between preparations.

TABLE 7
Tetanus Prophylaxis (See also p. 383)

History of Absorbed Tetanus Toxoid Immunization	Clean, Minor Wounds		All Other Wounds[a]	
	Td[b]	TIG[c]	Td[d]	TIG[c]
Unknown or < 3 doses	Yes	No	Yes	Yes
= 3 doses	No[e]	No	No[f]	No

[a] Such as, but not limited to, wounds contaminated with dirt, feces, soil, saliva, etc.; puncture wounds; avulsions; and wounds resulting from missiles, crushing, burns, and frostbite.

[b] Td = tetanus-diphtheria toxoid (adult type), 0.5 mL IM.
- For children < 7 y, DPT (DT, if pertussis vaccine is contraindicated) is preferred to tetanus toxoid alone.
- For persons > 7 y, Td is preferred to tetanus toxoid alone.
- DT = diphtheria-tetanus toxoid (pediatric), used for those who cannot receive pertussis.

[c] TIG = tetanus immune globulin, 250 units IM.

[d] If only 3 doses of fluid toxoid have been received, then a fourth dose of toxoid, preferably an adsorbed toxoid, should be given.

[e] Yes, if >10 y since last dose.

[f] Yes, if > 5 y since last dose.

Data from Guidelines from the Centers for Disease Control and Prevention and reported in *MMWR* (*MMWR*, December 1, 2006; 55(RR-15):1-48).

TABLE 8
Oral Anticoagulant Standards of Practice (See also warfarin pp. 411–412)

Thromboembolic Disorder	INR	Duration
Deep Venous Thrombosis & Pulmonary Embolism		
Treatment of single episode		
Transient risk factor	2–3	3 mo
Idiopathic[a]	2–3	long-term
Recurrent systemic embolism	2–3	long-term
Prevention of Systemic Embolism		
Atrial fibrillation (AF)[b]	2–3	long-term
AF: cardioversion	2–3	3 wk prior; 4 wk post sinus rhythm
Mitral valvular heart dx[c]	2–3	long-term
Cardiomyopathy (usually ASA)[d]	2–3	long-term
Acute Myocardial Infarction		
High risk[e]	2–3 + low-dose aspirin	long-term
All other infarcts (usually ASA)[f]		

(Continued)

TABLE 8
Oral Anticoagulant Standards of Practice (See also warfarin pp. 411–412) (continued)

Thromboembolic Disorder	INR	Duration
Prosthetic Valves		
Bioprosthetic heart valves		
Mitral position	2–3	3 mo
Aortic position[g]	2–3	3 mo
Bileaflet mechanical valves in aortic position[h]	2–3	long-term
Other mechanical prosthetic valves[i]	2.5–3.5	long-term

[a] 3 mo if mod or high risk of bleeding or distal DVT; if low risk of bleeding, then long-term for proximal DVT/PE.

[b] Paroxysmal AF or ≥2 risk factors (age > 75, Hx, BP, DM, mod–severe LV dysfunction or CHF), then warfarin; 1 risk factor, warfarin or 75–325 mg ASA; 0 risk factors, ASA.

[c] Mitral valve Dz: rheumatic if Hx systemic embolism, or AF or LA thrombus or LA > 55 mm; MVP: only if AF, systemic embolism or TIAs on ASA; mitral valve calcification: warfarin if AF or recurrent embolism on ASA; aortic valve w/ calcification: warfarin not recommended.

[d] In adults only ASA; only indication for anticoagulation cardiomyopathy in children, to begin no later than their activation on transplant list.

[e] High risk = large anterior MI, significant CHF, intracardiac thrombus visible on TE, AF, and Hx of a thromboembolic event.

[f] If meticulous INR monitoring and highly skilled dose titration are expected and widely accessible, then INR 3.5 (3.0–4.0) w/o ASA or 2.5 (2.0–3.0) w/ ASA long-term (4 years).

[g] Usually ASA 50–100 mg; warfarin if Hx embolism, LA thrombus, AF, low EF, hypercoagulable state, 3 mo, or until thrombus resolves.

[h] Target INR 2.5–3.5 if AF, large anterior MI, LA enlargement, hypercoagulable state, or low EF.

[i] Add ASA 50–100 mg if high risk (AF, hypercoagulable state, low EF, or Hx of ASCVD).

ACCP guidelines-Antithrombotic Therapy and Prevention of Thrombosis: American College of *Chest* Physicians Evidence-Based: Clinical Practice Guidelines (9th Ed.) CHEST 2012; 141 (suppl 2) 1s-801s.

TABLE 9
Antiarrhythmics: Vaughn Williams Classification

Class I: *Sodium Channel Blockade*

A. **Class Ia:** Lengthens duration of action potential (↑ the refractory period in atrial and ventricular muscle, in SA and AV conduction systems, and Purkinje fibers)
   1. Amiodarone (also classes II, III, IV)
   2. Disopyramide (Norpace)
   3. Imipramine (MAO inhibitor)
   4. Procainamide (Pronestyl)
   5. Quinidine
B. **Class Ib:** No effect on action potential
   1. Lidocaine (Xylocaine)
   2. Mexiletine (Mexitil)
   3. Phenytoin (Dilantin)
   4. Tocainide (Tonocard)
C. **Class Ic:** Greater sodium current depression (blocks the fast inward Na⁺ current in heart muscle and Purkinje fibers, and slows the rate of ↑ of phase 0 of the action potential)
   1. Flecainide (Tambocor)
   2. Propafenone

Class II: *β-Blocker*

D. Amiodarone (also classes Ia, III, IV)
E. Esmolol (Brevibloc)
F. Sotalol (also class III)

Class III: *Prolong Refractory Period via Action Potential*

G. Amiodarone (also classes Ia, II, IV)
H. Sotalol

Class IV: *Calcium Channel Blocker*

I. Amiodarone (also classes Ia, II, III)
J. Diltiazem (Cardizem)
K. Verapamil (Calan)

TABLE 10
Cytochrome P-450 Isoenzymes and Common Drugs
They Metabolize, Inhibit, and Induce

Increased or decreased (primarily hepatic cytochrome P-450) metabolism of medications may influence the effectiveness of drugs or result in significant drug-drug interactions. Understanding the common cytochrome P-450 isoforms (eg, CYP2C9, CYP2D9, CYP2C19, CYP3A4) and common drugs that are metabolized by (aka "substrates"), inhibit, or induce activity of the isoform helps identify and minimize significant drug interactions.

CYP1A2

Substrates:	Acetaminophen, caffeine, cyclobenzaprine, clozapine, imipramine, mexiletine, naproxen, propranolol, theophylline
Inhibitors:	Amiodarone, cimetidine, most fluoroquinolone antibiotics, fluvoxamine, verapamil
Inducers:	Carbamazepine, charcoal-broiled foods, cruciferous vegetables, omeprazole, modafinil, tobacco smoking

CYP2C9

Substrates:	Most NSAIDs (including COX-2), glipizide, irbesartan, losartan, phenytoin, tamoxifen, warfarin
Inhibitors:	Amiodarone, fluconazole, isoniazid (INH), ketoconazole, metronidazole
Inducers:	Aprepitant, barbiturates, rifampin

CYP2C19

Substrates:	Amitriptyline, clopidogrel, cyclophosphamide, diazepam, lansoprazole, omeprazole, pantoprazole, phenytoin, rabeprazole
Inhibitors:	Fluoxetine, fluvoxamine, isoniazid, ketoconazole, lansoprazole, omeprazole, ticlopidine
Inducers:	Barbiturates, carbamazepine, prednisone, rifampin

CYP2D6

Substrates:	**Antidepressants:** Most tricyclic antidepressants, clomipramine, fluoxetine, paroxetine, venlafaxine **Antipsychotics:** Aripiprazole, clozapine, haloperidol, risperidone, thioridazine **Beta-blockers:** Carvedilol, metoprolol, propranolol, timolol

(Continued)

TABLE 10
Cytochrome P-450 Isoenzymes and Common Drugs
They Metabolize, Inhibit, and Induce (continued)

CYP2D6 (continued)

Opioids: Codeine, hydrocodone, oxycodone, tramadol
Others: Amphetamine, dextromethorphan, duloxetine, encainide, flecainide, mexiletine, ondansetron, propafenone, selegiline, tamoxifen

Inhibitors: Amiodarone, bupropion, cimetidine, clomipramine, doxepin, duloxetine, fluoxetine, haloperidol, methadone, paroxetine, quinidine, ritonavir

Inducers: Dexamethasone, rifampin

CYP3A

(involved in the metabolism of > 50% of drugs metabolized by the liver)

Substrates: **Anticholinergics:** Darifenacin, oxybutynin, solifenacin, tolterodine
Benzodiazepines: Alprazolam, diazepam, midazolam, triazolam
Calcium channel blockers: Amlodipine, diltiazem, felodipine, nifedipine, nimodipine, nisoldipine, verapamil
Chemotherapy: Cyclophosphamide, erlotinib, ifosfamide, paclitaxel, tamoxifen, vinblastine, vincristine
HIV protease inhibitors: Atazanavir, indinavir, nelfinavir, ritonavir, saquinavir
HMG-CoA reductase inhibitors: Atorvastatin, lovastatin, simvastatin
Immunosuppressive agents: Cyclosporine, tacrolimus
Macrolide-type antibiotics: Clarithromycin, erythromycin, telithromycin, troleandomycin
Opioids: Alfentanil, cocaine, fentanyl, methadone, sufentanil
Steroids: Budesonide, cortisol, 17-β-estradiol, progesterone
Others: Acetaminophen, amiodarone, carbamazepine, delavirdine, efavirenz, nevirapine, quinidine, repaglinide, sildenafil, tadalafil, trazodone, vardenafil

Inhibitors: Amiodarone, amprenavir, aprepitant, atazanavir, ciprofloxacin, cisapride, clarithromycin, diltiazem, erythromycin, fluconazole, fluvoxamine, grapefruit juice (in high ingestion), indinavir, itraconazole, ketoconazole, nefazodone, nelfinavir, norfloxacin, ritonavir, saquinavir, telithromycin, troleandomycin, verapamil, voriconazole

(Continued)

TABLE 10
Cytochrome P-450 Isoenzymes and Common Drugs
They Metabolize, Inhibit, and Induce (continued)

CYP3A (continued)

Inducers: Carbamazepine, efavirenz, glucocorticoids, modafinil, nevirapine, phenytoin, phenobarbital, rifabutin, rifapentine, rifampin, St. John's wort

Data from Katzung B, ed. *Basic and Clinical Pharmacology.* 12th ed. New York, NY: McGraw-Hill; 2012; *The Medical Letter.* July 4, 2004; 47; *N Engl J Med.* 2005;352:2211–2221. Flockhart DA. Drug Interactions: Cytochrome P450 Drug Interaction Table. Indiana University School of Medicine. http://medicine.iupui.edu/ clinpharm/ddis/table.aspx. Accessed August 31, 2013.

TABLE 11
SSRIs/SNRIs/Triptans and Serotonin Syndrome

A life-threatening condition, serotonin syndrome, results when selective serotonin reuptake inhibitors (SSRIs) and 5-hydroxytryptamine receptor agonists (triptans) are used together. However, many other drugs have been implicated (see below). Signs and symptoms of serotonin syndrome include the following:

Restlessness, coma, N/V/D, hallucinations, loss of coordination, overactive reflexes, hypertension, mydriasis, rapid changes in BP, increased body temperature

Class	Drugs
Antidepressants	MAOIs, TCAs, SSRIs, SNRIs, mirtazapine, venlafaxine
CNS stimulants	Amphetamines, phentermine, methylphenidate, sibutramine
5-HT$_1$ agonists	Triptans
Illicit drugs	Cocaine, methylenedioxymethamphetamine (ecstasy), lysergic acid diethylamide (LSD)
Opioids	Tramadol, oxycodone, morphine, meperidine
Others	Buspirone, chlorpheniramine, dextromethorphan, linezolid, lithium, selegiline, tryptophan, St. John's wort

Management includes removal of the precipitating drugs and supportive care. To control agitation, the serotonin antagonist cyproheptadine can be used. When symptoms are mild, discontinuation of the medication or medications and the control of agitation with benzodiazepines may be needed. Critically ill patients may require sedation and mechanical ventilation as well as control of hyperthermia. (Ables AZ, Nagubilli R. Prevention, recognition, and management of serotonin syndrome. *Am Fam Physician.* May 1, 2010;81(9):1139–1142.)
MOAI = monoamine oxidase inhibitor.
TCA = tricyclic antidepressant.
SNRI = serotonin-norepinephrine reuptake inhibitors.

TABLE 12
Selected Multivitamin Supplements

This table lists common multivitamins available without a prescription, and most chains have generic versions. Many specialty vitamin combinations are available and are not included in this table. (Examples are B vitamins plus C; disease-specific supplements; pediatric and infant formulations; prenatal vitamins, etc.) A check (✓) indicates the component is found in the formulation; NA indicates it is not in the formulation. Details of the specific composition of these multivitamins can be found at www.eDrugbook.com or on the product site.

	Fat-Soluble Vitamins		Water-Soluble Vitamins[a]		Minerals[b]								Trace Elements[b]				Other
	A, D, E	K	C, B₁, B₂, B₃, B₅, B₆, B₁₂, Folate	Biotin	Ca	P	Mg	Fe	Zn	I	Se	K	Mn	Cu	Cr	Mo	
Centrum	✓	✓	✓	✓	✓	✓	✓	✓	✓	✓	✓	✓	✓	✓	✓	✓	
Centrum Performance	✓	✓	✓	✓	✓	✓	✓	✓	✓	✓	✓	✓	✓	✓	✓	✓	lycopene Ginseng, Ginkgo
Centrum Silver	✓	✓	✓	✓	✓	✓	✓	NA	✓	✓	✓	✓	✓	✓	✓	✓	
NatureMade Multi Complete	✓	NA	✓	NA	✓	NA	NA	✓	✓	✓	✓	✓	✓	✓	✓	✓	lycopene
NatureMade Multi Daily	✓	NA	✓	✓	✓	NA	NA	✓	✓	✓	NA	NA	NA	NA	NA	NA	Lycopene
NatureMade Multi Max	✓	✓	✓	✓	✓	✓	✓	✓	✓	✓	✓	✓	✓	✓	✓	NA	Lutein

(Continued)

TABLE 12 (continued)
Selected Multivitamin Supplements

This table lists common multivitamins available without a prescription, and most chains have generic versions. Many specialty vitamin combinations are available and are not included in this table. (Examples are B vitamins plus C; disease-specific supplements; pediatric and infant formulations; prenatal vitamins; etc.) A check (✓) indicates the component is found in the formulation; NA indicates it is not in the formulation. Details of the specific composition of these multivitamins can be found at www.eDrugbook.com or on the product site.

	Fat-Soluble Vitamins[a]		Water-Soluble Vitamins[a]		Minerals[b]								Trace Elements[b]				Other
	A, D, E	K	C, B_1, B_2, B_3, B_5, B_6, B_{12}, Folate	Biotin	Ca	P	Mg	Fe	Zn	I	Se	K	Mn	Cu	Cr	Mo	
NatureMade Multi 50+	✓	✓	✓	✓	✓	✓	✓	NA	✓	✓	✓	✓	✓	✓	✓	✓	
One-A-Day 50 Plus	✓	✓	✓	✓	✓	✓	NA	✓	✓	✓	✓	✓	✓	✓	✓	✓	Lutein
One-A-Day Essential	✓	NA	✓	NA	NA	NA	NA	✓	✓	NA	NA	NA	NA	NA	NA	NA	
One-A-Day Maximum	✓	✓	✓	✓	✓	✓	✓	✓	✓	✓	✓	✓	✓	✓	✓	✓	
Therapeutic Vitamin	✓	NA	✓	✓	✓	NA	NA	✓	✓	NA	NA	NA	NA	NA	NA	NA	

Product														
Theragran-M Advanced Formula High Potency	✓		✓		✓	✓	✓	✓	✓	✓		✓	✓	
Theragran-M Premier High Potency	✓		✓		✓	✓	✓	✓	✓	✓		✓	✓	Lutein
Theragran-M Premier 50 Plus High Potency	✓	NA	✓		✓	✓	NA	✓	✓	✓	low	✓	✓	Lutein
Therapeutic Vitamin + Minerals Enhanced	✓		✓		✓	✓	✓	✓	✓	✓		✓	✓	
Unicap M	✓	NA	✓	NA	✓	✓	NA	✓	✓	✓	NA	✓	NA NA	
Unicap Senior	✓	NA	✓	NA	✓	✓	✓	✓	✓	✓	low	✓	NA NA	
Unicap T	✓	NA	✓	NA	NA NA	✓	NA	✓	✓	✓	low	✓	NA NA	

a Vitamin B₁ = thiamine; B₂ = riboflavin; B₃ = niacin; B₅ = pantothenic acid; B₆ = pyridoxine; B₁₂ = cyanocobalamin.

b Ca = calcium; Cr = chromium; Cu = copper; Fe = iron; Fl = fluoride; I = iodine; K = potassium; Mg = magnesium; Mn = manganese; Mo = molybdenum; P = phosphorus; Se = selenium; Zn = zinc.

TABLE 13
Influenza Vaccine Strains for 2014–2015 (See also pp. 219–221)

The 2013–2014 trivalent influenza vaccine is made from the following three viruses:

- A/California/7/2009 (H1N1)-like virus
- A/Texas/50/2012 (H3N2)-like virus
- B/Massachusetts/2/2012-like virus.

It is recommended that quadrivalent vaccines containing two influenza B viruses contain the above three viruses and a B/Brisbane/60/2008-like virus. (http://www.cdc.gov/flu/about/season/flu-season-2014-2015.htm Accessed 29 August 2014)

Age	Brand Name Product	Dosage Form/Strength
6–35 mo	Fluzone	0.25 mL prefilled syringe
	Fluzone Quadrivalent	0.25 mL prefilled syringe
2–49 y	FluMist Quadrivalent	0.2 mL prefilled intranasal sprayer
≥ 36 mo	Fluarix	0.5 mL prefilled syringe
	Fluzone	0.5 mL prefilled syringe & single-dose vial; 5 mL multi-dose vial
	Fluarix Quadrivalent	0.5 mL prefilled syringe
	Fluzone Quadrivalent	0.5 mL prefilled syringe & single-dose vial
≥ 4 y	Fluvirin	0.5 mL prefilled syringe & 5 mL multi-dose vial
≥ 9 y[a]	Afluria	0.5 mL prefilled syringe & 5 mL multi-dose vial
≥ 18 y	Flucelvax	0.5 mL prefilled syringe
	FluLaval	5 mL multi-dose vial
18–49 y	FluBlok[b]	0.5 mL single-dose vial
18–64 y	Fluzone Intradermal	0.1 mL prefilled microinjection system
≥ 65 y	Fluzone High-Dose	0.5 mL prefilled syringe

[a] Age indication per package labeling is ≥ 5 y; ACIP (http://www.cdc.gov/vaccines/hcp/acip-recs/vacc-specific/flu.html Accessed August 18, 2014) recommends *Afluria* not be used in children 6–8 y due to increased risk of febrile Rxn.

[b] Adolescents of age 18 y and older with egg allergy of any severity can receive the recombinant influenza vaccine (RIV) (*FluBlok*). RIV does not contain any egg protein.

Index